Modeling and Simulation in Science, Engineering and Technology

Series Editor
Nicola Bellomo
Politecnico di Torino
Italy

Advisory Editorial Board

Selected Topics in Cancer Modeling

Genesis, Evolution,
Immune Competition, and Therapy

Nicola Bellomo
Mark Chaplain
Elena De Angelis
Editors

Birkhäuser
Boston • Basel • Berlin

Nicola Bellomo
Dipartimento di Matematica
Politecnico di Torino
Corso Duca degli Abruzzi 24
10129 Torino
Italy
`nicola.bellomo@polito.it`

Mark Chaplain
The SIMBIOS Centre
Division of Mathematics
University of Dundee
Dundee DD1 4HN
Scotland
`chaplain@maths.dundee.ac.uk`

Elena De Angelis
Dipartimento di Matematica
Politecnico di Torino
Corso Duca degli Abruzzi 24
10129 Torino
Italy
`elena.deangelis@polito.it`

ISBN: 978-0-8176-4712-4   e-ISBN: 978-0-8176-4713-1
DOI: 10.1007/978-0-8176-4713-1

Library of Congress Control Number: 2008925859

Mathematics Subject Classification (2000): 92B05, 92C50

Printed on acid-free paper.

9 8 7 6 5 4 3 2 1

www.birkhauser.com

Contents

8 Modeling Diffusely Invading Brain Tumors: An Individualized Approach to Quantifying Glioma Evolution and Response to Therapy
Russell Rockne, Ellsworth C. Alvord Jr., Mindy Szeto, Stanley Gu,

9 Multiphase Models of Tumour Growth
Sergey Astanin, Luigi Preziosi 223

10 The Lymphatic Vascular System in Lymphangiogenesis, Invasion and Metastasis: A Mathematical Approach
Michael S. Pepper, Georgios Lolas 255

11 M for Invasion: Morphology, Mutation and the Microenvironment
Alexander R. A. Anderson 277

Preface

"To live is to change, and to be perfect is to have changed often"[1]

"Evil has no substance of its own, but is only the defect, <u>excess</u>, perversion, or corruption of that which has substance."[1]

Medically, a tumour may be defined as follows:

"A mass of tissue formed as the result of abnormal, <u>excessive</u> and inappropriate (i.e., purposeless) proliferation of cells, the growth of which continues indefinitely and regardless of the mechanisms which control normal cellular proliferation"[2]

In a very real sense, a tumour lives to change and changes often in order to be perfect (from the point of view of the tumour itself). A tumour's successful growth and development depends crucially on its ability to proliferate excessively, to undergo mutations, to adapt to its local environment and to spread from its initial location in the host tissue to distant colonies elsewhere in the body. In this respect, a malignant tumour (i.e., a cancer) is a paradigmatic microcosm for the whole of biology, and offers applied mathematicians of all shapes and sizes (modellers, applied analysts, numerical analysts, computational scientists) many exciting and challenging problems.

In the context of the current book, perhaps one can trace the origins of modelling solid tumours back to the seminal work of Greenspan.[3] It goes without saying that since the publication of this paper in 1976, many things have

---

[1] J.H. Newman

[2] *Muir's Textbook of Pathology*, 12th Edition (1985), Anderson, J.R., Ed., E. Arnold Publishers

[3] Greenspan, H.P. (1976) On the growth and stability of cell cultures and solid tumours. *J. Theor. Biol.* **65**, 229-242

changed. Much more is known biologically, and there have been many new developments in applied mathematics. Perhaps looking back from a distance of over 30 years and with the benefit of advances in biological understanding, one may find faults in some of the modelling assumptions, but not with the spirit of the paper, which still stands out as a beautiful example of the benefit of applying mathematics to a biological problem to gain a deeper understanding of the system.

The past decade has witnessed enormous advances in our understanding of the molecular basis of cell structure and function. Scientists recognize the spectacular success of the human genome project and the consequent burgeoning interest in the related field of proteomics. Biochemists and cell biologists have made similarly impressive strides in elucidating the mechanisms mediating cell signalling and its consequences for the control of cell proliferation, motility and gene expression. Therefore, at the present point in time, with the recent explosion of biological data, the task of accurately modelling solid tumour growth may seem daunting to say the least:

"Nothing would be done at all if one waited until one could do it so well that no one could find fault with it." [1]

"Let us take things as we find them: let us not attempt to distort them into what they are not... We cannot make facts. All our wishing cannot change them. We must use them." [1]

It is, however, abundantly clear that reductionist logic using this impressive "sub-cell-level" information base is not sufficient to deduce an understanding of phenomena operative at the next higher level of biological organisation: the tissue. Employing a literary analogy, the vast "-omic" databases of catalogued genes and proteins, taken together with our growing understanding of the inner workings of individual cells, provide a "dictionary" and a "grammatical syntax" required for the next great challenge, i.e., understanding the "sentences" and "paragraphs" characteristic of emergent tissue-level phenomena. This book, therefore, has an overall aim of quantitative, predictive mathematical modelling of solid tumour growth at all scales, from genetics through to treatment therapy of patients. The different chapters are linked to one another in various ways and at various different biological scales (from intra-cellular to tissue level), and the overall theme of the book may be termed "multi-scale mathematical modelling" or, from a biological perspective, "quantitative systems biology," of solid tumour growth. To use the previous literary analogy, the ultimate goal is to build a "mathematical book of the cancer cell," composed of individual chapters made from the sentences and paragraphs of the specific models.

Nicola Bellomo, Mark Chaplain, Elena De Angelis
April 2008

List of Contributors

Natalia L. Komarova
University of California, Department
of Mathematics, 103 Multipurpose
Science & Technology Bldg, Irvine,
CA 92697, USA
komarova@math.uci.edu

Dominik Wodarz
University of California, Department
of Ecology and Evolution, Irvine, CA
92697, USA
dwodarz@uci.edu

C. Richard Boland
Baylor University Medical Center,
Department of Internal Medicine,
Division of Gastroenterology and
Charles A. Sammons Cancer Center,
Dallas, TX 75246, USA
RickBo@BaylorHealth.com

Ajay Goel
Baylor University Medical Center,
Department of Internal Medicine,
Division of Gastroenterology and
Charles A. Sammons Cancer Center,
Dallas, TX 75246, USA

Abdelghani Bellouquid
University Cadi Ayyad, Ecole
Nationale des Sciences Appliquées,
Safi, Maroc
bellouquid@gmail.com

Marcello Delitala
Politecnico di Torino, Dipartimento
di Matematica, Corso Duca Degli
Abruzzi 24, 10129 Torino, Italy
marcello.delitala@polito.it

Mirosław Lachowicz
University of Warsaw, Institute
of Applied Mathematics and Mechanics, Faculty of Mathematics,
Informatics and Mechanics,
ul. Banacha 2, PL-02-097 Warsaw,
Poland
lachowic@mimuw.edu.pl

Benoît Perthame
École Normale Supérieure,
Département de Mathématiques et
Applications, 45 rue d'Ulm,
75230 Paris, France
perthame@dma.ens.fr

Suman Kumar Tumuluri
École Normale Supérieure,
Département de Mathématiques et
Applications, 45 rue d'Ulm,
75230 Paris, France
suman@dma.ens.fr

David Basanta
Technische Universität Dresden,
Zentrum für Informationsdien-
ste und Hochleistungsrechnen,
Nöthnitzer-str. 46, 01187, Dresden,
Germany
david.basanta@tu-dresden.de

Andreas Deutsch
Technische Universität Dresden,
Zentrum für Informationsdien-
ste und Hochleistungsrechnen,
Nöthnitzer-str. 46, 01187 Dresden,
Germany
andreas.deutsch@tu-dresden.de

Vittorio Cristini
University of Texas Health Science
Center at Houston, School of Health
Information Sciences, TX 77030,
USA
vittorio.cristini@uth.tmc.edu

Hermann B. Frieboes
University of Texas Health Science
Center at Houston, School of Health
Information Sciences, TX 77030,
USA

Xiaongrong Li
University of California, Department
of Biomedical Engineering, Irvine,
CA 92697, USA

John S. Lowengrub
University of California, Department
of Mathematics, Irvine, CA 92697,
USA
lowengrb@math.uci.edu

Paul Macklin
University of Texas Health Science
Center at Houston, School of Health
Information Sciences, TX 77030,
USA
Paul.Macklin@uth.tmc.edu

Sandeep Sanga
University of Texas Health Science
Center at Houston, School of Health
Information Sciences, TX 77030,
USA
sandeep.sanga@uth.tmc.edu

Steven M. Wise
University of California, Department
of Mathematics, Irvine, CA 92697,
USA
swisea@math.uci.edu

Xiaoming Zheng
University of California, Department
of Mathematics, Irvine, CA 92697,
USA
xzheng@math.uci.edu

Alessandro Bertuzzi
Istituto di Analisi dei Sistemi ed
Informatica "A. Ruberti" - CNR,
Viale Manzoni 30, 00185 Roma, Italy
bertuzzi@iasi.cnr.it

Antonio Fasano
Università di Firenze, Diparti-
mento di Matematica "U. Dini",
Viale Morgagni 67/A, 50134 Firenze,
Italy
fasano@math.unifi.it

Alberto Gandolfi
Istituto di Analisi dei Sistemi ed
Informatica "A. Ruberti" - CNR,
Viale Manzoni 30, 00185 Roma, Italy
gandolfi@iasi.cnr.it

Carmela Sinisgalli
Istituto di Analisi dei Sistemi ed
Informatica "A. Ruberti" - CNR,
Viale Manzoni 30, 00185 Roma, Italy
sinisgalli@iasi.cnr.it

Russell Rockne
University of Washington, Department of Pathology, 1959 NE Pacific St., Box 357470, Seattle, WA 98195, USA
rockne@u.washington.edu

E. C. Alvord Jr.
University of Washington, Department of Pathology, 1959 NE Pacific St. Box 357470, Seattle, WA 98195, USA

Mindy Szeto
University of Washington, Department of Pathology, 1959 NE Pacific St., Box 357470, Seattle, WA 98195, USA
bluesilk@u.washington.edu

Stanley Gu
University of Washington, Department of Pathology, 1959 NE Pacific St., Box 357470, Seattle, WA 98195, USA
stanleyg@u.washington.edu

Gargi Chakraborty
University of Washington, Department of Pathology, 1959 NE Pacific St., Box 357470, Seattle, WA 98195, USA
gargi@u.washington.edu

Kristin R. Swanson
University of Washington, Department of Pathology, 1959 NE Pacific St., Box 357470, Seattle, WA 98195, USA
swanson@amath.washington.edu

Sergey Astanin
Politecnico di Torino, Dipartimento di Matematica, Corso Duca Degli Abruzzi 24, 10129 Torino, Italy
sergey.astanin@polito.it

Luigi Preziosi
Politecnico di Torino, Dipartimento di Matematica, Corso Duca Degli Abruzzi 24, 10129 Torino, Italy
luigi.preziosi@polito.it

Michael S. Pepper
University of Pretoria, Department of Immunology, Faculty of Health Sciences, and Netcare Institute of Cellular and Molecular Medicine, Lifestyle Management Park, 223 Clifton Avenue, 0157 Lyttleton, South Africa
mpepper@doctors.netcare.co.za

Georgios Lolas
Technological and Educational Institute of Athens, Department of Mathematics, Ag. Spyridonos, 12210 Aigaleo, Athens, Greece
georgioslolas@hotmail.com

Alexander R. A. Anderson
University of Dundee, Division of Mathematics, Dundee DD1 4HN, UK
anderson@maths.dundee.ac.uk

Vincenzo Capasso
Università degli Studi di Milano, Dipartimento di Matematica, Via C. Saldini 50, 20133 Milano, Italy
Vincenzo.Capasso@unimi.it

Elisabetta Dejana
Università degli Studi di Milano, Dipartimento di Scienze Biomolecolari e Biotecnologie, via Celoria 26, 20133 Milano, Italy
elisabetta.dejana@
ifom-ieo-campus.it

Alessandra Micheletti
Università degli Studi di Milano,
Dipartimento di Matematica, Via C.
Saldini 50, 20133 Milano, Italy
Alessandra.Micheletti@unimi.it

Heiko Enderling
Tufts University School of Medicine,
Center of Cancer Systems Biology,
Caritas St. Elizabeth's Medical
Center, 736 Cambridge Street,
Boston, MA 02135, USA
heiko.enderling@tufts.edu

Jayant S Vaidya
University of Dundee, Division of
Surgery and Molecular Oncology,
Ninewells Hospital and Medical
School, Dundee DD1 9SY, UK
j.s.vaidya@dundee.ac.uk

Pier-Luigi Lollini
Università di Bologna, Sezione
di Cancerologia, Dipartimento di
Patologia Sperimentale, Italy
pierluigi.lollini@unibo.it

Arianna Palladini
Università di Bologna, Sezione
di Cancerologia, Dipartimento di
Patologia Sperimentale, Italy
arianna.palladini@unibo.it

Francesco Pappalardo
Università di Catania, Dipartimento
di Matematica e Informatica, Viale
A.Doria n. 6, 95125 Catania, Italy
francesco@dmi.unict.it

Santo Motta
Università di Catania, Dipartimento
di Matematica e Informatica, Viale
A.Doria n. 6, 95125 Catania, Italy
motta@dmi.unict.it.

Steven R. McDougall
Heriot-Watt University, Institute of
Petroleum Engineering, Edinburgh,
EH14 4AS, Scotland
Steve.Mcdougall@pet.hw.ac.uk.

Anastasios Matzavinos
Ohio State University, Department
of Mathematics, Columbus, OH
43210, USA
tatos@math.ohio-state.edu

Helen M. Byrne
University of Nottingham, Centre for
Mathematical Medicine and Biology,
School of Mathematical Sciences,
Nottingham NG7 2RD, UK
helen.byrne@nottingham.ac.uk

I.M.M. van Leeuwen
University of Nottingham, Centre for
Mathematical Medicine and Biology,
School of Mathematical Sciences,
Nottingham NG7 2RD, UK
i.m.m.vanleeuwen@
maths.nottingham.ac.uk

Markus R. Owen
University of Nottingham, Centre for
Mathematical Medicine and Biology,
School of Mathematical Sciences,
Nottingham NG7 2RD, UK
markus.owen@nottingham.ac.uk

Tomás Alarcón
Imperial College, Department of
Mathematics, 180 Queen's Gate,
London SW7 2AZ, UK
a.tomas@imperial.ac.uk

Philip K. Maini
University of Oxford, Centre for
Mathematical Biology, Mathematical
Institute, 24–29 St Giles', Oxford
OX1 3LB, UK
maini@maths.ox.ac.uk

1

Genetic and Epigenetic Pathways to Colon Cancer: Relating Experimental Evidence with Modeling

Natalia L. Komarova,[1] Dominik Wodarz,[2] C. Richard Boland,[3] and Ajay Goel[3]

[1] Department of Mathematics, University of California, Irvine, CA 92697, USA
[2] Department of Ecology and Evolution, University of California, Irvine, CA 92697, USA
[3] Department of Internal Medicine, Division of Gastroenterology and Charles A. Sammons Cancer Center, Baylor University Medical Center, Dallas, TX 75246, USA

1.1 Introduction

Colorectal cancer (CRC) for many years has provided a prototypic model to study the genetic basis of human cancer. Current understanding suggests that CRC is not a single disease, but encompasses a number of heterogeneous complex diseases caused by distinctive genetic/epigenetic mechanisms. It is now believed that CRC results from the progressive accumulation of genomic alterations that lead to the transformation of normal colonic epithelium to colon adenocarcinoma. Comprehensive analyses of the molecular genesis of CRC have revealed several unifying tenets that underlie the pathogenesis of this disease process. First, it is clear that CRC emerges via a multistep progression at both the molecular and the morphologic levels [23]. Second, genetic and epigenetic alterations that trigger colon cancer formation provide the much-needed growth advantage to a pool of colonic cells that get clonally selected in subsequent cell divisions and acquire the malignant phenotype. Third, and most importantly, loss of genomic stability is the key molecular step in the emergence and progression of colon cancer [59].

A common trait of most cancer cells is their altered karyotype. It is conjectured that the unifying principle of tumor development is loss of genomic stability. CRC arises from inherited mutations, de novo somatic mutations or through epigenetic modifications of growth-regulatory tumor suppressor genes. Approximately 30% of the genes in the human genome encode for proteins that regulate DNA fidelity. Not only does this imply that the maintenance of the integrity of genomic DNA is important in eukaryotic cells, but it also indicates that there are likely to be a variety of different mechanisms

N. Bellomo et al. (eds.), *Selected Topics in Cancer Modeling*,
DOI: 10.1007/978-0-8176-4713-1_1, © Springer Science+Business Media, LLC 2008

that can lead to loss of genomic DNA stability. In the majority of cancers, the mechanisms responsible for emergence of aneuploidy are not known. This has led some investigators to even propose that genomic instability can arise in the absence of genetic mutations and is self-propagating in cancer [20]. Under normal circumstances, DNA tends to maintain remarkable stability. Therefore it appears that the incessant process of evolution and natural selection would not be possible without a means to deregulate the stability of the genome. It would seem that once such genomic instability is established, it allows selection and enrichment of advantageous cells with somatic alterations that favor cellular proliferation [12].

In recent years data have emerged to suggest that, at least in a subset of cancers, a specific etiology argues for specific genetic and epigenetic alterations that mediate the loss of genomic stability in colon cancer. In this article, we will briefly discuss the experimental data suggesting distinct underlying molecular mechanisms of genomic instability in colonic tumorigenesis. Subsequently, we will present mathematical models to predict the rate kinetics for the appearance of these molecular alterations to better appreciate and understand the contribution of these individual processes in the genesis of CRC.

The rest of this paper is organized as follows. In Section 1.2 we review the three distinct molecular phenotypes of CRC and discuss chromosomal instability, microsatellite instability and CpG island methylator phenotype. In Section 1.3 we describe the stochastic modeling framework based on mutation: selection networks. In Section 1.4 we apply this framework to study the initiation of CRC, and discuss the chromosomal and microsatellite instability phenotypes as well as two familial CRC syndromes. In Section 1.5 we discuss the biological relevance of our findings.

1.2 Genomic Instability in CRC: The Three Molecular Phenotypes

One of the important features of CRC is a high degree of genomic instability [23, 59, 56, 57]. This genomic instability can be observed by the heterogeneity in karyotypes within each tumor of the same type, and in different parts of the same tumor. However, whether genomic instability is a cause or a consequence of tumorigenesis has been debated for years.

In the context of CRC, theoretically, every tumor arises and behaves in a unique fashion which cannot exactly be recapitulated by any other CRC. Yet, we believe that tumors with similar characteristics most likely arise or behave in a similar way. This is partly because we have gained enough insight into the pathogenesis of CRC to allow us to classify individual tumors based upon similar characteristics, in order to empirically predict pathogenesis and biological behavior and to understand the underlying molecular mechanisms in these neoplasms.

Tumor classification is historically based on various clinical (e.g., proximal vs. distal) and pathological (e.g., mucinous vs. non-mucinous; well-moderated vs. poorly differentiated) features. However, in recent years, the molecular classification of CRC is becoming increasingly important because it reflects the underlying mechanisms of carcinogenesis. Nonetheless, even though clinical and pathological features are largely phenotypical, they are equally important because some of those features are associated with particular molecular defects, and are thus useful in estimating the likelihood of a particular molecular subtype.

There are different approaches to molecular classification. One can theoretically divide tumors into different groups by the presence or absence of any molecular feature(s). However, as a primary discriminator in classification, emphasis should be put on molecular classification based on global cellular events. In this context, three mechanisms that increase genomic diversity in CRC include: chromosomal instability (CIN), microsatellite instability (MSI) and the CpG island methylator phenotype (CIMP) [33, 29]. It would be prudent to classify all CRCs based upon any of these genetic and epigenetic alterations, rather than a single molecular event (such as TP53 mutation, KRAS mutation, MLH1 methylation, etc.). Tumors classified into one group by any single molecular event will still contain a very heterogeneous group of tumors, in contrast to tumors classified by a global molecular phenomenon.

1.2.1 Chromosomal Instability (CIN)

Chromosomal instability (CIN) is defined as continuous and conspicuous changes in chromosome structure and number. These genetic events produce either gains or losses of complete or large portions of chromosomes at an accelerated rate [75]. CIN was the first form of genomic instability discovered in human cancers. It appears to be a distinct and the most frequent phenotype in colorectal cancers, and is characterized by abnormal karyotypes [33]. CIN is considered to promote carcinogenesis through losses of tumor suppressor genes and copy number gains of oncogenes. These cancer cells can either show heterogeneous karyotypes within a single tumor mass, or include areas with homogeneous karyotypes, suggesting both a constant genetic change and clonal evolution of selected cells. The mutation rates are thought to be accelerated in cells with CIN, which dramatically alters the expression of thousands of genes and increases the likelihood of cellular differentiation and malignancy. Although the occurrences of chromosomal abnormalities are essentially a random process, the selection process can also create a non-random pattern of chromosomal aberrations in tumor cells.

CIN has been commonly assessed by DNA ploidy analysis or loss of heterozygosity (LOH) analyses of microsatellite markers. In CRC, frequently lost chromosomal arms have been found to be the loci of some important tumor suppressor genes, including p53 (17p), SMAD4/DCC (18q), and APC (5q), [46, 63, 86]. In addition to somewhat crude LOH analysis methods, recently, array-based comparative genomic hybridization (array-CGH) and single nucleotide polymorphism (SNP) arrays have been used to study quantitative copy number gains/losses and LOH, respectively, in various cancers. Compared to conventional LOH analyses, both of these techniques have higher resolution in genome-wide analysis of DNA copy number gains and losses.

CIN may be present in as many as 50% or more of all CRCs, and tends to occur in a mutually exclusive manner with MSI cancers [29, 21]. Even though CIN is so frequently present in colon cancers, and despite the fact that aneuploidy has long been appreciated as a hallmark of cancer, the mechanisms underpinning CIN and aneuploid karyotypes are still unclear. It is believed that causes of CIN are likely to be heterogeneous. Mutations in genes encoding mitotic checkpoint proteins such as BUB1 and BUB1B (BUBR1) may cause CIN in a subset of CRCs [13]. In addition, abnormal centrosome number and function has been a candidate mechanism for CIN. Amplification of AURKA (Aurora kinase A, STK15/BTAK), a centrosome-associated serine threonine kinase, has been found in colon cancer cell lines [10], and is correlated with CIN in colon cancer [68]. Indeed, overexpression of AURKA can induce aneuploidy in various cell lines [27, 39, 28]. Other candidate genes that may be involved in the development of CIN include APC [24, 25] and FBXW7 (CDC4 ubiquitin ligase) [74]. In addition, there is also evidence suggesting that a human polyomavirus, JC Virus (JCV) that ubiquitously infects humans, is frequently present in the gastrointestinal tract and encodes a transforming oncogene (large T-antigen, or T-Ag), and may be the cause of CIN in a subset of CRCs [54, 80, 79, 30].

1.2.2 Microsatellite Instability (MSI)

Microsatellite instability (MSI) refers to altered allelic lengths ("instability") of short nucleotide repeat sequences, referred to as "microsatellites", in tumor DNA compared to normal DNA [95]. It has also been referred to as RER (replication error), mutator phenotype, and MIN (microsatellite instability). A high degree of MSI occurs as the consequence of inactivation of the DNA mismatch repair (MMR) system that consists of a complex of proteins that recognize and repair base pair mismatches that occur during DNA replication. Inactivation of the MMR system due to germline mutations in MSH2, MLH1, MSH6 and PMS2 genes is the cause of 2–5% of all colon cancers, giving rise to what is called the Lynch syndrome (also referred to as hereditary non-polyposis colorectal cancer or HNPCC) [15]. In contrast, somatic inactivation of the MMR system additionally gives rise to approximately 12% of sporadic CRC where functional loss of MLH1 due to promoter methylation and gene silencing is the most common cause of MSI [48].

MSI resulting from loss of MMR activity predominantly affects mono- and di-nucleotide tandem repeat sequences. Genes that possess such microsatellite repeats in their coding regions appear to be the targets in MSI colon cancers. Mutations of coding mono-nucleotide repeats in tumor suppressor genes such as TGFBR2 (the TGF-β receptor type 2), BAX, hMSH3, hMSH6, RIZ1 and CDX2 have been shown to be important in carcinogenesis [62, 76, 108, 72, 106, 65]. Importantly, MSI and the subsequent target gene mutations appear to occur throughout the adenoma-to-carcinoma progression. Thus MSI creates a favorable state for accumulating mutations in vulnerable genes that control critical biological activities of the cell, and these alterations can be predicted to ultimately lead to the generation of colon cancers.

MSI is typically assessed by analyzing five microsatellite markers (D2S123, D5S346, D17S250, BAT25 and BAT26) referred to as the NCI consensus panel [11] by comparing allelic lengths at each of these markers in tumor DNA to that of normal non-neoplastic cells. More recently a new panel of five quasi-monomorphic microsatellite markers has been proposed that utilizes a multiplex-PCR amplification of only tumor DNA, eliminating the need for normal DNA [94]. Typically, tumors that demonstrate instability at more than 2 of 5 markers are categorized as MSI or MSI-H (high frequency MSI); the ones with 1 or 2 markers mutated as MSI-L (low frequency MSI); and the ones with no instability as MSS (microsatellite stable). In contrast to MSI-H tumors, it has been controversial whether MSI-L exists as a distinct phenotype from MSS tumors. A study has shown that virtually all CRCs show some degree of microsatellite instability when a large number of markers are tested. The study concluded that the difference between MSI-L and MSS is merely quantitative and that it is unlikely that there are different genetic pathways to MSI-L tumors and MSS tumors [97]. In clinical settings, MSI testing has been performed as a screening test for the identification of Lynch syndrome, and sometimes as a prognostic marker (generally MSI tumors imply a better prognosis compared with non-MSI tumors) or a marker for predicting efficacy of chemotherapy (generally MSI-H implies resistance) [78].

MSI has been suggested as a carcinogenic mechanism alternative to the CIN pathway [95]. The corresponding distinct phenotype is found in approximately 15% of sporadic CRCs [33]. Although most MSI sporadic CRCs primarily arise as a consequence of hypermethylation of hMLH1 promoter, these tumors typically demonstrate frequent methylation of multiple other genes. This observation suggests that this subset of tumors is actually part of the CIMP tumors [48, 42, 98, 31, 89]. Reversal of methylation-induced silencing and restoration of gene expression for various genes has been demonstrated using demethylating agents such as 5-deoxy-5-azacytidine (5-Aza). As inactivation of hMLH1 presumably plays an initiating role in the pathogenesis of sporadic MSI CRCs, it seems plausible that demethylating treatments in the future may hold promise for the chemoprevention of these neoplasms.

A number of pathologic and molecular features of MSI cancers provide them with a clear distinction from CIN neoplasms, indicating that these two CRCs arise from two different molecular pathways [29]. The features of MSI CRC include more frequent occurrence in women, proximal location, diploid DNA content, highly mucinous structure, signet ring cell morphology, Crohn's-like lymphoid reaction, abundant tumor infiltrating lymphocytes, tumor necrosis and poor differentiation [92, 3, 45]. Additionally, patients with MSI CRC exhibit longer overall and cancer-specific survival than stage-matched patients with CIN cancers [35]. Mutations of the p53 gene are less common in MSI tumors, compared to CIN neoplasms [90]. Lastly, adjuvant chemotherapy with fluorouracil seems to benefit patients with CIN exhibiting tumors, but apparently not those with MSI CRC [78]. Collectively, it is now established that CRC with MSI follows a pathway different from that typified by CIN.

1.2.3 CpG Island Methylator Phenotype (CIMP)

DNA methylation has been recognized as a crucial epigenetic modification of the genome that is involved in regulating several cellular processes including embryonic development, transcription, chromatin structure, X-chromosome inactivation, genomic imprinting and chromosome stability [84]. Epigenetic modification of DNA in mammals consists of methylation at cytosine residues in CpG dinucleotide sequences [8]. Since 5-methylcytosine (m5C) is the only methylated nucleotide in human DNA, and it produces a modification of genetic information without an associated change in DNA sequence, this is referred to as an "epigenetic" alteration. In the past few years tremendous advances have been made in our understanding of the functional consequences of epigenetic alterations. It has been shown that dense methylation at CpG-rich sequences within gene promoters (also referred to as "CpG islands") is associated with compacted chromatin structure, and accompanies transcriptional silencing of the associated gene [85, 60].

Following the initial discoveries for hypermethylation-induced silencing of the retinoblastoma (Rb) gene and Von Hippel–Lindau (VHL) genes, it became increasingly evident that promoter hypermethylation may be a common mechanism for the inactivation of tumor suppressor genes, and that this might be a much broader issue in human tumorigenesis [38]. Since CpG islands are present in more than 50% of human tumor suppressor genes, and because multiple tumor suppressor genes are concurrently silenced by promoter methylation in CRC, this "epigenetic process" was later defined as the CpG island methylator phenotype, or CIMP [42, 98, 52, 77]. CIMP represents an abnormal degree of hypermethylation that occurs in the context of CpG islands only, and is very different from the methylation observed at dinucleotide sequences outside of these regions (primarily in repetitive Alu and LINE sequences) which are ordinarily methylated in normal cells [109].

Since the initial discovery of CIMP in CRC, concordant methylation of multiple genes has also been suggested in gastric cancers [99], liver cancers [91], pancreatic cancers [101], esophageal cancers [41] and several other malignancies outside of the gastrointestinal tract. Despite these suggestions, the concept of CIMP was not well embraced until recently when data from large-scale population-based studies clearly indicated that CIMP represents a unique epigenetic phenotype in CRC [89, 70]. It is now evident that these tumors have a distinct clinical, pathologic and molecular profile, such as associations with older age, proximal tumor location, female sex, poor differentiation, MSI, and high V600E BRAF and low TP53 mutation rates [89, 70, 100, 105, 47, 66, 81, 36, 104]. Using analyses on a large number of CpG island methylation markers, CIMP-high tumors are shown to form a distinct group by an unsupervised cluster analysis [104].

Although the panel of methylation markers and the method for assessment of CIMP are not yet standardized, recent studies have found a fairly sensitive and specific identification of CIMP tumors using various quantitative methods and evaluation of panels of 4 to 8 CpG islands (RUNX3, CACNA1G, IGF2, MLH1, NEUROG1, CRABP1, SOCS1 and CDKN2A (p16) [104]. Any of these panels may be useful to examine CRCs with CIMP; however, there is a lack of consensus criteria to reliably estimate true CIMP frequencies. As a consequence, there is a lack of clear understanding as to what proportion of CRCs may have this underlying epigenetic defect. A recent study suggested that CIN and CIMP may represent two major independent and inversely related mechanisms of genetic and epigenetic instability in sporadic CRCs, and that sporadic MSI cancers are merely a consequence of CIMP due to associated methylation of the hMLH1 gene [31].

Analogous to CIN tumors, the precise molecular mechanisms underlying CIMP are not clear, although empirical observations suggest that methylation per se blocks the binding of transcription factors in the vicinity of methylated CpG islands, or that methylation modifies chromatin structure in a manner that inhibits access to transcription factors [61]. Recent findings, however, indicate that DNA methylation, histone acetylation and changes in chromatin organization may collectively conspire to repress transcription, although the fundamental processes remain, for the most part, enigmatic [84, 9].

From a clinical perspective, limited evidence suggests that CIMP-positive MSI CRCs tend to have a better prognosis, compared to CIMP-positive MSS lesions, which have relatively poorer outcomes [89, 103]. It has also been suggested that the serrated pathway of tumorigenesis may be instrumental in the development of CIMP colon cancers, rather than the traditional adenoma-to-carcinoma sequence [43, 44]. The serrated lesions include a subset of large hyperplastic polyps, and tend to have a high degree of CIMP, and harbor frequent mutations in BRAF and K-Ras genes [47, 14].

The knowledge of epigenetic defects in CRC could be potentially useful for cancer diagnosis and treatment. It is established that epigenetic alterations occur very early during carcinogenesis, and low levels of methylation can be detected in the normal epithelium of some patients. This presents an opportunity to identify methylation markers that demonstrate a gradual increase in methylation and the associated risk of neoplastic transformation. Additionally, since methylation alterations can be easily detected in clinical specimens such as sputum, serum and urine, these approaches offer promise for early diagnosis, risk assessment and follow-up in individuals with suspected underlying colonic disease [93]. An even more exciting aspect of these epigenetic alterations is that, unlike genetic defects, restoring gene function that had been silenced by epigenetic changes using demethylating agents in cancer has the potential for an "epigenetic therapy" by reversing the malignant potential of cancer cells. This could have a large impact on prevention and treatment of CRC. Taken together, aberrant DNA methylation of a subset of genes marks a distinct alternative epigenetic pathway to CRC, with a promise for the development of early detection and prevention strategies, and for CRC treatment.

1.3 Mathematical Modeling of Pathways to Cancer

1.3.1 Mutation-Selection Networks

Here we review mathematical tools of modeling pathways to cancer. The notion of a mutation-selection network has been developed in [69, 51]. A mutation-selection network is a systematic way to present the current state of knowledge about the sequence of molecular events leading to cancer. It may also include hypothetical pathways whose probability can be calculated; see an example in Fig. 1.1. A mutation-selection network consists of nodes, which are different cellular types, connected by arrows. An arrow means that one genetic (or epigenetic) event can transform a given type into a different one. For instance, it could indicate a small-scale inactivating mutation in a certain gene, or an LOH event or a methylation event. Each arrow is equipped with the probability of the corresponding event, such as the mutation rate, or the rate of chromosome loss, or the methylation rate. Depending on the particular system of interest, such rates can be measured per cell division. Otherwise, if the molecular event is independent of cell divisions, the rates are per a time unit.

Each type can also be equipped with some fitness values. Fitness is a term coming from ecological and evolutionary research which describes reproductive success of a species. In the context of somatic evolution of cells in an organ, it refers to the cell's ability to divide and die. In some simple models, the relative cell fitness can be characterized by just one number. In other models, two numbers, the rate of division and the rate of death, characterize the (initial) growth rate of a cell type in a population.

To summarize, a mutation-selection network provides the following information on the cellular processes leading to cancer. The topology of the network tells us which cell types are relevant and which molecular processes could be possible. The fitness parameters tell us about the relative reproductive rates of various types, and the mutation rates characterize the likelihood of transformations.

1.3.2 Rates and Probabilities

In order to proceed with modeling, we need to know the rate parameters. Some of them have been measured, others are unknown.

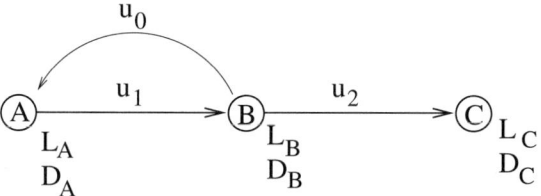

Fig. 1.1. An example of a mutation-selection network. The three types, A, B and C, are connected by arrows corresponding to possible mutation processes; there is a possibility of a back-mutation from B to A, but not from C to B. The division rates of each type are denoted by L with the corresponding subscript; the death rates are D with corresponding subscripts.

For example, the rates of small-scale mutations in cells have been measured in many circumstances, usually resulting in a rate of 10^{-7} per cell division per gene, see e.g. [19, 71, 2, 26]. The somatic mutation rate in human cells has been estimated to be about 10^{-6} per cell division [4]. A mutation rate of about 2×10^{-9} per base pair per year was found on average for mammalian genomes in [53]; it was argued that a large contributing factor here is reproduction-independent mutation processes.

Rates of cell divisions and deaths have also been measured by many authors. The net value of cell growth (the cell division minus cell death) can be measured quite easily by calculating the slope of the log plot of the cell population size vs. time. A more difficult task is to measure the cell division (or cell death) rate independently, in vitro and in vivo. The kinetics of cell death have been quantified in various systems, starting several decades ago [7, 37, 16]. In [82], the cell division rates were measured in vitro by a radioisotopic method. Another technique is to measure cell division rates by DNA synthesis, based on the incorporation of labeled biosynthetic precursors into replicating polydeoxyribonucleotide chains [34, 102]. Several other measures of proliferation such as mitotic index, S-phase fraction and Ki-67 labeling, have been employed [17, 32, 88, 96]. The papers [67] and [64] describe a direct method of measuring breast epithelial cell proliferation rates in vivo in women using heavy water labeling coupled with mass spectrometric analysis.

1.3.3 Stochastic Dynamics on Mutation-Selection Networks

The mutation-selection network itself does not completely specify the dynamics for the system. We need to make further assumptions on the timing of the underlying processes.

A reasonable model is a multispecies stochastic birth-death process with mutations [107]. Depending on the context, one could use the linear birth-death process which describes an exponentially increasing (decreasing) population of cells, or a nonlinear logistic-type process which captures growth with saturation. For our purposes, that is, in order to describe the initiation of CRC, the most suitable models are those that keep the population size constant. Before the first malignant cell is created, homeostatic cell number control is intact, and the total number of cells remains unchanged.

A common example of a stochastic process which preserves the total system size is the Moran process. At each step, a cell is randomly picked for death, and then at the same time a cell is chosen for reproduction (possibly with mutations). While all cells have an equal probability to die, reproduction occurs according to the cells' fitness. (Alternatively, fitness could define the probability of death, or the probabilities of both death and reproduction.)

For example, if the mutation-selection network is just $A \to B$, that is, the type A mutating to type B, then the state of the system is characterized by one integer, j, the number of cells of type B (the number of cells of type A is given by $N - j$, where N is the total, constant population size). There are only three types of transitions that are possible in this system: $j \to j - 1$, $j \to j + 1$ and $j \to j$. The first transition happens if a cell of type B is chosen for death, a cell of type A is chosen for reproduction and the reproduction is faithful. The transition $j \to j + 1$ corresponds to a death of a type A cell and a division of a type B cell, or, alternatively, to a death of a type A cell and a division with a mutation of a type A cell. The transition $j \to j$ corresponds to all other possibilities.

The transition rates can be written as, for example, $P_{j \to j-1} = \frac{j}{N} \times \frac{r_A(N-j)(1-u)}{r_A(N-j)+r_B j}$, where the first factor represents a death of a type B cell, and the second factor represents the faithful reproduction of a type A cell. Constants r_A and r_B are the fitness parameters of types A and B, and u is the mutation rate. A detailed description of the dynamics of the Moran process can be found in [51, 107]. Once the rates are known, a continuous-type Markov process can be formulated, whereby the probability of a $j \to j-1$ event during an infinitesimally small time interval, Δt, is given by $P_{j \to j-1} \Delta t$; the probability of transitioning $j \to j+1$ is $P_{j \to j+1} \Delta t$ and the probability of no change is $1 - (P_{j \to j+1} + P_{j \to j-1}) \Delta t$.

The usual formalism of stochastic processes yields in this case a very large coupled system for probabilities, which is difficult to handle. In the next section we will use an approximate method which allows us to reduce such systems to only a few equations for long-lived states. Then a complete analytical treatment is possible. More details can be found in [50].

1.4 Modeling Sporadic and Familial CRC Initiation

1.4.1 A Simple Model for the Initiation of Sporadic Colorectal Cancers

The colonic epithelium is organized in crypts covered with a self-renewing layer of cells. The total number of crypts is of the order of $M = 10^7$ in a human. Each crypt contains of the order of 10^3 cells. A crypt is renewed by a small number of stem cells (perhaps 1–10) [83, 110]. The life cycle of stem cells is of the order of 1–20 days [73, 5]. Stem cells give rise to differentiated cells which divide at a faster rate, and travel to the top of the crypt where they undergo apoptosis.

Table 1.1. Parameters, notation and possible numerical values; the mutation and LOH rates are given per gene per cell division.

Quantity	Definition	Range
M	Number of crypts in a colon	10^7
N	Effective number of cells in a crypt	1–100
τ	Effective time of cell cycle, days	1–20
u	Probability of mutation in normal (non-MSI) cells	10^{-7}
$\tilde{u}$	Probability of mutation in MSI cells	10^{-4}
p_0	Rate of LOH in normal (non-CIN) cells	10^{-7}
p	Rate of LOH in CIN cells	10^{-2}
n_m	Total number of MSI genes	2–5
n_c	Total number of CIN genes	?

We start with the basic model of sporadic colorectal cancer initiation. All the relevant parameters with their respective values are summarized in Table 1.1. Let us assume that the *effective population size* of a crypt is N; this means that N cells are at risk of developing mutations which can lead to cancer. If only the stem cells are at risk of developing cancer, then $N \sim 1$–10, and the average turnover rate is $\tau = 1$–20 days. Let us denote by X_0, X_1 and X_2 the probability that the whole crypt consists of cells with 0, 1 and 2 copies of the APC gene inactivated, respectively. The relevant mutation-selection network leading from X_0 to X_1 to X_2 is shown in Fig. 1.2.

At the beginning (see Fig. 1.2), all cells are wild type. The first copy of the APC gene can be inactivated by a mutation event. Because the mutation rate per gene per cell division, $u \approx 10^{-7}$, is very small and the number of cells, N, is not large, it is safe to assume that once a mutation occurs, the population typically has enough time to become homogeneous again before the next mutation occurs. The condition is that the mutation rate, u, is much smaller than $1/N$, as was derived in [51]. This means that most of the time the effective population of cells in a crypt can be considered as homogeneous with respect to APC mutations. Under this assumption we have $X_0 + X_1 + X_2 = 1$.

Initially, all the N cells of a crypt have two copies of the APC gene. The first copy of the APC gene can be inactivated by means of a point mutation. The probability of mutation is given by N (a mutation can occur in any of the N cells) times the mutation rate per cell division, u, times 2, because either of the two copies of the APC gene can be mutated. Because inactivation of one copy of the APC does not lead to any phenotypic changes, the rate of fixation of the corresponding (neutral) mutant is equal to

$$\rho = \lim_{r \to 1} \frac{1 - 1/r}{1 - 1/r^N} = 1/N,$$

see [51]. "Fixation" means that the mutant cells take over the crypt. Therefore, the rate of change from X_0 to X_1 is $2uN \times 1/N = 2u$. Once the first allele of the APC gene has been inactivated, the second allele can be inactivated either by another point mutation or by an LOH event. This process occurs with rate $N(u + p_0)$, where p_0 is the rate of LOH in normal (non-CIN) cells. We assume that mutants with both copies of the APC gene inactivated have a large selective advantage.

The mutation-selection network of Fig. 1.2 is equivalent to a linear system

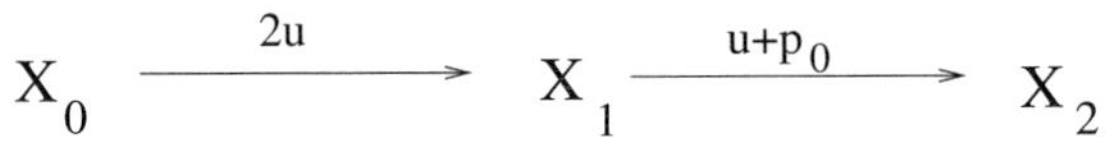

$$X_0 \xrightarrow{\quad 2u \quad} X_1 \xrightarrow{\quad u+p_0 \quad} X_2$$

Fig. 1.2. Mutation-selection network of sporadic colorectal cancer initiation. Initially, the crypt is at the state X_0, i.e. all cells are wild type. A point mutation in one of the copies of the APC gene leads to type X_1. The first allele of the APC gene is inactivated at a rate $2u$, the factor 2 comes from the fact that there are two intact alleles at first. The inactivation of the second allele of the APC gene (the transition to X_2) can happen by a point mutation (at the rate u), or by an LOH event (rate p_0).

of ordinary differential equations (ODEs), where the rates by the arrows refer to the coefficients and the direction of the arrows to the sign of the terms. One (non-dimensional) time unit ($t/\tau = 1$) corresponds to a generation turn-over. The calculations leading to the mutation-selection network are performed for a Moran process where the population size is kept constant by removing one cell each time a cell reproduces, see [107]. Our biological time unit again corresponds to N "elementary events" of the Moran process, where an elementary event includes one birth and one death. We have

$$\dot{X}_0 = -2uX_0,$$
$$\dot{X}_1 = 2uX_0 - N(u + p_0)X_1,$$

with the constraint $X_0 + X_1 + X_2 = 1$ and the initial condition

$$X_0(0) = 1, \quad X_1(0) = 0.$$

With the rate $2u$, cells with one copy of the APC gene mutated will take over the crypt (state X_1). This rate of change is calculated as N times the probability (per cell division) to produce a mutant of X_1 ($2u$ because either of the two alleles can be mutated) times the probability of *one* mutant of type X_1 to get fixed ($1/N$ since there is no phenotypic change). From state X_1 the system can go to state X_2 (both copies of the APC gene inactivated) with the rate $N(u + p_0)$. This rate is calculated as N times the probability per cell division to produce a mutant of X_2 (u for an independent point mutation plus p_0 for an LOH event) times the probability of the *advantageous* mutant of type X_2 to take over (this is 1). In the equations above, we use the fact that the intermediate mutant is neutral and that the population size is small, so that the probability to jump directly from state X_0 to state X_2 can be neglected (see [51] for the exact condition). Calculations for larger values of N can also be performed.

Using $ut/\tau \ll 1$ and $N(p_0 + u)t/\tau \ll 1$, we can approximate the solution for X_2 as

$$X_2(t) = Nu(u + p_0)(t/\tau)^2.$$

The quantity $X_2(t)$ stands for the probability that a crypt is dysplastic (i.e. consists of cells with both copies of the APC gene inactivated) at time t measured in days. There are two steps that separate the state X_0 from the state X_2, and thus the expected number of dysplastic crypts in a person of age t is proportional to the product of the two rates and the second power of time. This reminds us of the general Armitage–Doll model where the power dependence of the probability of cancer is equal to the number of mutations in the multistage process. In our case, the number of mutations needed to create a dysplastic crypt is two.

The probability to have i dysplastic crypts by the age t is given by a simple binomial, $\binom{M}{i} X_2(t)^i (1 - X_2(t))^{M-i}$. The expected number of dysplastic crypts in a person of age t is then given by the following quantity:

$$MNu(u + p_0)(t/\tau)^2. \tag{1.1}$$

Some estimates of the expected number of dysplastic crypts, based on equation (1.1), are given in Fig. 1.3. We plot the logarithm of the expected number of dysplastic crypts as a function of τ, the effective time of cell cycle, for two different values of the rate of LOH in stable cells, p_0. When comparing these calculations with data, one has to keep the following considerations in mind. It is possible that dysplastic crypts can be lost. The model presented here gives the number of dysplastic crypts that are being *produced* over time, which could be larger than the actual number of dysplastic crypts that patients have at a particular time point. Exact measurements of the incidence of dysplastic crypts will provide important information about the crucial parameters of CRC initiation.

1.4.2 Sporadic Colorectal Cancers, CIN and MSI

Next we consider the possibility of developing genetic instabilities during cancer initiation. Starting from a population of normal cells, three different events can occur: (i) inactivation of the first copy of the APC gene, (ii) inactivation of the first copy of one of n_m MSI genes and (iii) mutation of one copy of one of n_c CIN genes.

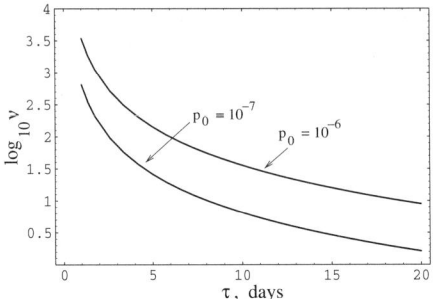

Fig. 1.3. The simple model of CRC initiation: the logarithm of the expected number of dysplastic crypts at the age 70 years, as a function of τ. $N = 5$, $M = 10^7$, $u = 10^{-6}$.

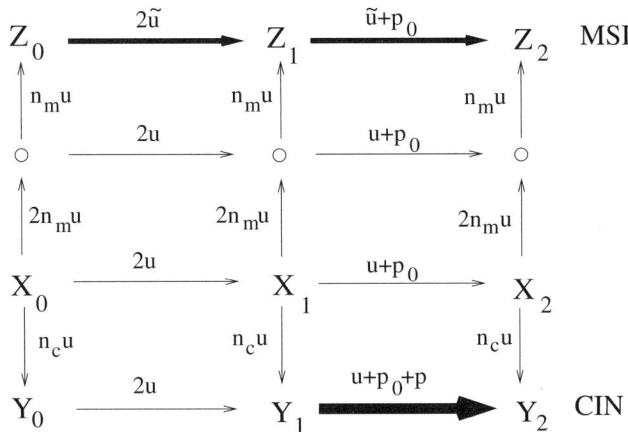

Fig. 1.4. Mutation-selection network of sporadic CRC initiation including CIN and MSI. From the initial wild type state, X_0, the crypt can change to state X_1 as in Fig. 1.2, acquire a CIN mutation (the arrow down) or an MSI mutation (the arrow up). The line $X_0 \to X_1 \to X_2$ is identical to the process in Fig. 1.2 of developing a dysplastic crypt with no genetic instabilities. The bottom row of the diagram corresponds to CIN cells acquiring the first, and then the second, mutation (loss) of the APC gene; the second copy can be lost by a point mutation or by an LOH event whose rate is much larger for CIN cells than it is for normal or MSI cells. The state Y_2 corresponds to a CIN dysplastic crypt. The top row is the development of an MSI dysplastic crypt. The MSI phenotype is characterized by an increased point mutation rate, $\tilde{u}$. The state Z_2 is an MSI dysplastic crypt. Thick arrows denote faster steps. Note that it takes only one leap (down) to go to a CIN state from a state with no genetic instability, because CIN genes are dominant-negative. It takes two steps to acquire MSI (up) because both copies of an MSI gene need to be inactivated before any phenotypic changes occur.

We use the notation X_i, Y_i and Z_i, respectively, for the probability that a crypt consists of normal cells, CIN cells or MSI cells with i copies of the APC gene inactivated, see Table 1.2. Fig. 1.4 shows the mutation-selection network of colorectal cancer initiation including CIN and MSI. All the transition rates are calculated as the relevant mutation rate times the probability that the mutant will take over the crypt.

Table 1.2. The three major classes of homogeneous states.

Quantity	Definition	Point mutation rate	Rate of LOH
X_0, X_1, X_2	non-CIN, non-MSI	u	p_0
Y_0, Y_1, Y_2	CIN	u	$p > p_0$
Z_0, Z_1, Z_2	MSI	$\tilde{u} > u$	p_0

Let us denote the rate of LOH in CIN cells as p. We assume that the crucial effect of CIN is to increase the rate of LOH [58, 6], which implies $p > p_0$. Intuitively, the advantage of CIN for the cancer cell is to accelerate the loss of the second copy of a tumor suppressor gene. Similarly, the advantage of MSI is to increase the point-mutation rate, which means that $\tilde{u} > u$.

We are interested in the probability to find the crypt in the state X_2, Y_2 and Z_2 as a function of t. In other words, we want to know the probability for the dysplastic crypt to have CIN (Y_2), MSI (Z_2) or no genetic instability (X_2). The mutation-selection network of Fig. 1.4 is more complicated than the one-dimensional network of Fig. 1.2, but the solutions for X_2, Y_2 and Z_2 can still be written.

The diagram of Fig. 1.4 corresponds to a system of 11 linear ODEs describing the time evolution of the probabilities to find the system in any of the 12 possible homogeneous states. Let us use the fact that the quantities ut/τ and $N(u+p_0)t/\tau$ are very small compared to 1 for $t \sim 70$ years, and the quantity $Npt/\tau \gg 1$. This tells us that the steps in the diagram characterized by the rates u and p_0 are slow (rate limiting) compared to the steps with the rate p. Taking the Taylor expansion of the solution in terms of ut/τ and $N(u+p_0)t/\tau$, we obtain the following result:

$$X_2(t) = Nu(u + p_0)(t/\tau)^2, \qquad Y_2(t) = 4n_c u^2 (t/\tau)^2. \qquad (1.2)$$

The rate $\tilde{u}$ is neither fast nor slow, so the solution for Z_2 is more complicated. We have

$$Z_2(t) = \frac{n_m u(u + p_0)}{(ab\tilde{u})^2(a - b)} \Big(2(b^3 E_a - a^3 E_b + a^3 - b^3$$

$$+ ab(b^2 - a^2)\tilde{u}t/\tau) + a^2 b^2 (a - b)\tilde{u}^2 (t/\tau)^2 \Big) \qquad (1.3)$$

where $a = 2$, $b = N(\tilde{u} + p_0)/\tilde{u}$ and $E_x = e^{-x\tilde{u}t/\tau}$. Note that if the $\tilde{u}$-steps are fast (i.e. if $\tilde{u}t/\tau \gg 1$), the limit of this expression is given by $Z(t) =$

$n_m u(u + p_0)(t/\tau)^2$. In the opposite limit where $\tilde{u}t/\tau \ll 1$, we have $Z(t) = n_m N u(u + p_0)\tilde{u}(\tilde{u} + p_0)(t/\tau)^4/6$.

The key idea of this analysis is to identify how many slow (rate-limiting) steps separate the initial state (X_0) from the state of interest. The slow steps in our model are the ones whose rates scale with u or p_0. The step from Y_1 to Y_2 is fast, because it is proportional to the rate of LOH in CIN cells, p, which is much larger than u and p_0. The steps with the rate $\tilde{u}$ are neither fast nor slow. For all possible pathways from the initial state to the final state of interest, we have to multiply the slow rates together times the appropriate power of t/τ, and divide by the factorial of the number of slow steps. Summing over all possible paths we will obtain the probability to find the crypt in the state in question.

Applying this rule, we can see that $X_2(t)$ and $Y_2(t)$ are both quadratic in time, because it takes two rate-limiting steps to go from X_0 to X_2 and from X_0 to Y_2. The state Z_2 is separated from X_0 by two rate-limiting steps and two "intermediate" steps (whose rate is proportional to $\tilde{u}$), so the quantity $Z_2(t)$ grows as the fourth power of time for $\tilde{u}t/\tau \ll 1$ and as the second power of time in the opposite limit.

The probability that a crypt is dysplastic at time t is given by $P(t) = X_2(t) + Y_2(t) + Z_2(t)$. Therefore, the expected number of dysplastic crypts in a person of age t, $\nu(t)$, is given by $MP(t)$,

$$\nu(t) = M(X_2(t) + Y_2(t) + Z_2(t)).$$

Of these dysplastic crypts, $MY_2(t)$ have CIN and $MZ_2(t)$ have MSI. This suggests that the fraction of CIN cancers is at least $Y_2(t)/P(t)$ and the fraction of MSI cancers is at least $Z_2(t)/P(t)$. Some numerical examples of such computations are presented in Fig. 1.5, where the logarithm of the expected number of dysplastic crypts is plotted against τ, for three different values of n_c, the number of CIN genes. We can see that n_c leads to much elevated numbers of dysplastic crypts which may be unrealistic.

Fig. 1.6(a) presents relative fractions of dysplastic crypts with CIN (gray lines) and MSI (black lines) as functions of of n_c. Larger values of n_c lead to an increased percentage of dysplastic crypts with CIN. The fraction of MSI crypts as predicted by this model is quite low (for $n_c = 10$ we get only 0.1% of dysplastic crypts with MSI). This could mean that MSI develops at later stages of cancer. However, there is indirect evidence that the replication error phenotype precedes, and is responsible for, APC mutations in MSI cancers [40]. At the same time, according to observations, 13% of all sporadic CRCs have MSI [59]. Our model is consistent with this data if we assume higher rates of MSI induction in a cell. These could be a consequence of epigenetic mechanisms of MSI gene inactivation. DNA methylation of the hMLH1 gene is found at a high frequency in sporadic MSI tumors [1, 48, 18].

In the diagram of Fig. 1.4 this means that the rates from X_0 to the MSI type (vertical arrows), $2n_m u$ and $u + p_0$, should be replaced by $2n_m u_{met}$ and $u_{met} + p_0$, respectively, where u_{met} is the rate of methylation per gene

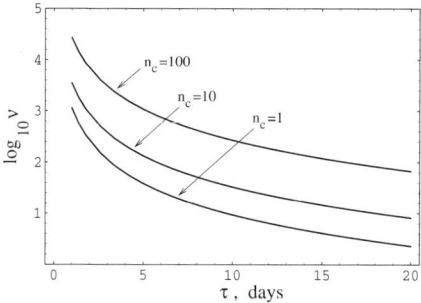

Fig. 1.5. Sporadic CRC: the logarithm of the expected number of dysplastic crypts as a function of τ at 70 years of age, in the model with CIN and MSI. The three curves correspond to three different values of n_c. $M = 10^7$, $N = 5$, $u = 10^{-7}$, $\tilde{u} = 10^{-4}$, $p_0 = 10^{-7}$, $n_m = 3$ and $t = 70$ years.

per cell division. In terms of our equations, we need to replace u by u_{met} in the expression for $Z_2(t)$, equation (1.3). De novo methylation rates have not been quantified; in Fig. 1.6(b) we assume that u_{met} is larger than the basic mutation rate, u ($u_{met} = 10^{-6}$), and plot the proportion of MSI crypts. We can see that the expected fraction of MSI crypts predicted by our model becomes larger. Fig. 1.6(b) should be compared with the observation that 13% of dysplastic crypts are MSI. We can see that this holds for values of n_c of the order of 10. As n_c becomes larger than about 20, the predicted fraction of CIN crypts becomes much higher, and the fraction of MSI crypts much lower than expected.

In our model, we assume that CIN is generated by means of a mutation in any of n_c dominant-negative CIN genes. In other words, a genetic hit in either of the two copies of a CIN gene will lead to the acquisition of the CIN phenotype. Alternatively, it could happen that the CIN phenotype requires the inactivation of both copies, like MSI genes or tumor suppressor genes. In terms of Fig. 1.4, this would mean that we have two steps separating the wild type (X_0) from the CIN phenotype (Z_0). If we assume that the CIN phenotype is neutral, the fraction of CIN dysplastic crypts in Fig. 1.6 would be negligible. This means that in this case, the CIN phenotype must be very advantageous in order to show up early in carcinogenesis.

1.4.3 Familial Adenomatous Polyposis (FAP)

This framework allows us to study familial cancers in a systematic manner, by modifying the basic mutation-selection diagram of Fig. 1.4. In FAP patients, one allele of the APC gene is inactivated in the germ line. In terms of our model this means that all crypts start in state X_1. The corresponding mutation-selection network is shown in Fig. 1.7(a).

Again, the mutation-selection diagram can be converted into a system of ODEs. The solutions are given by

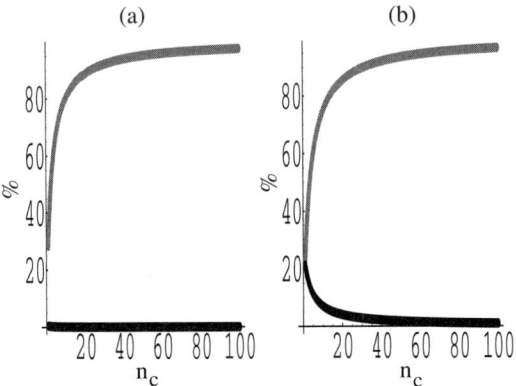

Fig. 1.6. Sporadic CRC: fractions of crypts with different instabilities, as a function of n_c; gray lines correspond to CIN and black lines to MSI. (a) The inactivation of MCI genes is by mutation, with the rate $u = 10^{-7}$. (b) The inactivation of MCI genes is by methylation, with the rate $u = 10^{-6}$. The rest of the parameters are as in Fig. 1.5.

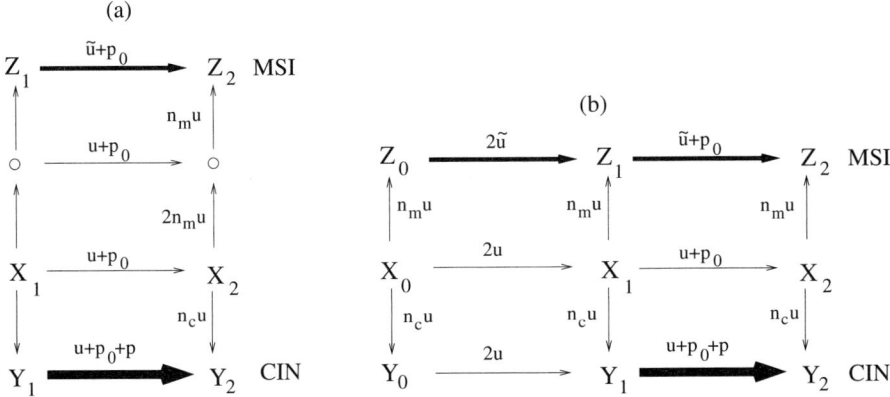

Fig. 1.7. (a) Mutation-selection network of FAP initiation. We start with the type X_1 because the first copy of the APC gene is inactivated in the germ line. (b) Mutation-selection network of HNPCC initiation. One mutation of an MSI gene is inherited, and therefore it takes only *one* step (inactivation of the second copy of the MSI gene, arrows up) to develop the MSI phenotype.

$$X_2(t) = N(u + p_0)t/\tau, \qquad Y_2(t) = 2n_c ut/\tau,$$

and

$$Z_2(t) = \frac{n_m u(u + p_0)[2 - 2\tilde{u}bt/\tau + (\tilde{u}bt/\tau)^2 - 2E_b]}{(\tilde{u}b)^2}.$$

In the limit where $\tilde{u}t/\tau \to \infty$, we have $Z_2(t) = n_m u(u+p_0)(t/\tau)^2$. If $\tilde{u}t/\tau \ll 1$, then $Z_2(t) = n_m Nu(u + p_0)(\tilde{u} + p_0)(t/\tau)^3/3$. $X_2(t)$ and $Y_2(t)$ are linear functions of time (there is one rate-limiting step), whereas $Z_2(t)$ grows more slowly than the second power of time (two rate-limiting steps plus one 'intermediate' step).

Some predictions of the model are shown in Fig. 1.8. The expected number of dysplastic crypts and the fraction of CIN crypts are calculated for $t = 16$ years. As the number of CIN genes, n_c, increases, we expect more dysplastic crypts, and a larger fraction of crypts with CIN. According to our model, the expected number of dysplastic crypts grows linearly with time, and by the age of 16 years is expected to be in the thousands to tens of thousands (see Fig. 1.8(a)). This should be compared with the observation that about 50% of FAP patients develop polyps (a more advanced stage of carcinogenesis compared with dysplastic crypts) by age 16.

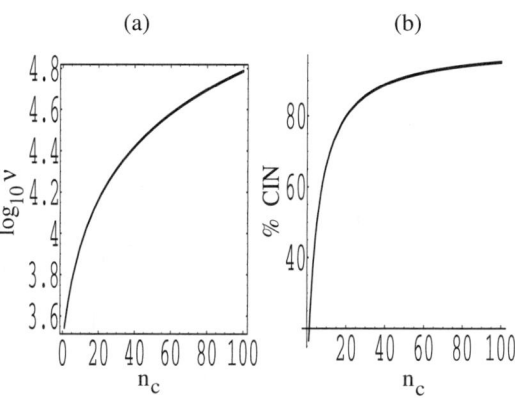

Fig. 1.8. FAP: (a) the logarithm of the expected number of dysplastic crypts and (b) the fraction of CIN crypts, at 16 years of age, as functions of n_c. Parameter values are as in Fig. 1.5. In (b), the fraction of MSI is nearly zero.

The number of polyps in FAP patients does not grow linearly with time. Instead, most polyps appear "suddenly" in the second decade of life. These observations are consistent with the predictions of our model. It is believed that polyps result from dysplastic crypts by means of further somatic mutations and clonal expansions. Therefore, the number of polyps is expected to be a higher than linear power of time, which looks like a steep increase in the number of lesions after a relatively non-eventful period. Also, the number of dysplastic crypts (10^3–10^4 in our model) is expected to be much larger than the number of polyps (10^2–10^3) consistent with the expectation that not all dysplastic crypts progress to polyps.

Another prediction of this model is that the fraction of MSI crypts in patients with FAP is negligible. This is consistent with an experimental study where MSI was found in none of the 57 adenomas from FAP patients [49].

Finally, we note that the logical possibility exists that the second copy of the APC gene in FAP patients may be inactivated by an epigenetic event, just like the second copy of an MSI gene can be silenced by methylation. Experimental investigations [22] however suggest that this is unlikely: out of the 84 FAP tumors, only 1 exhibited hypermethylation of the APC gene.

1.4.4 HNPCC

Patients with HNPCC inherit one mutation in an MSI gene. The corresponding mutation-selection network is presented in Fig. 1.7(b). The solutions for X_2 and Y_2 in this case are identical to those for sporadic CRCs and are given by equations (1.2). The solution for Z_2 is as follows:

$$Z_2(t) = \frac{(u + p_0)[a^2 E_b - b^2 E_a + (a - b)(\tilde{u}abt/\tau - (a + b))]}{ab\tilde{u}(a - b)} ;$$

in the limit where $\tilde{u}$ is a fast rate we have $Z_2(t) = (u + p_0)t/\tau$. In the opposite limit, where $\tilde{u}$ is a slow rate, $Z_2(t) = N(u + p_0)\tilde{u}(\tilde{u} + p_0)(t/\tau)^3/3$. If we assume that the second copy of the MSI gene is silenced by methylation, we need to replace u by u_{met} in the expression for $Z_2(t)$.

The solutions for X_2 and Y_2 in this case are quadratic in time (two rate-limiting steps), and the quantity $Z_2(t)$ grows slower than linear but faster than quadratic, because it requires one rate-limiting and two intermediate steps (note that we are talking about linear and quadratic functions of an argument smaller than one). In Fig. 1.9 we present the expected number of dysplastic crypts and the fraction of MSI crypts, calculated for $t = 40$. We have varied the rate at which inactivation of the second copy of an MSI gene occurs. This rate, u_{met}, ranges from 10^{-7}, which corresponds to the methylation rate equal to the mutation rate (or to inactivation happening by a point mutation), to 10^{-5}, where we assume that the methylation rate is a hundred times higher than the mutation rate.

Our model predicts that the majority of dysplastic crypts in HNPCC patients are expected to have MSI. However, we do not find that 100% of dysplastic crypts will contain MSI, if the inactivation of an MSI gene occurs by a point mutation (this corresponds to $u_{met} = 10^{-7}$. On the other hand, we know that virtually all tumors in HNPCC patients have MSI. This might suggest that the inactivation of MSI genes occurs by methylation, and its rate is significantly higher than that of point mutations.

Finally, we note that the total number of dysplastic crypts in HNPCC patients, as predicted by our model, is of the order 10 at age 40, which is only slightly larger than the expected number of dysplastic crypts in normal individuals and is not nearly as high as in the case of FAP (of the order $10,000$, Fig. 1.8). This is also consistent with observations.

1.5 Discussion

We have applied mathematical tools to study the dynamics of CRC initiation. We calculate the rate of dysplastic crypt formation as a consequence of inacti-

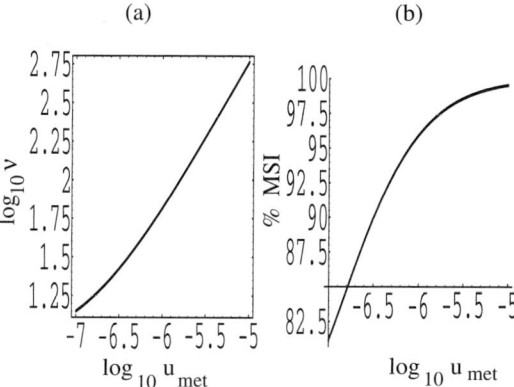

Fig. 1.9. HNPCC: (a) the logarithm of the expected number of dysplastic crypts and (b) the fraction of MSI crypts, at 40 years of age, as functions of $\log_{10} u_{met}$. Parameter values are as in Fig. 1.5, with $n_c = 10$.

vating both alleles of the APC tumor suppressor gene. This can either happen in normal cells or in cells that have already acquired one of the two genetic instabilities, MSI or CIN. If the rate of triggering genetic instability in a cell is high and if the cost of genetic instability is not too large, then inactivation of APC will frequently occur in cells that are genetically unstable. In this case, genetic instability is the first phenotypic modification of a cell on the way to cancer.

It is interesting to compare the two types of instability, MSI and CIN. MSI, being associated with subtle changes in the genome, is probably less of a liability for the cell than CIN. In other words, CIN cells are more likely to produce non-viable offspring than MSI cells. At the same time, it may be possible that CIN is easier to trigger (for instance, if it requires a change in a single allele of many genes). Our analysis shows that if inactivation of MSI genes (either by point mutation or by methylation) occurs at a sufficiently fast rate—around 10^{-6} per cell division—then MSI can precede APC inactivation in a significant number of cases. Regarding CIN, the crucial questions are (i) how many dominant CIN genes can be found in the human genome, (ii) how fast are CIN genes inactivated and (iii) what are the costs of CIN.

Our calculations show that important insights could be derived by carefully monitoring the incidence rate of dysplastic crypts in patients as a function of age. With or without early genetic instability, the abundance of dysplastic crypts should grow approximately as a second power of time. The two rate-limiting steps can either refer to two mutations of APC, or one mutation of APC and one CIN mutation. In the case of CIN, LOH of the second allele of APC is not rate-limiting. Hence, two rate-limiting steps for the inactivation of a tumor suppressor gene can be compatible with an additional genetic instability mutation.

Our analysis also gives rise to some quantitative estimates of biological parameters whose values are unknown. This comes by comparing the results of the calculations with experimental observations. For example, it is known that about 12–15% of sporadic CRCs have MSI. Assuming that CIN and MSI are irreversible, the maximum fraction of dysplastic crypts with CIN should be 88%, while the maximum fraction of dysplastic crypts with MSI should be 15%. This provides certain restrictions on the possible parameter values of our model.

In general, an analysis of this type creates a bridge between very different levels of description of the process of carcinogenesis. At the lowest, intracellular level, we have biological information about mutations and other molecular events that play a role in CRC. At the next (intercellular) scale we create our models which describe stochastic dynamics of populations of cells. Our models include the intracellular level of description in the form of rate parameters (mutation and methylation rates), as well as the geometry of the mutation-selection networks. Finally, the outcome of modeling can be compared with the highest level of cancer description, that is, the epidemiology of cancer. Data such as incidence curves and percentages of CRC with certain characteristics can be used for a meaningful comparison with the predictions of stochastic models. This is a simple but instructive example of a multiscale approach to cancer description.

Several further insights emerge from our analysis.

Epigenetic factors. If we assume that MSI genes in sporadic CRC are inactivated only by point mutation or LOH events, then the fraction of dysplastic crypts with MSI is very low. We get higher fractions of MSI if we assume that MSI genes can also be inactivated by methylation and if methylation of MSI genes is fast compared to point mutation or LOH. Thus, methylation events could play a crucial role in the formation of sporadic MSI cancers.

Competition among crypts. Another interesting possibility is that dysplastic crypts can be lost and replaced by normal crypts. In this case, many dysplastic crypts could be produced, but only a part of them retained, so that the actual number of dysplastic crypts stays low. To our knowledge, the competitive dynamics of crypts in a colon has not been investigated experimentally.

No MSI in FAP. Our model predicts that the fraction of MSI dysplastic crypts in FAP patients is close to zero. A significant number of dysplastic crypts will contain CIN. This is consistent with experimental observations.

The number of dysplastic crypts. We calculated both the absolute numbers and relative proportions of dysplastic crypts with or without genetic instabilities. An interesting empirical project is to measure the abundance of such dysplastic crypts as a function of age. This will provide crucial information on the dynamics of colorectal cancer initiation.

A more precise description of the mutation spectrum. The mutation spectrum of the APC gene is far from random (one reason being that the APC gene is long and multifunctional). The type of the second APC mutation may depend on where the first APC mutation took place [87, 55]. Our model is well suited to take this into account. Here is a simple way to differentiate between two kinds of point mutations. Let us assume that the total probability of a point mutation is u (as in the basic model), and there are two kinds of mutations. (i) With probability u_1, a mutation occurs such that the second allele can *only* be inactivated by a point mutation. (ii) With probability u_2, a mutation occurs which can be followed by another point mutation *or* an LOH event. We have $u_1 + u_2 = u$. These two scenarios can be incorporated in our calculations, adding a new level of complexity to the basic theory.

References

1. Ahuja, N., Mohan, A.L., Li, Q., Stolker, J.M., Herman, J.G., Hamilton, S.R., Baylin, S.B., Issa, J.P.: Association between CpG island methylation and microsatellite instability in colorectal cancer. Cancer Res **57**(16), 3370–3374 (1997)
2. Albertini, R.J., Nicklas, J.A., O'Neill, J.P., Robison, S.H.: In vivo somatic mutations in humans: measurement and analysis. Annu Rev Genet **24**, 305–326 (1990)
3. Alexander, J., Watanabe, T., Wu, T.T., Rashid, A., Li, S., Hamilton, S.R.: Histopathological identification of colon cancer with microsatellite instability. Am J Pathol **158**(2), 527–535 (2001)
4. Araten, D.J., Golde, D.W., Zhang, R.H., Thaler, H.T., Gargiulo, L., Notaro, R., Luzzatto, L.: A quantitative measurement of the human somatic mutation rate. Cancer Res **65**(18), 8111–8117 (2005)
5. Bach, S.P., Renehan, A.G., Potten, C.S.: Stem cells: the intestinal stem cell as a paradigm. Carcinogenesis **21**(3), 469–476 (2000)
6. Bardelli, A., Cahill, D.P., Lederer, G., Speicher, M.R., Kinzler, K.W., Vogelstein, B., Lengauer, C.: Carcinogen-specific induction of genetic instability. Proc Natl Acad Sci USA **98**(10), 5770–5775 (2001)
7. Bernheim, J.L., Mendelsohn, J., Kelley, M.F., Dorian, R.: Kinetics of cell death and disintegration in human lymphocyte cultures. Proc Natl Acad Sci USA **74**(6), 2536–2540 (1977)
8. Bird, A.: DNA methylation patterns and epigenetic memory. Genes Dev **16**(1), 6–21 (2002)
9. Bird, A.P., Wolffe, A.P.: Methylation-induced repression—belts, braces, and chromatin. Cell **99**(5), 451–454 (1999)
10. Bischoff, J.R., Anderson, L., Zhu, Y., Mossie, K., Ng, L., Souza, B., Schryver, B., Flanagan, P., Clairvoyant, F., Ginther, C., Chan, C.S., Novotny, M., Slamon, D.J., Plowman, G.D.: A homologue of Drosophila aurora kinase is oncogenic and amplified in human colorectal cancers. EMBO J **17**(11), 3052–3065 (1998). Comparative Study
11. Boland, C.R., Thibodeau, S.N., Hamilton, S.R., Sidransky, D., Eshleman, J.R., Burt, R.W., Meltzer, S.J., Rodriguez-Bigas, M.A., Fodde, R., Ranzani, G.N.,

Srivastava, S.: A National Cancer Institute Workshop on Microsatellite Instability for cancer detection and familial predisposition: development of international criteria for the determination of microsatellite instability in colorectal cancer. Cancer Res **58**(22), 5248–5257 (1998). Consensus Development Conference

12. Cahill, D.P., Kinzler, K.W., Vogelstein, B., Lengauer, C.: Genetic instability and darwinian selection in tumours. Trends Cell Biol **9**(12), 57–60 (1999)

13. Cahill, D.P., Lengauer, C., Yu, J., Riggins, G.J., Willson, J.K., Markowitz, S.D., Kinzler, K.W., Vogelstein, B.: Mutations of mitotic checkpoint genes in human cancers. Nature **392**(6673), 300–303 (1998)

14. Chan, A.O.O., Issa, J.P., Morris, J.S., Hamilton, S.R., Rashid, A.: Concordant CpG island methylation in hyperplastic polyposis. Am J Pathol **160**(2), 529–536 (2002)

15. de la Chapelle, A.: Genetic predisposition to colorectal cancer. Nat Rev Cancer **4**(10), 769–780 (2004)

16. Chu, K., Leonhardt, E.A., Trinh, M., Prieur-Carrillo, G., Lindqvist, J., Albright, N., Ling, C.C., Dewey, W.C.: Computerized video time-lapse (CVTL) analysis of cell death kinetics in human bladder carcinoma cells (EJ30) X-irradiated in different phases of the cell cycle. Radiat Res **158**(6), 667–677 (2002)

17. Clahsen, P.C., van de Velde, C.J., Duval, C., Pallud, C., Mandard, A.M., Delobelle-Deroide, A., van den Broek, L., van de Vijver, M.J.: The utility of mitotic index, oestrogen receptor and Ki-67 measurements in the creation of novel prognostic indices for node-negative breast cancer. Eur J Surg Oncol **25**(4), 356–363 (1999)

18. Cunningham, J.M., Christensen, E.R., Tester, D.J., Kim, C.Y., Roche, P.C., Burgart, L.J., Thibodeau, S.N.: Hypermethylation of the hMLH1 promoter in colon cancer with microsatellite instability. Cancer Res **58**(15), 3455–3460 (1998)

19. Drake, J.W., Charlesworth, B., Charlesworth, D., Crow, J.F.: Rates of spontaneous mutation. Genetics **148**(4), 1667–1686 (1998)

20. Duesberg, P., Rausch, C., Rasnick, D., Hehlmann, R.: Genetic instability of cancer cells is proportional to their degree of aneuploidy. Proc Natl Acad Sci USA **95**(23), 13,692–13,697 (1998)

21. Eshleman, J.R., Casey, G., Kochera, M.E., Sedwick, W.D., Swinler, S.E., Veigl, M.L., Willson, J.K., Schwartz, S., Markowitz, S.D.: Chromosome number and structure both are markedly stable in RER colorectal cancers and are not destabilized by mutation of p53. Oncogene **17**(6), 719–725 (1998). Comparative Study

22. Esteller, M., Fraga, M.F., Guo, M., Garcia-Foncillas, J., Hedenfalk, I., Godwin, A.K., Trojan, J., Vaurs-Barriere, C., Bignon, Y.J., Ramus, S., Benitez, J., Caldes, T., Akiyama, Y., Yuasa, Y., Launonen, V., Canal, M.J., Rodriguez, R., Capella, G., Peinado, M.A., Borg, A., Aaltonen, L.A., Ponder, B.A., Baylin, S.B., Herman, J.G.: DNA methylation patterns in hereditary human cancers mimic sporadic tumorigenesis. Hum Mol Genet **10**(26), 3001–3007 (2001)

23. Fearon, E.R., Vogelstein, B.: A genetic model for colorectal tumorigenesis. Cell **61**(5), 759–767 (1990)

24. Fodde, R., Kuipers, J., Rosenberg, C., Smits, R., Kielman, M., Gaspar, C., van Es, J.H., Breukel, C., Wiegant, J., Giles, R.H., Clevers, H.: Mutations in

the APC tumour suppressor gene cause chromosomal instability. Nat Cell Biol **3**(4), 433–438 (2001)

25. Fodde, R., Smits, R., Clevers, H.: APC, signal transduction and genetic instability in colorectal cancer. Nat Rev Cancer **1**(1), 55–67 (2001)

26. Foster, P.L.: Sorting out mutation rates. Proc Natl Acad Sci USA **96**(14), 7617–7618 (1999). Comment

27. Fraizer, G.C., Diaz, M.F., Lee, I.L., Grossman, H.B., Sen, S.: Aurora-A/STK15/BTAK enhances chromosomal instability in bladder cancer cells. Int J Oncol **25**(6), 1631–1639 (2004)

28. Giet, R., Petretti, C., Prigent, C.: Aurora kinases, aneuploidy and cancer, a coincidence or a real link? Trends Cell Biol **15**(5), 241–250 (2005)

29. Goel, A., Arnold, C.N., Niedzwiecki, D., Chang, D.K., Ricciardiello, L., Carethers, J.M., Dowell, J.M., Wasserman, L., Compton, C., Mayer, R.J., Bertagnolli, M.M., Boland, C.R.: Characterization of sporadic colon cancer by patterns of genomic instability. Cancer Res **63**(7), 1608–1614 (2003)

30. Goel, A., Li, M.S., Nagasaka, T., Shin, S.K., Fuerst, F., Ricciardiello, L., Wasserman, L., Boland, C.R.: Association of JC virus T-antigen expression with the methylator phenotype in sporadic colorectal cancers. Gastroenterology **130**(7), 1950–1961 (2006). Comparative Study

31. Goel, A., Nagasaka, T., Arnold, C.N., Inoue, T., Hamilton, C., Niedzwiecki, D., Compton, C., Mayer, R.J., Goldberg, R., Bertagnolli, M.M., Boland, C.R.: The CpG island methylator phenotype and chromosomal instability are inversely correlated in sporadic colorectal cancer. Gastroenterology **132**(1), 127–138 (2007)

32. Goodson, W.H., Moore, D.H., Ljung, B.M., Chew, K., Florendo, C., Mayall, B., Smith, H.S., Waldman, F.M.: The functional relationship between in vivo bromodeoxyuridine labeling index and Ki-67 proliferation index in human breast cancer. Breast Cancer Res Treat **49**(2), 155–164 (1998). Comparative Study

33. Grady, W.M.: Genomic instability and colon cancer. Cancer Metastasis Rev **23**(1-2), 11–27 (2004)

34. Gratzner, H.G.: Monoclonal antibody to 5-bromo- and 5-iododeoxyuridine: A new reagent for detection of DNA replication. Science **218**(4571), 474–475 (1982)

35. Gryfe, R., Kim, H., Hsieh, E.T., Aronson, M.D., Holowaty, E.J., Bull, S.B., Redston, M., Gallinger, S.: Tumor microsatellite instability and clinical outcome in young patients with colorectal cancer. N Engl J Med **342**(2), 69–77 (2000). Comparative Study

36. Hawkins, N., Norrie, M., Cheong, K., Mokany, E., Ku, S.L., Meagher, A., O'Connor, T., Ward, R.: CpG island methylation in sporadic colorectal cancers and its relationship to microsatellite instability. Gastroenterology **122**(5), 1376–1387 (2002)

37. Henderson, B.W., Waldow, S.M., Mang, T.S., Potter, W.R., Malone, P.B., Dougherty, T.J.: Tumor destruction and kinetics of tumor cell death in two experimental mouse tumors following photodynamic therapy. Cancer Res **45**(2), 572–576 (1985)

38. Herman, J.G., Latif, F., Weng, Y., Lerman, M.I., Zbar, B., Liu, S., Samid, D., Duan, D.S., Gnarra, J.R., Linehan, W.M.: Silencing of the VHL tumor-suppressor gene by DNA methylation in renal carcinoma. Proc Natl Acad Sci USA **91**(21), 9700–9704 (1994)

39. Hontz, A.E., Li, S.A., Lingle, W.L., Negron, V., Bruzek, A., Salisbury, J.L., Li, J.J.: Aurora a and B overexpression and centrosome amplification in early estrogen-induced tumor foci in the Syrian hamster kidney: implications for chromosomal instability, aneuploidy, and neoplasia. Cancer Res **67**(7), 2957–2963 (2007)

40. Huang, J., Papadopoulos, N., McKinley, A.J., Farrington, S.M., Curtis, L.J., Wyllie, A.H., Zheng, S., Willson, J.K., Markowitz, S.D., Morin, P., Kinzler, K.W., Vogelstein, B., Dunlop, M.G.: APC mutations in colorectal tumors with mismatch repair deficiency. Proc Natl Acad Sci USA **93**(17), 9049–9054 (1996). Comparative Study

41. Issa, J.P.: Methylation and prognosis: of molecular clocks and hypermethylator phenotypes. Clin Cancer Res **9**(8), 2879–2881 (2003). Comment

42. Issa, J.P.: CpG island methylator phenotype in cancer. Nat Rev Cancer **4**(12), 988–993 (2004)

43. Jass, J.R.: Serrated adenoma of the colorectum: a lesion with teeth. Am J Pathol **162**(3), 705–708 (2003). Comment

44. Jass, J.R.: Serrated adenoma of the colorectum and the DNA-methylator phenotype. Nat Clin Pract Oncol **2**(8), 398–405 (2005)

45. Jass, J.R.: Classification of colorectal cancer based on correlation of clinical, morphological and molecular features. Histopathology **50**(1), 113–130 (2007)

46. Jass, J.R., Biden, K.G., Cummings, M.C., Simms, L.A., Walsh, M., Schoch, E., Meltzer, S.J., Wright, C., Searle, J., Young, J., Leggett, B.A.: Characterisation of a subtype of colorectal cancer combining features of the suppressor and mild mutator pathways. J Clin Pathol **52**(6), 455–460 (1999)

47. Kambara, T., Simms, L.A., Whitehall, V.L.J., Spring, K.J., Wynter, C.V.A., Walsh, M.D., Barker, M.A., Arnold, S., McGivern, A., Matsubara, N., Tanaka, N., Higuchi, T., Young, J., Jass, J.R., Leggett, B.A.: BRAF mutation is associated with DNA methylation in serrated polyps and cancers of the colorectum. Gut **53**(8), 1137–1144 (2004)

48. Kane, M.F., Loda, M., Gaida, G.M., Lipman, J., Mishra, R., Goldman, H., Jessup, J.M., Kolodner, R.: Methylation of the hMLH1 promoter correlates with lack of expression of hMLH1 in sporadic colon tumors and mismatch repair-defective human tumor cell lines. Cancer Res **57**(5), 808–811 (1997)

49. Keller, J.J., Offerhaus, G.J., Drillenburg, P., Caspers, E., Musler, A., Ristimaki, A., Giardiello, F.M.: Molecular analysis of sulindac-resistant adenomas in familial adenomatous polyposis. Clin Cancer Res **7**(12), 4000–4007 (2001)

50. Komarova, N.L., Lengauer, C., Vogelstein, B., Nowak, M.A.: Dynamics of genetic instability in sporadic and familial colorectal cancer. Cancer Biol Ther **1**(6), 685–692 (2002)

51. Komarova, N.L., Sengupta, A., Nowak, M.A.: Mutation-selection networks of cancer initiation: tumor suppressor genes and chromosomal instability. J Theor Biol **223**(4), 433–450 (2003)

52. Kondo, Y., Issa, J.P.: Epigenetic changes in colorectal cancer. Cancer Metastasis Rev **23**(1-2), 29–39 (2004)

53. Kumar, S., Subramanian, S.: Mutation rates in mammalian genomes. Proc Natl Acad Sci USA **99**(2), 803–808 (2002)

54. Laghi, L., Randolph, A.E., Chauhan, D.P., Marra, G., Major, E.O., Neel, J.V., Boland, C.R.: JC virus DNA is present in the mucosa of the human colon and in colorectal cancers. Proc Natl Acad Sci USA **96**(13), 7484–7489 (1999)

55. Lamlum, H., Ilyas, M., Rowan, A., Clark, S., Johnson, V., Bell, J., Frayling, I., Efstathiou, J., Pack, K., Payne, S., Roylance, R., Gorman, P., Sheer, D., Neale, K., Phillips, R., Talbot, I., Bodmer, W., Tomlinson, I.: The type of somatic mutation at APC in familial adenomatous polyposis is determined by the site of the germline mutation: a new facet to Knudson's 'two-hit' hypothesis. Nat Med **5**(9), 1071–1075 (1999)

56. Lengauer, C.: Cancer. An unstable liaison. Science **300**(5618), 442–443 (2003). Comment

57. Lengauer, C., Kinzler, K.W., Vogelstein, B.: DNA methylation and genetic instability in colorectal cancer cells. Proc Natl Acad Sci USA **94**(6), 2545–2550 (1997)

58. Lengauer, C., Kinzler, K.W., Vogelstein, B.: Genetic instability in colorectal cancers. Nature **386**(6625), 623–627 (1997)

59. Lengauer, C., Kinzler, K.W., Vogelstein, B.: Genetic instabilities in human cancers. Nature **396**(6712), 643–649 (1998)

60. Li, E.: Chromatin modification and epigenetic reprogramming in mammalian development. Nat Rev Genet **3**(9), 662–673 (2002)

61. Macaluso, M., Giordano, A.: How does DNA methylation mark the fate of cells? Tumori **90**(4), 367–372 (2004)

62. Markowitz, S., Wang, J., Myeroff, L., Parsons, R., Sun, L., Lutterbaugh, J., Fan, R.S., Zborowska, E., Kinzler, K.W., Vogelstein, B.: Inactivation of the type II TGF-beta receptor in colon cancer cells with microsatellite instability. Science **268**(5215), 1336–1338 (1995). Comment

63. Matsuzaki, K., Deng, G., Tanaka, H., Kakar, S., Miura, S., Kim, Y.S.: The relationship between global methylation level, loss of heterozygosity, and microsatellite instability in sporadic colorectal cancer. Clin Cancer Res **11**(24 Pt 1), 8564–8569 (2005)

64. Misell, L.M., Hwang, E.S., Au, A., Esserman, L., Hellerstein, M.K.: Development of a novel method for measuring in vivo breast epithelial cell proliferation in humans. Breast Cancer Res Treat **89**(3), 257–264 (2005). Comparative Study

65. Mori, Y., Sato, F., Selaru, F.M., Olaru, A., Perry, K., Kimos, M.C., Tamura, G., Matsubara, N., Wang, S., Xu, Y., Yin, J., Zou, T.T., Leggett, B., Young, J., Nukiwa, T., Stine, O.C., Abraham, J.M., Shibata, D., Meltzer, S.J.: Instabilotyping reveals unique mutational spectra in microsatellite-unstable gastric cancers. Cancer Res **62**(13), 3641–3645 (2002). Comparative Study

66. Nagasaka, T., Sasamoto, H., Notohara, K., Cullings, H.M., Takeda, M., Kimura, K., Kambara, T., MacPhee, D.G., Young, J., Leggett, B.A., Jass, J.R., Tanaka, N., Matsubara, N.: Colorectal cancer with mutation in BRAF, KRAS, and wild-type with respect to both oncogenes showing different patterns of DNA methylation. J Clin Oncol **22**(22), 4584–4594 (2004)

67. Neese, R.A., Misell, L.M., Turner, S., Chu, A., Kim, J., Cesar, D., Hoh, R., Antelo, F., Strawford, A., McCune, J.M., Christiansen, M., Hellerstein, M.K.: Measurement in vivo of proliferation rates of slow turnover cells by ^2H_2O labeling of the deoxyribose moiety of DNA. Proc Natl Acad Sci USA **99**(24), 15,345–15,350 (2002). Comparative Study

68. Nishida, N., Nagasaka, T., Kashiwagi, K., Boland, C., Goel, A.: High copy amplification of the aurora-A gene is associated with chromosomal instability phenotype in human colorectal cancers. Cancer Biol Ther **6**(4) (2007)

69. Nowak, M.A., Komarova, N.L., Sengupta, A., Jallepalli, P.V., Shih, I.M., Vogel-stein, B., Lengauer, C.: The role of chromosomal instability in tumor initiation. Proc Natl Acad Sci USA **99**(25), 16,226–16,231 (2002)

70. Ogino, S., Cantor, M., Kawasaki, T., Brahmandam, M., Kirkner, G.J., Weisen-berger, D.J., Campan, M., Laird, P.W., Loda, M., Fuchs, C.S.: CpG island methylator phenotype (CIMP) of colorectal cancer is best characterised by quantitative DNA methylation analysis and prospective cohort studies. Gut **55**(7), 1000–1006 (2006)

71. Oller, A.R., Rastogi, P., Morgenthaler, S., Thilly, W.G.: A statistical model to estimate variance in long term-low dose mutation assays: testing of the model in a human lymphoblastoid mutation assay. Mutat Res **216**(3), 149–161 (1989)

72. Piao, Z., Fang, W., Malkhosyan, S., Kim, H., Horii, A., Perucho, M., Huang, S.: Frequent frameshift mutations of RIZ in sporadic gastrointestinal and endome-trial carcinomas with microsatellite instability. Cancer Res **60**(17), 4701–4704 (2000)

73. Potten, C.S., Kellett, M., Rew, D.A., Roberts, S.A.: Proliferation in human gastrointestinal epithelium using bromodeoxyuridine in vivo: data for different sites, proximity to a tumour, and polyposis coli. Gut **33**(4), 524–529 (1992)

74. Rajagopalan, H., Bardelli, A., Lengauer, C., Kinzler, K.W., Vogelstein, B., Velculescu, V.E.: Tumorigenesis: RAF/RAS oncogenes and mismatch-repair status. Nature **418**(6901), 934 (2002)

75. Rajagopalan, H., Lengauer, C.: Aneuploidy and cancer. Nature **432**(7015), 338–341 (2004)

76. Rampino, N., Yamamoto, H., Ionov, Y., Li, Y., Sawai, H., Reed, J.C., Perucho, M.: Somatic frameshift mutations in the BAX gene in colon cancers of the microsatellite mutator phenotype. Science **275**(5302), 967–969 (1997)

77. Rashid, A., Issa, J.P.: CpG island methylation in gastroenterologic neoplasia: a maturing field. Gastroenterology **127**(5), 1578–1588 (2004)

78. Ribic, C.M., Sargent, D.J., Moore, M.J., Thibodeau, S.N., French, A.J., Gold-berg, R.M., Hamilton, S.R., Laurent-Puig, P., Gryfe, R., Shepherd, L.E., Tu, D., Redston, M., Gallinger, S.: Tumor microsatellite-instability status as a predictor of benefit from fluorouracil-based adjuvant chemotherapy for colon cancer. N Engl J Med **349**(3), 247–257 (2003). Clinical Trial

79. Ricciardiello, L., Baglioni, M., Giovannini, C., Pariali, M., Cenacchi, G., Ri-palti, A., Landini, M.P., Sawa, H., Nagashima, K., Frisque, R.J., Goel, A., Boland, C.R., Tognon, M., Roda, E., Bazzoli, F.: Induction of chromosomal instability in colonic cells by the human polyomavirus JC virus. Cancer Res **63**(21), 7256–7262 (2003)

80. Ricciardiello, L., Laghi, L., Ramamirtham, P., Chang, C.L., Chang, D.K., Ran-dolph, A.E., Boland, C.R.: JC virus DNA sequences are frequently present in the human upper and lower gastrointestinal tract. Gastroenterology **119**(5), 1228–1235 (2000)

81. van Rijnsoever, M., Grieu, F., Elsaleh, H., Joseph, D., Iacopetta, B.: Char-acterisation of colorectal cancers showing hypermethylation at multiple CpG islands. Gut **51**(6), 797–802 (2002)

82. Rivkin, R.B.: Radioisotopic method for measuring cell division rates of indi-vidual species of diatoms from natural populations. Appl Environ Microbiol **51**(4), 769–775 (1986)

83. Ro, S., Rannala, B.: Methylation patterns and mathematical models reveal dynamics of stem cell turnover in the human colon. Proc Natl Acad Sci USA **98**(19), 10, 519–10,521 (2001). Comment

84. Robertson, K.D.: DNA methylation and human disease. Nat Rev Genet **6**(8), 597–610 (2005)

85. Robertson, K.D., Wolffe, A.P.: DNA methylation in health and disease. Nat Rev Genet **1**(1), 11–19 (2000)

86. Rowan, A., Halford, S., Gaasenbeek, M., Kemp, Z., Sieber, O., Volikos, E., Douglas, E., Fiegler, H., Carter, N., Talbot, I., Silver, A., Tomlinson, I.: Refining molecular analysis in the pathways of colorectal carcinogenesis. Clin Gastroenterol Hepatol **3**(11), 1115–1123 (2005)

87. Rowan, A.J., Lamlum, H., Ilyas, M., Wheeler, J., Straub, J., Papadopoulou, A., Bicknell, D., Bodmer, W.F., Tomlinson, I.P.: APC mutations in sporadic colorectal tumors: A mutational "hotspot" and interdependence of the "two hits." Proc Natl Acad Sci USA **97**(7), 3352–3357 (2000)

88. Rudolph, P., Alm, P., Heidebrecht, H.J., Bolte, H., Ratjen, V., Baldetorp, B., Ferno, M., Olsson, H., Parwaresch, R.: Immunologic proliferation marker Ki-S2 as prognostic indicator for lymph node-negative breast cancer. J Natl Cancer Inst **91**(3), 271–278 (1999)

89. Samowitz, W.S., Albertsen, H., Herrick, J., Levin, T.R., Sweeney, C., Murtaugh, M.A., Wolff, R.K., Slattery, M.L.: Evaluation of a large, population-based sample supports a CpG island methylator phenotype in colon cancer. Gastroenterology **129**(3), 837–845 (2005)

90. Samowitz, W.S., Holden, J.A., Curtin, K., Edwards, S.L., Walker, A.R., Lin, H.A., Robertson, M.A., Nichols, M.F., Gruenthal, K.M., Lynch, B.J., Leppert, M.F., Slattery, M.L.: Inverse relationship between microsatellite instability and K-ras and p53 gene alterations in colon cancer. Am J Pathol **158**(4), 1517–1524 (2001)

91. Shen, L., Ahuja, N., Shen, Y., Habib, N.A., Toyota, M., Rashid, A., Issa, J.P.: DNA methylation and environmental exposures in human hepatocellular carcinoma. J Natl Cancer Inst **94**(10), 755–761 (2002)

92. Shia, J., Ellis, N.A., Paty, P.B., Nash, G.M., Qin, J., Offit, K., Zhang, X.M., Markowitz, A.J., Nafa, K., Guillem, J.G., Wong, W.D., Gerald, W.L., Klimstra, D.S.: Value of histopathology in predicting microsatellite instability in hereditary nonpolyposis colorectal cancer and sporadic colorectal cancer. Am J Surg Pathol **27**(11), 1407–1417 (2003). Evaluation Studies

93. Sidransky, D.: Emerging molecular markers of cancer. Nat Rev Cancer **2**(3), 210–219 (2002)

94. Suraweera, N., Duval, A., Reperant, M., Vaury, C., Furlan, D., Leroy, K., Seruca, R., Iacopetta, B., Hamelin, R.: Evaluation of tumor microsatellite instability using five quasimonomorphic mononucleotide repeats and pentaplex PCR. Gastroenterology **123**(6), 1804–1811 (2002)

95. Thibodeau, S.N., Bren, G., Schaid, D.: Microsatellite instability in cancer of the proximal colon. Science **260**(5109), 816–819 (1993). Comment

96. Thor, A.D., Liu, S., Moore, D.H.n., Edgerton, S.M.: Comparison of mitotic index, in vitro bromodeoxyuridine labeling, and MIB-1 assays to quantitate proliferation in breast cancer. J Clin Oncol **17**(2), 470–477 (1999). Comparative Study

97. Tomlinson, I., Halford, S., Aaltonen, L., Hawkins, N., Ward, R.: Does MSI-low exist? J Pathol **197**(1), 6–13 (2002)

98. Toyota, M., Ahuja, N., Ohe-Toyota, M., Herman, J.G., Baylin, S.B., Issa, J.P.: CpG island methylator phenotype in colorectal cancer. Proc Natl Acad Sci USA **96**(15), 8681–8686 (1999)

99. Toyota, M., Ahuja, N., Suzuki, H., Itoh, F., Ohe-Toyota, M., Imai, K., Baylin, S.B., Issa, J.P.: Aberrant methylation in gastric cancer associated with the CpG island methylator phenotype. Cancer Res **59**(21), 5438–5442 (1999)

100. Toyota, M., Ohe-Toyota, M., Ahuja, N., Issa, J.P.: Distinct genetic profiles in colorectal tumors with or without the CpG island methylator phenotype. Proc Natl Acad Sci USA **97**(2), 710–715 (2000)

101. Ueki, T., Toyota, M., Skinner, H., Walter, K.M., Yeo, C.J., Issa, J.P., Hruban, R.H., Goggins, M.: Identification and characterization of differentially methylated CpG islands in pancreatic carcinoma. Cancer Res **61**(23), 8540–8546 (2001)

102. Waldman, F.M., Chew, K., Ljung, B.M., Goodson, W., Hom, J., Duarte, L.A., Smith, H.S., Mayall, B.: A comparison between bromodeoxyuridine and 3H thymidine labeling in human breast tumors. Mod Pathol **4**(6), 718–722 (1991). Comparative Study

103. Ward, R.L., Cheong, K., Ku, S.L., Meagher, A., O'Connor, T., Hawkins, N.J.: Adverse prognostic effect of methylation in colorectal cancer is reversed by microsatellite instability. J Clin Oncol **21**(20), 3729–3736 (2003)

104. Weisenberger, D.J., Siegmund, K.D., Campan, M., Young, J., Long, T.I., Faasse, M.A., Kang, G.H., Widschwendter, M., Weener, D., Buchanan, D., Koh, H., Simms, L., Barker, M., Leggett, B., Levine, J., Kim, M., French, A.J., Thibodeau, S.N., Jass, J., Haile, R., Laird, P.W.: CpG island methylator phenotype underlies sporadic microsatellite instability and is tightly associated with BRAF mutation in colorectal cancer. Nat Genet **38**(7), 787–793 (2006)

105. Whitehall, V.L.J., Wynter, C.V.A., Walsh, M.D., Simms, L.A., Purdie, D., Pandeya, N., Young, J., Meltzer, S.J., Leggett, B.A., Jass, J.R.: Morphological and molecular heterogeneity within nonmicrosatellite instability-high colorectal cancer. Cancer Res **62**(21), 6011–6014 (2002)

106. Wicking, C., Simms, L.A., Evans, T., Walsh, M., Chawengsaksophak, K., Beck, F., Chenevix-Trench, G., Young, J., Jass, J., Leggett, B., Wainwright, B.: CDX2, a human homologue of Drosophila caudal, is mutated in both alleles in a replication error positive colorectal cancer. Oncogene **17**(5), 657–659 (1998)

107. Wodarz, D., Komarova, N.L.: Computational biology of cancer: lecture notes and mathematical modeling. World Scientific, New Jersey, London, Singapore (2005)

108. Yamamoto, H., Sawai, H., Weber, T.K., Rodriguez-Bigas, M.A., Perucho, M.: Somatic frameshift mutations in DNA mismatch repair and proapoptosis genes in hereditary nonpolyposis colorectal cancer. Cancer Res **58**(5), 997–1003 (1998)

109. Yang, A.S., Estecio, M.R.H., Doshi, K., Kondo, Y., Tajara, E.H., Issa, J.P.: A simple method for estimating global DNA methylation using bisulfite PCR of repetitive DNA elements. Nucleic Acids Res **32**(3), e38 (2004)

110. Yatabe, Y., Tavare, S., Shibata, D.: Investigating stem cells in human colon by using methylation patterns. Proc Natl Acad Sci USA **98**(19), 10,839–10,844 (2001)

From Kinetic Theory for Active Particles to Modelling Immune Competition

Abdelghani Bellouquid[1] and Marcello Delitala[2]

[1] University Cadi Ayyad, Ecole Nationale des Sciences Appliquées, Safi, Maroc
   `bellouquid@gmail.com`
[2] Dipartimento di Matematica, Politecnico di Torino, Torino, Italy
   `marcello.delitala@polito.it`

2.1 Introduction

Methods of mathematical kinetic theory for active particles have been recently developed to describe the collective behavior of large populations of interacting individuals, where each individual is characterized not only by a mechanical variable (typically position and velocity), but also by a biological variable related to the organized, somehow intelligent, behavior of the whole population. The interest in this type of mathematical approach to modelling complex systems in biological sciences is documented in the review papers [1], [2], and in the book [3].

A generalization of the classical Boltzmann equation has been proposed in [4] showing that it includes, as a particular case, the well-known model of mathematical kinetic theory. Following [5], the interacting entities are called *active particles*. The state of each particle, called the *microscopic state*, is described by a variable related to the mechanical state of the particle, classically position and velocity, and by an additional variable, called the *activity*, related to specific biological functions of the particle. The overall behavior of the system is delivered by mathematical equations suitable to describe the evolution of the statistical distribution over the above microscopic states.

This chapter is focused on modelling of multicellular systems in biology by the above mathematical approach, which was first introduced in [6] with specific reference to the competition between tumor and immune cells. The method has been subsequently developed by various authors, e.g. [7]–[15]. The topic is referred to the broader environment of cancer modelling, as documented in the collections of surveys [16], [17], and in special issues devoted to the same argument [18], [19].

In this chapter, two models are studied on the basis of a qualitative and computational analysis. They are derived from the general approach proposed

N. Bellomo et al. (eds.), *Selected Topics in Cancer Modeling*,
DOI: 10.1007/978-0-8176-4713-1_2, © Springer Science+Business Media, LLC 2008

in Chapter 3 of the book [3], where two specific aspects of the tumor system-immune system competition are described. The models which will be studied cover the first stage of the competition, Model **C**, when no proliferation or destruction of cells occurs, while interactions only modify the biological functions, and the subsequent stage of the competition, Model **P**, when the proliferating or destructive events are predominant. After the latter stage, cells condense into a solid form, and the mathematical models need suitable equations, derived at the tissue level.

The contents of the chapter are organized as follows: Section 2.2 is related to modelling aspects, Section 2.3 develops a qualitative analysis, and Section 2.4 proposes some simulations finalized to visualize a few important phenomena of the immune competition, also with the aim of enlightening the description offered by the qualitative analysis. A critical analysis addressed to show how the proposed mathematical framework may be further developed towards relatively more accurate models of complex biological systems is proposed in Section 2.5.

2.2 Mathematical Frameworks and a General Model

Consider a large system of n interacting cells populations labelled by the index $i = 1, \ldots, n$. Each population is characterized by a different way of expressing its peculiar activities as well as by interactions with the other populations.

Modelling by methods of mathematical kinetic theory essentially means defining the microscopic state of the cells, describing the distribution function over that state and deriving an evolution equation for the distribution. The analysis is developed in the case of spatial homogeneity.

The variable used to describe the biological state of each cell is called the **activity**, and is assumed to be a scalar quantity. The distribution over the microscopic state is identified by the distribution function, and is written as follows:

$$f_i = f_i(t, u), \qquad i = 1, \ldots, n, \qquad (2.1)$$

where $f_i(t, u)\, du$ denotes the number of cells whose state, at time t, is in the interval $[u, u + du]$.

In more detail, the application proposed in this chapter deals with the modelling of the competition among two cellular populations, $n = 2$.

The first population is constituted by cells of a specific biological system, or *environmental* cells (i.e., endothelial cells), whose activity denotes how far cells are from the biological normality. The activity of the environmental cells is called the **progression**, and is defined by the scalar variable $u \in \mathbb{R}$, where $u \leq 0$ identifies the state of normal cells, and $u > 0$ the state of abnormal cells. The degree of malignancy increases with increasing progression: growth-autonomous, tissue-invasive, metastatically competent.

The second population is constituted by cells of the immune system, seen as a whole, whose activity denotes how far immune cells are active to contrast abnormal states of the cells of the first population. The activity of the immune cells is called the **activation**, and is defined by the scalar variable $u \in \mathbb{R}$, where $u \leq 0$ identifies the state of the inhibited immune cells, and $u > 0$ the state of the active immune cells. The degree of ability to contrast abnormal cells increases with increasing activation.

The following types of binary interactions are considered:

– **Conservative interactions**, between *candidate* or *test* cells and *field* cells, which modify the microscopic activity of the interacting cells, but not the size of the populations;

– **Proliferating or destructive interactions**, between *test cells* and *field cells*, which generate death or birth of test cells.

The evolution equation is obtained by equating, in the elementary volume of the state space, the rate of increase of particles with microscopic state u to the net flux of particles which attain such a state due to microscopic interactions. In the space homogeneous case, the result is as follows:

$$\partial_t f_i(t, u) = \sum_{j=1}^{2} \int_{-\infty}^{\infty} \eta_{ij} \mathcal{B}_{ij}(u_*, u^*; u) f_i(t, u_*) f_j(t, u^*) \, du_* \, du^*$$

$$ - f_i(t, u) \sum_{j=1}^{2} \int_{-\infty}^{\infty} \eta_{ij}[1 - \mu_{ij}(u, u^*)] f_j(t, u^*) \, du^* \,, $$

(2.2)

where

• The **interaction rate** between pairs of particles is denoted by η_{ij} and is assumed to be a constant independent of the activities of the interacting particles.

• The **transition probability density**, related to conservative interactions, $\mathcal{B}_{ij}(u_*, u^*; u)$ models the transition probability density of the candidate cell of the ith population, with state u_*, to fall into the state u after the interaction with the field cell of the jth population, with state u^*. The transition probability density functions have the structure of a probability density with respect to the variable u. It is assumed that $\mathcal{B}_{ij}$ is a delta function over the most probable output $m_{ij}(u_*, u^*)$, which depends on the microscopic states u_* and u^* of the interacting pairs,

$$\mathcal{B}_{ij}(u_*, u^*; u) = \delta(u - m_{ij}(u_*, u^*)) \,. \tag{2.3}$$

• The **net proliferation rate** $\mu_{ij}(u, u^*)$ models, in the continuous case, the proliferation density due to encounters, with rate η_{ij}, between the test cell of the ith population, with state u, with the field cell of the jth population, with state u^*.

If f_i is known, then macroscopic gross variables can be computed, under suitable integrability properties, as moments weighted by the above distribution function. For instance, the *size* of the ith population is given by

$$n_i[f_i](t) = \int_{-\infty}^{\infty} f_i(t, u) \, du \,. \tag{2.4}$$

In what follows, we will indicate with n_1^T the size of abnormal (tumor) cells, and with n_1^E the size of normal cells:

$$n_1^T[f_1](t) = \int_0^{\infty} f_1(t, u) \, du \,, \qquad n_1^E[f_1](t) = \int_{-\infty}^0 f_1(t, u) \, du \,, \tag{2.5}$$

while the size of active immune cells, n_2^A, and the size of inhibited immune cells, n_2^I will be

$$n_2^A[f_2](t) = \int_0^{\infty} f_2(t, u) \, du \,, \qquad n_2^I[f_2](t) = \int_{-\infty}^0 f_2(t, u) \, du \,. \tag{2.6}$$

First order moments provide the *linear biological macroscopic* quantities which will be called the **activation** at time t, and are computed as follows:

$$A_i = A[f_i](t) = \int_{-\infty}^{\infty} u f_i(t, u) \, du \,. \tag{2.7}$$

As already mentioned, the mathematical model was proposed in Chapter 3 of [3], and is written as follows:

$$\begin{cases} \partial_t f_1(t, u) = n_1[f_1](t)[f_1(t, u - \alpha_{11}) - f_1(t, u)] \\[2mm] \qquad + n_2^A[f_2](t) f_1(t, u + \alpha_{12}) U_{[0,\infty)}(u + \alpha_{12}) \\[2mm] \qquad + f_1(t, u) \left[\beta_{11} n_1^E[f_1](t) - (1 + \beta_{12}) n_2^A[f_2](t) \right] U_{[0,\infty)}(u) \,, \\[4mm] \partial_t f_2(t, u) = n_1^T[f_1](t) \left[f_2(t, u + \alpha_{21}) U_{[0,\infty)}(u + \alpha_{21}) \right. \\[2mm] \qquad \left. + (\beta_{21} - 1) f_2(t, u) U_{[0,\infty)}(u) \right] \,, \end{cases} \tag{2.8}$$

where $n_1[f_1](t)$, $n_1^T[f_1](t)$, $n_2^A[f_2](t)$ and $n_1^E(t)$ are the quantities defined in (2.4)–(2.6).

The model is characterized by six phenomenological parameters, where the α-type parameters are related to mass conservative encounters, while the β-type parameters are related to proliferating/destructive encounters. All parameters are positive quantities (eventually equal to zero) small with respect to unity. In detail:

α_{11} is related to the variation of the progression due to encounters between environmental cells. It describes the tendency of a normal cell to degenerate and to increase its progression;

α_{12} is related to the ability of the active immune cells to reduce the state of abnormal (neoplastic) environmental cells;

α_{21} is related to the ability of abnormal cells to inhibit the active immune cells;

β_{11} is related to the proliferation rate of abnormal cells due to their encounters with normal environmental cells;

β_{12} is related to the ability of immune cells to destroy abnormal cells;

β_{21} is related to the proliferation rate of immune cells due to their interaction with progressed cells.

The phenomenological assumptions by which cellular interactions have been modelled are reported in the Appendix.

The above mathematical model, although stated using a relatively simple structure, can possibly describe several stages of the immune competition. During the first stage, cells of the two interacting populations simply modify their respective biological functions, while later the onset of proliferating or destructive phenomena may end up with the growth or the destruction of the cells of the progressing population. The output of the competition depends primarily on the ability of immune cells to identify and destroy the abnormal cells. Two specific models are reported in what follows in view of the qualitative analysis and simulations.

• This first example, called Model **C**, is related to (prevalent) conservative interactions, and it is obtained by simply equating to zero all β-parameters. Thus, it corresponds to a competition where no proliferation or destruction occurs, and interactions only modify the biological functions of the cells of the two populations. The model is written as

$$\begin{cases} \partial_t f_1(t,u) = n_1[f_1](t)[f_1(t, u - \alpha_{11}) - f_1(t,u)] \\ \qquad + n_2^A[f_2](t) f_1(t, u + \alpha_{12}) U_{[0,\infty)}(u + \alpha_{12}) \\ \qquad - f_1(t,u) n_2^A[f_2](t) U_{[0,\infty)}(u), \\ \\ \partial_t f_2(t,u) = n_1^T[f_1](t)\big[f_2(t, u + \alpha_{21}) U_{[0,\infty)}(u + \alpha_{21}) \\ \qquad - f_2(t,u) U_{[0,\infty)}(u)\big]. \end{cases} \qquad (2.9)$$

Remark 2.1. Model **C** can be applied to analyze latent immune competitions, when cells degenerate before the onset of relevant proliferation phenomena which give evidence of the presence of a pathological state.

• A second example, called Model **P**, is related to a stage characterized by the fact that the distribution over the biological functions reaches a slowly varying value, while the proliferating or destructive events are predominant. This predominant proliferating-destructive model is obtained by setting the α-type parameters equal to zero. The evolution equation for the distribution function is written as follows:

$$\begin{cases} \partial_t f_1(t,u) = f_1(t,u)\left[\beta_{11}n_1^E[f_1](t) - \beta_{12}n_2^A[f_2](t)\right]U_{[0,\infty)}(u), \\ \\ \partial_t f_2(t,u) = \beta_{21}f_2(t,u)n_1^T[f_1](t)U_{[0,\infty)}(u). \end{cases} \tag{2.10}$$

Remark 2.2. This model can be used to analyze the last period of the competition, when both cell populations have reached a fixed stage of the biological functions, and only proliferating or destructive phenomena are relevant.

Both models, Model **C** and Model **P**, refer to the mathematical description of the immune competition when certain phenomena are prevalent with respect to others. Not only is the particularization useful to capture specific biological phenomena, but it can be used for the identification of the parameters of the model by comparison between theory and experiment, as documented in [3].

2.3 Qualitative Analysis

Predictions of the model are obtained by solving the initial value problem obtained through the addition of the initial conditions. The qualitative analysis is focused on the well-posedness and on the asymptotic behavior, which defines the trend of the biological system towards the prevalence of one of the two populations over the other.

Some theorems, followed by interpretations from a biological point of view, are reported in this section. For the proofs, the reader is addressed to the already cited book [3]. The analysis does not cover the whole panorama of all possible outcomes of the competition. The simulations offered in the next section are necessary to complete the predictability analysis.

2.3.1 Local and Global Existence

Consider the initial value problem obtained by linking the initial conditions $f_0 = (f_1(t,0), f_2(t,0))$ with $f_1(t,0) = f_{10}$ and $f_2(t,0) = f_{20}$ to the general model (2.8). Local and global existence of the solutions are obtained by application of the classical fixed point theorem, see Chapter 4 of [3].

The following function spaces must be defined:

- $L_1(\mathbb{R})$ is the Lebesgue space of measurable, real-valued functions which are integrable on $\mathbb{R}$. The norm is denoted by $\|\cdot\|_1$.
- $\mathcal{X} = L_1(\mathbb{R}) \times L_1(\mathbb{R}) = \{f = (f_1, f_2) : f_1 \in L_1(\mathbb{R}), f_2 \in L_1(\mathbb{R})\}$ is the Banach space equipped with the norm

$$\| f \| = \| f_1 \|_1 + \| f_2 \|_1.$$

- $\mathcal{X}_+ = \{f = (f_1, f_2) \in \mathcal{X} : f_1 \geq 0, f_2 \geq 0\}$ is the positive cone of $\mathcal{X}$.
- $\mathcal{Y} = C([0,T], \mathcal{X})$ and $\mathcal{Y}_+ = C([0,T], \mathcal{X}_+)$ is the space of the functions continuous on $[0,T]$ with values, respectively, in a Banach space $\mathcal{X}$ and $\mathcal{X}_+$, equipped with the norm

$$\| f \|_{\mathcal{Y}} = \sup_{t \in [0,T]} \| f \| .$$

Then, *local existence* of the solutions is stated by the following theorem.

Theorem 1. *There exists positive constants T and a_0, such that the initial value problem defined linking the general model (2.8) with initial conditions $f_0 \in \mathcal{X}_+$, has a unique solution $f \in C([0,T], \mathcal{X}_+)$. The solution f satisfies*

$$f(t) \in \mathcal{X}_+, \quad t \in [0,T], \tag{2.11}$$

and

$$\| f \| \leq a_0 \| f_0 \|, \quad \forall t \in [0,T] .$$

Theorem 2. $\forall T > 0$, *there exists a unique solution $f \in C([0,T], \mathcal{X})$ of (2.8) with the initial data, $f_0 \in \mathcal{X}_+$. The solution satisfies (2.11), and for some constant C_T depending on T and on the initial data,*

$$\sup_{t \in [0,T]} f(t) \leq C_T .$$

Global existence of the solutions and, in more detail, an analysis of the a-symptotic behavior are obtained by analyzing the influence of the parameters of the model on the qualitative behavior of the solutions. Both Model **C** and Model **P** are considered.

Theorem 3. *Model **C**: There exists a unique, nonnegative, strong solution $f(t)$ in $(L_1(\mathbb{R}))^2$ of the problem obtained linking (2.9) with the initial data $f_0 \in \mathcal{X}_+$, for $t \geq 0$, and for every $f_0 \geq 0$ in $(L_1(\mathbb{R}))^2$. Moreover, the equality $\| f \| = \| f_0 \|$ is satisfied.*

Theorem 4. *Model **P**: $\forall T > 0$ there exists a unique solution $f \in C([0,T], \mathcal{X})$ of (2.10) with the initial data, $f_0 \in \mathcal{X}_+$. The solution satisfies*

$$f(t) \in \mathcal{X}_+, \quad \forall t \in [0,T],$$

and, for some constant C_T depending on T and on the initial data,

$$\sup_{t \in [0,T]} f(t) \leq C_T .$$

2.3.2 Asymptotic Behavior

In general, it is interesting to analyze the influence of the parameters of the model and of the mathematical problem on the bifurcation separating two different behaviors:

i) Growth of progressing cells, while the immune cells are inhibited;

ii) Destruction of progressing cells due to the action of the immune system, which remains sufficiently active.

The analysis of the asymptotic behavior refers to the time evolution of the densities n_1^T, n_1^E and n_2^A, while simulations visualize the evolution of the distribution function.

Consider first the conservative model. The study of the asymptotic behavior has been focused on two particular cases, called Model **C1** and Model **C2**, obtained by Model **C**, Eq. (2.9), setting α_{12} and α_{11}, respectively, equal to zero. Therefore, Model **C1** is written as follows:

$$
\begin{cases}
\partial_t f_1(t, u) = n_1[f_1](t)[f_1(t, u - \alpha_{11}) - f_1(t, u)], \\[2ex]
\partial_t f_2(t, u) = n_1^T[f_1](t)\big[f_2(t, u + \alpha_{21})U_{[0,\infty)}(u) \\[2ex]
\qquad\qquad - f_2(t, u)U_{[0,\infty)}(u)\big],
\end{cases}
\tag{2.12}
$$

while Model **C2** is written as

$$
\begin{cases}
\partial_t f_1(t, u) = n_2^A[f_2](t)f_1(t, u + \alpha_{12})U_{[0,\infty)}(u + \alpha_{12}) \\[2ex]
\qquad\qquad - f_1(t, u)n_2^A[f_2](t)U_{[0,\infty)}(u), \\[2ex]
\partial_t f_2(t, u) = n_1^T[f_1](t)\big[f_2(t, u + \alpha_{21})U_{[0,\infty)}(u + \alpha_{21}) \\[2ex]
\qquad\qquad - f_2(t, u)U_{[0,\infty)}(u)\big].
\end{cases}
\tag{2.13}
$$

Remark 3.1. The assumption $\alpha_{12} = 0$ means that either the immune cells are able to destroy the progressing cells (destructive interaction), or they are unable to contrast the progression. In other words, the immune system is not able to partially "repair" the genetic degradation of the progressing cell.

Remark 3.2. The assumption $\alpha_{11} = 0$ means that the progressing cells do not show a natural trend to increase their progression. This means that either the cells do not show a trend to degenerate at all, or that the phenotypic changes occur so rarely that they are negligible with respect to the time scale of the model.

The study of the asymptotic behavior gives the following results.

Theorem 5. *Consider the initial value problem for Model* **C1**.
i) n_2^A is decreasing, and n_1^T is increasing.
ii) Moreover, $n_1^T(t)$ and $n_2^A(t)$ satisfy, in the limit $t \longrightarrow +\infty$, the following estimates:

$$\lim_{t \longrightarrow +\infty} n_1^T(t) \geq \int_{-\alpha_{11}}^{+\infty} f_{10}(u)du > n_1^T(0),$$

$$\lim_{t \longrightarrow +\infty} n_2^A(t) \leq \int_{\alpha_{21}}^{+\infty} f_{20}(u)du < n_2^A(0).$$

Remark 3.3. Note that the number density $n_1^T(t)$ at any time $t > 0$ is always greater than the initial number density $n_1^T(0)$. Likewise, the number density $n_2^A(t)$ at any time $t > 0$ is always less than the initial number density $n_2^A(0)$.

Theorem 6. *Consider the initial value problem for Model* **C2**.
i) n_2^A and n_1^T decrease.
ii) Moreover, $n_1^T(t)$ and $n_2^A(t)$ satisfy, in the limit $t \to +\infty$, the following estimates:

$$\lim_{t \to +\infty} n_1^T(t) \leq \exp\left(-\frac{n_2^A(0)}{n_1^T(0)}\right) \int_0^{\alpha_{12}} f_{10}(u)du + \int_{\alpha_{12}}^{+\infty} f_{10}(u)du < n_1^T(0),$$

$$\lim_{t \to +\infty} n_2^A(t) \leq \exp\left(-\frac{n_1^T(0)}{n_2^A(0)}\right) \int_0^{\alpha_{12}} f_{20}(u)du + \int_{\alpha_{21}}^{+\infty} f_{20}(u)du < n_2^A(0).$$

Remark 3.4. Note that the number densities $n_1^T(t)$ and $n_2^A(t)$ are always strictly smaller than the initial number densities $n_1^T(0)$ and $n_2^A(0)$ respectively.

Referring to the initial value problem corresponding to Model **P**, (2.10), it is useful to introduce the following parameter:

$$\delta = \beta_{11} n_1^E(0) - \beta_{12} n_2^A(0), \tag{2.14}$$

which plays a relevant role. Then we have the following.

Theorem 7. *Consider the initial value problem for Model* **P**, *as defined by Eqs. (2.10):*

- *If $\beta_{21} = 0$, then $n_2^A = Cst, n_1^E = Cst$ and n_1^T satisfies the equality*

$$n_1^T(t) = n_1^T(0) \exp(\delta t),$$

  thus, if $\delta \geq 0$ then n_1^T increases and if $\delta < 0$ then n_1^T decreases.
- *If $\beta_{21} \neq 0$, then:*
  - *If $\beta_{12} = 0$, then n_1^T increases, $n_1^E = Cst$ and n_2 increases.*
  - *If $\beta_{12} \neq 0$, then $n_1^E = Cst$, n_2^A increases and*

·   *If $\delta \leq 0$, then n_1^T decreases and satisfies the following estimate:*

$$n_1^T(t) \leq n_1^T(0)\exp(\delta t). \tag{2.15}$$

·   *If $\delta > 0$: if $n_1^T(0) \neq 0$, then $\exists t_0$ such that n_1^T increases in $[0, t_0]$ and n_1^T decreases in $[t_0, T]$ $\forall T > 0$.*

2.4 Simulations

In this section we focus on the computational analysis of Model **C** and of Model **P**, showing how simulations complete and enlarge the asymptotic scenario depicted by the theorems of the previous section.

2.4.1 Conservative Model

In Model **C**, (2.9), the number of cells is constant in time since the observation time is short and no proliferation phenomenon occurs, while the distribution function over the microscopic state shifts toward higher or lower values.

The evolution is ruled only by the evolution of the states, and the expected behavior strongly depends on the ability of the cells of a population to inhibit the competitor cells of the other population, and thus on the ratio between α_{21} and α_{12}. An additional role is played by the parameter related to the tendency to degenerate the cells of the first population, α_{11}. Thus, we expect a complex scenario, dependent on the values of the conservative parameters.

Consider first Model **C2**, defined in Eq. (2.13). It describes the situation in which no degeneration occurs, since $\alpha_{11} = 0$, and only the parameters α_{21} and α_{12} are different from zero. The qualitative scenario of the model is studied in Theorem 6, which states that

$$n_2^A \downarrow \qquad \text{and} \qquad n_1^T \downarrow .$$

As is expected, simulations show that both neoplastic and immune cells are reduced during the competition (since no proliferation may occur). However, the asymptotic scenario is such that only one cell population survives and the other is completely depleted. The ratio between the values of α_{21} and α_{12}, as well as the initial conditions, defines which of the populations will survive.

Consider the same initial condition for neoplastic and immune cells. If $\alpha_{21} > \alpha_{12}$, the ability of neoplastic cells to inhibit immune cells is greater than the ability of immune cells to reduce the state of neoplastic cells. The final output is a complete inhibition of immune cells and a final survival of neoplastic cells, as reported in Fig. 2.1.

If $\alpha_{21} < \alpha_{12}$, the final scenario is a reduction of the state of the neoplastic cells, until their complete depletion and the final survival of immune cells, as reported in Fig. 2.2.

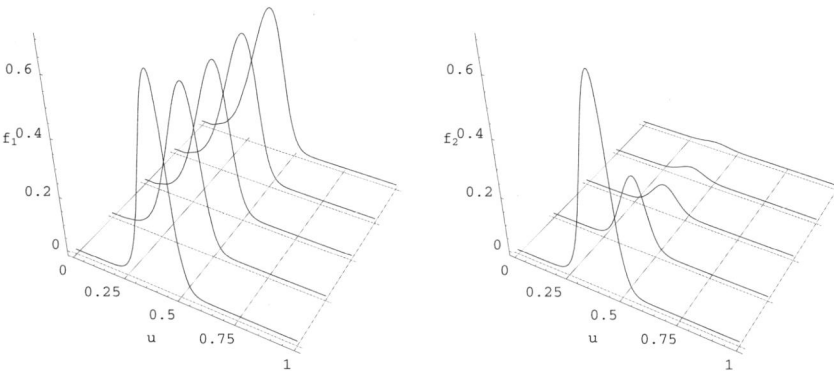

Fig. 2.1. $\alpha_{11} = 0$, $\alpha_{12} = 0.05$, $\alpha_{21} = 0.95$. Model C2. Evolution in time of the distribution functions. Evolution of neoplastic cells (on the left) and immune suppression (on the right).

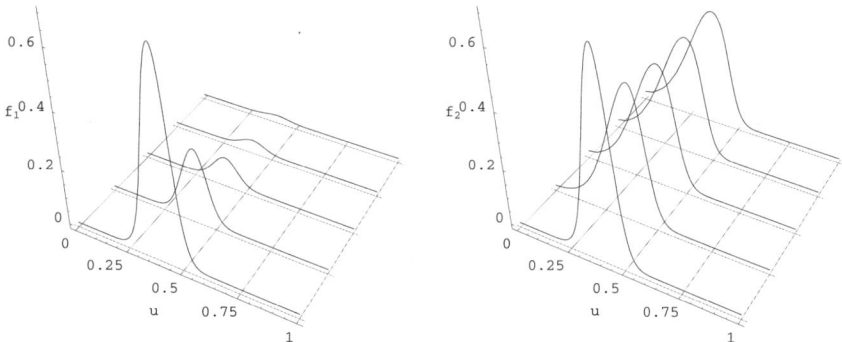

Fig. 2.2. $\alpha_{11} = 0$, $\alpha_{12} = 0.95$, $\alpha_{21} = 0.05$. Model C2. Evolution in time of the distribution functions. Reduction of neoplastic cells (on the left) and immune survival (on the right).

2.4.2 Proliferative Model

The Model **P**, (2.10), is such that proliferating/destructing events are predominant. The simulations proposed here aim to complete the qualitative analysis proposed in the previous section.

Let us define a ***critical immune density*** $n_{2_C}^A = \beta^*$ with

$$\beta^* = \frac{\beta_{11}}{\beta_{12}} n_1^E(0),$$

a product of the initial number of environmental cells and the ratio of the proliferation rate of abnormal cells and the ability of immune cells to destroy them. The results of Theorem 7 can be summarized as follows.

$$\text{If } n_2^A(0) \geq n_{2_C}^A = \beta^* \ (\delta \leq 0) \ : \ \begin{cases} n_2^A(t) \uparrow, \\ \\ n_1^T(t) \downarrow; \ \exists \delta \leq 0 : n_1^T(t) \leq n_1^T(0) \exp(\delta t). \end{cases}$$

$$\text{If } n_2^A(0) < n_{2_C}^A = \beta^* \ (\delta > 0) \ : \ \begin{cases} n_2^A(t) \uparrow, \\ \\ \exists t_0 \ : \ n_1^T \uparrow, \forall t \in [0, t_0] \text{ and} \\ \\ n_1^T \downarrow, \forall t \in [t_0, T], \forall T > 0. \end{cases}$$

Thus, the immune system is stimulated to grow by the presence of abnormal (aggressive) cells, and its density increases, while the following two behaviors are predicted by the model:

- If $n_2^A(0) \geq \beta^*$, i.e. $\delta \leq 0$, the number of abnormal cells decreases with the rate of decrease given by estimate (2.15).
- If $n_2^A(0) < \beta^*$, i.e. $\delta > 0$, at the beginning the number of abnormal cells grows, since the number of immune cells is not sufficient to contrast them. Nevertheless, since the immune cells are stimulated to proliferate, after a certain critical time t_0 their number will be large enough to reduce the number of abnormal cells.

Some computational analysis may be useful to complete the above interpretation. Indeed, simulations show the evolution of the distribution functions, thus providing a deeper insight on the inner structure of the system, giving additional information with respect to the theorems on the asymptotic behavior which refer to the evolution of the densities.

Thus, if $n_2^A(0) \leq \beta^*$, i.e. $\delta \leq 0$, we get a decrease from the beginning of the number of neoplastic cells and an increase of the number of immune ones, see Fig. 2.3.

The opposite behavior is obtained if $n_2^A(0) > \beta^*$, i.e. $\delta > 0$, where immune cells are stimulated to proliferate, while neoplastic ones increase at the beginning and after a certain critical time start to be depleted, see Fig. 2.4.

2.5 Looking Forward

This chapter has shown how methods of mathematical kinetic theory for active particles can be properly developed to model the competition between

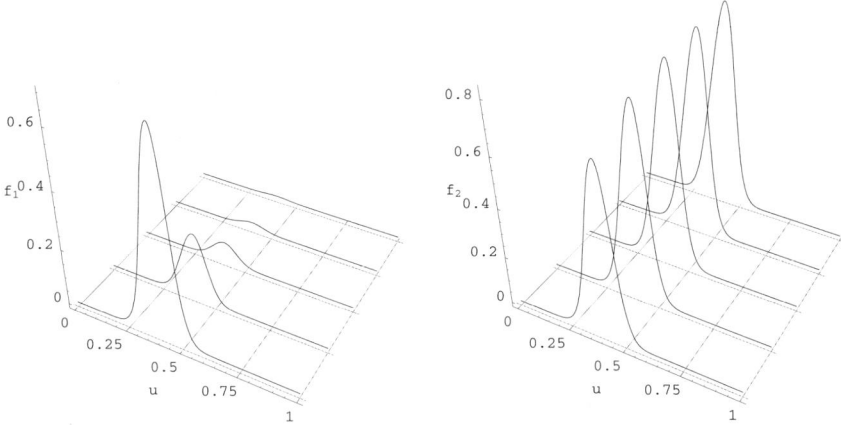

Fig. 2.3. $\beta_{11} = 0.15$, $\beta_{12} = 0.95$, $\beta_{21} = 0.15$, $\delta \leq 0$. Model P. Evolution in time of the distribution functions. Depletion of neoplastic cells (on the left) and immune cell proliferation (on the right).

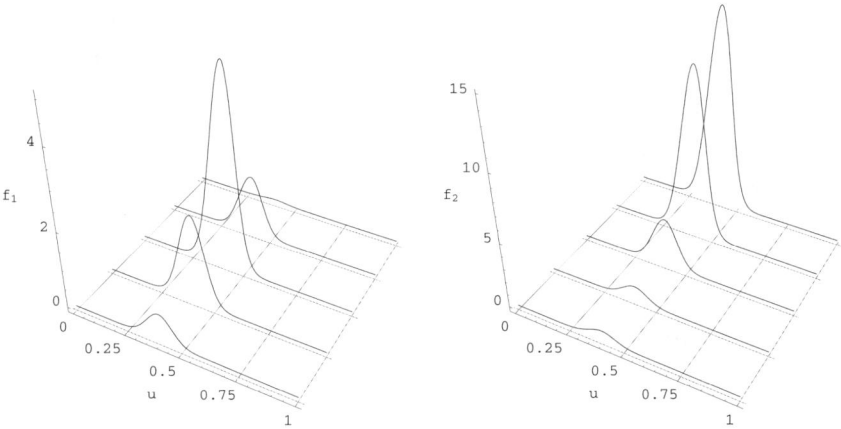

Fig. 2.4. $\beta_{11} = 0.95$, $\beta_{12} = 0.15$, $\beta_{21} = 0.15$, $\delta > 0$. Model P. Evolution in time of the distribution functions. Initial increase and final depletion of neoplastic cells (on the left) and immune proliferation (on the right).

neoplastic and immune cells. The contents have focused on qualitative and computational analyses of the early and final stages of the competition.

This final section presents some research perspectives, which have already received attention from applied mathematicians. It is also worthwhile to develop further speculations and research activity towards the ambitious objective of developing a mathematical theory of multicellular systems.

- The first topic discusses the mathematical structure (2.2) which acts as a paradigm for the derivation of models. Some technical developments are proposed in [20] and [21], while [22] and [23] discuss how the above structure may possibly evolve towards a proper mathematical-biological theory.

  The approach proposed in the last two cited papers is in two steps: first the populations which play the competition are identified on the basis of Hartwell's theory of modules [24]. Then, the project is completed by implementing the structure by expression of the terms which model cellular interactions using a biological theory instead of the approach reported in the Appendix.

  Hartwell's theory suggests identifying cell populations as **modules** characterized by a well-defined functional purpose. The difficulties dealing with the above topics are proposed in [25] and [26] from a mathematical and a biological sciences viewpoint, respectively. It is shown in [27] that a deeper understanding of cellular interactions can contribute to specific therapies.

- The second topic is related to the derivation of macroscopic equations from the underlying cellular description as a necessary step in developing a mathematical biological theory of multicellular systems.

  Asymptotic methods can be used to derive tissue-level equations. The approach models spatial phenomena by adding to the spatially homogeneous equations a stochastic perturbation corresponding to a velocity jump process [28]–[33].

  It is worth stressing again that the analysis needs to be implemented by a theoretical input from biology. It is shown [32] and [34] that suitable scaling leads either to diffusion models or to hyperbolic models. In both cases, the presence of source terms appears if the proliferation rate is sufficiently large. Moreover, as remarked in [23], the structure of the mathematical equations modelling tissues may evolve in time due to the aforementioned dynamics. So far, the formal approach provides a scenario of structurally different macroscopic equations to be identified using a biological sciences characterization.

- Finally, note that this chapter has proposed an analysis of models where genetic mutations are continuous from normal to progressing states. A recent paper [35] proposes a model which describes sequential genetic mutations of a neoplastic cell with increasing levels of malignancy. It is hoped that this approach, which requires a deep understanding of the dynamics at the molecular level [36]–[38], may offer a complete multiscale modelling, from the cellular level to the tissue level.

Appendix

This appendix reports the phenomenological assumptions on cellular interactions which have generated model (2.8). The list includes only the interactions which have an outcome which modifies the microscopic state of the interacting pairs, or generates proliferating/destructive events.

- **H.1:** The most probable output of conservative interactions between cells of the first population is

$$u_*, u^* \in \mathbb{R} : m_{11} = u_* + \alpha_{11},$$

  where α_{11} is a parameter related to the inner tendency of both normal and progressing cells to degenerate and progress.
- **H.2:** The proliferation rate of cells of the first populations with $u_* \geq 0$, stimulated by encounters with non-progressing cells $u_* < 0$, is:

$$\mu_{11}(u_*, u^*) = \beta_{11} U_{[0,\infty)}(u_*) U_{(-\infty,0)}(u^*),$$

  where β_{11} is a parameter which characterizes the proliferating ability of abnormal cells.
- **H.3:** The progression of an abnormal cell decreases due to encounters with an active immune cell, and the most probable output of the microscopic state after the interaction is given as follows:

$$u_*, u^* \geq 0 : \quad m_{12} = u_* - \alpha_{12},$$

  where α_{12} is a parameter which indicates the ability of the immune system to reduce the state of cells of the first population.
- **H.4:** The proliferation rate of non-progressing cells due to encounters with immune cells is equal to zero. On the other hand, when $u_* \geq 0$, cells are partially destroyed due to encounters with active immune cells:

$$\mu_{12}(u_*, u^*) = -\beta_{12} U_{[0,\infty)}(u_*) U_{[0,\infty)}(u^*),$$

  where β_{12} is a parameter which characterizes the destructive ability of active immune cells.
- **H.5:** The most probable output of the microscopic state of the immune cell after the interaction with progressing cells, with state u^*, is given as follows:

$$u_* \geq 0, u^* \geq 0 : \quad m_{21} = u_* - \alpha_{21},$$

  where α_{21} is a parameter which indicates the ability of abnormal cells to inhibit immune cells.
- **H.6:** The proliferation rate of inhibited immune cells due to encounters with cells of the first population is equal to zero. On the other hand, when $u^* \geq 0$, cells proliferate due to encounters with progressing cells:

$$\mu_{21}(u_*, u^*) = \beta_{21} U_{[0,\infty)}(u_*) U_{[0,\infty)}(u^*), \qquad \mu_{22} = 0,$$

  where β_{21} is a parameter which characterizes the proliferating ability of abnormal cells.

References

1. Bellomo, N., De Angelis, E., Preziosi, L.: Multiscale modelling and mathematical problems related to tumor evolution and medical therapy. J. Theor. Medicine, **5**, 111–136 (2003).
2. Bellomo, N., Bellouquid, A., Delitala, M.: Mathematical topics in the modelling complex multicellular systems and tumor immune cells competition. Math. Mod. Meth. Appl. Sci., **14**, 1683–1733 (2004).
3. Bellouquid, A., Delitala, M.: Mathematical Modeling of Complex Biological Systems. A Kinetic Theory Approach. Birkhäuser, Boston (2006).
4. Arlotti, L., Bellomo, N., De Angelis, E.: Generalized kinetic (Boltzmann) models: mathematical structures and applications. Math. Mod. Meth. Appl. Sci., **12**, 579–604 (2002).
5. Bellomo, N.: Modeling Complex Living Systems. A Kinetic Theory and Stochastic Game Approach. Birkhäuser, Boston (2008).
6. Bellomo, N., Forni, G.: Dynamics of tumor interaction with the host immune system. Math. Comp. Mod., **20**, 107–122 (1994).
7. Arlotti, L., Lachowicz, M., Gamba, A.: A kinetic model of tumor/immune system cellular interactions. J. Theor. Medicine, **4**, 39–50 (2002).
8. De Angelis, E., Jabin, P.E.: Qualitative analysis of a mean field model of tumor-immune system competition. Math. Meth. Appl. Sci., **28**, 2061–2083 (2005).
9. Kolev, M.: Mathematical modeling of the competition between acquired immunity and cancer. Appl. Math. Comp. Science, **13**, 289–297 (2003).
10. Bellouquid, A., Delitala, M.: Kinetic (cellular) models of cell progression and competition with the immune system. Z. Angew. Math. Phys., **55**, 295–317 (2004).
11. Derbel, L.: Analysis of a new model for tumor-immune system competition including long time scale effects. Math. Mod. Meth. Appl. Sci., **14**, 1657–1682 (2004).
12. Kolev, M.: A mathematical model of cellular immune response to leukemia. Math. Comp. Mod., **41**, 1071–1082 (2005).
13. Kolev, M., Kozlowska, E., Lachowicz, M.: Mathematical model of tumor invasion along linear or tubular structures. Math. Comp. Mod., **41**, 1083–1096 (2005).
14. Bellouquid, A., Delitala, M.: Mathematical methods and tools of kinetic theory towards modelling of complex biological systems. Math. Mod. Meth. Appl. Sci., **15**, 1619–1638 (2005).
15. Brazzoli, I., Chauviere, A.: On the discrete kinetic theory for active particles. Modelling the immune competition. Comput. and Math. Meth. in Medicine, **7**, 143–157 (2006).
16. Adam, J., Bellomo, N. (Eds.): A Survey of Models on Tumor Immune Systems Dynamics. Birkhäuser, Boston (1997).
17. Preziosi, L.: Modeling Cancer Growth. CRC Press-Chapman Hall, Boca Raton, FL (2003).
18. Bellomo, N., Maini, P.K.: Preface of the Special issue on cancer modeling (II). Math. Mod. Meth. Appl. Sci., **16**, iii)–vii) (2006).
19. Bellomo, N., Sleeman, B.D.: Preface of the Special issue on multiscale cancer modelling. Comput. and Math. Meth. in Medicine, **7**, 67–70 (2006).
20. Bellomo, N., De Lillo, S., Salvatori, C.: Mathematical tools of the kinetic theory of active particles with some reasoning on the modelling progression and heterogeneity. Math. Comp. Mod., **45**, 564–578 (2007).

21. De Angelis, E., Delitala, M.: Modelling complex systems in applied sciences methods and tools of the mathematical kinetic theory for active particles. Math. Comp. Mod., **43**, 1310–1328 (2006).
22. Bellomo, N., Forni, G.: Looking for new paradigms towards a biological-mathematical theory of complex multicellular systems. Math. Mod. Meth. Appl. Sci., **16**, 1001–1029 (2006).
23. Bellomo, N., Forni, G.: Complex multicellular systems and immune competition: new paradigms looking for a mathematical theory. Current Topics in Developmental Biology, **81**, 485–502 (2007).
24. Hartwell, H.L., Hopfield, J.J., Leibner, S., Murray, A.W.: From molecular to modular cell biology. Nature, **402**, c47–c52 (1999).
25. Reed, R.: Why is mathematical biology so hard? Notices of the American Mathematical Society, **51**, 338–342 (2004).
26. Woese, C.R.: A new biology for a new century. Microbiology and Molecular Biology Reviews, **68**, 173–186 (2004).
27. Lollini, P.L., Motta, S., Pappalardo, F.: Modelling the immune competition. Math. Mod. Meth. Appl. Sci., **16**, 1091–1124 (2006).
28. Hillen, T., Othmer, H.: The diffusion limit of transport equations derived from velocity jump processes. SIAM J. Appl. Math., **61**, 751–775 (2000).
29. Stevens, A.: The derivation of chemotaxis equations as limit dynamics of moderately interacting stochastic many-particle systems. SIAM J. Appl. Math., **61**, 183–212 (2000).
30. Bellomo, N., Bellouquid, A.: From a class of kinetic models to macroscopic equations for multicellular systems in biology. Discrete Contin. Dyn. Syst. B, **4**, 59–80 (2004).
31. Lachowicz, M.: Micro and meso scales of description corresponding to a model of tissue invasion by solid tumours. Math. Mod. Meth. Appl. Sci., **15**, 1667–1684 (2005).
32. Bellomo, N., Bellouquid, A.: On the mathematical kinetic theory of active particles with discrete states—The derivation of macroscopic equations. Math. Comp. Mod., **44**, 397–404 (2006).
33. Chalub, F., Dolak-Struss, Y., Markowich, P., Oeltz, D., Schmeiser, C., Soref, A.: Model hierarchies for cell aggregation by chemotaxis. Math. Mod. Meth. Appl. Sci., **16**, 1173–1198 (2006).
34. Bellomo, N., Bellouquid, A., Nieto, J., Soler, J.: Multicellular biological growing systems: hyperbolic limits towards macroscopic description. Math. Mod. Meth. Appl. Sci., **17**, 1675–1692 (2007).
35. Delitala, M., Forni, G.: From the mathematical kinetic theory of active particles to modelling genetic mutations and immune competition. Internal Report, Dept. Mathematics, Politecnico, Torino (2008).
36. Nowak, M.A., Sigmund, K.: Evolutionary dynamics of biological games. Science, **303**, 793–799 (2004).
37. Komarova, N.: Stochastic modelling of loss- and gain-of-function mutations in cancer. Math. Mod. Meth. Appl. Sci., **17**, 1647–1673 (2007).
38. Weinberg, R.A.: The Biology of Cancer. Garland Sciences-Taylor and Francis, New York (2007).

3

Towards Microscopic and Nonlocal Models of Tumour Invasion of Tissue

Mirosław Lachowicz

Institute of Applied Mathematics and Mechanics,
Faculty of Mathematics, Informatics and Mechanics,
University of Warsaw,
ul. Banacha, 2, 02-097 Warsaw, Poland
lachowic@mimuw.edu.pl

3.1 Introduction

Usually the description of biological populations is carried out on a macroscopic level of interacting subpopulations within the system. Such an approach is related to deterministic reaction-diffusion equations. They describe the (deterministic) evolution of densities of subpopulations of the system rather than the individual entities. However, in many cases the description on a microscale (or mesoscale) of interacting entities (e.g. cells) seems to be more appropriate, see [2, 3, 4, 5, 18, 19, 24] and the references therein. For example, in the case of tumour cells in competition with the immune system, the following steps of the evolution:

- Loss of differentiation and replication; reproducing of the cells in the form of identical descendants;
- Interaction (activation or inhibition) and competition at the cellular level with immune and environmental cells e.g. through the emission of cytokine signals;

are related to cellular and subcellular interactions between tumour cells and cells and factors of the immune system. The subcellular scale refers to processes that take place within the cells or at the cell membrane, e.g. synthesis of DNA and the activities of chemical signals between cells. The cellular scale refers to various types of interactions between cells, e.g. interactions between tumour cells and immune system cells. Therefore, those scales may be connected with a microscopic level of description, i.e. the level of interacting individual entities of the system or, with some suitable reduction of the description, to the mesoscopic scale of test entities. The important feature of the microscopic level is a nonlocal way of interacting: for example, one entity may interact with another one even if the distance between them is not negligible.

N. Bellomo et al. (eds.), *Selected Topics in Cancer Modeling*,
DOI: 10.1007/978-0-8176-4713-1_3, © Springer Science+Business Media, LLC 2008

A prototype of the mathematical setting and relationships between the three possible scales of description: micro, meso and macro can be the kinetic theory of rarefied gases, see [6, 2, 14] and the references therein. There is however an important difference: in the case of biological systems a basic microscopic theory, such as Newton's laws in the kinetic theory case, is not available. Therefore it is reasonable to apply the following strategy. One may start with a deterministic macroscopic model for which the identification of parameters by an experiment is easier. Then one provides the theoretical framework for modelling at the microscopic scale in such a way that the corresponding models at the macro- and microscales are asymptotically equivalent, i.e. the solutions are close to each other in a properly chosen norm. Then, if the parameters of the microscopic model are suitably chosen, one may hope that it covers not only macroscopic behaviour of the system in question, but also some of its microscopic features. The microscopic model by its nature can be richer and can describe a larger variety of phenomena.

This chapter reviews a general conceptual framework for our program ([15, 16, 17, 18, 19, 20]) of finding possible transitions between the different levels of description, i.e.

- **(Mi)** at the level of interacting entities ("microscale"),
- **(Me)** at the level of the statistical description of a testentity ("mesoscale"),
- **(Ma)** at the level of densities of subpopulations ("macroscale").

The levels **(Mi)** and **(Me)** are of a nonlocal character. The general framework will be related to modelling of tumour invasion of tissue—a very important process in the evolution of the tumour.

In mathematical terms we are interested in the links between the following mathematically defined structures:

- **(Mi)** the microscale of stochastically interacting entities (cells, individuals), in terms of jump Markov processes, that lead to continuous (linear) stochastic semigroups;
- **(Me)** the mesoscale of statistical entities, in terms of continuous nonlinear semigroups related to the solutions of bilinear Boltzmann-type nonlocal kinetic equations;
- **(Ma)** the macroscale of densities of interacting entities, in terms of dynamical systems related to bilinear reaction-diffusion-chemotaxis equations.

In Ref. [15, 16, 17, 18] and [20] such a conceptual framework was developed for various situations of biological interest. In particular, Ref. [18] deals with the mathematical theory for a large class of reaction-diffusion systems (with limited diffusion). Ref. [19] shows that the theory can be generalised to take into account reaction-diffusion-chemotaxis systems (i.e. reaction-diffusion equations with a chemotaxis-type term). These methods may lead to a new and more accurate modelling of complex processes.

There is a huge literature related to the rigorous derivation of chemotaxis equations from microscopic models. The interested reader is referred to Ref. [26, 27] and references therein.

In Ref. [12] the idea of hydrodynamic limit was used to derive hyperbolic models for chemosensitive movements as a hydrodynamic limit of a velocity jump process. In Ref. [24] the stochastic modelling of a spatially structured biological population was investigated. Based on a law of large numbers, the convergence of a system of stochastic differential equations describing the evolution of the mean-field spatial density of the population was proved. In Ref. [29] a large system of particles was studied and convergence of the empirical measures was proved as the number of particles tends to infinity.

A variety of macroscopic models have been developed for various aspects of solid tumour growth. For example, the reader is referred to Ref. [7, 8, 9, 23] and references therein.

The plan of the chapter is as follows. In Section 3.2 we consider a simple but illuminating example of the logistic equation at the macroscopic level and the corresponding microscopic and mesoscopic equations. Section 3.3 describes the macroscopic models of tumour invasion; Section 3.4 the definition of corresponding microscopic and nonlocal models; and Section 3.5 the mesoscopic model. The main theorem is formulated in Section 3.5. The chapter concludes with Section 3.6.

3.2 A Simple Example

In this section we consider a simple example of a macroscopic model and a corresponding class of models on the microscopic and mesoscopic levels.

Example 1. Consider one population of individuals with a logistic growth given by

$$\dot{\varrho} = \alpha \varrho - \beta \varrho^2 \,, \tag{3.1}$$

where $\dot{\varrho} = \frac{d\varrho}{dt}$ and $\alpha, \beta > 0$ are parameters of the model. Equation (3.1) describes a macroscopic model in terms of the density of population $\varrho = \varrho(t)$.

In order to introduce the corresponding microscopic model we need the following function:

$$A = A(u), \qquad A \geq 0, \qquad \int_0^R A(u)\,du = 1\,, \tag{3.2}$$

such that

$$\int_0^R u\,A(u)\,du = \frac{\alpha}{\beta}\,, \tag{3.3}$$

where $R > 0$ is chosen sufficiently large for given α and β. The function A describes the transition probability.

We consider now a large number N of individuals. Every individual n ($n \in \{1, \ldots, N\}$) is characterized by the parameter $u \in [0, R]$, the inner state (its activity or fitness).

The Markov jump process of N individuals is defined by the generator Λ_N

$$
\begin{aligned}
\Lambda_N \phi(u_1, \ldots, u_N) = \\
(N-1)\beta R \int_0^R \cdots \int_0^R \Big(\phi(v_1, \ldots, v_N) - \phi(u_1, \ldots, u_N) \Big) \\
\times \nu(dv_1, \ldots, dv_N; u_1, \ldots, u_N),
\end{aligned}
\tag{3.4}
$$

with the *transition function* ν

$$
\begin{aligned}
\nu\big(dv_1, \ldots, dv_N; u_1, \ldots, u_N \big) \\
= \Big(1 - \sideset{}{'}\sum_{\substack{1 \le n,m \le N \\ n \ne m}} \tfrac{u_m}{N(N-1)R} \Big) \delta_{u_1}(dv_1) \ldots \delta_{u_N}(dv_N) \\
+ \sum_{\substack{1 \le n,m \le N \\ n \ne m}} \tfrac{u_m}{N(N-1)R} A(v_n) \, dv_n \\
\times \ \delta_{u_1}(dv_1) \ldots \delta_{u_{n-1}}(dv_{n-1}) \delta_{u_{n+1}}(dv_{n+1}) \ldots \delta_{u_N}(dv_N),
\end{aligned}
$$

where ϕ is a test function (a real-valued, Borel measurable bounded function), and δ_u is the atom measure concentrated in u.

Λ_N is the generator for a Markov jump process in $[0, R]^N$ that can be constructed as in Ref. [11], Section 4.2.

If the stochastic system is initially distributed according to the probability density $F^N \in L_{1,N}$, where $L_{1,N}$ is the space equipped with the norm

$$
\|f\|_{L_{1,N}} = \int_0^R \cdots \int_0^R \Big| f\big(u_1, \ldots, u_N\big) \Big| \, du_1 \ldots du_N,
\tag{3.5}
$$

and the time evolution is described by the following linear equation:

$$
\partial_t f^N = \Lambda_N^* f^N,
\tag{3.6}
$$

where

$$
\begin{aligned}
\Lambda_N^* f(u_1, u_2, \ldots, u_N) = \\
\tfrac{1}{N} \sum_{\substack{1 \le n,m \le N \\ n \ne m}} \Big(A(u_n) \, u_m \int_0^R f\big(u_1, \ldots, u_{n-1}, v, u_{n+1}, \ldots, u_N\big) \, dv \\
- \ u_m \, f\big(u_1, \ldots, u_N\big) \Big),
\end{aligned}
$$

we consider now the following bilinear Boltzmann-type equation (the level of mesoscopic description):

$$\partial_t f(t,u) = \beta A(u)\bar{f}(t)\hat{f}(t) - \beta f(t,u)\hat{f}(t)\,, \qquad (3.7)$$

where

$$\bar{f} = \int_0^R f(u)\,\mathrm{d}u\,, \qquad\qquad \hat{f} = \int_0^R u f(u)\,\mathrm{d}u\,. \qquad (3.8)$$

Applying the methods of [15, 17, 18] we show the following.

Theorem 1. *We are given positive parameters α, β. Let F be a probability density on $[0, R]$. Then $\forall\, t_0 > 0\quad \exists N_0\quad \forall\, N > N_0$*

$$\sup_{t\in[0,t_0]} \int_0^R \left| f^{N,1}(t,u) - f(t,u)\right|\,\mathrm{d}u \le \frac{\mathfrak{c}}{N^\zeta}\,, \qquad (3.9)$$

where $f^N \in L_1^{(N)}$ is the unique solution of Eq. (3.6) corresponding to the factorized initial datum

$$f^N\Big|_{t=0} = \underbrace{F \otimes \ldots \otimes F}_{N\,\times} = F^{N\otimes}\,, \qquad (3.10)$$

$$f^{N,1}(t,u) = \int_0^R \ldots \int_0^R f^N(t,u,u_2,\ldots,u_N)\,\mathrm{d}u_2\ldots\mathrm{d}u_N\,, \qquad (3.11)$$

where $f \in L_1^{(1)}$ is the unique solution of Eq. (3.7) corresponding to initial datum F and ζ, $\mathfrak{c}$ are positive constants that depend on t_0.

The solution to Eq. (3.7) satisfies

$$\bar{f}(t) = 1 \qquad \text{and} \qquad \partial_t \hat{f} = \alpha\hat{f} - \beta\,\hat{f}^{\,2} \qquad \forall\, t > 0\,, \qquad (3.12)$$

i.e. $\varrho = \hat{f}$ satisfies Eq. (3.1) and therefore we have the following.

Corollary 1. *Under the assumptions of Theorem 1*

$$\sup_{[0,t_0]} \left| \hat{f}^{N,1} - \varrho \right| \le \frac{\mathfrak{c}}{N^\zeta}\,, \qquad (3.13)$$

where ϱ is the unique solution of Eq. (3.1).

3.3 Macroscopic Models of Tumour Invasion

Various models of the invasive spatial spread of solid tumours were considered in Ref. [7, 8, 9, 19, 23, 28]. See also the references therein. Following

Chaplain and Anderson [7] we consider a system of deterministic reaction--diffusion-chemotaxis equations that is able to capture some aspects of solid tumour growth and invasion at the tissue level at the macroscopic scale. The model is based on generic solid tumour growth at the avascular stage, and it describes the interactions between the tumour and the surrounding tissue. The variables of the model are: tumour cell density, denoted by ϱ_1, ECM (the surrounding tissue or extracellular matrix) density, denoted by ϱ_2, and MDE (certain factors produced by the tumour cells and known as *matrix degrading* or *degradative enzymes*) concentration, denoted by ϱ_3. The model describes one key aspect of tissue invasion, namely the ability of tumour cells to produce and secrete MDEs and their migratory response. Chaplain and Anderson made the assumptions that the tumour cells produce MDEs which degrade the ECM locally; the ECM degradation aids in tumour cells motility; the movement of tumour cells up to a gradient of ECM is referred to as haptotaxis; and tumour cell motion is driven only by random motility and haptotaxis. Additionally to the model of [7] the proliferation of tumour cells and of the ECM is taken into account (cf. [23] and [28]).

With these assumptions the model (in the dimensionless form) reads

$$
\partial_t \varrho_1 = \overbrace{d_1 \nabla^2 \varrho_1}^{\text{random motility}} - \overbrace{\gamma \nabla \cdot \left(\varrho_1 \nabla \varrho_2 \right)}^{\text{haptotaxis}}
$$

$$
+ \overbrace{\mu_1 \varrho_1}^{\text{proliferation}} - \overbrace{\mu_1 \varrho_1 \left(\varrho_1 + \varrho_2 \right)}^{\text{inhibition of proliferation}} ,
$$

$$
\partial_t \varrho_2 = - \overbrace{\eta \, \varrho_2 \, \varrho_3}^{\text{degradation}} + \overbrace{\mu_2 \varrho_2}^{\text{proliferation}} - \overbrace{\mu_2 \varrho_2 \left(\varrho_1 + \varrho_2 \right)}^{\text{inhibition of proliferation}} ,
$$

$$
\partial_t \varrho_3 = \overbrace{d_3 \nabla^2 \varrho_3}^{\text{diffusion}} + \overbrace{\alpha \, \varrho_1}^{\text{production}} - \overbrace{\beta \, \varrho_3}^{\text{decay}} ,
$$

(3.14)

where d_1, γ, μ_1, η, μ_2, d_3, α, β are given positive constants (the macroscopic parameters).

The proliferation terms in Eq. (3.14) are defined as the logistic-type terms in an analogous way as in the space homogeneous case (see Section 3.2), i.e using linear growth with inhibition terms.

The space variable x is in Ω—a domain in $\mathbb{R}^3$. Here, in order to avoid some additional technical difficulties, the periodic boundary conditions are assumed, i.e. the domain Ω is identified with the three-dimensional torus $\mathbb{T}^3$. Analogously, the case of $\Omega = \mathbb{R}^3$ may be considered.

It seems that more realistic proliferation terms than those defined in Eq. (3.14) could be nonlocal inhibition of the cell proliferation terms (cf. the discussion in [28])

$$\partial_t \varrho_1 = \overbrace{d_1 \nabla^2 \varrho_1}^{\text{random motility}} \overbrace{- \gamma \nabla \cdot \left(\varrho_1 \nabla \varrho_2 \right)}^{\text{haptotaxis}}$$
$$+ \overbrace{\mu_1 \varrho_1}^{\text{proliferation}} \overbrace{- \mu_1 \varrho_1 \left(k_{1,1} * \varrho_1 + k_{1,2} * \varrho_2 \right)}^{\text{inhibition of proliferation}},$$

$$\partial_t \varrho_2 = - \overbrace{\eta \varrho_2 \varrho_3}^{\text{degradation}} + \overbrace{\mu_2 \varrho_2}^{\text{proliferation}} \overbrace{- \mu_2 \varrho_2 \left(k_{2,1} * \varrho_1 + k_{2,2} * \varrho_2 \right)}^{\text{inhibition of proliferation}},$$

$$\partial_t \varrho_3 = \overbrace{d_3 \nabla^2 \varrho_3}^{\text{diffusion}} + \overbrace{\alpha \varrho_1}^{\text{production}} - \overbrace{\beta \varrho_3}^{\text{decay}},$$

(3.15)

where $*$ denotes the convolution with respect to the space variable

$$k * \varrho(t, x) = \int_\Omega k(x - y) \varrho(t, y) \, \mathrm{d}y, \qquad (3.16)$$

and $k_{i,j}$ $(i, j = 1, 2)$ are given probability densities (spatial kernels). The integrals with $k_{i,j}$ describe the inhibition of cell proliferation caused by the density of ECM and of MDE.

In a similar spirit another model can be proposed (see [28])

$$\partial_t \varrho_1 = \overbrace{d_1 \nabla^2 \varrho_1}^{\text{random motility}} \overbrace{- \nabla \cdot \left(\gamma(\varrho_2) \varrho_1 \nabla \varrho_2 \right)}^{\text{haptotaxis}}$$
$$+ \overbrace{\mu_1 \varrho_1}^{\text{proliferation}} \overbrace{- \mu_1 \varrho_1 \left(k_{1,1} * \varrho_1 + k_{1,2} * \varrho_2 \right)}^{\text{inhibition of proliferation}},$$

(3.17)

$$\partial_t \varrho_2 = - \overbrace{\eta \varrho_2 \, k * \varrho_1}^{\text{degradation}} + \overbrace{\mu_2 \varrho_2}^{\text{proliferation}} \overbrace{- \mu_2 \varrho_2 \left(k_{2,1} * \varrho_1 + k_{2,2} * \varrho_2 \right)}^{\text{inhibition of proliferation}},$$

where k is a given probability density (a spatial kernel) and γ is a smooth positive function of ϱ_2. In [28] the corresponding model in a general bounded domain was proposed and analysed.

The systems of equations (3.14), (3.15) and (3.17) define three macroscopic models of tumour invasion of tissue.

3.4 Microscopic Nonlocal Models of Tumour Invasion

In this section we construct the microscopic model that corresponds to the macroscopic model defined by Eq. (3.14). A similar idea can be applied for

Eq. (3.15) or Eq. (3.17) with $\gamma = $ const. The microscopic model is constructed in terms of a Markov jump process as in Section 3.2. We are going to introduce a linear generator that completely describes the evolution of the density probability at the microscopic scale that approximates the solution of Eq. (3.14).

In what follows, a (large) number N of entities (cells or factors) of 3 subpopulations is considered. We follow here the general framework [15, 16, 17, 18, 19].

Every entity n ($n \in \{1, \ldots, N\}$) is characterized by

$$\mathbf{u}_n = (j_n, u_n, x_n) \in \mathbf{U} = \mathcal{J} \times [0, R] \times \Omega , \qquad (3.18)$$

where $j_n \in \mathcal{J} = \{1, 2, 3, \}$ is its subpopulation, $u_n \in [0, R]$ its (inner) state (its "activity" or "fitness"), $R > 0$, and $x_n \in \Omega$ its position (of the centre of mass).

The n-entity interacts with the m-entity, and the interaction take place at random times. After the interaction both entities may change their populations and/or their states.

The rate of interaction between the entity of the jth population with state u at point x, and the entity of the kth population with state v at point y, is given by the measurable function a such that

$$0 \le a = a(\mathbf{u}, \mathbf{v}) \le a_+ < \infty , \qquad \forall \, \mathbf{u}, \mathbf{v} \in \mathbf{U} , \qquad (3.19)$$

where a_+ is a constant.

The transition into the jth population with state u at point x, of an entity of the kth population with state v at point y, due to the interaction with an entity of the lth population with state w at point z, is described by the measurable function

$$A = A(\mathbf{u}; \mathbf{v}, \mathbf{w}) \ge 0 , \qquad \forall \, \mathbf{u}, \mathbf{v}, \mathbf{w} \in \mathbf{U} , \qquad (3.20)$$

where A is the transition probability and therefore

$$\sum_{j=1}^{3} \int_{0}^{R} \int_{\Omega} A\Big((j, u, x); \mathbf{v}, \mathbf{w}\Big) \, dx \, du = 1 , \qquad (3.21)$$

for all $\mathbf{v}, \mathbf{w} \in \mathbf{U}$ such that $a(\mathbf{v}, \mathbf{w}) > 0$.

The stochastic model (at the microscopic level) will be completely determined by the choice of functions a and A. Different choices of a and A give rise to different—[15, 16, 17, 18, 19]. microscopic models (Markov processes) The definitions of a and A that lead to the microscopic model corresponding to the macroscopic model (3.14) may be given in a similar way as in [19].

If a and A are given, then we assume that the stochastic system is given by the Markov jump process of N individuals defined by the generator Λ_N

$$
\Lambda_N \phi(\mathbf{u}_1, \dots, \mathbf{u}_N) = (N-1)a_+ \int_{\mathbf{U}^N} \Big(\phi(\mathbf{v}_1, \dots, \mathbf{v}_N) - \phi(\mathbf{u}_1, \dots, \mathbf{u}_N) \Big)
$$
$$
\times \nu\big(d\mathbf{v}_1, \dots, d\mathbf{v}_N; \mathbf{u}_1, \dots, \mathbf{u}_N \big),
$$

$$(3.22)$$

with the transition function ν defined by

$$
\nu\big(d\mathbf{v}_1, \dots, d\mathbf{v}_N; \mathbf{u}_1, \dots, \mathbf{u}_N\big)
$$
$$
= \left(1 - \sum_{\substack{1 \le n,m \le N \\ n \ne m}} \frac{a(\mathbf{u}_n, \mathbf{u}_m)}{N(N-1)a_+}\right) \delta_{\mathbf{u}_1}(d\mathbf{v}_1) \dots \delta_{\mathbf{u}_N}(d\mathbf{v}_N)
$$
$$
+ \sum_{\substack{1 \le n,m \le N \\ n \ne m}} \frac{a(\mathbf{u}_n, \mathbf{u}_m)}{N(N-1)a_+} A(d\mathbf{v}_n ; \mathbf{u}_n, \mathbf{u}_m)
$$
$$
\times \delta_{\mathbf{u}_1}(d\mathbf{v}_1) \dots \delta_{\mathbf{u}_{n-1}}(d\mathbf{v}_{n-1}) \delta_{\mathbf{u}_{n+1}}(d\mathbf{v}_{n+1}) \dots \delta_{\mathbf{u}_N}(d\mathbf{v}_N),
$$

$$(3.23)$$

where ϕ is a test function (a real-valued, Borel measurable bounded function). We have adopted the convention that for $\mathbf{u} = (j, u, x)$, $\mathbf{v} = (k, v, y)$,

$$
\delta_{\mathbf{u}}(d\mathbf{v}) = \delta_{j,k}\, \delta_u(dv)\, \delta_x(dy), \tag{3.24}
$$

and

$$
\int_{\mathbf{G}} A(d\mathbf{u} ; \mathbf{v}, \mathbf{w}) = \sum_{j \in \mathcal{J}_1} \int_{\mathcal{U}} \int_{\mathcal{X}} A\big((j, u, x) ; \mathbf{v}, \mathbf{w}\big)\, du\, dx, \tag{3.25}
$$

for $\mathbf{G} = \mathcal{J}_1 \times \mathcal{U} \times \mathcal{X}$, where $\mathcal{J}_1 \in \mathcal{J}$, and $\mathcal{U}$, $\mathcal{X}$ are measurable sets in $[0, R]$, Ω, respectively, δ_u is the atom measure concentrated in u and $\delta_{j,k}$ is the Kronecker delta.

By [11] Λ_N is the generator for a Markov jump process in $\mathbf{U}^N$.

We assume now that the system is initially distributed according to the probability density $F^N \in L_{1,N}$, where $L_{1,N}$ is the space equipped with the norm

$$
\|f\|_{L_{1,N}} =
$$
$$
\sum_{j_1=1}^{3} \int_0^R \int_\Omega \dots \sum_{j_N=1}^{3} \int_0^R \int_\Omega \Big| f\big((j_1, u_1, x_1), \dots, (j_N, u_N, x_N)\big) \Big| dx_1\, du_1 \dots dx_N\, du_N,
$$

and the time evolution is described by the following linear equation:

$$
\partial_t f^N = \Lambda_N^* f^N ; \qquad f^N \big|_{t=0} = F^N, \tag{3.26}
$$

where Λ_N^* is the generator

$$
\Lambda_N^* f(\mathbf{u}_1, \mathbf{u}_2, \dots, \mathbf{u}_N)
$$
$$
= \frac{1}{N} \sum_{\substack{1 \le n,m \le N \\ n \ne m}} \left(\sum_{k=1}^{3} \int_0^R \int_\Omega A\big(\mathbf{u}_n; (k, v, y), \mathbf{u}_m\big) a\big((k, v, y), \mathbf{u}_m\big) \right.
$$
$$
\times f\big(\mathbf{u}_1, \dots, \mathbf{u}_{n-1}, (k, v, y), \mathbf{u}_{n+1}, \dots, \mathbf{u}_N\big) dy\, dv
$$
$$
\left. - a(\mathbf{u}_n, \mathbf{u}_m) f\big(\mathbf{u}_1, \dots, \mathbf{u}_N\big) \right)
$$

$$(3.27)$$

and $\mathbf{u}_n = (j_n, u_n, x_n)$ for any $n = 1, \ldots, N$.

The idea is to define a and A in such a way that the operator Λ_N^* is a bounded operator in the space $L_{1,N}$. In such a case the Cauchy problem (3.26) has the unique solution $f^N(t) \in L_{1,N}$ for all $t \geq 0$. Moreover, the solution is nonnegative and its $L_{1,N}$-norm is preserved,

$$\|f^N(t)\|_{L_{1,N}} = \|F^N\|_{L_{1,N}} = 1, \qquad \text{for } t > 0. \tag{3.28}$$

Thus $\exp\left(t\Lambda_N^*\right)$ defines a continuous linear semigroup of Markov operators (continuous stochastic semigroups) at the microscopic level.

The definition of the appropriate functions a and A can be analogous to those in [19].

In addition to the macroscopic parameters d_1, γ, η, d_3, α, β, the microscopic model contains the microscopic parameters N, $\varepsilon > 0$ and $R > 0$. The microscopic model has a nonlocal (in space) character: in fact the two entities may interact up to some distance as the interactions are defined by a jump process. The parameter ε describes a distance of possible interaction. Actually two characteristic distances of the order of ε and ε^3 are defined. The limit $\varepsilon \to 0$ leads to local (in space) interactions (as in (3.14)). The parameter R has a more technical meaning: it is introduced in order to make the operator Λ_N^* bounded. However, it may be related to the possible range of the activity variable.

The functions a and A defined in [19] on $(\{1,2,3\} \times [0,R] \times \Omega)^2$ and $(\{1,2,3\} \times [0,R] \times \Omega)^3$, respectively, satisfy (3.19)–(3.21). The operator Λ_N^* defined by (3.27) is a bounded operator in the space $L_{1,N}$ and the Cauchy problem (3.26) has the unique solution $f^N(t) \in L_{1,N}$ for all $t \geq 0$. The solution preserves the nonnegativity and $L_{1,N}$-norm (3.26) of the initial data. Therefore $\exp\left(t\Lambda_N^*\right)$ defines a continuous stochastic semigroup.

3.5 Mesoscopic Model

In order to derive a mesoscopic model from Eq. (3.26) we follow [17, 19], we assume that the function f^N is symmetric,

$$f^N(\mathbf{u}_1, \mathbf{u}_2, \ldots, \mathbf{u}_N) = f^N(\mathbf{u}_{r_1}, \mathbf{u}_{r_2}, \ldots, \mathbf{u}_{r_N}), \tag{3.29}$$

for any permutation $\{r_1, r_2, \ldots, r_N\}$ of the set $\{1, 2, \ldots, N\}$, and we introduce the s-entity marginal density ($1 \leq s < N$)

$$f^{N,s}(\mathbf{u}_1, \ldots, \mathbf{u}_s) = \tag{3.30}$$

$$\sum_{j_{s+1}=1}^{3} \int_0^R \int_\Omega \cdots \sum_{j_N=1}^{3} \int_0^R \int_\Omega f^N\Big(\mathbf{u}_1, \ldots \mathbf{u}_s, (j_{s+1}, u_{s+1}, x_{s+1}) \ldots, (j_N, u_N, x_N)\Big)$$

$$\times dx_{s+1}\, du_{s+1} \ldots dx_N\, du_N,$$

and $f^{N,N} = f^N$.

We assume that the process starts with the chaotic (i.e. factorized) probability density

$$F^{N,s} = (F)^{s\otimes} = \underbrace{F \otimes \ldots \otimes F}_{s\times}, \qquad s = 1, \ldots, N, \qquad (3.31)$$

i.e. an s-fold outer product of a probability density F.

In the limit $N \to \infty$ the linear equation (3.26) results ([17]) in a bilinear system of Boltzmann-like integro-differential equations (generalized kinetic models) that can be related to the mesoscopic description

$$\partial_t f(t, \mathbf{u}) = \Gamma[f](\mathbf{u}), \qquad t > 0, \quad \mathbf{u} \in \{1, 2, 3\} \times [0, R] \times \Omega, \qquad (3.32)$$

where

$$\Gamma[f](t, \mathbf{u}) = \sum_{k=1}^{3} \int_0^R \int_\Omega \sum_{l=1}^{3} \int_0^R \int_\Omega A\left(\mathbf{u}; (k, v, y), (l, w, z)\right)$$
$$\times a\left((k, v, y), (l, w, z)\right) f(t, k, v, y) f(t, l, w, z) \, \mathrm{d}z \, \mathrm{d}w \, \mathrm{d}y \, \mathrm{d}v \qquad (3.33)$$
$$- f(t, \mathbf{u}) \sum_{k=1}^{3} \int_0^R \int_\Omega a\left(\mathbf{u}, (k, v, y)\right) f(t, k, v, y) \, \mathrm{d}y \, \mathrm{d}v.$$

In the context of biological or medical processes various Boltzmann-like equations were considered by various authors; see [1, 2, 3, 4, 5, 17, 20, 22] (and references therein).

The existence and uniqueness theory for Eq. (3.32) is standard [22, 2].

Introducing

$$\tilde{f}_j = \int_0^\infty u f(j, u) \, \mathrm{d}u, \qquad (3.34)$$

for any $f(j, \, .\,) \in L_1(0, \infty)$ as in [19] we obtain

$$\partial_t \tilde{f}_1(t, x) = \frac{10\, d_1}{\varepsilon^2\, \kappa_1} \int_\Omega \chi\left(|y - x| < \varepsilon\right) \tilde{f}_1(t, y) \, \mathrm{d}y - \frac{10\, d_1}{\varepsilon^2} \tilde{f}_1(t, x)$$
$$+ \frac{20\, \gamma}{\varepsilon^2\, \kappa_3\, \kappa_1} \int_\Omega \int_\Omega \chi\left(\left|\frac{y+z}{2} - x\right| < \varepsilon^3\right) \chi\left(|z - y| < \varepsilon\right) \tilde{f}_1(t, y) \tilde{f}_2(t, z) \, \mathrm{d}z \, \mathrm{d}y \qquad (3.35)$$
$$- \frac{20\, \gamma}{\varepsilon^2\, \kappa_1} \tilde{f}_1(t, x) \int_\Omega \chi\left(|y - x| < \varepsilon\right) \tilde{f}_2(t, y) \, \mathrm{d}y,$$

$$\partial_t \tilde{f}_2(t, x) = -\frac{\eta}{\kappa_3} \int_\Omega \int_\Omega \chi\left(|x - y| < \varepsilon^3\right) \tilde{f}_2(t, x) \tilde{f}_3(t, y) \, \mathrm{d}y \, \mathrm{d}y$$
$$+ \frac{\eta}{2\, \kappa_3^2} \int_\Omega \int_\Omega \chi\left(|y - x| < \varepsilon^3\right) \chi\left(|z - y| < \varepsilon^3\right) \tilde{f}_2(t, y) \tilde{f}_3(t, z) \, \mathrm{d}y \, \mathrm{d}z, \qquad (3.36)$$

$$\partial_t \tilde{f}_3(t, x) = \frac{10\, d_3}{\varepsilon^2\, \kappa_1} \int_\Omega \chi\left(|y - x| < \varepsilon\right) \tilde{f}_3(t, y) \, \mathrm{d}y - \frac{10\, d_3}{\varepsilon^2} \tilde{f}_3(t, x)$$
$$+ \frac{\alpha}{\kappa_3} \int_\Omega \chi\left(|y - x| < \varepsilon^3\right) \tilde{f}_1(t, y) \, \mathrm{d}y, \qquad (3.37)$$

where $\kappa_i = \frac{\varepsilon^{3i}}{3}|\mathbb{S}^2|$, for $i = 1, 3$; $\mathbb{S}^2 = \{y \in \Omega : |y| = 1\}$.

Expanding in Taylor's series we obtain (see [19])

$$\begin{aligned}
\partial_t \tilde{f}_1(t, x) &= d_1 \nabla^2 \tilde{f}_1(t, x) - \gamma \nabla \cdot \left(\tilde{f}_1(t, x) \nabla \tilde{f}_2(t, x) \right) + \mathcal{O}(\varepsilon^3), \\
\partial_t \tilde{f}_2(t, x) &= \eta \tilde{f}_2(t, x) \tilde{f}_3(t, x) + \mathcal{O}(\varepsilon^3), \\
\partial_t \tilde{f}_3(t, x) &= d_3 \nabla^2 \tilde{f}_3(t, x) + \alpha \tilde{f}_1(t, x) - \beta \tilde{f}_3(t, x) + \mathcal{O}(\varepsilon^3).
\end{aligned} \tag{3.38}$$

One may compare Eq. (3.38) with Eq. (3.14). It follows that Eq. (3.35) are nonlocal versions of the local equations (3.14).

In this chapter we assume that

$$\sigma_i = \varepsilon^2 \sigma_i^*, \quad i = 1, 3, \qquad \gamma = \varepsilon^2 \gamma^*, \tag{3.39}$$

where σ_i^* and γ^* are given ε-independent positive constants. The parameter $\varepsilon \in]0, 1[$ is assumed to be small and therefore assumption (3.39) refers to weak diffusion and haptotaxis processes. In other words, the diffusion and haptotaxis are small in comparison with other processes (the parameters α, β, η are assumed to be ε independent). This was actually the case in the situation considered in Ref. [7, 8, 23].

We may note that the parameters σ_i, γ that are ε independent may be considered (at the formal level) analogously with Ref. [18].

Following [19] we state the theorems that define links between the solutions to various equations (descriptions) presented in the previous sections.

We start with the transition from the microscopic level to the mesoscopic level. By Ref. [17] we have the following.

Theorem 2. *Let F be a probability density on $\{1, 2, 3\} \times [0, R] \times \Omega$. Then, for each $t_0 > 0$, there exists N_0 such that for $N \geq N_0$*

$$\sup_{t \in [0, t_0]} \sum_{j=1}^{3} \int_0^R \int_\Omega |f^{N,1}(t, j, u, x) - f(t, j, u, x)| \, \mathrm{d}x \, \mathrm{d}u \leq \frac{\mathfrak{c}_1}{N^\zeta}, \tag{3.40}$$

where $f^N \in L_{1,N}$ is the unique, nonnegative solution of Eq. (3.26) corresponding to the initial datum (3.31); $f \in L_{1,1}$ is the unique, nonnegative solution of Eq. (3.32) corresponding to the initial datum F; and ζ, $\mathfrak{c}_1$ are positive constants that depend on t_0.

We need an existence theorem for Eq. (3.14). This is actually an open problem and it will be studied elsewhere. The reader is referred to [10] for general methods (see also references therein). The local existence and uniqueness of regular solutions for the model of tissue invasion without the proliferation terms, i.e. Eq. (3.14) with $\mu_1 = \mu_2 = 0$, were proved by Morales-Rodrigo [25]. The global existence and uniqueness of regular solutions for Eq. (3.17) were proved in [28]. Here we restrict ourselves to a conditional result with the following assumption.

Assumption A. *Given positive parameters* d_1^*, γ^*, η, d_3^*, α, β *independent of* ε *and initial data*

$$\left(\varrho_1^{(0)}, \varrho_2^{(0)}, \varrho_3^{(0)}\right) \in C^m\left(\Omega; [0, \infty[^3\right), \qquad \text{with some } m \geq 6, \tag{3.41}$$

we assume that $t_1 > 0$ *is such that the unique classical solution* $(\varrho_1, \varrho_2, \varrho_3)$ *to the Cauchy problem for system* (3.14) *with* (3.39) *exists in* $[0, t_1]$.

Let F be a probability density on $\{1, 2, 3\} \times [0, \infty[\times \Omega$ such that

$$\tilde{F}_j = \varrho_j^{(0)}, \qquad j = 1, 2, 3, \tag{3.42}$$

$$F(j, u, x) = 0, \qquad \text{for } j = 1, 2, 3, \quad u > R_0, \quad x \in \Omega, \tag{3.43}$$

for some $R_0 > 0$, R_0 is fixed and $R > R_0$.

In much the same way as in the proof of Theorem 4.1 in [22], and using (3.40), we obtain the main result.

Theorem 3. *Let* Assumption A *be satisfied and let* $F \in X_2^{m,1}$ *be a probability density such that* (3.42) *and* (3.43) *are satisfied. Then for sufficiently large* N, R *and small* $\varepsilon > 0$

$$\sup_{t \in [0, t_1]} \sum_{j=1}^{3} \int_{\Omega} \left| \tilde{f}_j^{N,1}(t, x) - \varrho_j(t, x) \right| dx \leq \frac{\mathfrak{c}_1}{N^\zeta} + \frac{\mathfrak{c}_2}{R} + \mathfrak{c}_3 \varepsilon^3, \tag{3.44}$$

where the nonnegative function $f^N \in L_{1,N}$ *is the unique solution of Eq.* (3.26) *and corresponds to the initial datum* $F^{N \otimes}$; ζ *and* $\mathfrak{c}_1$ *are positive constants that depend on* R *and* ε; $\mathfrak{c}_2$ *is a positive constant that depends on* ε; $\mathfrak{c}_3$ *is a constant.*

Theorem 3 shows that if the solution to the nonlinear Eq. (3.14) exists then it may be approximated by the solutions of the linear equation (3.26). On the other hand, the linear equation (3.26) related to the microscopic description, and the nonlinear equation (3.14) at the mesoscopic scale, may play independently an important role in the mathematical description of the process in question, even if Eq. (3.14) does not possess smooth solutions.

3.6 Conclusions

In Section 3.4 we proposed the microscopic linear model (3.26) corresponding to the macroscopic bilinear model (3.14). In Section 3.5 the mesoscopic bilinear model (3.32) was introduced and was related to the nonlocal version (3.35), (3.36), (3.37) of the macroscopic model (3.14). The main result is Theorem 3, which states the relationship between the solutions of the microscopic linear model (3.26) and the solutions of the macroscopic bilinear model (3.14). We gave the explicit error estimates in (3.44).

Acknowledgments

The author acknowledges research support from the EU project *"Modeling, Mathematical Methods and Computer Simulations of Tumour Growth and Therapy"*-M3CSTuTh, Contract No. MRTN–CT–2004–503661 and the Polish SPUB-M Grant.

References

1. Arlotti, L., Bellomo, N., Lachowicz, M.: Kinetic equations modelling population dynamics. Transport Theory Statist. Phys., **29**, 125–139 (2000)
2. Arlotti, L., Bellomo, N., De Angelis, E., Lachowicz, M.,: Generalized Kinetic Models in Applied Sciences, World Sci., River Edge, NJ (2003)
3. Bellomo, N., Bellouquid, A., Delitala, M.: Mathematical topics on the modelling complex multicellular systems and tumor immune cells competition. Math. Models Methods Appl. Sci., **14**, 1683–1733 (2004)
4. Bellomo, N., Forni, G.: Dynamics of tumor interaction with the host immune system. Math. Comput. Modelling, **20**, 107–122 (1994)
5. Bellomo, N., Forni, G.: Looking for new paradigms towards a biological-mathematical theory of complex multicellular systems. Math. Models Methods Appl. Sci., **16**, 1001–1029 (2006)
6. Cercignani, C., Illner, R., Pulvirenti, M.: The Mathematical Theory of Dilute Gases, Springer, New York (1994)
7. Chaplain, M.A.J., Anderson, A.R.A.: Mathematical modelling of tissue invasion. In: Preziosi, L. (ed): Cancer Modelling and Simulation, 269–297, Chapman & Hall/CRT, London (2003)
8. Chaplain, M.A.J., Lolas, G.: Spatio-temporal heterogeneity arising in a mathematical model of cancer invasion of tissue. Math. Models Methods Appl. Sci., **15**, 1685–1734 (2005)
9. Chaplain, M.A.J.: Modelling tumour growth. In Multiscale Problems in Life Sciences. From Microscopic to Macroscopic. Eds. Capasso, V., Lachowicz, M., CIME Courses, Springer Lecture Notes in Mathematics (2008), to appear.
10. Corrias, L., Perthame, B., Zaag, H.: Global solutions of some chemotaxis and angiogenesis systems in high space dimensions. Milan J. Math., **72**, 1–28 (2004)
11. Ethier, S.N., Kurtz, T.G.: Markov Processes, Characterization and Convergence. Wiley, New York (1986)
12. Filbert, F., Laurençot, P., Perthame, B.: Derivation of hyperbolic models for chemosensitive movement. J. Math. Biol., **50**, 189–207 (2005)
13. Jäger, E., Segel, L.: On the distribution of dominance in a population of interacting anonymous organisms. SIAM J. Appl. Math., **52**, 1442–1468 (1992)
14. Lachowicz, M.: From microscopic to macroscopic description for generalized kinetic models. Math. Models Methods Appl. Sci., **12**, 985–1005 (2002)
15. Lachowicz, M.: Describing competitive systems at the level of interacting individuals. In: Proceedings of the Eight Nat. Confer. Appl. Math. Biol. Medicine, Łajs, Poland (25–28 Sept.), 95–100 (2002)
16. Lachowicz, M.: From microscopic to macroscopic descriptions of complex systems. Comp. Rend. Mecanique (Paris), **331**, 733–738 (2003)

17. Lachowicz, M.: On bilinear kinetic equations. Between micro and macro descriptions of biological populations. Banach Center Publ., **63**, 217–230 (2004)
18. Lachowicz, M.: General population systems. Macroscopic limit of a class of stochastic semigroups. J. Math. Anal. Appl., **307**, 585–605 (2005)
19. Lachowicz, M.: Micro and meso scales of description corresponding to a model of tissue invasion by solid tumours. Math. Models Methods Appl. Sci., **15**, 1667–1683 (2005)
20. Lachowicz, M.: Links Between Microscopic and Macroscopic Descriptions. In Multiscale Problems in Life Sciences. From Microscopic to Macroscopic. Eds. Capasso, V., Lachowicz, M., CIME Courses, Springer Lecture Notes in Mathematics (2008), to appear.
21. Lachowicz, M., Pulvirenti, M.: A stochastic particle system modeling the Euler equation. Arch. Rational Mech. Anal., **109**, 81–93 (1990)
22. Lachowicz, M., Wrzosek, D.: Nonlocal bilinear equations. Equilibrium solutions and diffusive limit. Math. Models Methods Appl. Sci., **11**, 1375–1390 (2001)
23. Lolas, G.: Mathematical modelling of the urokinase plasminogen activation system and its role in cancer invasion of tissue. Ph.D. Thesis, Department of Mathematics, University of Dundee (2003)
24. Morale, D., Capasso, V., Oelschläger, K.: An interacting particle system modelling aggregation behaviour: from individuals to populations. J. Math. Biol., **50**, 49–66 (2005)
25. Morales-Rodrigo, C.: Local existence and uniqueness of regular solutions in a model of tissue invasion by solid tumours. Math. Comput. Model., to appear
26. Perthame, B.: PDE models for chemotactic movements: Parabolic, hyperbolic and kinetic. Appl. Math., **49**, 539–564 (2004)
27. Stevens, A.: The derivation of chemotaxis equations as limit dynamics of moderately interacting stochastic many-particle systems. SIAM J. Appl. Math., **61**, 183–212 (2000)
28. Szymańska, Z., Morales Rodrigo, C., Lachowicz, M., Chaplain, M.A.J.: Mathematical modelling of cancer invasion of tissue: Nonlocal interactions, to appear.
29. Wagner, W.: A functional law of large numbers for Boltzmann type stochastic particle systems. Stochastic Anal. Appl., **14**, 591–636 (1996)

4

Nonlinear Renewal Equations

Benoît Perthame[1,2,3] and Suman Kumar Tumuluri[1,2]

[1] Département de Mathématiques et Applications, École Normale Supérieure, 75230 Paris, France
{perthame, suman}@dma.ens.fr
[2] INRIA-Rocquencourt B.P. 105, Projet BANG, F78153, Le Chesnay Cedex
[3] Institut Universitaire de France, 75005 Paris, France

4.1 Introduction

In this chapter we consider a common nonlinear age-structured population model which arises in many different contexts. One of them is the description of cell proliferation and thus tumor growth, another is metastatisis size distribution. It can be written as a partial differential equation (PDE) on the unknown function $n(x, t) \geq 0$ which represents the population density of individuals of age x, at time t,

$$\begin{cases} \frac{\partial}{\partial t}n(t, x) + \frac{\partial}{\partial x}n(t, x) + d(x, S(t))n(t, x) = 0, \ t \geq 0, \ x \geq 0, \\ n(t, 0) = \int_0^\infty B(x, S(t))n(t, x)dx, \\ n(0, x) = n_0(x) \geq 0. \end{cases} \tag{4.1}$$

The vector-valued function $S(t) = \big(S_1(t), S_2(t), \ldots, S_k(t)\big)$ represents the environmental factors which depend on the solution $n(x, t)$ itself, with a coupling, which we take as simply as possible,

$$S_i(t) = \int_0^\infty \psi_i(x)n(t, x)dx, \qquad 1 \leq i \leq k. \tag{4.2}$$

Also $B \geq 0$, $d \geq 0$ represent the birth and death rates respectively. Throughout this chapter our interest is on cells, cell cycles and related topics, therefore we consider a single population living isolated, in an invariant habitat, with all individuals equal and where there is no sex difference.

The model (4.1)–(4.2) arises in many examples from population biology. Historically, it is the first PDE introduced in biology, and the linear equation (when d and b do not depend on S) is usually known after McKendrick [32] who introduced it for epidemiology and Feller [21] who made an extensive study through Markov processes. The linear equation is also known as the Von Foerster equation because he was first to use it for modeling cell cultures.

N. Bellomo et al. (eds.), *Selected Topics in Cancer Modeling*,
DOI: 10.1007/978-0-8176-4713-1_4, © Springer Science+Business Media, LLC 2008

It is well understood and there are several mathematical ways to express the main behavior of its solutions: they exhibit exponential growth or decay of the population with a rate and profile that can be entirely characterized. For example, using the general relative entropy (GRE) inequalities ([37, 38, 43]), one can prove that solutions to the linear model satisfy the long time asymptotics

$$\int \phi(x) \left| n(x,t) \, e^{-\lambda t} - \rho N(x) \right| dx \xrightarrow[t \to \infty]{} 0, \qquad (4.3)$$

for some real number $\rho > 0$ and appropriate functions ϕ and N (see Sect. 4.3). Hence depending on the sign of λ, we conclude that either the population will grow forever or become extinct.

As for nonlinear models, the most famous was proposed by Kermack and McKendrick for epidemiology with continuous state (age in the disease), [30]. Nowadays, these models are used in various domains ranging from epidemiology to ecology, medicine and cell cultures. We give several examples and references in Sect. 4.2. The first mathematical study of such nonlinear equations is due to Gurtin and MacCamy [23], and thus (4.1)–(4.2) is sometimes referred to as the Gurtin–MacCamy model, in the case $\psi_1 = \psi_2 \equiv 1$ at least. Existence, uniqueness and stability results of solutions of this model were discussed in [11, 22, 23]. Afterwards it was extensively studied by several mathematicians using various techniques such as semigroup theory, entropy GRE methods and Laplace transforms. To deal with this model, the basic technique which many people (including Gurtin and MacCamy) used was to apply the method of characteristics to convert this problem to systems of Volterra integral equations (see [23, 26, 27, 48, 8]). The papers [14, 15] and the book [46] contain a recent account of the theory. Here we will try to avoid this artefact and deal with PDE methods, some of which can be extended to more elaborate models, e.g., size-structured models [34, 43, 44, 37, 36].

An important aspect in the linear model leading to the behavior (4.3) is that it does not take resources into account. This is the main drawback of the linear model. In the system (4.1)–(4.2) we overcome this and consider the consumption of resources like nutrients, by introducing nonlinearity in the birth and death terms. In many of the examples we will consider later, these terms limit the possible growth and induce extra growth when the solution becomes too small. In other words, these models contain the classical assumption of Verhulst (for a mere ODE) as a basic ingredient. However due to the delay induced by the boundary condition in (4.1), this limitation can have dramatic effects such as the existence of chaotic solutions, periodic solutions and "oscillating" solutions, see [18, 39, 35]. Traveling waves have also been studied [17], and periodic forcing is treated in [12]. Of course stability questions are also a major issue, and are studied by many authors, see [7, 33]. In this chapter we pay special interest to global a priori bounds and cases where we can prove that there is an exponentially attractive nonzero steady state.

We begin with several examples of nonlinearities taken from the literature (Sect. 4.2). Then, we introduce our main assumptions (Sect. 4.3). Existence theory and uniform bounds on the solutions require some work which we perform in Sects. 4.4 and 4.5. Our first original result concerns a case where we can prove the asymptotic behavior as $n(x,t) \sim N(x)\tilde{n}(t)$, see Sect. 4.6. Then, we recall in Sect. 4.7, the long time asymptotics result of Michel [35] on "concave type" nonlinearities on the birth term. After these general cases we conclude in Sect. 4.8 with special nonlinearities for which we can reduce the system to ODE systems and prove again their exponential stability.

4.2 Examples of Age-Structured Models

Many variants of the system (4.1)–(4.2) have been proposed in the literature in various area of biology, leading to different choices of the model parameters d, B and ψ. In this section we present some specific examples. Of course this presentation is incomplete, but we hope it can give a general view of the broad use of such models. We begin with examples from epidemiology, ecology and bacterial cell culture and conclude with the cell population models which arise in medical applications. This section is far from exhaustive and we refer for instance to [41] for an original modeling of the actin-cytoskeleton in symmetric lamellipodial fragments, to [42] for an application to neuroscience and to [5] for a cannibalism model (this is one of the most interesting phenomena in population studies, see [13] for an evolutionary point of view); here the authors arrive at equation (4.1) with $\psi = 1$.

Metastasis size distribution. A linear version of equation (4.1) arises in modeling oncology. In [28], the authors propose it as a dynamical model for the growth and size distribution of multiple metastatic tumors. The density $n(t,x)$ represents tumors of size x and the birth term represents metastatic tumors that grow (with an x-dependent velocity to take into account Gompertz's law).

Epidemiology. As mentioned earlier, the first age-structured model in epidemiology goes back to Kermack and McKendrick [30, 32]. It has been widely studied by many mathematicians as well as biologists (see [26, 27, 48]). Here we briefly introduce a model which describes the propagation of a virus in a population. Let $\Sigma(t)$, $n(t,x)$, $R(t)$ denote the total susceptible population, infective population and total recovered population at time t respectively, reflecting the effect of the virus. Here the age structure is incorporated into the density of infective population n and x represents the age in the disease. Let B_Σ, d_Σ denote the birth rate and mortality rate of the susceptible population, and let $B_R(x)$, d_n denote the rate of conversion of infected cells into recovered cells and the mortality rate of infected cells. It is very natural to assume that $d_n > d_\Sigma$. Another main assumption in this model is that individuals are infected from encounters between susceptibles and infected individuals with age x in the disease with the rate $\psi(x)$. Therefore the total infection rate is $S(t)$ defined by

$$S(t) = \int_0^\infty \psi(x)n(t,x)dx,$$

and thus the Kermack–Mckendrick model is defined, for $t > 0$, $x > 0$, by

$$\frac{d}{dt}\Sigma(t) = B_\Sigma - d_\Sigma\Sigma(t) - S(t)\Sigma(t),$$

$$\begin{cases} \frac{\partial}{\partial t}n(t,x) + \frac{\partial}{\partial x}n(t,x) + \left[d_n(x) + B_R(x)\right]n(t,x) = 0, \\ n(t,0) = S(t)\Sigma(t), \end{cases}$$

$$\frac{d}{dt}R(t) = \int_0^\infty B_R(x)n(t,x)dx.$$

In the book [16] one can find a recent account of the subject. At this point we note that if we make a quasistatic hypothesis on $\Sigma(t)$, we arrive at

$$0 = B_\Sigma - d_\Sigma\Sigma(t) - S(t)\Sigma(t), \qquad \Sigma(t) = \frac{B_\Sigma}{d_\Sigma + S(t)}.$$

This model falls in the class studied by Michel [35] that we recall in Sect. 4.7.

Ecology. Our next examples concern models in ecology. To begin with, we refer the reader to the book [40] which contains a full analysis of a crocodile population based on age-structured equations. Bees et al. (see [4]) studied *Deroceras reticulatum* population dynamics (this species of slug causes the majority of the damage to agricultural crops and turns out to be a pest of global economic importance. Another example of an application in ecology can be found in [20] where a similar model describes the density $n(t,x)$ of a particular tree (*Pinus cembra*) in a forest. Let $S(t)$ describe the population of a certain bird (*Nucifraga caryocatactes*) that helps disseminate the seeds. The authors arrive to a variant where the equation on $S(t)$ is

$$\frac{d}{dt}S(t) + \mu(S(t))S(t) = S(t)\int_{-\infty}^t k(t-x)P(s,t)ds,$$

where $P(s,t)$ is the total population of trees at time t which were born at time s, $s \le t$. If the time scale for bird reproduction is faster than that of *Pinus cembra* (these trees don't produce seeds for the first forty years!) then we arrive to a model as in (4.1)–(4.2), transforming this delay integral into an age-structured equation.

Cell proliferation. As mentioned earlier, modeling cell cultures by age-structured equations is an old subject, see [47, 10, 3] for instance. Gyllenberg proposed a nonlinear age-structured model for bacterial culture growth in a continuous fermentation process (see [25]). He studied the existence, uniqueness, positivity and boundedness of solutions, the existence of equilibrium solutions and the stability of equilibria of the model. In his model, the growth, death and fission rates of the cells are nonlinear functions of the substrate concentration in the reactor tank.

More general and realistic age-structured models were obtained by different authors. We recall now some of them because they use PDEs in higher dimensions. The first one was proposed by Rotenberg [45], still for cells, who introduces a maturation velocity variable $\mu \in [0,1]$. It is the ratio between biological age and physical age. Let $n(t, x, \mu)$ be the density of a population, then it satisfies

$$
\begin{cases}
\frac{\partial}{\partial t}n(t,x,\mu) + \frac{\partial}{\partial x}n(t,x,\mu) + d(x,\mu)n(t,x,\mu) = \int K(x,\mu,\mu')n(t,x,\mu')d\mu', \\
n(t,0,\mu) = \int b(x',\mu,\mu')n(t,x',\mu')d\mu'dx', \\
n(0,x,\mu) = n_0(x,\mu).
\end{cases}
$$

Here $K(x,\mu,\mu')$ is the probability of a change of maturation velocity from μ to μ'. For stability and long time asymptotics results via the GRE method and the existence of periodic solutions see [39].

Medical sciences, tumor growth. Another model proposed by Mackey and Rey [31] to study the production of red blood cells (hematopoiesis) has attracted several people. In this model the main biological assumption is that the life period of any cell is divided into quiescent and proliferating phases. The cells in the quiescent phase can't divide, but they mature and if they don't die, then they will enter the proliferating phase. There, when they don't die by apoptosis, they will divide and give birth to two daughter cells which are in the quiescent phase. Hence this age-structured model takes into account maturity m and is the following coupled system of two nonlinear equations. For $t \geq 0$, $x \geq 0$, $m \geq 0$,

$$
\begin{cases}
\frac{\partial}{\partial t}p(t,x,m) + \frac{\partial}{\partial x}p(t,x,m) + \frac{\partial}{\partial m}\big[V(m)p(t,x,m)\big] + d_1(m)p(t,x,m) = 0, \\
p(t,0,m) = b_2(m, N(t,m)), \\
N(t,m) = \int_0^\infty n(t,x,m)dx,
\end{cases}
$$

$$
\begin{cases}
\frac{\partial}{\partial t}n(t,x,m) + \frac{\partial}{\partial x}n(t,x,m) + \frac{\partial}{\partial m}\big[V(m)n\big] + \big[d_2(m) + b_2(m, N(t,m))\big]n \\
\hspace{10cm} = 0, \\
n(t,0,m) = 2\int_0^\infty b_1(x,m)p(t,x,G^{-1}(m))dx.
\end{cases}
$$

Here $p(t,x,m)$ and $n(t,x,m)$ denote the population density of proliferating cells and resting cells at time t, having age x, with maturity m, with mortality rates d_1, d_2 respectively. The cell division rate or birth rate is b_1. The main assumption in this model are that $V(0) = 0$ and $\forall m$, $\int_0^m \frac{dm'}{V(m')} = \infty$, $V(\cdot)$ is increasing. The second assumption is $G : \mathbb{R}^+ \to \mathbb{R}^+$ such that $G \in C^1(\mathbb{R}^+)$, G is increasing, $G(0) = 0$ and $G(m) < m$. Moreover $b_2(., N)$ is decreasing in N. This model is related to cancer modeling, it has nonvanishing steady states and possesses periodic solutions (which might represent a classical blood disease called chronic myeloid leukemia). Adimy and Pujo-Menjouet simplified this model by assuming that all cells in the proliferating phase divide exactly at age

τ (see [2]) and obtained existence, uniqueness results and global exponential stability. A more general case was considered by Adimy and Crauste in which cells in the proliferating phase divide at an age distributed between $\underline{\tau}$ and $\overline{\tau}$ with continuous density function $x \mapsto k(x, m)$ supported in $[\underline{\tau}, \overline{\tau}]$ (see [1]). An important observation made in [1, 2] is if the time of replication is large enough, then the destruction of a population of stem cells affects the total population to a greater extent and the total population goes extinct in finite time.

A further example in higher dimensions is a coupled nonlinear model which takes the content of cyclin/cyclin-dependent kinases (CDKs) into account. It has been studied by Perthame et al. in [6] for comparing healthy tissues and tumoral tissues. Any tissue comprises two compartments, proliferative and quiescent compartments. The first one represents a complete cell cycle with G_1, S, G_2, M phases. Cyclins/CDK complexes are the most crucial control molecules in phase transitions. Each phase has its particular cyclins/CDK. The main idea behind the modeling is that the proliferating cells grow and divide whereas quiescent cells don't undergo physiological evolution. Let $p(t, x, c)$, $q(t, x, c)$ be the densities of proliferating and quiescent cells at time t with age a and content c in cyclin/CDKs. Let $L(x, c)$, $F(x, c)$ denote the demobilization rate from proliferation to quiescence and the rate of cell division. Let d_1, d_2 be the rates of apoptosis of proliferating cells and quiescent cells respectively. Let $\Gamma_1(x, c)$ be the evolution speed of cyclin/CDKs and let $\Gamma_0 > 0$ be a constant. With this information the model reads as an age-structured model

$$
\begin{cases}
\frac{\partial}{\partial t}\, p(t, x, c) + \frac{\partial}{\partial x} p(t, x, c) + \frac{\partial}{\partial c}\big(\Gamma_1 p(t, x, c)\big) \\
\qquad\qquad - \big[L(x, c) + F(x, c) + d_1\big]\, p(t, x, c) + G(S(t))\, q(t, x, c), \\
p(t, 0, c) = \int b(x, c, c') p(t, x, c') dc', \\
\frac{\partial}{\partial t}\, q(t, x, c) = L(x, c)\, p(t, x, c) - \big[G(S(t)) + d_2\big]\, q(t, x, c)\,.
\end{cases}
$$

Here $G(S)$ is the rate at which quiescent cells reenter the proliferative phase. $S(t)$ denotes the total weighted population given by

$$
S(t) = \int_0^\infty \int_0^\infty \psi_1(x, c) p(t, x, c) + \psi_2(x, c) q(t, x, c) dx dc.
$$

Typical boundary data and appropriate initial data have been given to close the model. Finally let us mention an original model describing the ovulatory process. Clément et al. [19] have derived an age and maturity structured model, with either proliferative or differentiated phases, depending on the cell maturity level and in which cells in the differentiated phase will never reenter the proliferative phase. In [19], nonlocal nonlinearities also arise through hormone production. For instance follicule-stimulating hormone acts on follicular cells and is described by a biochemical dynamical model.

4.3 Assumptions and Eigenelements

In this section, we present our basic assumptions and definitions which will be used from now on. We always assume that the functions d, B, ψ are continuous in S, nonnegative and locally bounded. Then, we also need the assumptions

$$B(.,0) \in L^\infty(0,\infty) \cap L^1(0,\infty), \; B(x,.) \in L^\infty_{loc}(0,\infty) \text{ for all } x \geq 0, \quad (4.4)$$

$$1 < \int_0^\infty B(x,0)e^{-\int_0^x d(y,0)dy}dx < \infty, \quad (4.5)$$

$$0 < \int_0^\infty B(x,\infty)e^{-\int_0^x d(y,\infty)dy}dx < 1, \quad (4.6)$$

$$1 < \lim_{a\to\infty}\int_0^\infty B(x,\infty)e^{ax-\int_0^x d(y,\infty)dy}dx = \beta_\infty < \infty. \quad (4.7)$$

There exists $L > 0$ such that for all x, S_1, $S_2 \geq 0$ we have

$$|B(x,S_1) - B(x,S_2)| \leq L|S_1 - S_2|, \; |d(x,S_1) - d(x,S_2)| \leq L|S_1 - S_2|. \quad (4.8)$$

$$\frac{\partial d(.,.)}{\partial S} > 0, \quad (4.9)$$

$$d(.,\infty) \in L^\infty(0,\infty), \; d(x,.) \in L^\infty_{loc}(0,\infty) \text{ for all } x \geq 0, \quad (4.10)$$

$$\frac{\partial B(.,.)}{\partial S} < 0. \quad (4.11)$$

There exist two maps $\widehat{D}_0$, $\widehat{D}_\infty : \mathbb{R}^+ \to \mathbb{R}$ defined by

$$\widehat{D}_0(S) = \inf_x \left\{ (d(x,0) - d(x,S) + \frac{\phi_0(0)}{\phi_0(x)}\left(B(x,S) - B(x,0)\right) \right\}, \quad (4.12)$$

$$\widehat{D}_\infty(S) = \sup_x \left\{ (d(x,\infty) - d(x,S) + \frac{\phi_\infty(0)}{\phi_\infty(x)}\left(B(x,S) - B(x,\infty)\right) \right\}. \quad (4.13)$$

Finally for the competition weight $\psi(\cdot)$, we assume that there are two positive constants C^0_{min} and C^0_{max} such that

$$C^0_{min}\phi_0(x) \leq \psi(x) \leq C^0_{max}\phi_0(x). \quad (4.14)$$

Also there are two positive constants C^∞_{min} and C^∞_{max} such that

$$C^\infty_{min}\phi_\infty(x) \leq \psi(x) \leq C^\infty_{max}\phi_\infty(x). \quad (4.15)$$

Our last two assumptions use notation that is introduced later on. However we use it now in order to gather all the assumptions. The eigenelements $\lambda_0, \lambda_\infty, N_0, N_\infty, \phi_0, \phi_\infty$ are defined as follows.

Consider the eigenvalue problem corresponding to $S = 0$

$$\begin{cases} \frac{d}{dx}N_0(x) + (d(x,0) + \lambda_0)N_0(x) = 0, & \forall\, x \geq 0, \\ N_0(0) = \int_0^\infty B(y,0)N_0(y)dy \;=\; 1, \\ N_0(\cdot) \geq 0, \; N_0 \in L^1(\mathbb{R}^+) \cap L^\infty(\mathbb{R}^+). \end{cases} \qquad (4.16)$$

The corresponding adjoint equations for the above equations are

$$\begin{cases} -\frac{d}{dx}\phi_0(x) + (d(x,0) + \lambda_0)\phi_0(x) = \phi_0(0)B(x,0), & \forall\, x \geq 0, \\ \int_0^\infty \phi_0(x)N_0(x)dx = 1, \quad \phi_0(\cdot) \geq 0, \; \phi_0 \in L^\infty(\mathbb{R}^+). \end{cases} \qquad (4.17)$$

The eigenvalue problem corresponding to $S = \infty$ is also written as

$$\begin{cases} \frac{d}{dx}N_\infty(x) + (d(x,\infty) + \lambda_\infty)N_\infty(x) = 0, & \forall\, x \geq 0, \\ N_\infty(0) = \int_0^\infty B(y,\infty)N_\infty(y)dy \;=\; 1, \\ N_\infty(\cdot) \geq 0, \quad N_\infty \in L^\infty_{\mathrm{loc}}(\mathbb{R}^+). \end{cases} \qquad (4.18)$$

Similarly for this set of equations at $S = \infty$, we have the following adjoint equation:

$$\begin{cases} -\frac{d}{dx}\phi_\infty(x) + (d(x,\infty) + \lambda_\infty)\phi_\infty(x) = \phi_\infty(0)B(x,\infty), & \forall\, x \geq 0, \\ \int_0^\infty \phi_\infty(x)N_\infty(x)dx = 1, \quad \phi_\infty(\cdot) \geq 0, \; \phi_\infty \in L^\infty(\mathbb{R}^+). \end{cases} \qquad (4.19)$$

We conclude this section with a result concerning existence and uniqueness of solutions to eigenvalue problems, corresponding adjoint problems and signs of eigenvalues.

Theorem 1. *Under assumptions* (4.4)–(4.7), *the problems* (4.16)–(4.19) *have unique solutions, and we have the inequalities* $\lambda_0 > 0$, $\lambda_\infty < 0$. *Moreover there exists* $C > 0$, *and for all* $r > 0$ *we have*

$$N_0(x) \leq e^{-\lambda_0 x}, \; N_\infty(x) \leq e^{-\lambda_\infty x}, \; \phi_0(x) \leq C, \; \phi_\infty(x) \leq \beta_\infty \phi_\infty(0)e^{(\lambda_\infty - r)x}$$

for all $x \geq 0$.

Proof. We first consider the direct problems on N_0 and N_∞. A direct computation shows that $N_0(x)$ is given by

$$N_0(x) = e^{-\int_0^x (\lambda_0 + d(y,0))dy}.$$

Consider the map $\lambda \longmapsto \displaystyle\int_0^\infty B(x,0)e^{-\lambda x}e^{-\int_0^x d(y,0)dy}dx$ and observe that it is integrable for all $\lambda > 0$, continuous and decreasing. Moreover by (4.5)

$$\lim_{\lambda\to 0} \int_0^\infty B(x,0)e^{-\lambda x}e^{-\int_0^x d(y,0)dy}dx > 1,$$

$$\lim_{\lambda\to\infty} \int_0^\infty B(x,0)e^{-\lambda x}e^{-\int_0^x d(y,0)dy}dx = 0.$$

Therefore there exists a unique λ_0 satisfying (4.16) which is positive.

A similar argument using (4.6) and (4.7) proves that λ_∞ is negative. Next we turn to the adjoint problem. One can also compute ϕ_0 explicitly to get

$$\phi_0(x) = \frac{\phi_0(0)}{e^{-\int_0^x (\lambda_0 + d(y,0))dy}} \int_x^\infty B(y,0)e^{-\int_0^y (\lambda_0 + d(x',0))dx'}dy, \quad (4.20)$$

$$\phi_\infty(x) = \frac{\phi_\infty(0)}{e^{-\int_0^x (\lambda_\infty + d(y,\infty))dy}} \int_x^\infty B(y,\infty)e^{-\int_0^y (\lambda_\infty + d(x',\infty))dx'}dy. \quad (4.21)$$

Clearly ϕ_0, $\phi_\infty \geq 0$. Using (4.4) we have $B(.,0) \in L^1(0,\infty)$, therefore $\phi_0 \in L^\infty(0,\infty)$. Moreover we can choose $\phi_0(0)$ in order to normalize as follows:

$$\int_0^\infty N_0(x)\phi_0(x)dx = \phi_0(0)\int_0^\infty xB(x,0)e^{-\int_0^x (\lambda_0 + d(x',0))dx'}dx = 1.$$

This normalization is possible because $B(.,0) \in L^\infty(0,\infty)$ and $\lambda_0 > 0$. Now we prove a similar result on ϕ_∞. According to (11), we denote an upper bound by L', $d(x,\infty) \leq L' < \infty$. From the explicit formula (4.21) for $\phi_\infty(x)$, we get

$$\phi_\infty(x) \leq \phi_\infty(0)e^{(\lambda_\infty + L')x} \int_x^\infty B(y,\infty)e^{-\int_0^y (\lambda_\infty + d(x',\infty))dx'}dy$$

and thus

$$\phi_\infty(x) \leq \phi_\infty(0)e^{(\lambda_\infty - r)x} \int_x^\infty e^{(-\lambda_\infty + L' + r)y}B(y,\infty)e^{-\int_0^y d(x',\infty)dx'}dy.$$

Now due to (4.7), we obtain $\phi_\infty(x) \leq \beta_\infty \phi_\infty(0)e^{(\lambda_\infty - r)x}$, for any $r > 0$, with $\lambda_\infty < 0$. Again it can be normalized because N_∞ has growth as $e^{-\lambda_0 x}$. $\square$

4.4 Existence of Solutions to the Linear Problem

In this section we consider that $S(t)$ is a given locally bounded function. We recall quickly basic facts, which are used later on, about the linear renewal equation

$$\begin{cases} \frac{\partial}{\partial t}n(t,x) + \frac{\partial}{\partial x}n(t,x) + d(x,S(t))n(t,x) = 0, \quad t \geq 0, x \geq 0, \\ n(t,0) = \int_0^\infty B(x,S(t))n(t,x)dx, \\ n(0,x) = n_0(x) \in L^1_{loc}(\mathbb{R}^+). \end{cases} \quad (4.22)$$

We define the notion of weak (distributional) solutions as usual.

Definition 1. *A function $n \in L^1_{loc}(\mathbb{R}^+ \times \mathbb{R}^+)$ satisfies the renewal equation (4.22) in the weak sense if $\int_0^\infty B(t,x)|n(t,x)|dx \in L^1_{loc}(\mathbb{R}^+)$ and for all $T > 0$, for all test functions $\Psi \in C^1_{comp}\big([0,T] \times [0,\infty)\big)$ such that $\Psi(T,x) \equiv 0$, we have*

$$-\int_0^T \int_0^\infty n(t,x)\left\{\frac{\partial}{\partial t}\Psi(t,x) + \frac{\partial}{\partial x}\Psi(t,x) - d(x,S(t))\Psi(t,x)\right\}dx\ dt$$

$$= \int_0^\infty n_0(x)\Psi(0,x)dx + \int_0^T \Psi(t,0)\int_0^\infty B(x,S(t))n(t,x)dx\ dt.$$

General uniqueness results can be proved, which means that other notions of solutions are all equivalent.

Theorem 2. *Let there exist $M > 0$ such that $B(.,.), d(.,.) < M$, $S(t) \geq 0$, $S(t) \in L^\infty_{loc}(\mathbb{R}^+)$, $n_0 \in L^\infty(0,\infty) \cap L^1(0,\infty)$. Then there is a unique weak solution $n \in C(\mathbb{R}^+; L^1(\mathbb{R}^+))$ solving (4.22). Moreover $n(t,x) \geq 0$ whenever $n_0 \geq 0$, and*

$$\int_0^\infty |n(t,x)|dx \leq e^{||(B-d)_+||_\infty t}\int_0^\infty |n_0(x)|dx. \tag{4.23}$$

We refer to [43] for proofs of such results. In particular the GRE method allows for more precise results than the long time asymptotics (4.3) when $S(t) \equiv S$ is independent of time.

4.5 Nonlinear Problem, Uniform Bounds

In this section we prove existence and uniqueness along with a priori bounds on $S(t)$. First we state our main theorem.

Theorem 3. *Assume (4.4)–(4.15), $n_0 \in L^\infty(0,\infty) \cap L^1(0,\infty)$, and also assume $\int_0^\infty \phi_0(x)n_0(x)dx > 0$. Then there exists a unique weak or distributional solution $n \in C(\mathbb{R}^+; L^1(\mathbb{R}^+))$ to (4.1)–(4.2). Moreover, because $\lambda_0 > 0$, $\lambda_\infty < 0$ (see Theorem 1) there exist two positive constants m, M such that*

$$m \leq S(t) \leq M, \qquad \forall\ t > 0.$$

This theorem is a consequence of Theorem 4 and Proposition 1 below. In the hypothesis, $\int_0^\infty \phi_0(x)n_0(x)dx > 0$ is a technical one, it tells us that the initial population density should be positive on a subset having nonzero measure, of $[0,\infty)$. Under this condition the estimate we present here tells us that the weighted population continues forever and it neither blows up, nor goes extinct even at infinite time. Hence these bounds open the question of long time behavior which is treated later.

Before proving the main theorem we give a statement with a stronger hypothesis on B, d.

Theorem 4. *Let us assume (4.8), and there exists $M > 0$ such that $B(.,.)$, $d(.,.)$, $\psi(\cdot) < M$ and $n_0 \in L^\infty(0,\infty) \cap L^1(0,\infty)$. Then there exists a unique weak solution $n \in C(\mathbb{R}^+; L^1(\mathbb{R}^+))$ to (4.1)–(4.2).*

Proof. We prove this result by the Banach fixed point theorem. First, we set $X = C([0, T])$ with the sup norm, later we choose T (very small). Let X_+ be the set of all nonnegative continuous functions on $[0, T]$ and define $\Lambda = ||(B - d)_+||_\infty$. For $S(t) \in C([0, T])$, due to Theorem 2, we have $n(t, x) \in C\big([0, T]; L^1(\mathbb{R}^+)\big)$ solving

$$\begin{cases} \frac{\partial}{\partial t}n(t, x) + \frac{\partial}{\partial x}n(t, x) + d(x, S(t))n(t, x) = 0, \quad t \in [0, T], \ x \geq 0, \\ n(t, 0) = \int_0^\infty B(x, S(t))n(t, x)dx, \\ n(0, x) = n_0(x) \geq 0. \end{cases} \tag{4.24}$$

Now define a map $\mathrm{T} : X_+ \to X_+$ by

$$S(t) \longmapsto \int_0^\infty \psi(x)n(t, x)dx. \tag{4.25}$$

To prove Theorem 4, it is enough to prove T is a contraction map.

Let $n_1(t, x)$, $n_2(t, x)$ be the solutions of (4.24) corresponding to $S_1(t)$, $S_2(t)$, then $n := n_1 - n_2$ satisfies

$$\begin{cases} \frac{\partial}{\partial t}n(t, x) + \frac{\partial}{\partial x}n(t, x) + d(x, S_1(t))n(t, x) + \big[d(x, S_1) - d(x, S_2)\big]n_2 = 0, \\ \qquad t \in [0, T], \ x \geq 0, \\ n(t, 0) = \int_0^\infty B(x, S_1(t))n(t, x) + \big[B(x, S_1) - B(x, S_2)\big]n_2 \ dx, \\ n(0, x) \equiv 0. \end{cases}$$

Now $|n(t, x)|$ satisfies

$$\begin{cases} \frac{\partial}{\partial t}|n| + \frac{\partial}{\partial x}|n| + d(x, S_1(t))|n| \leq |d(x, S_1(t)) - d(x, S_2(t))|n_2, \\ \qquad t \in [0, T], \ x \geq 0, \\ |n(t, 0)| \leq \int_0^\infty \big(B(x, S_1(t))n(t, x) + |B(x, S_1(t)) - B(x, S_2(t))|n_2\big)dx, \\ |n(0, x)| \equiv 0. \end{cases}$$

$$\tag{4.26}$$

Therefore by integration in age, we have

$$\frac{d}{dt}\int_0^\infty |n(t, x)|dx = \int_0^\infty \frac{\partial}{\partial t}|n| \ dx$$

$$\leq \int_0^\infty -\frac{\partial}{\partial x}|n| - d(x, S_1(t))|n| + |d(x, S_1(t)) - d(x, S_2(t))|n_2 \ dx$$

$$\leq |n(t, 0)| - \int_0^\infty d(x, S_1(t))|n| \ dx + L|S_1(t) - S_2(t)|\int_0^\infty n_2(t, x) \ dx$$

$$\leq \int_0^\infty \big(B(x, S_1(t))n(t, x) + |B(x, S_1(t)) - B(x, S_2(t))|\big)n_2 \, dx$$

$$- \int_0^\infty d(x, S_1(t))|n|dx + L|S_1(t) - S_2(t)| \int_0^\infty n_2(t, x) \, dx.$$

$$\leq \Lambda \int_0^\infty |n(t, x)| \, dx + 2L|S_1(t) - S_2(t)| \int_0^\infty n_2(t, x)dx$$

$$\leq \Lambda \int_0^\infty |n(t, x)|dx + 2L\Big(\sup_{0 \leq t \leq T} |S_1(t) - S_2(t)|\Big)|n_0|_{L^1}e^{\Lambda t}.$$

Gronwall's lemma gives

$$\int_0^\infty |n(t, x)|dx \leq 2Lt|n_0|_{L^1}e^{2\Lambda t}\Big(\sup_{0 \leq t \leq T} |S_1(t) - S_2(t)|\Big),$$

and thus

$$\sup_{0 \leq t \leq T} \int_0^\infty |n(t, x)|dx \leq 2LT|n_0|_{L^1}e^{2\Lambda T}\Big(\sup_{0 \leq t \leq T} |S_1(t) - S_2(t)|\Big). \qquad (4.27)$$

From this we deduce that

$$\sup_{0 \leq t \leq T} |TS_1 - TS_2| = \sup_{0 \leq t \leq T} \Big| \int_0^\infty \psi(x)(n_1(t, x) - n_2(t, x))dx\Big|$$

$$\leq M \sup_{0 \leq t \leq T} \int_0^\infty |n(t, x)|dx$$

$$\leq 2MLT|n_0|_{L^1}e^{2\Lambda T}\Big(\sup_{0 \leq t \leq T} |S_1(t) - S_2(t)|\Big).$$

Now we choose T small enough such that T becomes a contraction map. Hence we proved the existence and uniqueness of solutions of (4.1)–(4.2). $\qquad \square$

Proposition 1. *Under assumptions (4.4)–(4.7), (4.9)–(4.15) and $\int_0^\infty \phi_0(x)$ $n_0(x) > 0$ there exists $m, M > 0$ for $S(t)$ which is an unknown in the coupled system (4.1)–(4.2) such that $m \leq S(t) \leq M \quad \forall t > 0$.*

Proof. To prove this proposition we use a technique developed by Carrillo et al. in [9] based on an adjoint problem. First we treat the lower bound. We define an auxiliary function

$$S_0(t) = \int_0^\infty \phi_0(x)n(t, x)dx. \qquad (4.28)$$

A duality computation (related to the GRE method) using (4.1), (4.17) leads to

$$\frac{d}{dt}S_0(t) = \lambda_0 S_0(t) + \int_0^\infty \Big(d(x,0) - d(x,S(t))\Big)\phi_0(x)n(t,x)\ dx$$

$$+ \int_0^\infty \phi_0(0)[B(x,S(t)) - B(x,0)]n(t,x)dx.$$

$$\geq \lambda_0 S_0(t) + \widehat{D}_0(S(t))S_0(t)$$

$$\geq \lambda_0 S_0(t) + \widehat{D}_0(C_{\max}^0 S_0(t))S_0(t). \tag{4.29}$$

The last inequality holds because $\widehat{D}_0$ is decreasing with $\widehat{D}_0(0) = 0$. As long as $C_{\max}^0 S_0(t)$ is smaller than $\widehat{D}_0^{-1}(-\lambda_0)$, S_0 is increasing. Therefore we obtain

$$S_0(x) \geq \min\Big\{S_0(0), \frac{\widehat{D}_0^{-1}(-\lambda_0)}{C_{\max}^0}\Big\}, \quad \forall t \geq 0.$$

Finally we exploit the assumption (4.14) to get

$$S(x) \geq m := \min\Big\{C_{\min}^0 S_0(0), \frac{C_{\min}^0}{C_{\max}^0}\widehat{D}_0^{-1}(-\lambda_0)\Big\}, \quad \forall t \geq 0.$$

To prove the other inequality we use the same technique by defining another auxiliary function

$$S_\infty(t) = \int_0^\infty \phi_\infty(x)n(t,x)dx. \tag{4.30}$$

We follow the same methodology to get an upper bound for $S(\cdot)$. A particular choice of M we get after repeating a similar exercise is given by

$$M = \max\Big\{C_{\max}^\infty S_\infty(0), \frac{C_{\max}^\infty}{C_{\min}^\infty}\widehat{D}_\infty^{-1}(-\lambda_\infty)\Big\}.\ \square$$

4.6 A Case with Asymptotic Decoupling

For this section, we consider particular variants of the above birth and death rates. In this case we reduce the renewal equation to a single ODE where we can easily conclude about the convergence of the solution to the steady state. It occurs when

$$d(x,S) = d_1(x) + d_2(S), \qquad d_1(x) \geq 0, \tag{4.31}$$

$$B(x,S) \equiv B(x) \geq 0, \tag{4.32}$$

$$\int_0^\infty B(x)e^{-D(x)} = 1, \qquad D(x) = \int_0^x d_1(x)dx. \tag{4.33}$$

Here, the mortality rate d is the sum of the mortality rate due to inherent species aging $d_1(x) \geq 0$ and fluctuations (extra birth or death) d_2. In particular d_2 has no sign but it is natural to keep $d_1(x) + d_2(S)$ nonnegative.

Our method relies on the study of the following linearized state given by

$$\begin{cases} \frac{d}{dx}\tilde{N}(x) + d_1(x)\tilde{N}(x) = 0, \ x > 0, \\ \tilde{N}(0) = \int_0^\infty B(x)\tilde{N}(x)dx = 1. \end{cases} \tag{4.34}$$

In other words $\tilde{N} = e^{-D(x)}$. As usual we introduce the adjoint problem for (4.34)

$$\begin{cases} -\frac{d}{dx}\tilde{\phi}(x) + d_1(x)\tilde{\phi}(x) = \tilde{\phi}(0)B(x), \ x > 0, \\ \int_0^\infty \tilde{\phi}(x)\tilde{N}(x)dx = 1. \end{cases} \tag{4.35}$$

4.6.1 A Particular Solution

Before going to the main convergence result which we prove in the next subsection we prove the following.

Proposition 2. *With assumptions* (4.32)–(4.33), *the system* (4.1)–(4.2) *admits the particular solution* $n(t,x) = \tilde{n}(t)\tilde{N}$ *with* $\tilde{n}(t)$ *given by the differential equation*

$$\tilde{n}(t) + d_2(k\tilde{n}(t))\tilde{n}(t) = 0, \tag{4.36}$$

with

$$k = \int_0^\infty \psi(x)\tilde{N}(x)dx. \tag{4.37}$$

Therefore the nonlinear problem admits this particular family of solutions to (4.36) (parametrized by the initial value $\tilde{n}(0)$) which can be solved by standard ODE methods.

In particular from this example we can gain insight into the long time asymptotics of the solution. The conditions $\lambda_0 > 0$, $\lambda_\infty < 0$ here mean $d_2(0) < 0$, $d_2(\infty) > 0$. Assuming also $d_2'(\cdot) > 0$ as usual we see that $\tilde{n}(t) \longrightarrow \bar{n} > 0$ as $t \longrightarrow \infty$ with $\bar{n}$ the unique solution to $d_2(k\bar{n}) = 0$.

4.6.2 Long Time Decoupling

Now let us turn our attention towards a long time asymptotics result for the general solutions to the nonlinear system (4.1)–(4.2). We prove exponential convergence to the solution obtained by the separation of variables method. We use L^1 convergence with a proper weight function which will be introduced later.

This can be done introducing $\tilde{n}(t) = \int_0^\infty n(t,x)\tilde{\phi}(x)$, which satisfies (we leave the calculation to the reader)

$$\frac{d}{dt}\tilde{n}(t) + \tilde{n}(t)d_2(S(t)) = 0. \tag{4.38}$$

In this subsection we explain why these solutions obtained previously attract all other trajectories. Here we adapt a classical argument for parabolic systems, which can be found for instance in [29]. Namely, we prove the long time asymptotics result for this model.

Theorem 5. *Under the assumptions* (4.31)–(4.33) *and if there exists* $\mu \geq 0$, $\delta > 0$ *such that* $B(x) \geq \mu\tilde{\phi}(x)$, $\mu + d_2(S(t)) \geq \delta$, *then the solution of age-structured equations* (4.1)–(4.2) *satisfies*

$$\int_0^\infty |n(t,x) - \tilde{n}(t)\tilde{N}(x)|\tilde{\phi}(x)dx \leq e^{-\delta t}\int_0^\infty |n_0(x) - \tilde{n}(0)N(x)|\tilde{\phi}(x)dx$$

with $\tilde{n}(t) = \int_0^\infty n(t,x)\tilde{\phi}(x)$.

Proof. We prove this convergence result with the help of a combination of a perturbation argument and the duality method. One can easily compute

$$\frac{\partial}{\partial t}\tilde{n}(t)\tilde{N}(x) + \frac{\partial}{\partial x}\tilde{n}(t)\tilde{N}(x) + \big(d_1(x) + d_2(S(t))\big)\tilde{n}(t)\tilde{N}(x) = 0.$$

We subtract this expression from (4.1) to get

$$\begin{cases} \frac{\partial}{\partial t}(n - \tilde{n}\tilde{N}) + \frac{\partial}{\partial x}(n - \tilde{n}\tilde{N}) + \big(d_1(x) + d_2(S(t))\big)(n - \tilde{n}\tilde{N}) = 0, \\ (n - \tilde{n}\tilde{N})(t,0) = \int_0^\infty B(x)(n - \tilde{n}\tilde{N})dx. \end{cases}$$

Let us denote $h(t,x) = n(t,x) - \tilde{n}(t)\tilde{N}(x)$. With this notation we have by construction

$$\int_0^\infty h(t,x)\tilde{\phi}(x)dx = 0, \tag{4.39}$$

further

$$\begin{cases} \frac{\partial}{\partial t}|h(t,x)| + \frac{\partial}{\partial x}|h(t,x)| + \big(d_1(x) + d_2(S(t))\big)|h(t,x)| = 0, \\ |h(t,0)| = |\int_0^\infty B(x)h(t,x)dx|. \end{cases}$$

We integrate with respect to $\tilde{\phi}dx$ and use (4.39) to arrive at

$$\begin{aligned} 0 &= \frac{d}{dt}\int_0^\infty |h(t,x)|\tilde{\phi}dx - \tilde{\phi}(0)\Big|\int_0^\infty B(x)h(t,x)dx\Big| \\ &\quad + \int_0^\infty \tilde{\phi}(0)B(x)|h(t,x)|dx + d_2(S(t))\int_0^\infty |h(t,x)|\tilde{\phi}dx, \\ &= \frac{d}{dt}\int_0^\infty |h(t,x)|\tilde{\phi}dx - \tilde{\phi}(0)\Big|\int_0^\infty \big(B(x) - \mu\tilde{\phi}(x)\big)h(t,x)dx\Big| \\ &\quad + \int_0^\infty \tilde{\phi}(0)B(x)|h(t,x)|dx + d_2(S(t))\int_0^\infty |h(t,x)|\tilde{\phi}dx, \\ &= \frac{d}{dt}\int_0^\infty |h(t,x)|\tilde{\phi}dx + \big(\mu + d_2(S(t))\big)\int_0^\infty |h(t,x)|\tilde{\phi}dx\,. \end{aligned}$$

From hypothesis we have $\mu + d(S(t)) \geq \delta$, therefore

$$\frac{d}{dt} \int_0^\infty |n - \tilde{n}\tilde{N}|\tilde{\phi}dx + \delta \int_0^\infty |n - \tilde{n}\tilde{N}|\tilde{\phi}dx \leq 0.$$

From this the announced result follows. □

4.7 A Concave Nonlinearity on the Birth Term

Here we recall the result of Michel [35] based on ideas from the GRE method. He considers a particular nonlinearity in the age-structured equation which still contains several interesting applications, and in particular the Kermack–McKendrick model of epidemiology (see Sect. 4.2) in the quasi static case

$$0 = B_\Sigma - d_\Sigma \Sigma(t) - S(t)\Sigma(t).$$

His result describes the long time asymptotics of solutions: the nontrivial steady state is globally attractive.

The problem is given by

$$\begin{cases} \frac{\partial}{\partial t}n(t,x) + \frac{\partial}{\partial x}n(t,x) + d(x)n(t,x) = 0, \ t \geq 0, \ x \geq 0, \\ n(t,0) = g\left(\int_0^\infty B(x)n(t,x)dx\right), \\ n(0,x) = n_0(x) \geq 0. \end{cases} \tag{4.40}$$

Here and as usual, d and B are nonnegative functions and $g(\cdot)$ is a continuous and nonlinear function that satisfies assumptions which are described later on. Now our goal is to obtain that the solution to (4.1)–(4.2) converges to the nonzero steady state.

Changing the notation for $g(\cdot)$ by $g(r\cdot)$ and B in rB if necessary, we may assume

$$\int_0^\infty B(x)e^{-D(x)}dx = 1, \quad \text{with} \quad D(x) = \int_0^x d(y)dy.$$

Moreover let us make the following assumption on the nonlinearity g (which is more general but contains increasing and concave functions)

$$\begin{cases} \exists \ N_0 > 0, \quad g(N_0) = x_0, \\ x < g(x) < N_0, \quad \text{for } x < N_0, \\ x_0 < g(x) < x, \quad \text{for } N_0 < x. \end{cases} \tag{4.41}$$

With this hypothesis it is clear that the corresponding steady state problem

$$\begin{cases} \frac{d}{dx}N(x) + d(x)N(x) = 0, \ x \geq 0, \\ N(0) = g\left(\int_0^\infty B(x)N(x)dx\right), \end{cases} \tag{4.42}$$

admits the unique solution $N(x) = N_0 e^{-D(x)}$. As an immediate consequence we obtain that

$$g\left(\int_0^\infty B(x)N(x)dx\right) = N_0 = \int_0^\infty B(x)N(x)dx.$$

Once interpreted in this way, the corresponding adjoint problem is given by

$$\begin{cases} -\frac{d}{dx}\phi(x) + d(x)\phi(x) = \phi(0)B(x), & x \geq 0, \\ \int_0^\infty \phi(x)N(x)dx = 1, & \phi(\cdot) \geq 0. \end{cases} \quad (4.43)$$

We are now able to state the nonlinear stability result of [35].

Theorem 6. *Under the assumption* (4.41), *as* $t \to \infty$, *any solution* $n(t, x)$ *to* (4.40), *with nonzero initial data, converges to the solution* $N(x)$ *to* (4.42), *i.e.,*

$$\int_0^\infty |n(t, x) - N(x)|\phi(x)dx \longrightarrow 0 \quad \text{as} \quad t \longrightarrow \infty.$$

Proof. As we did in previous sections we try to get a contraction inequality and write

$$\frac{\partial}{\partial t}[n(t, x) - N(x)]_+ + \frac{\partial}{\partial x}[n(t, x) - N(x)]_+ + d(x)[n(t, x) - N(x)]_+ = 0,$$

$$[n(t, 0) - N(0)]_+ = \left[g\left(\int_0^\infty B(x)n(t, x)dx\right) - g\left(\int_0^\infty B(x)N(x)dx\right)\right]_+.$$

After integrating with respect to $\phi(x)dx$ we obtain

$$\frac{d}{dt}\int_0^\infty [n(t, x) - N(x)]_+ \phi dx$$

$$= -\int_0^\infty \left(\frac{\partial}{\partial x}[n(t, x) - N(x)]_+ \phi(x) - d(x)[n(t, x) - N(x)]_+ \phi\right)dx$$

$$= \phi(0)\left[g\left(\int_0^\infty B(x)n(t, x)dx\right) - g\left(\int_0^\infty B(x)N(x)dx\right)\right]_+$$

$$+ \int_0^\infty (\frac{d}{dx}\phi(x) - d(x))[n(t, x) - N(x)]_+ dx$$

$$= \phi(0)\left[g\left(\int_0^\infty B(x)n(t, x)dx\right) - g\left(\int_0^\infty B(x)N(x)dx\right)\right]_+$$

$$- \int_0^\infty \phi(0)B(x)[n(t, x) - N(x)]_+ dx.$$

Let us consider the times t where $\int_0^\infty B(x)n(t, x)dx \geq \int_0^\infty B(x)N(x)dx$; then from (4.41) we notice that

$$g\left(\int_0^\infty Bndx\right) - g\left(\int_0^\infty BNdx\right) \leq \int_0^\infty Bndx - \int_0^\infty BNdx \leq \int_0^\infty B[n - N]_+ dx.$$

Therefore

$$\left[g\left(\int_0^\infty Bn dx \right) - g\left(\int_0^\infty BN dx \right) \right]_+ \leq \int_0^\infty B[n - N]_+ dx.$$

For the other values of t, i.e., $\int_0^\infty B(x)n(t,x)dx \leq \int_0^\infty B(x)N(x)dx$, the above inequality is straightforward and hence we have obtained

$$\frac{d}{dt} \int_0^\infty [n(t,x) - N(x)]_+ \phi dx \leq 0.$$

Using similar arguments we get

$$\frac{d}{dt} \int_0^\infty [n(t,x) - N(x)]_- \phi dx \leq 0.$$

Finally we get

$$\frac{d}{dt} \int_0^\infty |n(t,x) - N(x)| \phi dx \leq 0. \qquad (4.44)$$

Using a standard compactness argument (for instance see [36], [39], [43]) we obtain the convergence of the solution to (4.40) towards the steady state $N(x)$. □

To conclude this section, we point out that the assumption (4.41) is nearly optimal for the above stated stability result. In [35], the reader may find many extensions, more precise results and counterexamples.

4.8 Stability for Nonlinearities Reducing to ODE Systems

In general, the problem of long time asymptotics for system (4.1)–(4.2) is not completely solved. Any approach takes advantage of inbuilt special properties of the system and proceeds by giving sufficient conditions to conclude the long time behavior. One of the well-known techniques to deal with such problems is to reduce the original equation or system to a system of ODEs. For instance Iannelli [27] reduced both linear and nonlinear renewal equations having a particular structure. In the nonlinear case he studied local behavior around the nonzero steady state. In this section first we discuss a case in which we can get nonlinear stability and the solution of (4.1)–(4.2) converges to the nonzero steady state. Finally we give some examples in which we reduce (4.1)–(4.2) to a 2×2 system of ODEs. We pay special attention to this problem because it serves as a simplified background before studying the more general problem.

4.8.1 Reduction to a System of ODEs (Example 1)

A classical case that can be reduced to a differential system has been studied by Iannelli (see [23, 27]). Here in Example 1, we slightly modify that case to study its linear and nonlinear stability. We have for some $\alpha > 0$,

$$B(x, S) = b_1(S)e^{-\alpha x} + b_2(S) \tag{4.45}$$

with

$$b_i > 0, \quad \frac{db_i}{dS}(\cdot) < 0 \text{ for } i = 1, 2. \tag{4.46}$$

Also we assume that the death rate is independent of age

$$d(x, S) = d(S), \quad \frac{d}{dS}d(\cdot) > 0. \tag{4.47}$$

Then we define two quantities

$$S(t) = \int_0^\infty n(t, x)dx, \qquad Q(t) = \int_0^\infty e^{-\alpha x}n(t, x)dx, \tag{4.48}$$

which means that the competition weight is assumed to be constant

$$\psi \equiv 1. \tag{4.49}$$

Now (4.1) becomes

$$\begin{cases} \frac{\partial}{\partial t}n(t, x) + \frac{\partial}{\partial x}n(t, x) + d(S(t))n(t, x) = 0, \ t \geq 0, \ x \geq 0, \\ n(t, 0) = b_1(S(t))Q(t) + b_2(S(t))S(t), \\ n(0, x) = n_0(x) \geq 0. \end{cases} \tag{4.50}$$

Integrating (4.50) with respect to dx and $e^{-\alpha x}dx$, we obtain the system on $S(\cdot)$ and $Q(\cdot)$

$$\begin{cases} \frac{dS}{dt}(t) = [b_2(S(t)) - d(S(t))]S(t) + b_1(S(t))Q(t), \\ \frac{dQ}{dt}(t) = b_2(S(t))S(t) + [b_1(S(t)) - d(S(t)) - \alpha]Q(t), \\ 0 < Q(0) < S(0). \end{cases} \tag{4.51}$$

Remark 1. With this notation if $\alpha = 0$, then (4.1)–(4.2) reduces to $S = Q$ and

$$\frac{dS}{dt}(t) = [b(S(t)) - d(S(t))]S(t), \qquad b = b_1 + b_2.$$

If $d(S) - b(S)$ is independent of the total population, i.e. S, then we get the classical Malthusian equation with parameter $d - b$. If $d(S) - b(S) = k_1 - k_2 S$

for constants k_1, $k_2 > 0$, then our model (4.1)–(4.2) turns out to be another classical model of Verhulst with intrinsic growth constant k_1 and carrying capacity $\frac{k_1}{k_2}$ (see Sect. 4.1). In general from (4.46), (4.47) one can see that $S(t) \longrightarrow \bar{S}$ as $t \longrightarrow \infty$, with $\bar{S}$ being the unique solution of $b(\bar{S}) = d(\bar{S})$ if it exists, moreover $n(t,x) \longrightarrow b(\bar{S})\bar{S}e^{-d(\bar{S})x}$ as $t \longrightarrow \infty$. Even though the system (4.1)–(4.2) is reduced to a single equation we note that it is still more elaborate than the example of Sect. 4.6.1.

In order to prove that $S(t)$ and $Q(t)$ are comparable, we have the following.

Lemma 1. *If $S(t), Q(t)$ are solutions of (4.51) then there exists $\rho > 0$ depending on $(S(0), Q(0))$, such that $\rho S(t) < Q(t) < S(t)$.*

Proof. One can easily compute

$$\frac{d}{dt}\left(\frac{Q(t)}{S(t)}\right) = \left(b_2(S) + b_1(S)\frac{Q}{S}\right)\left(1 - \frac{Q}{S}\right) - \alpha\frac{Q}{S}. \qquad (4.52)$$

As $b_2(0) > 0$, for fixed initial data $(S(0), Q(0))$, from (4.52) it follows that the quantity $\dfrac{Q(t)}{S(t)}$ cannot be arbitrarily close to zero. This implies that there exists ρ such that $\rho S(t) < Q(t)$. In (4.52) we observe that as soon as $\frac{Q(t)}{S(t)} > 1$, the quantity $\frac{Q(t)}{S(t)}$ starts decreasing and since the initial data satisfies $0 < Q(0) < S(0)$, then $Q(t) < S(t)$. This proves our assertion. $\square$

Now we study the long time behavior of the nonzero steady state of (4.51).

Lemma 2. *Assume, similar to the conditions $\lambda_0 > 0$, $\lambda_\infty < 0$ (see Theorem 1), that*

$$\frac{b_2(0)}{d(0)} + \frac{b_1(0)}{d(0) + \alpha} > 1, \qquad \frac{b_2(\infty)}{d(\infty)} + \frac{b_1(\infty)}{d(\infty) + \alpha} < 1. \qquad (4.53)$$

Then there exists a unique positive steady state $(\bar{S}, \bar{Q})$.

Proof. It is enough to prove that there exists $(\bar{S}, \bar{Q}) \neq (0,0)$ which solves

$$\begin{cases} (b_2(\bar{S}) - d(\bar{S}))\bar{S} + b_1(\bar{S})\bar{Q} = 0, \\ b_2(\bar{S})\bar{S} + [b_1(\bar{S}) - d(\bar{S}) - \alpha]\bar{Q} = 0, \end{cases}$$

and thus

$$\begin{cases} \bar{Q} = \dfrac{d(\bar{S}) - b_2(\bar{S})}{b_1(\bar{S})}\bar{S}, \\ b_1(\bar{S})b_2(\bar{S}) = (b_2(\bar{S}) - d(\bar{S}))(b_1(\bar{S}) - d(\bar{S}) - \alpha). \end{cases}$$

We finally reduce these equations to

$$\begin{cases} \bar{Q} = \dfrac{d(\bar{S}) - b_2(\bar{S})}{b_1(\bar{S})} \bar{S}, \\[3mm] \dfrac{b_2(\bar{S})}{d(\bar{S})} + \dfrac{b_1(\bar{S})}{d(\bar{S}) + \alpha} = 1. \end{cases} \tag{4.54}$$

First we show that there exists a unique positive solution to the second equation in (4.54). Now consider $F : \mathbb{R}^+ \to \mathbb{R}^+$ defined by

$$F(S) = \frac{b_2(S)}{d(S)} + \frac{b_1(S)}{d(S) + \alpha}. \tag{4.55}$$

Observe that F is a decreasing function. By (4.53) there exists a unique $\bar{S} > 0$ satisfying the second equation of (4.54). Again from the second equation of (4.54) we have $b_2(\bar{S}) < d(\bar{S})$; this assures $\bar{Q} > 0$.   □

4.8.2 Stability of the Linearized System (Example 1)

By a first order Taylor's expansion around $(\bar{S}, \bar{Q})$ we get the linearized system associated with (4.51). The Jacobian matrix for that system is given by

$$J = \begin{pmatrix} b_2 - d + b_2' \bar{S} - d' \bar{S} + b_1' \bar{Q} & b_1 \\ b_2 + b_2' \bar{S} + b_1' \bar{Q} - d' \bar{Q} & b_1 - d - \alpha \end{pmatrix}_{\text{at } S = \bar{S}}. \tag{4.56}$$

We compute

$$\text{Tr}(J) = b_1(\bar{S}) + b_2(\bar{S}) - 2d(\bar{S}) - \alpha + (b_2'(\bar{S}) - d'(\bar{S}))\bar{S} + b_1'(\bar{S})\bar{Q}.$$

From (4.54) we have

$$b_2(\bar{S}) < d(\bar{S}), \quad b_1(\bar{S}) < d(\bar{S}) + \alpha. \tag{4.57}$$

Combining this with (4.46),(4.47) we conclude that

$$\text{Tr}(J) < 0. \tag{4.58}$$

On the other hand we can compute

$$\text{Det}(J) = \big(b_2(\bar{S}) - d(\bar{S})\big)\big(b_1(\bar{S}) - d(\bar{S}) - \alpha\big) - b_1(\bar{S})b_2(\bar{S})$$
$$+ \big(b_2'(\bar{S})\bar{S} - d'(\bar{S})\bar{S} + b_1'(\bar{S})\bar{Q}\big)\big(b_1(\bar{S}) - d(\bar{S}) - \alpha\big)$$
$$- b_1(\bar{S})\big(b_2'(\bar{S})\bar{S} + b_1'(\bar{S})\bar{Q} - d'(\bar{S})\bar{Q}\big).$$

From (4.54) we can reduce this expression to

$$\text{Det}(J) = 0 + \big(b_2'(\bar{S})\bar{S} - d'(\bar{S})\bar{S} + b_1'(\bar{S})\bar{Q}\big)\big(b_1(\bar{S}) - d(\bar{S}) - \alpha\big)$$
$$- b_1(\bar{S})\big(b_2'(\bar{S})\bar{S} + b_1'(\bar{S})\bar{Q} - d'(\bar{S})\bar{Q}\big).$$

By (4.46), (4.47) and (4.57) we have

$$\text{Det}(J) > 0. \tag{4.59}$$

Therefore both eigenvalues of the linearized version of (4.51) have negative real parts. Hence (4.51) is linearly stable around the steady state $(\bar{S}, \bar{Q})$.

4.8.3 Nonlinear Stability (Example 1)

We recall the definition of steady state in (4.54) and assume

$$\theta := \frac{b_2(\bar{S})}{d(\bar{S})} > \frac{b_1(\bar{S})}{d(\bar{S}) + \alpha} := 1 - \theta. \tag{4.60}$$

Theorem 7. *Under the assumptions* (4.46)–(4.48), (4.53), (4.60), *the steady state* $(\bar{S}, \bar{Q})$ *is globally and exponentially attractive for the system* (4.51).

Our proof is based on a Lyapunov function for the system which shows a contraction inequality. We do not have a global Lyapunov function in the case when the opposite inequality in (4.60), however the numerical results in Sect. 4.8.7 seem to indicate that global exponential stability can hold true in general.

Proof. First let us fix initial point $(S(0), Q(0))$. As a first step, from (4.51) we compute

$$\frac{d}{dt}(S - \bar{S}) + d(\bar{S})(S - \bar{S}) + (d(S) - d(\bar{S}))S = b_2(\bar{S})(S - \bar{S})$$
$$+ (b_2(S) - b_2(\bar{S}))S + b_1(\bar{S})(Q - \bar{Q}) + (b_1(S) - b_1(\bar{S}))Q,$$

$$\frac{d}{dt}(Q - \bar{Q}) + (d(\bar{S}) + \alpha)(Q - \bar{Q}) + (d(S) - d(\bar{S}))Q = b_2(\bar{S})(S - \bar{S})$$
$$+ (b_2(S) - b_2(\bar{S}))S + b_1(\bar{S})(Q - \bar{Q}) + (b_1(S) - b_1(\bar{S}))Q.$$

This gives

$$\frac{d}{dt}|S - \bar{S}| + d(\bar{S})|S - \bar{S}| + |d(S) - d(\bar{S})|S = b_2(\bar{S})|S - \bar{S}|$$
$$- |b_2(S) - b_2(\bar{S})|S + b_1(\bar{S})(Q - \bar{Q})\mathrm{sgn}(S - \bar{S})$$
$$- |b_1(S) - b_1(\bar{S})|Q,$$

$$\frac{d}{dt}|Q - \bar{Q}| + (d(\bar{S}) + \alpha)|Q - \bar{Q}| + (d(S) - d(\bar{S}))Q\mathrm{sgn}(Q - \bar{Q})$$
$$= b_2(\bar{S})(S - \bar{S})\mathrm{sgn}(Q - \bar{Q}) + (b_2(S) - b_2(\bar{S}))S\mathrm{sgn}(Q - \bar{Q})$$
$$+ b_1(\bar{S})|Q - \bar{Q}| + (b_1(S) - b_1(\bar{S}))Q\mathrm{sgn}(Q - \bar{Q}).$$

At this stage we have two possibilities, either $\mathrm{sgn}(S - \bar{S}) = \mathrm{sgn}(Q - \bar{Q})$ or $\mathrm{sgn}(S - \bar{S}) \neq \mathrm{sgn}(Q - \bar{Q})$. In both cases by (4.54), (4.64) we have

$$\frac{d}{dt}\left(\tilde{\theta}|S - \bar{S}| + (1 - \theta)|Q - \bar{Q}|\right) < 0. \tag{4.61}$$

Therefore

$$\left(\tilde{\theta}|S(t) - \bar{S}| + (1 - \theta)|Q(t) - \bar{Q}|\right) \searrow L \geq 0 \text{ as } t \longrightarrow \infty. \tag{4.62}$$

As a second step we notice that for fixed initial data $(S(0), Q(0))$, the curve $(S(t), Q(t))$ cannot come arbitrarily close to zero. Indeed (4.61), together with Lemma 1, implies that $S(t)$, $Q(t)$ increase if they are close enough to zero. Hence we get

$$S(t), Q(t) \geq \Sigma_{\min} > 0.$$

In the third step we prove exponential convergence. We notice that the solutions are bounded due to (4.62) and thus there is a γ depending on $(S(0), Q(0))$ such that

$$|d(S) - d(\bar{S})| + |b_2(S) - b_2(\bar{S})| \geq \gamma|S - \bar{S}|. \tag{4.63}$$

Now we choose $\tilde{\theta}$ such that

$$1 - \theta < \tilde{\theta} < \theta, \qquad \theta(1 - \theta) < \left(1 - \theta + \frac{\gamma \Sigma_{\min}}{d(\bar{S})}\right)\tilde{\theta}. \tag{4.64}$$

Finally we compute to obtain

$$\frac{d}{dt}\left(\tilde{\theta}|S(t) - \bar{S}| + (1 - \theta)|Q(t) - \bar{Q}|\right) < -c\left(\tilde{\theta}|S(t) - \bar{S}| + (1 - \theta)|Q(t) - \bar{Q}|\right),$$

where

$$c = \min\left\{(d(\bar{S}) + \alpha)(\theta - \tilde{\theta}), \frac{d(\bar{S})}{\tilde{\theta}}\left(\left(1 - \theta + \frac{\gamma \Sigma_{\min}}{d(\bar{S})}\right)\tilde{\theta} - \theta(1 - \theta)\right), (1 - \theta)d(\bar{S})\right\}.$$

Finally we get the exponential convergence

$$\left(\tilde{\theta}|S(t) - \bar{S}| + (1 - \theta)|Q(t) - \bar{Q}|\right) < -c\left(\tilde{\theta}|S(0) - \bar{S}| + (1 - \theta)|Q(0) - \bar{Q}|\right)e^{-ct}. \tag{4.65}$$

Hence we proved the announced result. $\square$

4.8.4 Nonlinear Stability (Example 2)

With the notation (S, Q) used in the last example, we now consider another case in which we can reduce the equation (4.1) to a 2×2 system. This is when

$$B(x, t) = b_1\left(\frac{Q(t)}{S(t)}\right)e^{-\alpha x} + b_2\left(\frac{Q(t)}{S(t)}\right), \qquad \alpha > 0, \tag{4.66}$$

$$b_i > 0, \qquad \frac{d}{dP}b_i(P) < 0 \qquad \text{for } i = 1, 2. \tag{4.67}$$

$$d = d\Big(S(t), Q(t)\Big), \tag{4.68}$$

with

$$\frac{d}{dS}d(S,.) > 0, \qquad \frac{d}{dQ}d(.,Q) > 0. \qquad (4.69)$$

Finally the competition weight is chosen as

$$\psi \equiv 1. \qquad (4.70)$$

Now let us define a new variable $P(t) := \frac{Q(t)}{S(t)}$. Notice that $P(\cdot) < 1$. With this notation (4.1) becomes, with the help of the system in the previous example,

$$\begin{cases} \dfrac{d}{dt}S(t) = S(t)\Big(b_2(P(t)) - d\big(S(t), P(t)S(t)\big) + P(t)b_1(P(t))\Big), \\ \dfrac{d}{dt}P(t) = (1 - P(t))\big[P(t)b_1(P(t)) + b_2(P(t))\big] - \alpha P(t). \end{cases} \qquad (4.71)$$

Lemma 3. *Assume* (4.67)–(4.69),

$$d(0,0) \le b_2(1) \quad and \quad d(\infty,\infty) \ge b_1(0) + b_2(0),$$

then the system (4.71) *has a unique nonzero steady state* $(\bar{S}, \bar{P})$.

Proof. First let us focus on the second equation of (4.71). We prove that there exists a unique positive root to the function

$$F(P) = (1 - P)(Pb_1(P) + b_2(P)) - \alpha P.$$

We have $F(0) = b_2(0) > 0$, $F(1) = -\alpha < 0$, therefore F vanishes at least once in (0,1). We can write F as

$$F(P) = \begin{cases} b_2(0) & \text{if } P = 0, \\ PG(P) & \text{if } P \ne 0, \end{cases}$$

where G is given by

$$G(P) = b_1(P)(1 - P) - b_2(P) + \frac{b_2(P)}{P} - \alpha.$$

The zeros of F are precisely those of G and G is decreasing. Observe that $G(P)$ is positive for small values of P and $G(1) = F(1)$ which is negative. This proves the existence and uniqueness of a zero of G, and consequently the same for the function F. As a conclusion we characterize the steady state by

$$b_1(\bar{P})(1 - \bar{P}) - b_2(\bar{P}) + \frac{b_2(\bar{P})}{\bar{P}} = \alpha. \qquad (4.72)$$

Now we turn towards the first equation of (4.71). Observe that $d(S, \bar{P}S)$ increases as S increases. This fact together with our hypothesis on d confirms the existence and uniqueness of steady state $\bar{S}$, i.e.,

$$b_2(\bar{P}) - d\big(\bar{S}, \bar{P}\bar{S}\big) + \bar{P}b_1(\bar{P}) = 0. \qquad (4.73)$$

This proves our claim. $\square$

Now we introduce the notation $\bar{b}_1 = b_1(\bar{P})$ and $\bar{b}_2 = b_2(\bar{P})$, in order to simplify expressions. We are ready to prove the stability result for (4.71).

Theorem 8. *Under the assumptions of Lemma 3, the steady state $(\bar{S}, \bar{P})$ for (4.71) is globally and exponentially attractive.*

Proof. Again we prove a contraction inequality. First we fix initial values $S(0) > 0$, $P(0) > 0$. We begin in the same manner as we did in Example 1, by considering the Lyapunov functional

$$\frac{d}{dt}|P - \bar{P}| = -|b_1 - \bar{b}_1|P(t) + \bar{b}_1|P - \bar{P}| + |b_1 - \bar{b}_1|(P(t))^2 - \bar{b}_1(P + \bar{P})$$

$$|P - \bar{P}| - |b_2 - \bar{b}_2| + |b_2 - \bar{b}_2|P(t) - \bar{b}_2|P - \bar{P}| - \alpha|P - \bar{P}|$$

$$= \left[|b_2 - \bar{b}_2| + |b_1 - \bar{b}_1|P\right](P - 1) + (\bar{b}_1(1 - \bar{P}) - \bar{b}_2 - \alpha)|P - \bar{P}|.$$

By (4.72) we have

$$\frac{d}{dt}|P - \bar{P}| < -\frac{\bar{b}_2}{\bar{P}}|P - \bar{P}|, \tag{4.74}$$

and thus

$$|P(t) - \bar{P}| \le |P(0) - \bar{P}|\, e^{-\beta t}, \tag{4.75}$$

where $\beta = \frac{\bar{b}_2}{\bar{P}}$. This shows that $P(t) \longrightarrow \bar{P}$ as $t \longrightarrow \infty$. Next we treat the unknown $S(t)$. One can easily calculate, using (4.73),

$$\frac{d}{dt}S(t) = S\left(b_2 - \bar{b}_2 + Pb_1 - \bar{P}\bar{b}_1 + d(S, \bar{P}S) - d(S, PS)\right)$$

$$+ S\left(d(\bar{S}, \bar{P}\bar{S})| - d(S, \bar{P}S)\right).$$

For sufficiently large t, the sign of $\frac{d}{dt}S(t)$ is the same as the sign of $d(\bar{S}, \bar{P}\bar{S})| - d(S, \bar{P}S)$ because $P(t) \longrightarrow \bar{P}$ as $t \longrightarrow \infty$. Since we have uniqueness of the steady state $\bar{S}$ and $d(S, \bar{P}S)$ is increasing with S, then using (4.67), (4.69), (4.75) one can find C_1, $C_2 > 0$ such that

$$\frac{d}{dt}|S - \bar{S}| \le C_1 e^{-\beta t} - C_2|S - \bar{S}|, \qquad \forall t > 0.$$

With this, we get the announced result.   □

4.8.5 Nonlinear Stability (Example 3)

In this example we consider a more general situation. Here the death term depends only on total population S, the birth term depends on total population S and P, which is the ratio between weighted total population Q and total population S. As usual we assume the death term increases with its argument.

Regarding monotonicity of the birth term, our assumption in this example is different from the assumptions we had in previous examples. That is,

$$B(x, S(t)) = b_1(S(t), P(t))e^{\alpha t} + b_2(S(t), P(t)), \qquad (4.76)$$

$$b_3(S(t), P(t)) := P(t)b_1(S(t), P(t)) + b_2(S(t), P(t)), \qquad (4.77)$$

$$b_3(S(t), P(t)) > 0, \quad \frac{d}{dS}b_3(S, .) > 0, \quad \frac{d}{dP}b_3(., P) > 0, \qquad (4.78)$$

$$d = d(S(t)) > 0, \quad \frac{d}{dS}d(S) > 0. \qquad (4.79)$$

As usual we choose the competition weight

$$\psi \equiv 1.$$

For future use, we introduce the notation

$$\hat{S} := \log S, \ \hat{P} := -\log(1 - P). \qquad (4.80)$$

Due to (4.71), we get

$$\begin{cases} \dfrac{d}{dt}\hat{S}(t) = b_3\big(S(t), P(t)\big) - d(S(t)), \\[2mm] \dfrac{d}{dt}\hat{P}(t) = b_3\big(S(t), P(t)\big) - \alpha\dfrac{P(t)}{1-P(t)}. \end{cases} \qquad (4.81)$$

Lemma 4. *Assume (4.76)–(4.79) and asume that there exists* $\Sigma > 0$ *such that*

$$b_3\Big(\Sigma, \frac{d(0)}{d(0) + \alpha}\Big) < d(0) < b_3\Big(0, \frac{d(0)}{d(0) + \alpha}\Big).$$

Then the system (4.81) has the unique steady state $(\bar{S}, \bar{P}) > (0, 0)$.

Proof. Let $(\bar{S}, \bar{P})$ be a steady state. It is characterized by the solution of

$$b_3(\bar{S}, \bar{P}) = d(\bar{S}) = \alpha\frac{\bar{P}(t)}{1 - \bar{P}(t)}.$$

From a later equality we obtain $\bar{P} = \frac{d(\bar{S})}{d(\bar{S})+\alpha}$. Hence $d(\bar{S}) = b_3(\bar{S}, \frac{d(\bar{S})}{d(\bar{S})+\alpha})$ which has a unique solution from the hypothesis. Positivity and uniqueness of the steady state are straightforward. Hence we proved our assertion. □

Theorem 9. *Under the assumptions of Lemma 4 the steady state* $(\bar{S}, \bar{P})$ *for the system (4.81) is globally exponentially attractive.*

Proof. We build a Lyapunov functional as follows. After a small computation one can get

$$\frac{d}{dt}|\hat{S}(t) - \bar{S}| = -|b_3(S, \bar{P}) - b_3(\bar{S}, \bar{P})| - |b_3(S, P) - b_3(S, \bar{P})|\mathrm{sgn}(\hat{S} - \bar{S})\mathrm{sgn}$$
$$(\hat{P} - \bar{P}) - |d(S) - d(\bar{S})|,$$

$$\frac{d}{dt}|\hat{P}(t) - \bar{P}| = -|b_3(S, \bar{P}) - b_3(\bar{S}, \bar{P})|\mathrm{sgn}(\hat{S} - \bar{S})\mathrm{sgn}(\hat{P} - \bar{P}) - |b_3(S, P)$$

$$- b_3(S, \bar{P})| - \frac{\alpha|P - \bar{P}|}{(1 - P)(1 - \bar{P})}.$$

For given initial data $(S(0), P(0))$, by adding the last two equations we obtain that $S(t), P(t)$ are bounded. Therefore there exists $\delta > 0$ depending on $(S(0), P(0))$ such that $\delta \leq d'(S(t)) < \infty$. Finally we have proved the contraction inequality

$$\frac{d}{dt}\left(|\hat{S}(t) - \bar{S}| + |\hat{P}(t) - \bar{P}|\right) \leq -|d(S) - d(\bar{S})| - \frac{\alpha|P - \bar{P}|}{(1 - P)(1 - \bar{P})}$$

$$\leq -\delta(|\hat{S}(t) - \bar{S}| + \alpha|\hat{P}(t) - \bar{P}|)$$

$$\leq -C\left(|\hat{S}(t) - \bar{S}| + |\hat{P}(t) - \bar{P}|\right),$$

where $C = \min\{\delta, \alpha\}$. Our assertion easily follows from this. □

4.8.6 Nonlinear Stability (Kermack–McKendrick model)

We come back to the Kermack–McKendrick model ([30, 32]) already presented in Sect. 4.2. Recall that in Sect. 4.7, we proved a stability result for this system when $\Sigma(t)$ is quasistatic.

Now we present a simple and particular case in which this model can be reduced to a 2×2 system. In this subsection we prove, with a different method, a global and exponential stability result for the nontrivial steady state. This is a case which is not motivated by epidemiologic applications, but by its simplicity:

$$d_\Sigma(x) = d_n(x) + B_R \equiv d, \; B > d^2, \qquad (4.82)$$

$$\psi(x) \equiv 1. \qquad (4.83)$$

With these assumptions we may integrate the equation on $n(t, x)$ of the Kermack–McKendrick model, see Sect. 4.2. And it reduces to the system of ODEs with $S(t), \Sigma(t)$ as unknowns, and is given by

$$\begin{cases} \frac{d}{dt}\Sigma(t) = B - d\Sigma(t) - S(t)\Sigma(t), \\ \frac{d}{dt}S(t) = -dS(t) + S(t)\Sigma(t). \end{cases} \qquad (4.84)$$

Let us denote the nonzero steady state of system (4.84) by $(\bar{\Sigma}, \bar{S})$. With this notation we have $(\bar{\Sigma}, \bar{S}) = \left(d, \frac{B}{d} - d\right)$ (this is where we need $B > d^2$).

Proposition 3. *Under the assumptions* (4.82)–(4.83) *and with initial data satisfying* $\Sigma(0), S(0) > 0$, *the "nonzero" steady state* $(\bar{\Sigma}, \bar{S})$ *for the system* (4.84) *is globally exponentially stable.*

We recall that the chemostat problem leads to much more complicated systems, see for instance [43] and the references therein.

Proof. We introduce $H(t) := \Sigma(t) + S(t)$ and $\bar{H} := \bar{\Sigma} + \bar{S}$. With this notation we have

$$\frac{d}{dt}\big(H(t) - \bar{H}\big) = -d\big(H(t) - \bar{H}\big),$$

which implies

$$\big|H(t) - \bar{H}\big| = \big|H(0) - \bar{H}\big|e^{-dt}. \qquad (4.85)$$

We use the fact that $\bar{\Sigma} = d$ to obtain

$$\frac{d}{dt}\big(S(t) - \bar{S}\big) = S(t)\big(\Sigma - \bar{\Sigma}\big) = S(t)\big(H(t) - \bar{H} - S(t) + \bar{S}\big).$$

For simplicity, we denote $h := \big|H(0) - \bar{H}\big|$. With this notation, by straightforward computation we obtain

$$\frac{d}{dt}\big(S(t) - \bar{S}\big) \leq \big(S(t) - \bar{S}\big)\big(-\bar{S} + he^{-dt}\big) + h\bar{S}e^{-dt}.$$

Gronwall's lemma gives exponential convergence of $S(t)$ to the steady state $\bar{S}$, i.e., there exist two positive constants c, C such that

$$\big|S(t) - \bar{S}\big| < Ce^{-ct} \text{ for all } t > 0. \qquad (4.86)$$

The announced result follows from (4.85) and (4.86). $\quad\square$

4.8.7 Some Numerical Results

In this section we present some numerical evidences concerning the stability results we have discussed in the previous section and in particular the first example discussed in Sect. 4.8.1. As stated in Sect. 4.8.3, the proof of the global convergence result relies on the condition (4.60). However we have proved in Sect. 4.8.2 that the nonzero steady state is always stable under more general conditions. Therefore the question left open is to know if condition (4.60) is really necessary for exponential convergence to the nonzero steady state. Our numerical results indicate that this condition might not be necessary and are based on two examples we describe below.

As a first example, we choose

$$b_1(S) = \frac{1}{1+S}, \qquad b_2(S) = \frac{k}{1+S}, \qquad d(S) = \frac{S}{1+S}, \qquad (4.87)$$

with $k > 0$ a constant. One can easily check that a choice of α which violates the condition (4.60) is given by

$$0 < \alpha < \min\left\{\frac{1 - 2k}{k}, \frac{k - 2 + \sqrt{(k+2)^2 + 4}}{2}\right\}. \qquad (4.88)$$

We have computed numerically the trajectories of solutions of (4.51), where b_1, b_2, d are given by (4.87) with various choices of parameters α, k satisfying (4.88). All the cases we have computed turned out to exhibit global convergence. Two cases are depicted in the Fig. 4.1.

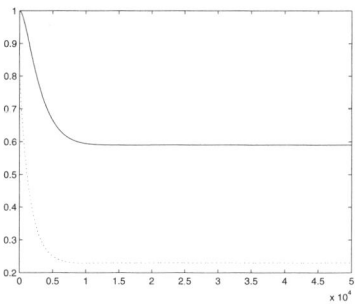 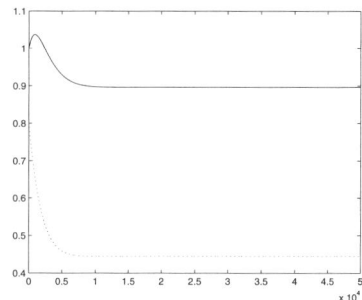

Fig. 4.1. Solutions of (4.51) with the choice of b_1, b_2, d given by (4.87); Left: $S(t)$ (continuous line) and $Q(t)$ (dashed line) with parameters $k = 0.2$, $\alpha = 0.58$, Right: S(t) (continuous line) and $Q(t)$ (dashed line) with parameters $k = 0.4$, $\alpha = 0.48$. These indicate that condition (4.60) might be too strong, and global convergence to the steady state holds true more generally.

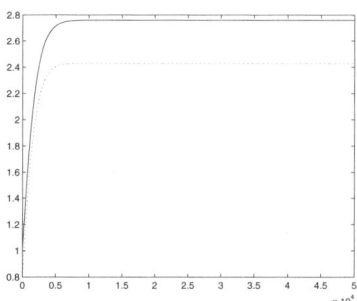 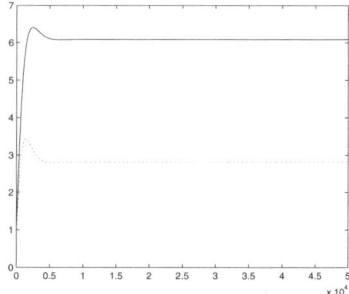

Fig. 4.2. Solutions of (4.51) with the choice of b_1, b_2, d given by (4.89); Left: $S(t)$ (continuous line) and $Q(t)$ (dashed line) with parameters $k = 1$, $\alpha = 0.1$, Right: S(t) (continuous line) and $Q(t)$ (dashed line) with parameters $k = 10$, $\alpha = 1$.

As a second example

$$b_1(S) = \frac{1+k}{1+S}, \qquad b_2(S) = \frac{1}{1+S}, \qquad d(S) = \frac{S}{1+S}. \tag{4.89}$$

A straightforward computation shows that the condition

$$\alpha < \frac{2k}{3} \tag{4.90}$$

is sufficient to violate (4.60). To conclude this section we show two more cases with different choices of the parameters k, α satisfying the condition (4.90), see Fig. 4.2.

Acknowledgment

Suman Kumar Tumuluri has been supported by Indo French CEFIPRA Project 3401-2.

References

1. Adimy, M., Crauste, F., Global stability of a partial differential equation with distributed delay due to cellular replication, Nonlinear Analysis, 54, p1469–1491 (2003).
2. Adimy, M., Pujo-Menjouet, L., Asymptotic behavior of a singular transport equation modelling cell division, Dis. Cont. Dyn. Sys. Ser. B 3, 3, p439–456 (2003).
3. Arino, O., Sanchez, E., Webb, G.F., Necessary and sufficient conditions for asynchronous exponential growth in age structured cell populations with quiescence, J. Math. Anal. Appl. 215 p499–513 (1997).
4. Bees, M.A., Angulo, O., López-Marcos, J.C., Schley, D., Dynamics of a structured slug population model in the absence of seasonal variation, Mathematical Models and Methods in Applied Sciences, Vol. 16, No. 12, p1961–1985, (2006).
5. Bekkal Brikci, F., Boushaba, K., Arino, O., Nonlinear age structured model with cannibalism, Discrete and Continuous Dynamical Systems, 2, Volume 7, p251–273, March (2007).
6. Bekkal Brikci, F., Clairambault, J., Perthame, B., Analysis of a molecular structured population model with possible polynomial growth for the cell division cycle, Mathematical and Computer Modelling, (2007), doi:10.1016/j.mcm.2007.06.008.
7. Busenberg, S., Iannelli, M., Class of nonlinear diffusion problems in age dependent population dynamics, Nonlinear Analy. Theory Meth. & Applic., Vol. 7, No. 5, p501–529 (1983).
8. Calsina, À., Cuadrado, S., Asymptotic stability of equilibria of selection-mutation equations. J. Math. Biol., 54, no. 4, p489–511, (2007).
9. Carrillo, J.A., Cuadrado, S., Perthame, B., Adaptive dynamics via Hamilton-Jacobi approach and entropy methods for a juvenile-adult model, Mathematical Biosciences, vol. 205(1), p137–161 (2007).
10. Chiorino, G., Metz, J.A.J., Tomasoni D., Ubezio, P., Desynchronization rate in cell populations: mathematical modeling and experimental data, J. Theor. Biol. 208, p185–199 (2001).
11. Chipot, M., On the equations of age dependent population dynamics, Arch. Rational Mech. Anal., 82, p13–25 (1983).
12. Clairambault, J., Gaubert, S., Perthame, B., An inequality for the Perron and Floquet eigenvalues of monotone differential systems and age structured equations. Preprint (2007).
13. Diekmann, O., A beginner's guide to adaptive dynamics. In Rudnicki, R. (Ed.), *Mathematical modeling of population dynamics*, Banach Centre Publications, Warsaw, Poland, Vol. 63, p47–86 (2004).
14. Diekmann, O., Gyllenberg, M., Metz, J.A.J., Steady state analysis of structured population models, Theoretical Population Biology, 63, p309–338 (2003).

15. Diekmann, O., Gyllenberg, M., Metz, J.A.J., Physiologically structured population models: towards a general mathematical theory. In *Mathematics for ecology and environmental sciences* Springer, New York, p5–20 (2007).
16. Diekmann, O., Heesterbeck, J.A.P., *Mathematical epidemiology of infectious diseases*, Wiley, New York (2000).
17. Ducrot, A., Travelling wave solutions for a scalar age structured equation, Discrete and Continuous Dynamical Systems, 2, Volume 7, p251–273, March (2007).
18. Dyson, J., Villella-Bressan, R. and Webb, G., A nonlinear age and maturity structured model of population dynamics. II. Chaos, J. Math. Anal. Appl., 242, No. 2, p255–270 (2000).
19. Echenim, N., Monniaux, D., Sorine, M., Clément F., Multi-scale modeling of the follicle selection process in the ovary, Math. Biosci., 198, No. 1, 57–79 (2005).
20. Fasano, A., Yashima, H.F., Equazioni integrali per un modello di simbiosi di età: caso di pino cembro e nocciolaia, Rend. Sem. Mat. Univ. Padova, Vol. 111, p205–238 (2004).
21. Feller, W., *An introduction to probability theory and applications*. Wiley, New York (1966).
22. Gopalsamy, K., Age-specific coexistence in two-species competition, Mathematical Biosciences, 61, p101–122 (1982).
23. Gurtin, M.E., MacCamy, R.C., Nonlinear age-dependent population dynamics, Arch. Rational Mech. Anal., 54, p281–300 (1974).
24. Gwiazda, P., Perthame, B., Invariants and exponential rate of convergence to steady state in renewal equation, Markov Processes and Related Fields (MPRF) 2, p413–424 (2006).
25. Gyllenberg, M., Nonlinear age-dependent population dynamics in continuously propagated bacterial cultures, Math. Bios., 62, p45–74 (1982).
26. Hoppensteadt, F., *Mathematical theories of populations: Demographics genetics and epidemics*, SIAM Reg. Conf. Series in Appl. Math. (1975).
27. Iannelli, M., *Mathematical theory of age-structured population dynamics*, Applied Mathematics Monograph C.N.R. Vol. 7, In Pisa: Giardini editori e stampatori (1995).
28. Iwata, K., Kawasaki, K., Shigesada, N., A dynamical model for the growth and size distribution of multiple metastatic tumors, J. Theor. Biol., 203, p177–186 (2000).
29. Jost, J., Mathematical Methods in Biology and Neurobiology, Lecture Notes given at ENS, http://www.mis.mpg.de/jjost/publications/mathematical_methods.pdf (2006).
30. Kermack, W.O., McKendrick, A.G., A contribution to the mathematical theory of epidemics, Proc. Roy. Soc., A 115, p700–721 (1927). Part II, Proc. Roy. Soc., A 138, p55–83 (1932).
31. Mackey, M. C., Rey, A., Multistability and boundary layer development in a transport equation with retarded arguments, Can. Appl. Math. Quart. 1, p1–21 (1993).
32. McKendrick, A.G., Applications of mathematics to medical problems, Proc. Edinburgh Math. Soc., 44, p98–130 (1926).
33. Marcati, P., On the global stability of the logistic age-dependent population growth, J. Math. Biology, 15, p215–226 (1982).
34. Metz, J.A.J., Diekmann, O., *The dynamics of physiologically structured population*, LN in Biomathematics 68, Springer-Verlag, New York (1986).

35. Michel, P., General Relative Entropy in a Nonlinear McKendrick Model, Stochastic Analysis and Partial Differential Equations, Editors: Gui-Qiang Chen, Elton Hsu, and Mark Pinsky. Contemp. Math (2007).

36. Michel, P. Existence of a solution to the cell division eigenproblem. M3AS, Vol. 16, suppl. issue 1, p1125–1153 (2006).

37. Michel, P., Mischler, S., Perthame, B., General entropy equations for structured population models and scattering, C.R. Acad. Sc Paris, Sér.1, 338, p697–702 (2004).

38. Michel, P., Mischler, S., Perthame, B., General relative entropy inequality: an illustration on growth models, J. Math. Pures et Appl., 84, Issue 9, p1235–1260 (2005).

39. Mischler, S., Perthame, B., Ryzhik, L., Stability in a nonlinear population maturation model, Math. Models Meth. Appli. Sci., 12, No. 12, p1751–1772 (2002).

40. Murray, J.D., *Mathematical biology*, Vol. 1 and 2, Second edition. Springer, New York (2002).

41. Öelz, D., Schmeiser, C. Modelling of the actin-cytoskeleton in symmetric lamellipodial fragments. Preprint 2007.

42. Pakdaman, K., Personal communication.

43. Perthame, B., *Transport Equations in Biology* (LN Series Frontiers in Mathematics), Birkhauser (2007).

44. Perthame, B., Ryzhik, L., Exponential decay for the fragmentation or cell-division equation, Journal of Differential Equations, 210, Issue 1, p155–177 (March 2005).

45. Rotenberg, M., Transport theory for growing cell populations, J. Theor. Biology, 103, p181–199 (1983).

46. Thieme, H.R. *Mathematics in population biology*. Woodstock Princeton University Press. Princeton, NJ (2003).

47. VonFoerster, H., Some remarks on changing populations. *The kinetics of cellular proliferation* (ed. F. Stohlman), Grune and Strutton, New York (1959).

48. Webb, G. F., *Theory of nonlinear age-dependent population dynamics*, Monographs and Textbooks in Pure and Applied Mathematics, 89, Marcel Dekker Inc., New York and Basel (1985).

A Game Theoretical Perspective on the Somatic Evolution of Cancer

David Basanta and Andreas Deutsch

Technische Universität Dresden, Zentrum für Informationsdienste und Hochleistungsrechnen, Nöthnitzer-str. 46, 01187, Dresden, Germany
{david.basanta, andreas.deutsch}@tu-dresden.de

5.1 Introduction

Environmental and genetic mutations can transform the cells in a co-operating healthy tissue into an ecosystem of individualistic tumour cells that compete for space and resources [1, 2, 3]. If we consider a tumour as an ecosystem it is possible to utilise tools traditionally used by ecologists to study the evolution of a population in which there is some degree of phenotypical diversity. One such tool is evolutionary game theory (EGT) which merges traditional game theory with population biology [4]. It allows the prediction of successful phenotypes and their adaptation to environmental selection forces. EGT is considered as a promising tool in which to frame oncological problems [5] and has been recently made more relevant by phenotypic studies of carcinogenesis such as the ones by Hanahan, Weinberg and colleagues [6, 7].

Game theory (GT) was introduced by von Neumann and Morgenstern as an instrument to study human behaviour [8, 9]. A game describes the interactions of two or more players that follow two or more well-defined strategies in which the benefit of each player (payoff) results from these interactions [10]. GT can be employed to study situations in which several players make decisions in order to maximise their own benefit. GT was initially introduced to model problems in economics, social and behavioural sciences and is used as a formal way to analyse interactions between agents that behave strategically. Evolutionary game theory is the application of conventional GT as used by economists and sociologists to study evolution and population ecology [4]. As opposed to conventional GT, in EGT the behaviour of the players is not assumed to be based on rational payoff maximisation but it is thought to have been shaped by trial and error—adaptation through natural selection or individual learning [11]. In the context of the evolution of populations there are two GT concepts that have to be interpreted in a different light. First, a strategy is not a deliberate course of action but a phenotypic trait. The payoff is Darwinian fitness, that is, average reproductive success. Second, the

N. Bellomo et al. (eds.), *Selected Topics in Cancer Modeling*,
DOI: 10.1007/978-0-8176-4713-1_5, © Springer Science+Business Media, LLC 2008

players are members of a population that compete or cooperate to obtain a larger share of the population [4].

To illustrate some of the ideas in EGT let us consider the following example named the Hawk-Dove game [11]. In this game we study an imaginary population of individuals and a resource V which affects the reproductive success of the individuals in this population. The population contains two phenotypes that represent two different strategies to access the resource. When two individuals compete for the resource the outcome will depend on the phenotypic strategies involved. The first phenotype, called Hawk in the game, always escalates the fight until injured (at a cost in fitness equal to C) or until the rival retreats. The second phenotype, known as Dove in the game, will retreat if the opponent escalates, that is, if the opponent seems determined to fight. The interactions between the different phenotypes are shown in the payoff table (Table 5.1).

Table 5.1. Payoff table for the change in fitness in the Hawk-Dove game.

	Hawk	Dove
Hawk	$\frac{V-C}{2}$	0
Dove	V	$\frac{V}{2}$

Table 5.1 presents the interactions between the different phenotypes considered in the game. The table should be read following the columns such that the payoff for a Hawk playing another Hawk is $\frac{V-C}{2}$ expressing the fact that they both have to share the resource and that they stand an equal chance of getting injured. The payoff of a Hawk playing a Dove is V since the Dove will withdraw from the competition. A Dove playing a Hawk gets no payoff since it withdraws and when playing another Dove it will get the resource V in half of the occasions. With this information it is possible to predict that if the population is mainly composed of individuals with the Dove phenotype then a Hawk individual will have a significant fitness advantage (because in most of the interactions, the rival is likely to be a Dove and thus retreat from a full scale fight for the resource). On the other hand if the fitness cost of injury is more than twice as high as the benefit provided by the contested resource then a Dove would be quite successful in a population dominated by Hawks (since a Hawk that interacts frequently with other Hawks is likely to be eventually wounded and a Dove will always avoid costly wounds). Using this example Maynard Smith introduced the concept of an evolutionarily stable strategy (ESS) [11]. An ESS is defined as a phenotype that, if adopted by the vast majority of a population, will not be displaced by any other phenotype

that could appear in the population as a result of evolution [11]. Under this definition the Dove phenotype cannot be an ESS and only under some specific circumstances (when the fitness benefit of getting the resource outweighs the fitness cost of an injury) would a Hawk phenotype be evolutionarily stable. are normally mixed strategies, that is, those strategies that play a group of pure strategies (Hawk and Dove in this example) with a given probability.

GT has been used to address many problems in biology in which different species or phenotypes within one species compete. Examples of this are the evolution of sex ratios [12], the emergence of animal communication [13] and fighting behaviour and territoriality [11]. A recent focus on the capabilities that cells acquire as tumours evolve [6] has shown how the interplay between different phenotypes with different capabilities can lead to different evolutionary paths. This stresses the importance of GT as a modelling tool in cancer. The most important capabilities which cells have to acquire in a neoplasm that will become a malignant tumour are shown in Fig. 5.1. They include: unlimited replicative potential, environmental independence for growth, evasion of apoptosis, angiogenesis and invasion. The circumstances in which these capabilities evolve and spread through the tumour population can be studied using GT. Some of the most important milestones in the transformation of healthy tissue cells into malignant cancer such as tumourigenesis, angiogenesis and invasion, have already been approached with GT.

The remainder of this chapter will provide, to the best of our knowledge, all the relevant examples of the application of GT to the study of the somatic cancer evolution and finally hint at some of the possible future venues of this method in the context of cancer research.

5.2 Tumourigenesis

Tumour initiation requires the acquisition of a number of phenotypic capabilities such as evasion of apoptosis and independence from environmental signals (see Fig. 5.1). The evolution of these capabilities, normally acquired when the tumour is still in the avascular stage, has been studied in research by Tomlinson and Bodmer [14, 15] and by Gatenby and Vincent [16].

5.2.1 Evasion of Apoptosis

Problem. Apoptosis or programmed cell death is a mechanism that hinders tumour progression. Cells with a working apoptotic machinery die when genetic abnormalities are detected [6]. Thus cells in a malignant cancer have to evolve mechanisms to disable the apoptotic machinery.

Model. Tomlinson and Bodmer [14] present a model in which three different apoptosis evasion related strategies are considered:

1. Cells that produce a paracrine growth factor to prevent apoptosis of neighbouring cells.

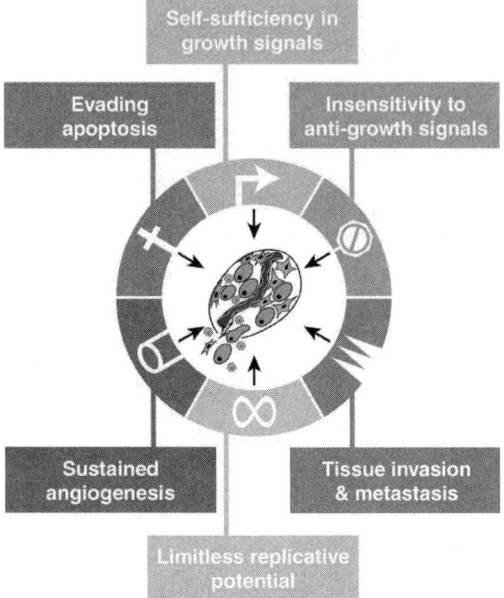

Fig. 5.1. Acquired capabilities of cancer: Hanahan and Weinberg suggest that most if not all cancers have acquired the same set of capabilities during their evolution. These capabilities are: unlimited replicative potential, environmental independence from anti-growth signals, production of own growth signals, evasion of apoptosis, angiogenesis and invasion (from [6] with permission).

2. Cells that produce an autocrine growth factor to prevent apoptosis of themselves.
3. Cells that are susceptible to paracrine growth factors but incapable of production of factors.

The aim of the model is to study the possibility of stable coexistence of the different phenotypes (polymorphism) that could be possible in a tumour when only these three phenotypes are considered.

Table 5.2. Payoff table for the game of programmed cell death. Parameter a represents the cost of producing a paracrine factor, b is the cost of the factor produced in an autocrine fashion, c is the fitness benefit of evading apoptosis.

	1	2	3
1	$1 - a + b$	$1 + b + c$	$1 + b$
2	$1 - a$	$1 + c$	1
3	$1 - a$	$1 + c$	1

In Table 5.2, a is the cost of producing the paracrine factor, b the benefit of receiving the paracrine factor and c the benefit of producing the autocrine factor.

Results. If a is positive then the third strategy displaces the first one from the population. If only the other two strategies are considered then if the benefit of the autocrine factor, provided by c, is positive the second strategy will displace the third one. In most relevant situations the model shows a strong selection for the autocrine factor-producing phenotype and under the assumptions of the model the altruistic strategy (the first one) will always be displaced.

Remarks. The model is very simple and easy to understand while at the same time it captures the relevant features necessary to study the evolution of the mechanisms to avoid apoptosis. However the authors do not explain the mechanisms by which these phenotypes could appear in a tumour and what would be the biological explanation of the costs and benefits of the different growth factors.

5.2.2 Environmental Poisoning

Problem. Tomlinson introduced a further model in which he considers the hypothesis that tumour cells might boost their own replicative potential at the expense of other tumour cells by evolving the capability of producing cytotoxic substances [15].

Model. Tomlinson speculates with different strategies that cells may adopt to produce or cope with toxic factors. The main model aims to study the polymorphic equilibria when cells can adopt one of the three following strategies:

1. Cells producing cytotoxic substances against other cells.
2. Cells producing resistance to external cytotoxic substances.
3. Cells producing neither cytotoxins nor resistance.

Table 5.3 shows the payoff table of the game with these phenotypes.

Table 5.3. Payoff table for the change in fitness for cells in a tumour in which the base payoff is z, e is the cost of producing the cytotoxin, f the fitness cost of being affected by the cytotoxin, g the advantage of subjecting another cell to the cytotoxin and h the cost of developing resistance to the cytotoxin.

	1	2	3
1	$z - e - f + g$	$z - h$	$z - f$
2	$z - e$	$z - h$	z
3	$z - e + g$	$z - h$	z

Results. Game theoretical analysis and simulations show that production of cytotoxic substances against other tumour cells can evolve in a tumour population and that several cytotoxin related strategies may be present at a given time (polymorphism).

Remarks. Although the author admits that there is little experimental evidence for mutations that cause tumour cells to harm their neighbours, the Warburg effect could fit nicely in the framework presented in this work. The Warburg effect describes the switch of tumour cells from the conventional aerobic metabolism to the glycolytic metabolism. This metabolism is less efficient but produces, as a by-product, acid that can harm neighbouring cells [17, 18, 19, 20]. Thus, in the game described by Tomlinson, e could correspond to the fitness loss of the less efficient glycolytic metabolism, f could be the fitness loss of a normal cell in an acid environment and g the fitness benefit received by glycolytic cells that can take advantage of the harm done to their non-glycolytic neighbours.

5.3 Angiogenesis

Problem. A very important capability that has to be acquired by tumours on the path to cancer is angiogenesis. Without access to the circulatory system tumours do not grow to sizes bigger than 2mm in diameter [21]. Cells capable of angiogenesis produce growth factors that promote the creation of new blood vessels that can provide nutrients and oxygen to previously unreachable areas in a growing tumour. Presumably the factors will be produced at a cost to the tumour cell.

Model I. In their interpretation of an angiogenic game Tomlinson and Bodmer [14] consider two strategies: cells denoted as A+ can produce angiogenic factors at a fitness cost i and cells denoted as A- that produce no angiogenic factors. In any case cells will get a benefit j when there is an interaction involving an angiogenic factor producing cell. The payoffs for the interactions between these cells are shown in Table 5.4.

Table 5.4. Payoff table for the change in fitness for a cell in a tumour with cells capable of producing angiogenic factors (A+) and cells susceptible to benefit from growth factors (A−).

	A+	A−
A+	$1 - i + j$	$1 + j$
A−	$1 - i + j$	1

Results. The model shows that as long as the benefit j of angiogenesis is greater than the cost i of producing angiogenic factors then both types of strategies will be present in a tumour in proportion to these costs.

Remarks. This model of angiogenesis is rather simplistic but constitutes a nice foundation for later models that take into account spatial considerations. A more significant drawback is that the model does not attempt to suggest a link between the different fitness costs and benefits and the underlying biological mechanisms.

Model II. The first extension to this model was proposed by Bach et al. [22] suggesting a game with interactions between three players. In this game the benefit j of angiogenesis is obtained only when at least two of the three players produce the angiogenic factor. The new payoff table is shown as Table 5.5.

Table 5.5. Payoff table for the change in fitness for a cell in a tumour with cells capable of producing angiogenic factors (A+) and cells susceptible to benefit from growth factors (A−). In this version the interactions involve three players. The payoff of a player is given by the columns (i.e. the payoff of an A+ cell interacting with an A+ and an A− cell is $1 - i + j$ but an A+ interacting with two A− cells is $1 - j$).

	A+	A−
A+, A+	$1-i+j$	$1+j$
A+, A−	$1 - i + j$	1
A−, A−	$1 - i$	1

Results. The authors produce simulations using Table 5.5 and show (see Fig. 5.2) that this game yields results that differ from the original ones introduced by Tomlinson and Bodmer. In this case even when the cost i is smaller than the benefit j there are many scenarios for which the angiogenic strategy will be displaced from the population. The existence of a polymorphic equilibrium containing the angiogenic strategy depends, intuitively, on the cost of producing angiogenic factors in comparison to the benefit they give but also on the relative frequency of cells playing the angiogenic strategy in the population. These results suggest that a gene therapy against the reparation of tumour supressor genes would only need to change a fraction of the mutated cells before the dynamics of the system drives them to extinction.

Model III. In a separate research Bach et al. [23] studied how a spatial version of the angiogenesis game could produce different results from those of the original model by Tomlinson and Bodmer. In this game players inhabit a 100×100 lattice. Each player can follow either the angiogenic (A+) or the non-angiogenic (A−) strategy. Time is discrete and in each time step a number of cells is removed from the lattice at random. Neighbouring cells compete (using Table 5.4) to occupy unallocated space. The candidate cell that achieves the

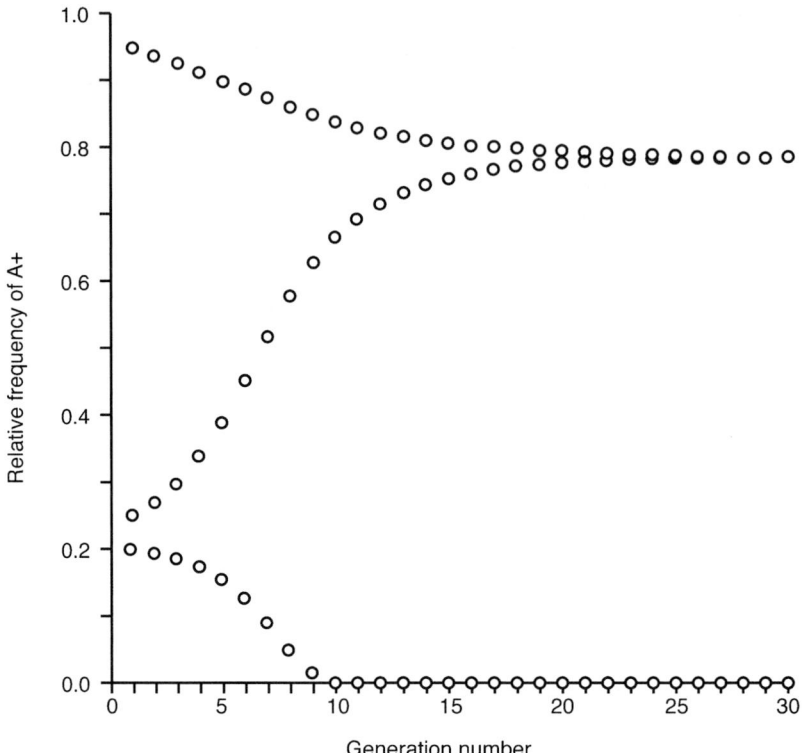

Fig. 5.2. Simulations of the threshold model in which the benefit of angiogenesis (j) is three times the cost of producing the growth factors (i). The plot shows the results of three simulations with varying A+/A− players in the starting population. The ordinate is the frequency of A+ cells and the abscissa is the number of cell generations (from [22] with permission).

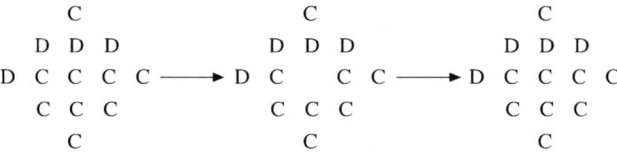

Fig. 5.3. A diagrammatic representation of the cell update process in the spatial model of the angiogenesis game by Bach and colleagues [23]. First a cell is selected to be removed (in this case the C marked in bold in the configuration on the left). Then the four neighbouring cells all assess their fitness (middle configuration). The cell with the highest fitness then reproduces into the empty space (right) (from [23] with permission).

highest score interacting with the neighbours determines the strategy that will be followed by the new cell in the vacant slot (see Fig. 5.3).

Results. The authors found the results of the new formulation of the model markedly different from those of the non-spatial counterpart. In spatial models, space tends to favour growth promoters in ways that cannot be seen in the non-spatial model. In any case polymorphic equilibria do exist and in both spatial and non-spatial cases the proportion of angiogenic players increases as the benefits of angiogenesis increase or as the cost of producing the growth factors decreases. The authors also conclude that, contrary to other evolutionary models [24], space does not significantly favour co-operative strategies in populations of cells.

5.4 Motility/Invasion

A tumour in which cells develop the capability of invading other tissues becomes a malignant tumour and thus significantly worsens the prognosis of a patient. EGT is a tool that could greatly improve our understanding of the circumstances that influence the successful evolution of invasive phenotypes.

Model I. Mansury and colleagues have recently introduced a rather unconventional EGT formulation that they used on top of a previous cellular automaton model in the context of brain tumours [25, 26]. This GT module allows the original model to deal with cell-cell interactions in a tumour consisting of cells with different phenotypes. The model was designed to investigate the genotype to phenotype link in a polymorphic tumour cell population. This model covers two distinct strategies. Strategy P is characterised by a highly proliferative genotype and a high number of gap junctions. Strategy M is characterised by a highly migratory phenotype and a low number of gap junctions (which are used for cell-to-cell communication). As opposed to other game theoretical models in which a payoff table determines the fitness change of players when they interact, in this model three tables are used not to compute fitness change but to encode the rules of the cellular automata. See Tables 5.6, 5.7 and 5.8.

Table 5.6 shows how the cell-to-cell communication capabilities change according to the strategies followed by the interacting cells. Since the authors assume that there is a negative correlation between the extent of communication and proliferation then the proliferative capability of a cell with the proliferative strategy P will be lower if it interacts with another cell with the same strategy. On the other hand it will be higher if it interacts with a cell with the motile strategy M. Table 5.7 shows that cells will have a higher proliferative potential when they interact with cells that have the motile strategy. Table 5.8 shows that interacting with cells with the motile strategy will also increase the probability of motility of the interacting cell. These tables are used to guide the behaviour of the cells on a 500×500 lattice containing initially 5 cells of each type and two unequal sources of nutrients in two different

Table 5.6. Payoff table that describes the rate of change in cell-to-cell communication skills depending on the phenotype of the interacting cell in the model by Mansury et al. [26].

	P	M
P	↑↑↑	↑↑
M	↑↑	↑

Table 5.7. Payoff table that describes how the proliferation capability of a cell is influenced by its interaction with cells with other phenotypes (proliferative or motile) in the model by Mansury et al. [26].

	P	M
P	↓↓↓	↓↓
M	↓↓	↓

Table 5.8. Payoff table that describes how the motility of a cell with a given phenotype changes depending on what other cells the cell is interacting with. Model by Mansury et al. [26].

	P	M
P	↑	↑↑
M	↑↑	↑↑↑

locations. In each time step the interactions of a cell with its neighbours are used to adjust the probabilities of proliferation and motility.

Results. The authors used this model to study how varying the payoffs for $A-A$ interactions affects a number of features of the tumour such as the speed (see Fig. 5.4) at which it reaches the nutrient sources or the fractality of the resulting spatial patterns.

Remarks. Although the model is interesting it is not as simple as other models reviewed in this chapter. A significant drawback is that the model is not evolutionary in the sense that it does not take into account the possibility of mutations introducing new phenotypes or tumour cells producing offspring different from their progenitors. This has been identified by the authors as something to be addressed in a future version of the model although they still claim the model to be based on EGT. Moreover, the authors do not take advantage of the tools provided by GT analysis to study the different steady state situations that could arise for different values of the payoff tables. This is probably due to the fact that the model is not a conventional GT model and the conventional game theoretical tools would not be easy to use in this

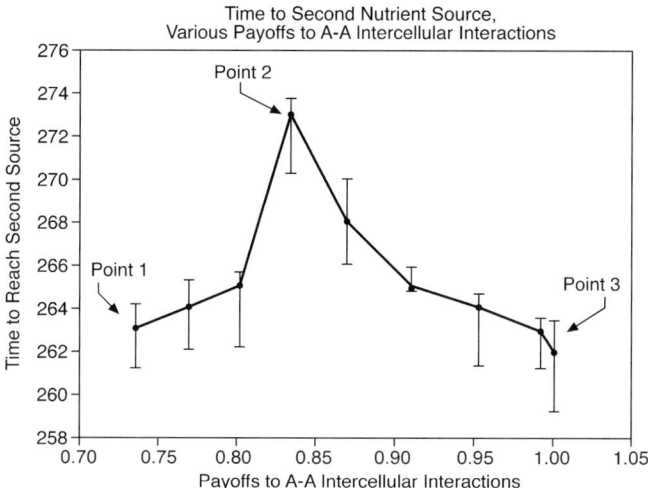

Fig. 5.4. Plot of the time to reach a nutrient source (i.e. the inverse of the tumour's average velocity) versus various payoff values conferred to P-P intercellular interactions (where A is the label for the proliferative phenotype in the paper). The error bars indicate the standard deviations from performing 10 Monte Carlo simulations for each value of payoffs for P-P interactions (from [26] with permission).

context. Also, the model provides a view on the dynamics of the tumour growth that is rarely found in most other GT analysis whose focus is on the study of equilibria.

Model II. The emergence of invasive phenotypes is influenced not only by its interaction with one phenotype or the other but by the complex interplay of several phenotypes which, in many cases has an indirect effect. Basanta et al. [27] hypothesise a number of scenarios in which three types of phenotypes interact in games with two and three players. They place these phenotypes in the context of an evolutionary non-spatial game theoretical model to test the hypothesis by Gatenby and colleagues that tumour invasion is promoted by the emergence of cells with a glycolytic metabolism [20]. The model represents a glioma tumour populated by cells with enhanced proliferative capabilities, known as autonomous growth (AG) cells, which can mutate into cells whose phenotype can make them follow either a more motile strategy (INV) or the glycolytic metabolism strategy (GLY).

Results. Table 5.9 defines the interactions between the three phenotypes. The authors investigate a number of scenarios in which subgames based on two strategies are used to study how one phenotype could emerge in a tumour populated by cells that use a different strategy. The results show that cells with a higher replicative potential (AG) and invasive cells (INV) can coexist in a tumour as long as the fitness cost of motility is not too high. They also reveal that autonomous growth (AG) cells cannot coexist with glycolytic

Table 5.9. Payoff table that represents the change in fitness of a tumour cell with a given phenotype interacting with another cell. Three different strategies are considered, those with higher replicative potential (AG), enhanced motility (INV) and glycolytic metabolism (GLY). The base payoff in a given interaction is equal to 1 and the cost of moving to another location with respect to the base payoff is c. The fitness cost of acidity is n and k is the fitness cost of having a less efficient glycolytic metabolism. The table should be read following the columns, thus the fitness change for an INV cell interacting with an AG would be $1 - c$.

	AG	INV	GLY
AG	$\frac{1}{2}$	$1-c$	$\frac{1}{2}+n-k$
INV	1	$1-\frac{c}{2}$	$1-k$
GLY	$\frac{1}{2}-n$	$1-c$	$\frac{1}{2}-k$

(GLY) cells. An interesting result of the model when all three strategies are considered simultaneously is that the appearance of the invasive phenotype is facilitated by the existence of glycolytic cells. Figure 5.5 shows how the proportion of invasive cells (X axis) increases as the cost of having a glycolytic metabolism (k) decreases and the cost of living in an acid environment (n) increases. In other words, the success of the invasive phenotype depends on the same factors that determine the fate of the glycolytic phenotype. The model suggests that any therapy that could increase the fitness cost of tumour cells switching to a glycolytic metabolism or the susceptibility of normal cells to acid environments might decrease the probability of the emergence of more invasive phenotypes.

5.5 Outlook

The examples described in this chapter treat tumour populations as ecosystems of potentially co-operating and/or competing cells. In these ecosystems, the success of one phenotype depends on its interactions with other existing phenotypes. Such an approach has been shown to be a helpful and useful way to study cancer evolution. Most of the applications use GT to study the steady state of a population of tumour cells that follow different strategies dictated by their phenotypes, acquired as a result of genetic and epigenetic mutations. This can be very relevant to study the different ways in which a tumour population may evolve under different model parameters and assumptions of their interplay. Such studies could lead to cancer therapies that would alter the dynamics of cancer evolution towards benign tumours. One limitation of EGT/GT is that all relevant potential phenotypes/strategies have to be known a priori if a good understanding of cancer evolution is to be obtained. Knowing all the potential relevant phenotypes might be difficult and even if the phenotypes and their interactions are well known the EGT

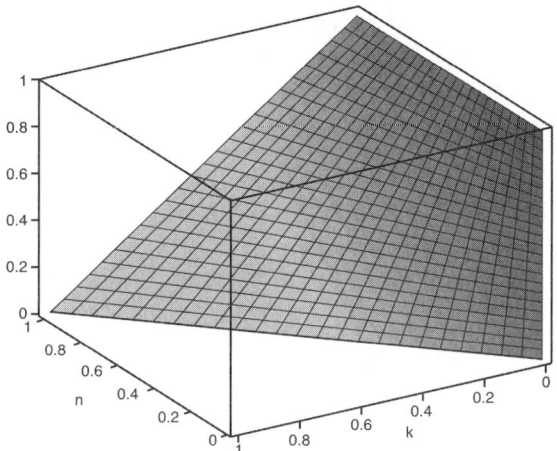

Fig. 5.5. Proportion of invasive cells in a tumour with three phenotypes (autonomous growth, invasive and glycolytic). k is the cost in terms of fitness of adopting the glycolytic metabolism whereas n is the fitness cost of a normal cell when staying with a glycolytic cell.

model might be too complicated to be analysed. Moreover, with more strategies/phenotypes the composition of the population may not converge to an equilibrium and the frequencies of the phenotypes could keep oscillating in a regular or chaotic fashion [4].

One more limitation of the GT models shown in this chapter is that they do not study the dynamics in a tumour population (dynamics which may or may not lead to an equilibrium). GT models that make use of population biology have the potential to overcome this limitation and also ease the connection between a quantitative model and experimental data as the payoff tables used in more conventional EGT models tend to make the assumption that the fitness values are independent of space or time. One promising venue is to couple conventional GT with population dynamics which is also based on the assumption that successful strategies spread [28, 4]. This trend is shown in the work of Gatenby and Vincent [16] whose EGT model uses methods from population biology in order to study how the phenotypes of cells in a population evolve towards ESS. Gatenby and Vincent adopted a GT approach influenced by population dynamics to study the influence of the tumour-host interface in colorectal carcinogenesis. The authors formulated an extended system of Lotka–Volterra equations to model the effect of nutrients and sensitivity to growth constraints in the proliferation of tumour cells. The cells in the tumour population are characterised by the number of substrate transporters (a higher number of them allow more nutrients in the cell) on the cell surface and by the cell response to normal growth constraints. Initially all the tumour cells are assumed to have normal values for both parameters but these values are allowed to change and the authors study their evolution. Their work demonstrates that normal cells in a multicellular organism occupy a ridge-shaped maximum of the fitness landscape that allows the heterogeneous coexistance of multiple cells. (See Fig. 5.6.) This fact makes them susceptible to mutations that are fitter and thus allow the somatic evolution that characterises cancer. The authors also conclude that any therapy that reduces the population density would be counterproductive s

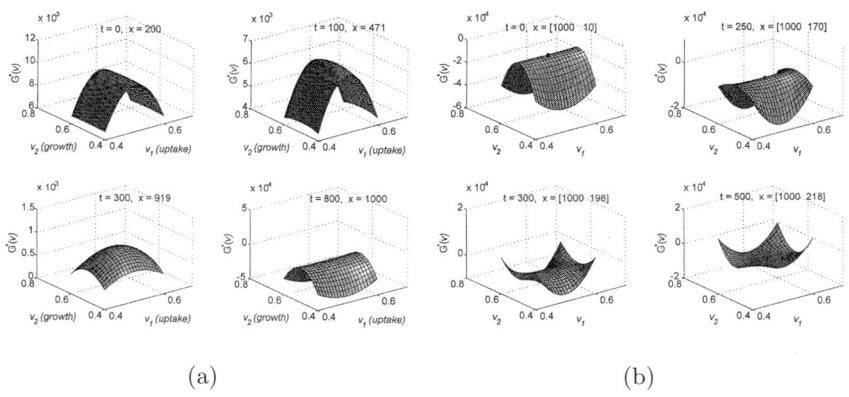

(a)   (b)

Fig. 5.6. (a) Upon reaching equilibrium, normal cells sit on the ridge-shaped maximum in the in vivo adaptive landscape. This provides a tissue structure that allows coexistence of multiple distinct non-competing populations, a necessary condition for the formation of multicellular organisms. (b) The presence of tumour cells deforms the tissue adaptive landscape over time so that normal cells arrive at a local minimum and are then readily subject to invasion by the mutant phenotypes (from [16] with permission).

GT is also a suitable tool to frame co-operative effects. Evolution of co-operation is a subfield of GT pioneered by Robert Axelrod [31]. Researchers in this field study the circumstances under which selfish agents will spontaneously co-operate. An example of how evolution of co-operation could be used to study cancer evolution was provided by Axelrod and collaborators in a recent paper [32] in which they show how tumour cells can co-operate sharing skills and capabilities (such as the production of angiogenic factors or paracrine growth factors needed to escape the homeostatic regulation of the tissue).

EGT has a relatively short history in the field of theoretical oncology. However with an increasingly better understanding of the role of the microenvironment in tumour evolution [33] and with the recent interest in studying cancer from ecological [2, 3] and phenotypic [6] viewpoints, the role of this tool in understanding the interactions between all the relevant agents within a tumour and their role in driving cancer evolution will surely rise.

Acknowledgments

We would like to acknowledge the help and suggestions from our colleagues at TU Dresden: Lutz Brusch, Haralambos Hatzikirou and Michael Kücken. The work in this chapter was supported in part by funds from the EU Marie Curie Network "Modeling, Mathematical Methods and Computer Simulation of Tumour Growth and Therapy" (EU-RTD-IST-2001-38923). We also acknowledge the support provided by the systems biology network HepatoSys of the German Ministry for Education and Research through grant 0313082C. Andreas Deutsch is a member of the DFG-Center for Regenerative Therapies Dresden - Cluster of Excellence - and gratefully acknowledges support by the Center.

References

1. P.C. Nowell. The clonal evolution of tumor cell populations. *Science*, 4260, 194:23–28, 1976.
2. B. Crespi and K. Summers. Evolutionary biology of cancer. *Tr. Ecol. Evol.*, 20(10):545–52, Oct. 2005.
3. L. Merlo, J. Pepper, B. Reid, and C. Maley. Cancer as an evolutionary and ecological process. *Nat. Rev. Cancer*, 6:924–935, Dec. 2006.
4. K. Sigmund and M. Nowak. Evolutionary game theory. *Curr. Biol.*, 9:503–5, 1999.
5. R. Gatenby and P. Maini. Cancer summed up. *Nature*, 421:321, Jan. 2003.
6. D. Hanahan and R. Weinberg. The hallmarks of cancer. *Cell*, 100:57–70, Jan. 2000.
7. W.C. Hahn and R. Weinberg. Rules for making human tumor cells. *N. Eng. J. Med.*, 347(20):1593–1603, Nov. 2002.
8. J. von Neumann and O. Morgernstern. *Theory of games and economic behaviour*. Princeton University Press, Princeton, NJ, 1953.
9. M. Nowak. *Evolutionary dynamics*. Belknap, Cambridge, MA, 2006.
10. M. Merston-Gibbons. *An introduction to game-theoretic modelling*. AMS, 2nd edition, Providence, RI, 2000.
11. J. Maynard Smith. *Evolution and the theory of games*. Cambridge University Press, Cambridge, 1982.
12. R.A. Fisher. *The genetical theory of natural selection*. Clarendon, Oxford, 1930.
13. J. Maynard Smith and D. Harper. *Animal signals*. Oxford University Press, Oxford, 2003.
14. I.P.M. Tomlinson and W.F. Bodmer. Modelling the consequences of interactions between tumour cells. *Brit. J. Cancer*, 75(2):157–60, 1997.
15. I.P.M. Tomlinson. Game theory models of interactions between tumour cells. Eur. J. Cancer, Vol 33, N9, pp. 1495–1500, 1997.

16. R. Gatenby and T. Vincent. An evolutionary model of carcinogenesis. *Cancer Res.*, 63:6212–6220, Oct. 2003.

17. O. Warburg. *The metabolism of tumors* (English translation by F. Dickens). Constable, London, 1930.

18. R.A. Gatenby and E.T. Gawlinski. The glycolytic phenotype in carcinogenesis and tumor invasion. Cancer Res. 63, 3847–3854, July 15, 2003.

19. R. Gatenby and R. J. Gillies. Why do cancers have high aerobic glycolysis? *Nat. Rev. Cancer*, 4:891–899, 2004.

20. R. Gatenby, E. Gawlinski, A. Gmitro, B. Kaylor, and R. Gillies. Acid-mediated tumor invasion: a multidisciplinary study. *Cancer Res.*, 66(10):5216–23, May 2006.

21. J. Folkman. The role of angiogenesis in tumor growth. *Semin. Cancer Biol.*, 3:65–71, 1992.

22. L.A. Bach, S.M. Bentzen, J. Alsner, and F.B. Christiansen. An evolutionary game model of tumour cell interactions: possible relevance to gene therapy. *Eur. Jour. Cancer*, 37:2116–2120, 2001.

23. L.A. Bach, D.J.T. Sumpter, J. Alsner, and V. Loeschke. Spatial evolutionary games of interaction among generic cancer cells. *Jour. Theo. Med.*, 5(1):47–58, 2003.

24. M. Nowak and R. May. Evolutionary games and spatial chaos. *Nature*, 18(359):826–29, 1992.

25. Y. Mansury and T. Deisboeck. The impact of 'search-precision' in an agent based tumor model. *Jour. Theo. Biol.*, 224:325–337, 2003.

26. Y. Mansury, M. Diggory, and T.S. Deisboeck. Evolutionary game theory in an agent based brain tumor model: exploring the genoype phenotype link. *Jour. Theo. Biol.*, 238:146–156, 2006.

27. D. Basanta, M. Simon, H. Hatzikirou, and A. Deutsch. An evolutionary game theory perspective elucidates the role of glycolysis in tumour invasion. Submitted to Cell Proliferation, 2008.

28. F. Hoppensteadt. *Mathematical methods of population biology.* Cambridge University Press, Cambridge, MA, 1982.

29. T. Vincent. Carcinogenesis as an evolutionary game. *Adv. in Compl. Sys.*, 9(4):369–382, 2006.

30. T. Vincent and R. Gatenby. Somatic evolution of cancer. *Int. Game Th. Rev.*, 9(4), 2007.

31. R. Axelrod and W. Hamilton. The evolution of cooperation. *Science*, 211:1390–1396, 1981.

32. R. Axelrod, D. Axelrod, and K. Pienta. Evolution of cooperation among tumor cells. *PNAS*, 103(36):13474–79, Sept. 2006.

33. C. Park, M. Bissell, and M. Barcellos-Hoff. The influence of the microenvironment on the malignant phenotype. *Mol. Med. Today*, 6:324–329, Aug. 2000.

6

Nonlinear Modeling and Simulation of Tumor Growth

Vittorio Cristini,[1,4,5] Hermann B. Frieboes,[1,2] Xiaongrong Li,[3] John S. Lowengrub,[2,3] Paul Macklin,[1] Sandeep Sanga,[1,4] Steven M. Wise,[2] and Xiaoming Zheng[2]

[1] School of Health Information Sciences, University of Texas Health Science Center at Houston, TX 77030, USA
`vittorio.cristini@uth.tmc.edu`
[2] Department of Mathematics, University of California, Irvine, CA 92697, USA
`lowengrb@math.uci.edu`
[3] Department of Biomedical Engineering, University of California, Irvine,
[4] Department of Biomedical Engineering, University of Texas, Austin, TX 78712, USA
[5] MD Anderson Cancer Center, University of Texas, Houston, TX 77030, USA

6.1 Introduction

The effects of the interaction between cellular- and tumor-scale processes on cancer progression and treatment response remain poorly understood (for instance, the crucial role of the microenvironment in cancer growth and invasion [94, 64, 183, 182, 159, 109, 65, 165]). Three-dimensional tissue morphology, cell phenotype, and molecular phenomena are intricately coupled; they influence cancer invasion potential by controlling tumor-cell proliferation and migration [77, 186, 197]. Hypoxia [87, 209, 185, 69, 90], acidosis [90, 198, 95], and associated diffusion gradients, caused by heterogeneous delivery of oxygen and nutrients and removal of metabolites [103, 102] due to highly disorganized microvasculature [91, 105] and often exacerbated by therapy (e.g., anti-angiogenic [159, 176]), can induce heterogeneous spatial distribution and invasiveness of tumor cells through a variety of molecular [174, 208, 207, 43, 164, 172, 144, 117, 27, 28, 189, 155, 184, 119, 121, 23, 159, 176, 173, 60] and tissue-scale [58, 126, 71] mechanisms corresponding to different tissue-scale invasive patterns [77, 163, 193, 166, 110, 186, 197, 203, 116, 205, 63, 178, 74, 76, 52, 171]. Such complex systems, dominated by large numbers of processes and highly nonlinear dynamics, are difficult to approach by experimental methods alone and can typically be better understood only by using appropriate mathematical models and sophisticated computer simulations, complementary to laboratory and clinical observations. Mathematical modeling has the potential to provide insight into these interactions through studies based on physical

N. Bellomo et al. (eds.), *Selected Topics in Cancer Modeling*,
DOI: 10.1007/978-0-8176-4713-1_6, © Springer Science+Business Media, LLC 2008

processes that treat cancer as a system. Our basic hypothesis, supported by an integrative approach combining sophisticated mathematical models with in vitro and in vivo experiments, is that the characteristics of the tumor-host interface can be used to predict the underlying dynamical interactions between tumor cell proliferation and adhesion, which, in turn, reflect both microenvironmental factors and cellular gene expression.

Over the past 10 years, activity in mathematical modeling and computational (in silico) simulation of cancer has increased dramatically (see, e.g., reviews such as [3, 25, 15, 36, 180, 167]). A variety of modeling strategies have been developed, each focusing on one or more aspects of cancer. Cellular automata and agent-based modeling, where individual cells are simulated and updated based upon a set of biophysical rules, have been developed to study genetic instability, natural selection, carcinogenesis, and interactions of individual cells with each other and the microenvironment. Because these methods are based on a series of rules for each cell, it is simple to translate biological processes (e.g., mutation pathways) into rules for the model. However, these models can be difficult to study analytically, and computational costs can increase rapidly with the number of cells. Because a 1-mm tumor spheroid may have several hundred thousand cells, these methods could become unwieldy when studying tumors of any significant size. See [10, 4, 137] for examples of cellular automata modeling, and [138, 1] for examples of agent-based modeling. In larger-scale systems where the cancer cell population is on the order of 1,000,000 or more, continuum methods may provide a more suitable modeling technique. Early work including [89, 38, 39] used ordinary differential equations to model cancer as a homogeneous population, as well as partial differential equation models restricted to spherical geometries. Linear and weakly nonlinear analyses have been performed to assess the stability of spherical tumors to asymmetric perturbations [48, 41, 58, 126, 15, 36] in order to characterize the degree of aggression. Various interactions of a tumor with the microenvironment, such as stress-induced limitations to growth, have also been studied [107, 6, 7, 175, 16, 17, 5]. Most of the modeling has considered single-phase (e.g., single cell species) tumors, although multiphase mixture models have also been developed to provide a more detailed account of tumor heterogeneity [7, 42, 49].

Recently, nonlinear modeling has been performed to study the effects of morphology instabilities on both avascular and vascular solid tumor growth. Results from this research will be the focus of this chapter, subdivided into four sections. Cristini et al. (2003) [58] used boundary integral methods (Sect. 6.2) to perform the first fully nonlinear simulations of a continuum model of tumor growth in the avascular and vascularized growth stages with arbitrary boundaries. These investigations of the nonlinear regime of shape instabilities predicted encapsulation of external, noncancerous tissue by morphologically unstable tumors. Li et al. (2007) [126] extended upon [58] in three dimensions (3-D) via an adaptive boundary integral method. Zheng et al. (2005) [211] (Sect. 6.3) built upon the model in [58] to include angiogenesis and an extratumoral microenvironment by developing and coupling a level set implementation with a hybrid continuum-discrete angiogenesis model originally developed by Anderson and Chaplain (1998) [11]. As in [58], Zheng et al. found that low-nutrient (e.g., hypoxic) conditions could lead to morphological instability. Their work served as a building block for recent studies of the effect of chemotherapy on tumor growth by Sinek et al. (2004) [187] and for studies of morphological instability and invasion by Cristini et al. (2005) [54] and Frieboes et al. (2006) [73]. Hogea et al. (2006) [96] have also begun exploring tumor growth and angiogenesis using a level set method coupled with a continuum model of angiogenesis. Macklin and Lowengrub (2007) (Sect. 6.4) used a ghost cell/level set method [135] for evolving interfaces to study tumor growth in heterogeneous tissue and further studied tumor growth as a function of the microenvironment [134]. Finally, Wise et al. (in review) [201] and Frieboes et al. (in review) [72] have developed a diffuse interface implementation of solid tumor growth to study the evolution of multiple tumor cell species, which was employed in Frieboes et al. (2007) [71] to model the 3-D vascularized growth of malignant gliomas (brain tumors) (Sect. 6.5).

6.2 Solid Tumor Growth Using a Boundary Integral Method[5]

6.2.1 Overview

In [58] and [126] we studied solid tumor growth in the nonlinear regime using boundary integral simulations in 2-D and 3-D to explore complex morphologies. A new formulation of classical models [89, 141, 39, 40] demonstrated that nonnecrotic tumor evolution could be described by a reduced set of two parameters that characterize families of solutions. The parameter G describes the relative rate of mitosis to the relaxation mechanisms (cell mobility and cell-to-cell adhesion). The parameter A describes the balance between apoptosis and mitosis. Both parameters also include the effect of vascularization. The analysis revealed that tumor evolution is qualitatively unaffected by the number of spatial dimensions. The 2-D simulations presented in [58] were the first fully nonlinear simulations of a continuum model of tumor growth, although there had been prior work on cellular automata-based simulations of tumor growth (e.g., see [108] and references therein).

Results reveal that the two new dimensionless parameters uniquely subdivide tumor growth into three regimes associated with increasing degrees

---

[5] Portions of this section are reprinted from *Journal of Mathematical Biology*, Cristini et al., Vol. 46, pp. 191–224, Copyright 2003 Springer (with kind permission of Springer Science and Business Media), and with permission from *Discrete and Continuous Dynamical Systems - Series B*, Li et al., Vol. 7, pp. 581–604, Copyright 2007 American Institute of Mathematical Sciences.

of vascularization: low (diffusion dominated), moderate, and high vascularization. Critical conditions exist for which the tumor evolves to nontrivial dormant states or grows self-similarly (i.e., shape invariant). Away from these critical conditions, evolution may be unstable leading to invasive fingering into the external tissues and to topological transitions such as tumor breakup and reconnection. Interestingly, the shape of highly vascularized tumors always stays compact and invasive fingering does not occur, even while growing unbounded. This is in agreement with experimental observations [150] of in vivo tumor growth and suggests that invasive growth of highly vascularized tumors is associated to vascular and elastic anisotropies (such as substrate inhomogeneities). Existence of nontrivial dormant states was recently proved [80], but no examples of such states were given until this work. The self-similar behavior described here is analogous to that recently found in diffusional crystal growth [57], and leads to the possibility of shape control and of controlling the release of tumor angiogenic factors by restricting the tumor volume-to-surface-area ratio. This could restrict angiogenesis during growth.

In the model, a tumor is treated as an incompressible fluid, and tissue elasticity is neglected. Cell-to-cell adhesive forces are modeled by a surface tension at the tumor-tissue interface. Growth of tumor mass is governed by a balance between cell mitosis and apoptosis (programmed cell death). The rate of mitosis depends on concentration of nutrient and growth inhibitor factors that obey reaction-diffusion equations in the tumor volume. The bulk source of factors is the blood. The concentration of capillaries in the tumor is assumed to be uniform, as are concentrations of factors in the external tissues. This work focused on the case of nonnecrotic tumors [37] with no inhibitor factors. These conditions apply to small-sized tumors or when nutrient concentrations in the blood and in external tissues are high. Such a model should over-predict growth away from these conditions.

To simulate solid tumor growth in 3-D [126], we developed a new, adaptive boundary integral method by extending to 3-D the continuum model in [58]. The 3-D problem is considerably more difficult owing to the singularities of the integrals and the 3-D surface geometry. In 2-D, it is possible to develop a spectrally accurate numerical algorithm together with a nonstiff time updating scheme for the tumor-host interface position. The numerical method relies on accurate discretizations of singular surface integrals, a spatial rescaling, and the use of an adaptive surface mesh originally developed in [53]. In both 2-D and 3-D, discretized boundary integral equations are solved iteratively using GMRES, and a discretized version of the Dirichlet–Neumann map is used to determine the normal velocity of the tumor surface. In 3-D, a version of the Dirichlet–Neumann map is used that relies on a vector potential formulation rather than a more standard double-layer potential. The vector potential has the advantage that singularity subtraction can be used to increase the order of accuracy of the numerical quadrature. Because of the difficulties in implementing an implicit time-stepping algorithm in 3-D, we instead used explicit time stepping with numerical fitting, which allows us to achieve acceptably large time steps.

Although the mathematical tumor model considered here is highly simplified, this work provides a benchmark to assess the effects of additional biophysical processes not considered, such as necrosis, multiple tumor cell types, tissue stress, angiogenesis and a developing neovasculature, as well as other microenvironmental features and inhomogeneities. In addition, the boundary integral results serve as a benchmark for validating other numerical methods (e.g., level set, mixture models) that are capable of simulating more complex biophysical processes.

6.2.2 Model Formulation

The model has only one intrinsic length scale, the diffusional length L_D, and three intrinsic time scales corresponding to the relaxation rate λ_R (associated to L_D, cell mobility, and cell-to-cell adhesion), the characteristic mitosis rate λ_M, and the apoptosis rate λ_A. The dimensional problem can be reformulated in terms of two nondimensional decoupled problems:

$$\nabla^2 \Gamma - \Gamma = 0, \quad (\Gamma)_\Sigma = 1 \tag{6.1}$$

$$\nabla^2 p = 0, \quad (p)_\Sigma = \kappa - AG \frac{(\mathbf{x} \cdot \mathbf{x})_\Sigma}{2d} \tag{6.2}$$

in a d-dimensional tumor. Time and space have been normalized with the intrinsic scales L_D and λ_R^{-1}, the interface Σ separates tumor volume from external tissue, and variables Γ and p represent a modified nutrient concentration and a modified pressure (see [58] for definitions). Tumor surface Σ (of local total curvature κ) is evolved using normal velocity

$$V = -\mathbf{n} \cdot (\nabla p)_\Sigma + G\mathbf{n} \cdot (\nabla \Gamma)_\Sigma - AG \frac{\mathbf{n} \cdot (\mathbf{x})_\Sigma}{d}, \tag{6.3}$$

where $\mathbf{n}$ is the outward normal to Σ and $\mathbf{x}$ is the position in space. The instantaneous problem as stated has only two dimensionless parameters:

$$G = \frac{\lambda_M}{\lambda_R}(1 - B), \quad A = \frac{\lambda_A/\lambda_M - B}{1 - B}. \tag{6.4}$$

The former describes the relative strength of cell mitosis to the relaxation mechanisms, and the latter describes the relative strength of cell apoptosis and mitosis. Effects of vascularization are in the parameter B (defined in [58]). Note that in the context of steady solutions, parameter A is related to parameter Λ (introduced in [37]) by $A = 3\Lambda$. The rescaled rate of change of tumor volume $H = \int_\Omega dx^d$ is defined as the mass flux $J = \frac{d}{dt}H = \int_\Sigma V dx^{d-1}$. By using (6.1) and (6.2) we obtain from (6.3):

$$J = -G \int_\Omega \Gamma dx^d - AGH. \tag{6.5}$$

6.2.3 Regimes of Growth

Considering evolution of a radially symmetric tumor identifies regimes of growth. The interface Σ is an infinite cylinder for $d = 2$ or a sphere for $d = 3$, with radius $R(t)$. All variables have only r-dependence, where r is the polar coordinate. Equations (6.1)–(6.2) have the nonsingular solutions

$$
\Gamma(r,t) = \begin{cases} \frac{I_0(r)}{I_0(R)}, & d = 2, \\[2mm] \left(\frac{\sinh(R)}{R}\right)^{-1}\left(\frac{\sinh(r)}{r}\right), & d = 3 \end{cases} \tag{6.6}
$$

and $p(r,t) = (d-1)R^{-1} - AGR^2/(2d)$. Note that $p(r,t) \equiv p(R,t)$, i.e., p is uniform across the tumor volume. From (6.3) the evolution equation for the tumor radius R is

$$
\frac{dR}{dt} = V = -AG\frac{R}{d} + G \begin{cases} \frac{I_1(R)}{I_0(R)}, & d = 2, \\[2mm] \left(\frac{1}{\tanh(R)} - \frac{1}{R}\right), & d = 3 \end{cases}. \tag{6.7}
$$

For a radially symmetric tumor, $|G|$ rescales time. In all dimensions, unbounded growth ($R \to \infty$) occurs if and only if $AG \le 0$. Growth velocity is plotted for $d = 2$ in Fig. 6.1. Note that, for $d = 3$, results are qualitatively similar and were reported in Fig. 9 in [37], although in the framework of the original formulation the growth regimes had not been identified. The figure is included here to identify the growth regimes. For given A, evolution from initial condition $R(0) = R_0$ occurs along the corresponding curve. Three regimes are identified, and the behavior is qualitatively unaffected by the number of spatial dimensions d.

1. *Low vascularization*: $G \ge 0$ and $A > 0$ (i.e., $B < \lambda_A/\lambda_M$). Note that the special case of avascular growth ($B = 0$) belongs to this regime. Evolution is monotonic and always leads to a stationary state R_∞, that corresponds to the intersection of the curves in Fig. 6.1 with the dotted line $V = 0$. This behavior is in agreement with experimental observations of in vitro diffusional growth [88] of avascular spheroids to a dormant steady state [146, 191]. In the experiments, however, tumors always develop a necrotic core that further stabilizes their growth [38].

2. *Moderate vascularization*: $G \ge 0$ and $A \le 0$ (i.e., $1 > B \ge \lambda_A/\lambda_M$). Unbounded growth occurs from any initial radius $R_0 > 0$. The growth tends to exponential for $A < 0$ with velocity $V \to -AGR/d$ as $R \to \infty$, and to linear for $A = 0$ with velocity $V \to G$ as $R \to \infty$.

3. *High vascularization*: $G < 0$ (i.e., $B > 1$). For $A > 0$, growth ($V > 0$) may occur, depending on the initial radius, and is always unbounded; for

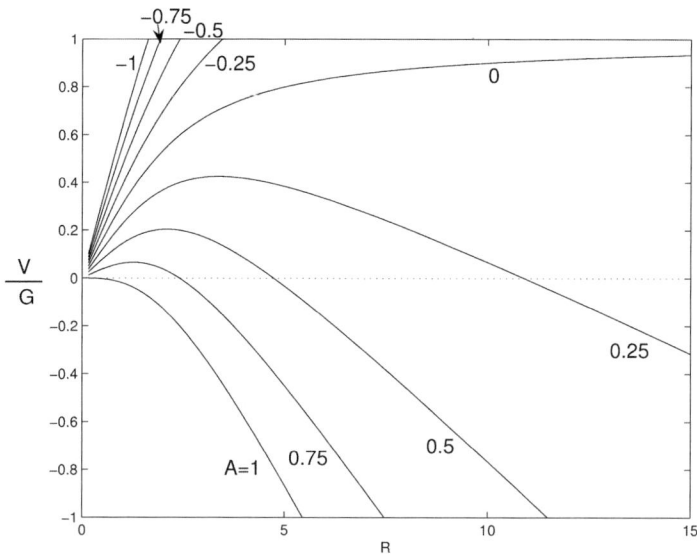

Fig. 6.1. Rescaled rate of growth $G^{-1}V$ from (6.7) as a function of rescaled tumor radius R for radially symmetric tumor growth and $d = 2$; A labeled. Reprinted from *Journal of Mathematical Biology*, Cristini et al., Vol. 46, p. 195, Copyright 2003 Springer. With kind permission of Springer Science and Business Media.

$A < 0$ (for which cell apoptosis is dominant: $\lambda_A/\lambda_M > B$), the evolution is always to the only stationary solution $R_\infty = 0$. This stationary solution may also be achieved for $A > 0$. The stationary radius R_∞ is independent of G, and is a solution of $V = 0$ with V from (6.7). The stationary radius has limiting behaviors

$$
\begin{aligned}
R_\infty &\to dA^{-1}, & A &\to 0, \\
R_\infty &\to d^{\frac{1}{2}}(d+2)^{\frac{1}{2}}(1-A)^{\frac{1}{2}}, & A &\to 1
\end{aligned}
\tag{6.8}
$$

where R_∞ vanishes. Note that the limit $A \to 1$ corresponds to $\lambda_A \to \lambda_M$.

Pressure P_C at the center of the tumor ($r \equiv 0$) can be calculated as (see [58]):

$$
\frac{P_C}{\gamma/L_D} = (d-1)/R + G - AGR^2/(2d) - G
\begin{cases}
1/I_0(R), & d = 2, \\[2mm]
R/\sinh(R), & d = 3
\end{cases}
\tag{6.9}
$$

which has asymptotic behavior $P_C(\gamma/L_D)^{-1} \to -AGR^2/(2d)$ as $R \to \infty$, indicating that if the tumor grows unbounded ($AG \leq 0$) the pressure at the center also does (unless $A = 0$). This is a direct consequence of the absence of a necrotic core in this model. In reality, increasing pressure may itself contribute to necrosis [149, 162]. It is known [45] that tumor cells continuously replace the loss of cell volume in a tumor because of necrosis, thus maintaining pressure finite.

6.2.4 Linear Analysis

Consider a perturbation of the spherical tumor interface Σ:

$$
R(t) + \delta(t) \begin{cases} \cos(l\theta), & d = 2, \\ \\ Y_{l,m}(\theta, \phi), & d = 3 \end{cases} \tag{6.10}
$$

where δ is the dimensionless perturbation size and $Y_{l,m}$ is a spherical harmonic, where l and θ are polar wavenumber and angle, and m and ϕ are azimuthal wavenumber and angle. By solving the system of (6.1)–(6.3) in the presence of a perturbed interface we obtain evolution (6.7) for unperturbed radius R and perturbation size δ using the shape factor δ/R:

$$
(\frac{\delta}{R})^{-1}\frac{d\frac{\delta}{R}}{dt} = \begin{cases} G - \frac{l(l^2-1)}{R^3} - G\frac{l+2}{R}\frac{I_1(R)}{I_0(R)} - G\frac{I_{l+1}(R)}{I_l(R)}\frac{I_1(R)}{I_0(R)} + l\frac{AG}{2}, & d = 2 \\ \\ G - \frac{l(l+2)(l-1)}{R^3} \\ \\ - (G\frac{l+3}{R} + G\frac{I_{l+3/2}(R)}{I_{l+1/2}(R)})(\frac{1}{\tanh(R)} - \frac{1}{R}) + l\frac{AG}{3}, & d = 3 \end{cases}
\tag{6.11}
$$

Note that linear evolution of the perturbation is independent of azimuthal wavenumber m and there is a critical mode l_c such that perturbations grow for $l < l_c$ and decay for $l > l_c$. The critical mode depends on the parameters A, G, and the evolving radius R. This agrees with the linear analyses presented in [89, 37, 40] for the special case where the unperturbed configuration is stationary (i.e., R constant).

6.2.5 Results

Unstable Growth in 2-D

We investigate unstable evolution in the low-vascularization (diffusion-dominated) regime, characterized by G, $A > 0$, for $d = 2$ using nonlinear boundary integral simulations. The linear analysis demonstrates that evolution in the other regimes is stable for $d = 2$. In Fig. 6.2, the evolution of the tumor surface from a nonlinear boundary integral simulation with $N = 1024$ and $\triangle t = 10^{-3}$ (solid curve) is compared to the result of the linear analysis (dotted). In this case $A = 0.5$, $G = 20$, and the initial shape of the tumor is

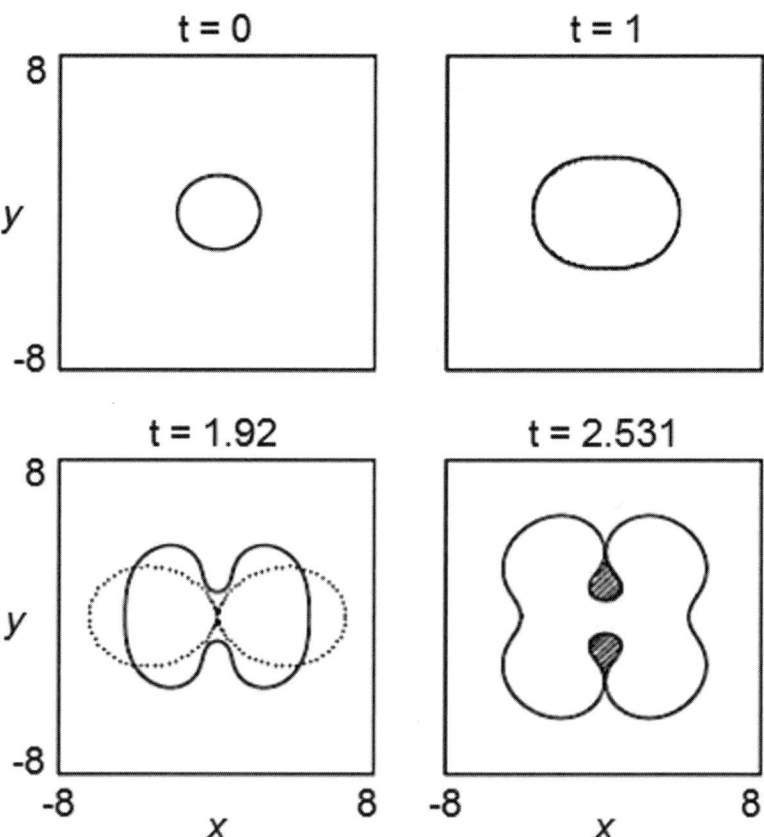

Fig. 6.2. Evolution of the tumor surface in the low-vascularization regime, for $d = 2$, $A = 0.5$, $G = 20$, and initial tumor surface as in equation (6.12). Dotted lines: solution from linear analysis; solid: solution from a nonlinear calculation with time step $\Delta t = 10^{-3}$ and a number of marker points $N = 1024$, reset, after time $t = 2.51$, to $\Delta t = 10^{-4}$ and $N = 2048$. Reprinted from *Journal of Mathematical Biology*, Cristini et al. Vol. 46, p. 202, Copyright 2003 Springer. With kind permission of Springer Science and Business Media.

$$(x(\alpha), y(\alpha)) = (2 + 0.1 \cos(2\alpha)(\cos(\alpha), \sin(\alpha))) . \tag{6.12}$$

According to linear theory ((6.7) and Fig. 6.1), the tumor grows. The radially symmetric equilibrium radius $R_\infty \approx 3.32$. Mode $l = 2$ is linearly stable initially, and becomes unstable at $R \approx 2.29$. The linear and nonlinear results in Fig. 6.2 are indistinguishable up to $t = 1$, and gradually deviate thereafter. Correspondingly, a shape instability develops and forms a neck. At $t \approx 1.9$ the linear solution collapses suggesting pinch-off; the nonlinear solution is stabilized by the cell-to-cell adhesive forces (surface tension) that resist development of high negative curvatures in the neck. This is not captured by the linear analysis. Instead of pinching off, as is predicted by linear evolution, the nonlinear tumor continues to grow and develops large bulbs that eventually reconnect thus trapping healthy tissue (shaded regions in the last frame in Fig. 6.2) within the tumor. The frame at $t = 2.531$ describes the onset of reconnection of the bulbs. We expect that reconnection would be affected by diffusion of nutrient outside the tumor, which is not included in the model used here. However, predictions of development of shape instabilities and of capture of healthy tissue during growth are in agreement with experimental observations [168].

We have found that during unstable evolution the linear and nonlinear solutions deviate from one another with the nonlinear solution being stabilized against pinch-off and leading instead to tumor reconnection and encapsulation of healthy tissue at later times as observed experimentally [168]. Reconnection occurs even when the amount of apoptosis is increased.

Unstable Growth in 3-D

We investigate the nonlinear, unstable evolution of 3-D tumors in the low-vascularization regime characterized by $G \geq 0$ and $A > 0$ by focusing on the parameters $G = 20$ and $A = 0.5$. Note that a spherical tumor with these parameters reaches a steady state with corresponding scale factor $S = 4.73$. The evolution is considered using three different initial conditions. In Fig. 6.3, the morphological evolution of a tumor is shown from the initial radius

$$r = 1 + 0.033 Y_{2,2}(\theta, \phi) \qquad (6.13)$$

with the initial scale factor $S(0) = 3.002$. Two 3-D views of the morphology are shown, as indicated. The tumor does not change volume in the simulation because spatial rescaling is used in the algorithm. The associated evolution of the scale factor $S(t)$ is shown in Fig. 6.4(a).

At early times, the perturbation decreases and the tumor becomes sphere-like. As the tumor continues to grow, the perturbation starts to increase around time $t \approx 0.4$ when the scale factor $S \approx 3.7$. The tumor then takes on a flattened ellipse-like shape. Around time $t \approx 2.2$ when $S \approx 4.6$, the perturbation growth accelerates dramatically, and dimples form around time $t \approx 2.42$. The dimples deepen, and the tumor surface buckles inwards. The instability and dimple formation allow the tumor to increase its surface area relative to its volume, thereby allowing the cells in the tumor bulk greater access to nutrient. This in turn allows the tumor to overcome the diffusional limitations on growth and to grow to larger sizes than would be possible if the tumor were spherical. For example, in Fig. 6.3d, the scale factor $S \approx 4.78$, which is larger than the corresponding value (4.73) for the steady state spherical tumor. (Note that the tumor is continuing to grow.) This provides additional support in 3-D for the hypothesis put forth by [58, 54, 55] based on 2-D simulations that morphologic instability allows an additional pathway for tumor

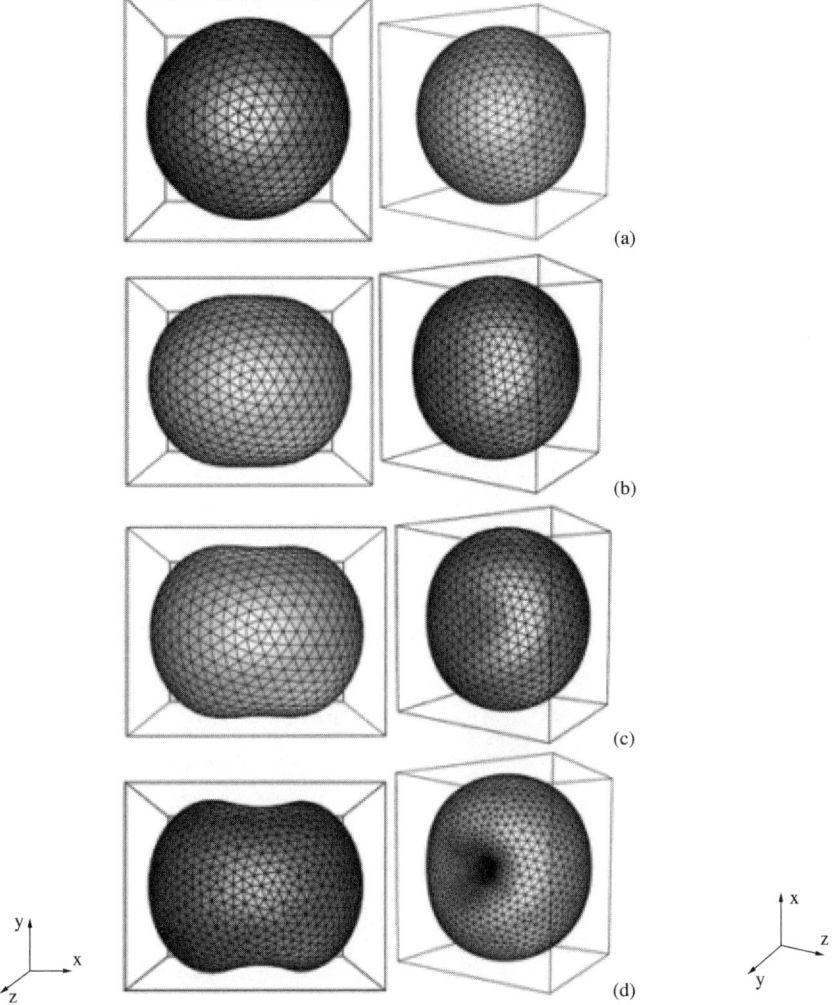

Fig. 6.3. Evolution of the tumor surface in the low-vascularization regime, $A = 0.5$, $G = 20$, and initial tumor surface as in (6.13). (a) $t = 0$, $\bar{\delta} = 0.0137$, $S = 3.0$; (b) $t = 2.21$, $\bar{\delta} = 0.12$, $S = 4.732$; (c) $t = 2.42$, $\bar{\delta} = 0.2$, $S = 4.745$; (d) $t = 2.668$, $\bar{\delta} = 0.496$, $S = 4.781$. Reprinted with permission from *Discrete and Continuous Dynamical Systems - Series B*, Li et al., Vol. 7, p. 599. Copyright 2007 American Institute of Mathematical Sciences.

invasion that does not require an additional nutrient source such as would be provided from a newly developing vasculature through angiogenesis.

In this simulation, the number of mesh points is $N = 1024$ initially. As seen in Fig. 6.3, the mesh adaptively clusters near the dimples where there is

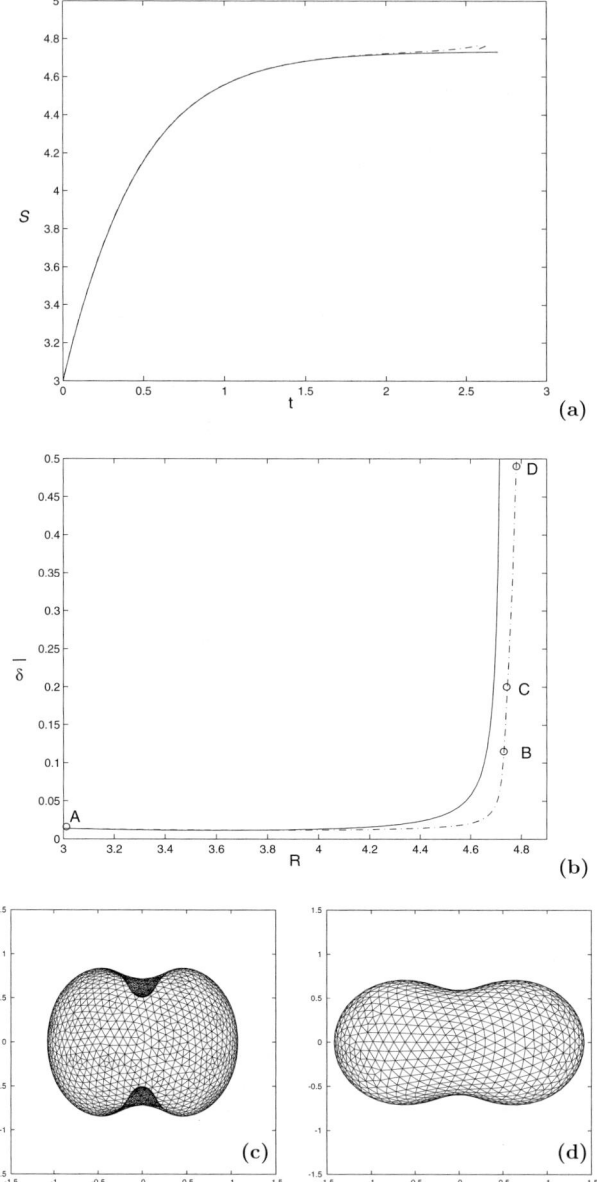

Fig. 6.4. Comparison of linear analysis (solid) and nonlinear results (dash-dotted) for the simulation in Fig. 6.3. (a) Scale factor $S(t)$; (b) Perturbation size $\overline{\delta}$; circles correspond to morphologies in Fig. 6.3 (a)–(d). (c) Nonlinear tumor morphology at $t = 2.668$, with $S = 4.78$ and $\overline{\delta} = 0.496$; (d). Linear solution morphology (shown with a triangulated mesh) at the same time, $S = 4.73$ and $\overline{\delta} = 0.42$. Positive z-axis view. Reprinted with permission from *Discrete and Continuous Dynamical Systems - Series B*, Li et al., Vol. 7, p. 600. Copyright 2007 American Institute of Mathematical Sciences.

large negative curvature thereby providing enhanced local resolution. At the final time $t_f = 2.67$ (with $S \approx 4.78$) there are $N = 2439$ nodes on the tumor surface. To compute for longer times, higher resolution is necessary.

We next compare the nonlinear results with the predictions of linear theory. To estimate the shape perturbation size $\bar{\delta}$ in the nonlinear simulation, we take

$$\bar{\delta} = \max_{\Sigma} |r_{\Sigma} - 1| \qquad (6.14)$$

since the overall bulk growth is scaled out of the nonlinear evolution by the scale factor $S(t)$ (the maximum is taken over all the computational nodes of the interface).

In Fig. 6.4b, the results of linear theory (solid) and nonlinear simulations (dashed-dot) for the perturbation size are shown as functions of $S(t)$ for the evolution from Fig. 6.3. Linear theory predicts that for $G = 20$, $A = 0.5$, the 2-mode is stable for $S < 3.54$. This is borne out by the nonlinear simulation, which agrees very well with the linear theory up until $S \approx 3.5$ where the linear theory predicts the perturbation starts to grow. In the nonlinear simulation, the perturbation continues to decay until $S \approx 3.7$. Although the linear and nonlinear results deviate at larger S with linear theory predicting larger perturbations, the qualitative behavior of the shape perturbation is very similar in both cases. In particular, there is rapid growth of the perturbation near $R \approx 4.6$. The circled points labeled A–D on the dashed-dot curve (nonlinear simulation) correspond to the morphologies shown in Figs. 6.3a–d. Note that at the final time, the nonlinear perturbation $\bar{\delta} \approx 0.5$, and so the evolution is highly nonlinear.

In Figs. 6.4c and 6.4d, the nonlinear and linear tumor morphologies, respectively, are shown at time $t = 2.668$ where $S \approx 4.78$ and $S_{\text{linear}} \approx 4.73$. The linear morphology is generated by evolving a sphere to the shape prescribed by linear theory. This is why the linear solution is shown with a triangulated mesh. The corresponding nonlinear and linear perturbation sizes are $\bar{\delta} = 0.496$ and $\delta/R = 0.42$ respectively. Note that the reason the linear result is smaller than the nonlinear value at this time is because the linear scale factor is slightly less than that from the nonlinear simulation which, when combined with the rapid growth of the perturbation around $S \approx 4.76$, gives rise to this behavior.

As seen in Figs. 6.4c and 6.4d, the nonlinear tumor morphology is more compact than the corresponding linear result. In fact, the linear perturbation eventually grows so large that the tumor pinches off in the center. In contrast, nonlinearity introduces additional modes that alter the growth directions, from primarily horizontal in Fig. 6.4d to more vertical in Fig. 6.4c, thereby avoiding pinch-off and resulting in more compact shapes. This is consistent with the 2-D results of [58].

Nontrivial Stationary States

We study the case of nontrivial nonlinear stationary states in the low-vascularization regime. That such states exist was recently proved [80] and is predicted by linear theory. To see this, let us consider the linear evolution of a perturbation of a stationary radius R_∞. The stationary radius is the solution of (6.7) with $V = 0$ (see also the related text) and is a function of $0 < A < 1$. Thus, the flux $J = 0$ and (6.11) indicates that there exists a critical

$$
G_l = \begin{cases}
R_\infty^{-3} \dfrac{2l(l^2-1)}{2-A[2+R_\infty I_{l+1}(R_\infty)/I_l(R_\infty)]}, & d = 2, \\[3mm]
R_\infty^{-3} \dfrac{3l(l-1)(l+2)}{3-A[3+R_\infty I_{l+3/2}(R_\infty)/I_{l+1/2}(R_\infty)]}, & d = 3
\end{cases}
\tag{6.15}
$$

such that for $G = G_l$ the perturbation also remains stationary. It can be shown that for both $d = 2$ and $d = 3$, $G_l > 0$ and a perturbed stationary shape always exists. The perturbation δ/R_∞ grows unbounded for $G > G_l$ and decays to zero for $G < G_l$. At large radii R_∞, $G_l \to 0$; thus, in this limit perturbations of stationary states always grow unbounded.

Next consider the nonlinear evolution for $d = 2$ of a mode l perturbation, which is predicted by the linear theory to be stationary. We let the value of G be equal to G_l, with $R = R_\infty$. Although the perturbations are linearly stationary, there is evolution due to nonlinearity. Our results (not shown) strongly suggest that for given l there exists a critical $G_l^{\mathrm{NL}} < G_l$ such that for $G = G_l^{\mathrm{NL}}$ a nonlinear, nontrivial steady shape exists. Thus, nonlinearity is destabilizing for the stationary shapes. This is in contrast with the results obtained earlier where nonlinearity stabilizes the pinch-off predicted by linear theory during unstable evolution. Finally, as expected, the deviation of G_l^{NL} from the linear G_l is second order (not shown).

Self-Similar Evolution

We investigate conditions for which the tumor grows self-similarly, thus maintaining its shape. This should have implications for angiogenesis, or tumor vascularization. It is known that angiogenesis occurs as tumor angiogenic factors are released, diffusing to nearby vessels and triggering chemotaxis of endothelial cells and thus the formation of a network of blood vessels that finally penetrates the tumor, providing nutrients. Assuming the flux of angiogenic factors to be proportional to the tumor/tissue interface area and the rate of production of angiogenic factors to be proportional to the tumor volume, we conclude that self-similar evolution divides tumor growth into two categories: one (stable growth) characterized by a decrease of the area-to-volume ratio during growth thus hampering or preventing angiogenesis, and the other (unstable growth) characterized by an increase of the area-to-volume ratio and thus favoring angiogenesis.

To maintain self-similar evolution during growth we may set $\frac{d}{dt}(\delta/R) = 0$ identically. This can be achieved by keeping G constant and varying A as a function of the unperturbed radius R by

$$A = \begin{cases} \frac{2(l^2-1)}{GR^3} + 2(l + \frac{2}{l})\frac{1}{R}\frac{I_1(R)}{I_0(R)} + \frac{2}{l}\frac{I_{l+1}(R)I_1(R)}{I_l(R)I_0(R)} - \frac{2}{l}, & d = 2, \\[2em] \frac{3(l-1)(l+2)}{GR^3} + 3(l + \frac{3}{l})\frac{1}{R}\left(\frac{1}{\tanh R} - \frac{1}{R}\right) \\[1em] \quad + \frac{3}{l}\frac{I_{l+3/2}(R)}{I_{l+1/2}(R)}\left(\frac{1}{\tanh R} - \frac{1}{R}\right) - \frac{3}{l}, & d = 3 \end{cases} \tag{6.16}$$

In Fig. 6.5 (top) apoptosis parameter $A(R)$ is shown for $d = 2$ (dashed lines) and $d = 3$ (solid). Growth velocity corresponding to self-similar evolution, obtained from (6.7) with A given by (6.16), is plotted in Fig. 6.5 (bottom). Curves of A divide the plot into regions of stable growth and regions of unstable growth of a given mode l. Figures 6.5 top and bottom indicate that in the low-vascularization (diffusion-dominated) regime ($G > 0, A > 0$) self-similar evolution towards a stationary state is not possible for G constant (stationary states R_∞ correspond to intersection of curves (6.16) in Fig. 6.5 (top) with the curves describing stationary radii). For instance, growth velocity $V < 0$ for initial radius $R_0 < R_\infty$, and thus self-similar shrinkage of the tumor to zero occurs. On the other hand, for $R_0 > R_\infty$, $V > 0$, and thus self-similar growth away from the stationary radius occurs. In the high-vascularization regime ($G < 0$), during self-similar evolution the velocity $V < 0$. Thus self-similar shrinkage of a tumor from arbitrary initial conditions to a point occurs, and self-similar unbounded growth is not possible.

To summarize, self-similar evolution, with the possiblity of shape control, is found in both low- and high-vascularization regimes with varying A and constant G. However, in the low-vascularization regime, self-similar evolution to a steady state does not occur under these conditions. Similarly, self-similar unbounded growth in the high- or moderate-vascularization regime does not occur. Further examinations [58] reveal the possibility of self-similar evolution to a steady state in the low-vascularization regime and of unbounded self-similar growth in the high-vascularization regime by varying G in addition to A.

Effect of Nonlinearity

We investigate the effect of nonlinearity on the self-similar evolution for $d = 2$ predicted by the linear analysis. As discussed above, self-similar evolution requires time-dependent apoptosis parameter $A = A(l, G, R)$ and is plotted in Fig. 6.5 (top). Radius R, used in the nonlinear simulation, is determined by the area of an equivalent circle: $R = \sqrt{H/\pi}$. In Fig. 6.6, the linear and nonlinear solutions are compared in the low-vascularization regime for $l = 5$,

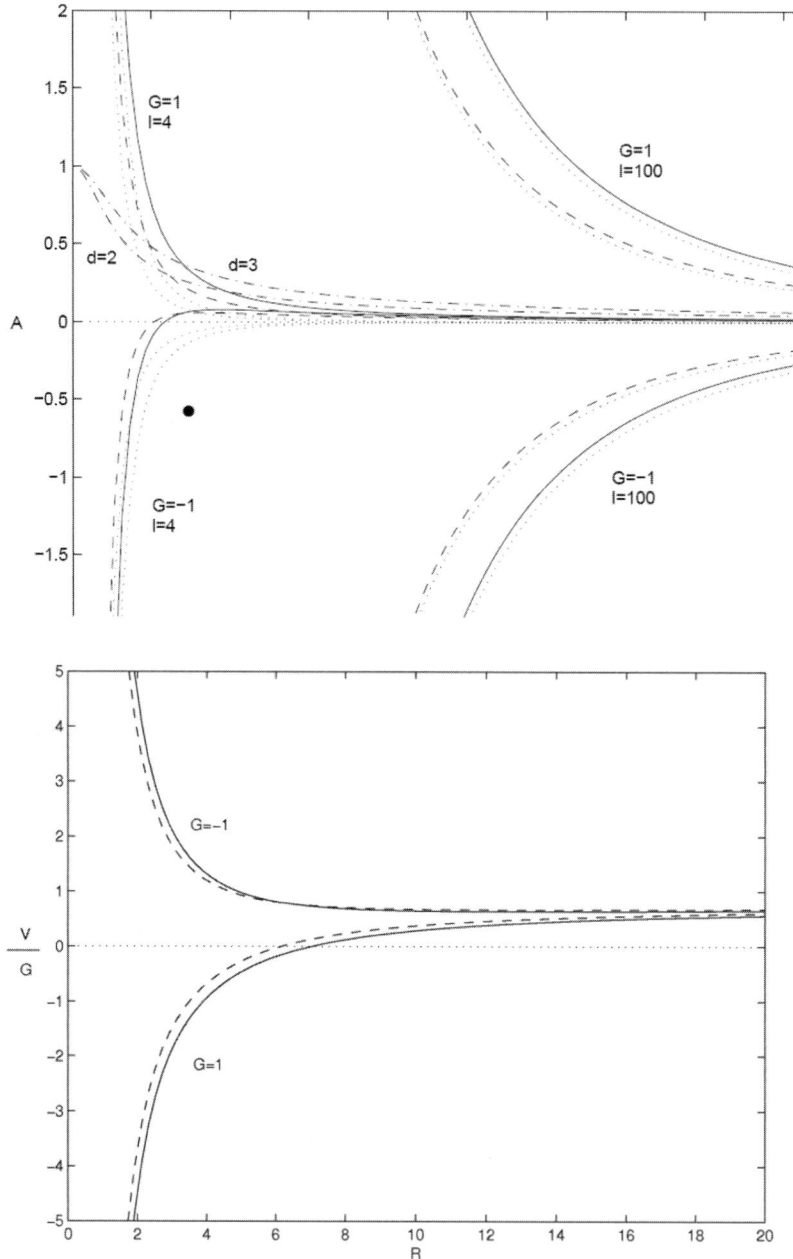

Fig. 6.5. Top: apoptosis parameter A as a function of unperturbed radius R from condition (6.16) for self-similar evolution; $d = 2$ (dashed) and $d = 3$ (solid); G and l labeled. Asymptotic behaviors are dotted (see [58]). The two solid curves labeled with values of d correspond to stationary radii. Reprinted with permission from *Discrete and Continuous Dynamical Systems - Series B,* Li et al., Vol. 7, p. 598. Copyright 2007 American Institute of Mathematical Sciences. **Bottom**: corresponding growth velocity $G^{-1}V$ for $l = 4$.

$G = 1$, $A = A(l, G, R)$ and $R_0 = 4$. Since $V < 0$, the tumors shrink and A increases. In the left frame, $\delta_0 = 0.2$ and in the right $\delta_0 = 0.4$. Results reveal that large perturbations are nonlinearly unstable and grow, leading to a topological transition. In the right frame, the onset of pinch-off is evident. This can have important implications for therapy. For example, one can imagine an experiment in which a tumor is made to shrink by therapy such that A is increased by increasing the apoptosis rate λ_A. This example shows that a rapid decrease in size can result in shape instability leading to tumor break-up and the formation of microscopic tumor fragments that can enter the blood stream through leaky blood vessels thus leading to metastases.

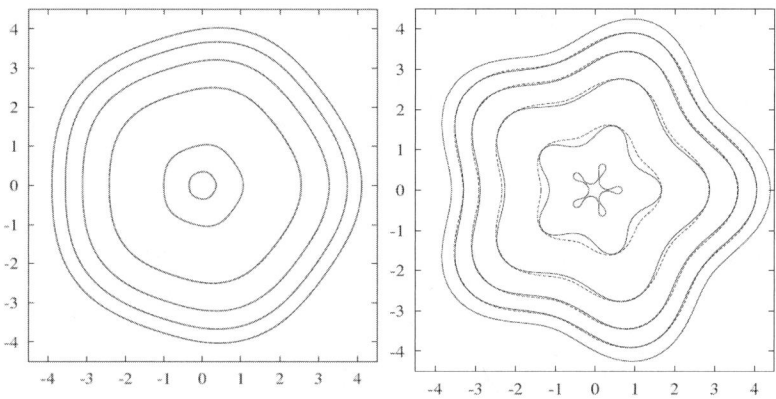

Fig. 6.6. Left: self-similar shrinkage for $R_0 = 4$ and $\delta_0 = 0.2$ ($t = 0$ to 0.96 shown). **Right**: unstable shrinkage for $R_0 = 4$ and $\delta_0 = 0.4$ ($t = 0$ to 0.99). The solid curves correspond to the nonlinear solution and the dashed curves to the linear. In both cases, $d = 2$, $G = 1$, $l = 5$, and the evolution is in the low-vascularization regime. $A = A(l, G, R)$ given in (6.16) and plotted in Fig. 6.5 (top). Reprinted from *Journal of Mathematical Biology*, Cristini et al. Vol. 46, p. 215, Copyright 2003 Springer. With kind permission of Springer Science and Business Media.

Evolution in the High-Vascularization Regime

In the high-vascularization regime ($G < 0$), both shrinkage and growth of tumors occur. Shrinkage ($A < 0$) may be stable, self-similar, and unstable. In contrast, unbounded growth ($A > 0$) is always characterized by a decay of the perturbation to zero with respect to the unperturbed radius and is thus stable for both $d = 2$ and $d = 3$. In the nonlinear regime, the self-similar and the unstable shrinkage are qualitatively very similar to that presented in Fig. 6.6. In fact, all the nonlinear simulations of growth in the high-vascularization regime lead to stable evolution, in agreement with the linear analysis. In contrast, it is known experimentally that highly vascularized cancers evolve invasively by extending branches into regions of the external tissue where mechanical resistance is lowest (see, e.g., [45]). Thus these results suggest that formation of invasive tumors should be due to anisotropies rather than to vascularization alone. Anisotropies (e.g., in the distribution of the resistance of the external tissue to tumor growth, or in the distribution of blood vessels) have been neglected in the model studied here. This conclusion has not been recognized before and is supported by experiments [150] of in vivo angiogenesis and tumor growth.

6.2.6 Summary

This work [58, 126] has studied solid tumor growth in the nonlinear regime using boundary integral simulations. In the model investigated [89, 141, 39, 40], the tumor core is assumed to be nonnecrotic and with no inhibitor factors present. A new formulation of this classical model was developed, and it was demonstrated that tumor evolution can be described by a reduced set of two dimensionless parameters and is qualitatively unaffected by the number of spatial dimensions. By constructing explicit examples using nonlinear simulations, it was demonstrated that critical conditions exist for which the tumor evolves to nontrivial dormant states or grows self-similarly. Self-similar growth separates stable tumors that grow maintaining a compact shape from unstable tumors, for which vascularization is favored and growth leads to invasive fingering into the healthy tissues. The possibility of tumor shape control during growth is suggested [58] by simulating a physical experiment in which the dimensionless parameters are varied in time to maintain stable or self-similar growth conditions, thus preventing invasive growth and hampering angiogenesis. It can also be shown that nonlinear unstable growth may lead to topological transitions such as tumor breakup and reconnection with encapsulation of healthy tissue [58]. The boundary integral methods reviewed here provide evidence that morphologic instability represents an additional means for tumor invasion.

6.3 Vascularized Tumor Growth Using an Adaptive Finite Element/Level Set Method[6]

6.3.1 Overview

In [211] we use a reformulation of several well-known continuum-scale models of growth and angiogenesis ([89, 37, 38, 45, 11, 79, 24, 15]). We build upon the

---

[6] Portions of this section are reprinted with permission from *Bull. Math. Biol.*, Zheng et al., Vol. 67, pp. 211–259, Copyright 2005 Springer (with kind permission of Springer Science and Business Media).

biological complexity of previous models that used boundary integral methods [58, 126] (described in Sect. 6.2), where tissue is represented as a constant-density fluid whose elasticity is neglected. Some cell-cell adhesion is modeled using a surface force at the tumor interface. A single vital nutrient is modeled, e.g., oxygen or glucose that is required for cell survival and mitosis. Nutrient diffuses through the extracellular matrix (ECM) and is taken up by tumor cells. Growth in this case is diffusion limited and necrosis may occur, unlike the methods in Sect. 6.2. Necrosis is represented as the region where nutrient is depleted below a certain level needed for cell viability. Once necrosis forms, the tumor releases tumor angiogenic factors (TAFs), such as vascular endothelial growth factor (VEGF), which stimulate vascular endothelial cells to migrate toward the tumor. TAF is described through a reaction-diffusion equation with a point boundary condition set on the necrotic rim, modeling the release of TAF. The endothelial cells density (ECD) obeys a reaction diffusion-convection equation. The problem is convection dominated, with the primary source of convection driven by chemotaxis of endothelial cells with respect to TAF concentration. The actual formation of capillaries from endothelial cells is modeled using a combined continuum-discrete model [11], coupling the vascular system with tumor growth for the first time.

This combined continuum/discrete-scale model demonstrates the capabilities for nonlinear simulation of in vivo cancer progression in two dimensions, for which state-of-the art numerical methods based on sophisticated finite element techniques are necessary. The level set method [153] is employed for capturing invasive fingering and complex topological changes such as tumor splitting and reconnection, and healthy tissue capture. An adaptive, unstructured mesh [53] is used that allows for finely resolving important regions of the computational domain such as the necrotic rim, the tumor interface, and the area around capillary sprouts. The adaptive mesh provides for enormous computational savings by greatly reducing the number of finite elements needed to resolve the finest length scale, when compared to a structured mesh having equal resolution.

6.3.2 Dimensional Formulation of the Model

The growth component of the model is inspired by the work of [89, 37, 38, 45, 79, 58]. The angiogenesis model is essentially that of [11] with some additions gleaned from [51, 158, 156]. Fig. 6.7 gives a basic description of these components, oversimplifying the underlying tumor physiology. The *growth* block is composed of nutrient transport, cell proliferation, and a constitutive equation that relates interstitial pressure and cell velocity. The *angiogenesis* block is composed of endothelial cell, fibronectin, and (TAF) transport equations. The schematic also illustrates how the two blocks are coupled throughout the evolution of a solid tumor. The instantaneous position of the necrotic rim $\Sigma_N(t)$ is determined by solving the growth problem and becomes an input to the angiogenesis problem by acting as a source of angiogenic factors.

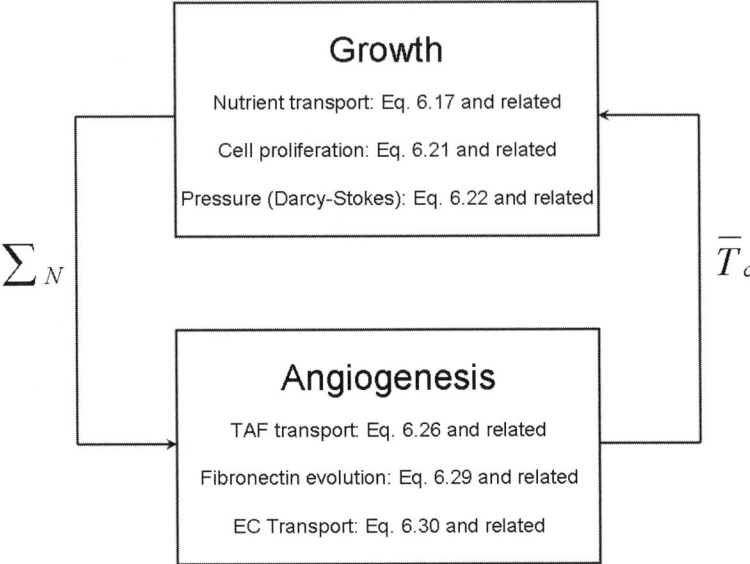

Fig. 6.7. Progression of a solid tumor is the result of coupling of growth and angiogenesis components that are mainly linked by the instantaneous position of the necrotic rim Σ_N and the blood-to-tissue nutrient transfer rate $\overline{T}_c$. Reprinted with permission from *Bull. Math. Biol.*, Zheng et al. Vol. 67, p. 214, Copyright 2005 Springer. With kind permission of Springer Science and Business Media.

Transfer of nutrients from capillaries to the tissue (characterized by the rate $\overline{T}_c$) depends on the instantaneous spatial distribution of capillaries determined by solving the angiogenesis problem and is an input to the *growth* block by acting as a source of nutrients. Rates (inverse time scales) are denoted by lowercase Greek letters with the following subscripts: (A) Apoptosis, (D) natural Degradation, (M) Mitosis, (N) Necrosis, (P) Production, or (U) Uptake. An overbar on a symbol indicates a dimensional parameter; the absence of an overbar indicates the corresponding nondimensional parameter. The field variables are

- concentration of tumor angiogenic factor (TAF) c
- endothelial cell's density (ECD) e
- density of fibronectin f
- concentration of (vital) nutrient n
- pressure p
- velocity $\mathbf{u}$

Both dimensional and nondimensional fields are expressed by the same symbol; the difference will be clear from the context.

Tumor Growth

Consider a computational tissue domain Ω that contains three disjoint sub-domains, viable tumor Ω_V, necrotic core Ω_N, and external healthy tissue Ω_H (cf. Fig. 6.8). The necrotic core contains cells that are not viable due to a lack of available nutrients and is defined as $\Omega_N = \{\mathbf{x}|\mathbf{n}(\mathbf{x}) \leq \overline{\mathbf{n}}_{\mathbf{N}}\} \setminus \Omega_H$, where $\overline{n}_N$ is the minimum nutrient level for cell viability. For simplicity, healthy cells are assumed to remain viable even when nutrient falls below $\overline{n}_N$. The tumor domain, which is defined as $\Omega_T = \Omega_V \cup \Omega_N$, contains both viable and necrotic cells. The nutrient concentration n obeys the following:

$$0 = \overline{D}_n \nabla^2 n + \begin{cases} \overline{T}_c - \overline{\nu}_U n & \text{if } x \in \Omega_V \\ \overline{T}_c & \text{if } x \in \Omega_H \\ 0 & \text{if } x \in \Omega_N \end{cases} \quad (6.17)$$

where $\overline{D}_n$ is a diffusion constant, $\overline{\nu}_U$ is nutrient consumption rate by the tumor cells, and $\overline{T}_c$ is the capillary-to-tissue nutrient transfer function. There is assumed to be no transfer of nutrients in the necrotic core. $\overline{T}_c$ may vary depending on the differences in nutrient and pressure levels between the capillaries and the surrounding tissue. We use the simple model $\overline{T}_c = \overline{T}_c^{\text{ang}} + \overline{T}_c^{\text{pre}}$ where

$$\overline{T}_c^{\text{ang}} = \overline{\nu}_p^{\text{ang}}(\overline{n}_c - n)b^{\text{ang}}(p)\delta_c \quad (6.18)$$

$$\overline{T}_c^{\text{pre}} = \overline{\nu}_p^{\text{pre}}(\overline{n}_c - n)b^{\text{pre}}(p), \quad (6.19)$$

where "ang" and "pre" denote new capillaries formed during angiogenesis and the uniformly distributed, preexisting capillaries, respectively. The $\overline{\nu}_p^*$ (* = ang, pre) are nutrient transfer (production) rates for new and old capillaries, $\overline{n}_c$ is nutrient concentration in capillaries, and p is tissue pressure. Pressure functions $b^*(p)$ have the form $b^*(p) = H(\overline{p}_c^* - p)(\overline{p}_c^* - p)/\overline{p}_T$, where $\overline{p}_c^*$ are new and preexisting capillary blood pressures, and $\overline{p}_T$ is a characteristic tissue pressure. δ_C is a dimensionless line delta function supported on the line domain Σ_C, where Σ_C describes the positions of all those capillaries that have formed loops in the new vasculature, hereby assuming that effective blood flow only occurs in capillaries that have formed loops (see Fig. 6.8). Integrating (6.17) gives line sources of nutrients emanating from the looped capillaries.

The nutrient concentration is fixed at the outer (far field) boundary Σ_∞, and is continuous (up to the first derivative) at interface Σ between the tumor and healthy tissue domains and at the necrotic interface $\Sigma_N = \{\mathbf{x}|\mathbf{n}(\mathbf{x}) = \overline{\mathbf{n}}_{\mathbf{N}}\} \setminus \Omega_H$ between the necrotic core and healthy tissue:

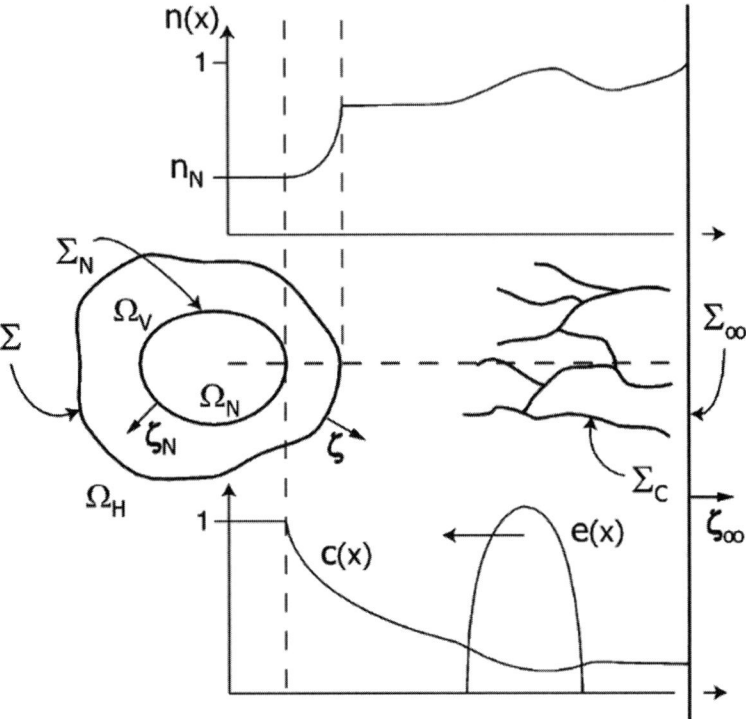

Fig. 6.8. Schematic (not to scale) of a necrotic tumor in transition from avascular to vascular growth gives a basic description of the model. Disjoint regions Ω_H, Ω_V, and Ω_N represent healthy tissue, viable tumoral tissue, and necrotic core domains, respectively. Tumor region is $\Omega_T = \Omega_V \cup \Omega_N$. Σ_∞ is far field boundary, Σ is tumor interface, and Σ_N is necrotic rim. Capillaries are defined on Σ_C. For illustration, nutrient concentration $n(x)$, TAF concentration $c(x)$, and endothelial cell density $e(x)$ are plotted along horizontal dashed line. Reprinted with permission from *Bull. Math. Biol.*, Zheng et al. Vol. 67, p. 215, Copyright 2005 Springer. With kind permission of Springer Science and Business Media.

$$n = \bar{n}_\infty \qquad \text{on } \Sigma_\infty$$

$$[n] = 0, \quad [\zeta \cdot \nabla n] = 0 \quad \text{on } \Sigma$$

$$n = \bar{n}_N, \quad [\zeta_N \cdot \nabla n] = 0 \qquad \text{on } \Sigma_N, \tag{6.20}$$

where ζ and ζ_N are unit normal vectors on Σ and Σ_N, respectively and $[\cdot]$ denotes the jump of the quantity across the interface (value inside minus value outside). Tumor cell proliferation leads to motion of the cells and growth of the overall tumor. The divergence of the cell velocity field obeys the equations

$$
\nabla \cdot \mathbf{u} = \begin{cases} \lambda_M n/\overline{n}_\infty - \overline{\lambda}_A & \text{if } \mathbf{x} \in \Omega_V \\ 0 & \text{if } \mathbf{x} \in \Omega_H \\ -\overline{\lambda}_N & \text{if } \mathbf{x} \in \Omega_N \end{cases} \tag{6.21}
$$

where cell mitosis is assumed proportional to local nutrient concentration and $\overline{\lambda}_M$ is the characteristic tumor cell mitosis rate. Parameter $\overline{\lambda}_A$ is the tumor cell apoptosis rate, and $\overline{\lambda}_N$ is a rate of volume loss in the necrotic core modeling cell necrosis and disintegration therein. Note that diffusion and chemotaxis of tumor cells is neglected, which have been taken into account in the model by [47], to emphasize tissue invasion due to uncontrolled proliferation of tumor cells. It should be noted that diffusion of cells is orders of magnitude smaller than advection, and that extent of chemotactic response of tumor cells is not universally agreed upon. Tumor cells are modeled at the continuum level as a viscous fluid (e.g., see [45]) flowing through a porous medium (ECM). Accordingly, the motion of tumor cells obeys the Darcy–Stokes law, [also called the Brinkman equation [195]: in Ω the velocity and pressure are related by

$$
\mathbf{u} - \overline{\varepsilon}\nabla^2\mathbf{u} = -\overline{\mu}\nabla\mathbf{p}\,, \tag{6.22}
$$

where $\overline{\varepsilon}$ is a constant and $\overline{\mu}$ is cell mobility. This is also called hydraulic conductivity [195] and represents in this case the extent of cell motion in response to a given pressure gradient, caused by nonhomogeneous cell proliferation. We introduce $\overline{\varepsilon}\nabla^2\mathbf{u}$ as a regularization term for the velocity and pressure and assume that $\overline{\varepsilon}$ is sufficiently small. This term helps keep the numerical scheme stable, especially with regard to the velocity calculation at the tumor interface. However, (6.22) can be regarded as physical (Batchelor, 1967, Chapter 3 [20])—whence $\overline{\varepsilon}$ becomes related to viscous stress associated to cell motion—upon introducing the physical pressure P, which is related to calculated (regularized) pressure p through $p = P - \frac{\overline{\varepsilon}}{3\overline{\mu}}\nabla \cdot \mathbf{u}$.

Velocity is assumed continuous across the necrotic rim, Σ_N, and tumor boundary Σ:

$$
[\mathbf{u}] = \mathbf{0} \text{ on } \Sigma_N, [\mathbf{u}] = \mathbf{0} \text{ on } \Sigma \tag{6.23}
$$

A regularized Laplace–Young jump condition is assumed at the tumor interface Σ to model cell-cell adhesion:

$$
((-p\mathbf{I} + \frac{\overline{\overline{\varepsilon}}}{\overline{\mu}}\nabla\mathbf{u}) \cdot \zeta) = -\overline{\gamma}\kappa\zeta \text{ on } \Sigma\,, \tag{6.24}
$$

where $\overline{\gamma}$ is the surface tension related to cell-to-cell adhesive forces, and κ is the local total curvature. Note that in this case the pressure may still experience a jump at the boundary when $\overline{\gamma} = 0$ and $\overline{\varepsilon} \neq 0$. At the outer boundary Σ_∞ we enforce the natural boundary condition:

$$(-p\mathbf{I} + \frac{\overline{\overline{\varepsilon}}}{\overline{\mu}}\nabla\mathbf{u}) \cdot \zeta_\infty = \mathbf{0} \text{ on } \mathbf{\Sigma}_\infty .\tag{6.25}$$

Angiogenesis

Once a tumor cell senses that the nutrient level has dropped below the minimum for viability, the cell releases TAFs that diffuse throughout the extracellular space. Endothelial cells become activated and migrate through the ECM towards the highest concentration of TAF at the necrotic rim of the tumor. As cell clusters move towards the tumor, the vasculature extends, using endothelial cells to construct the lining of capillaries (endothelium). This process is illustrated in Fig. 6.8. TAF molecules are much smaller than cells and diffuse quickly through the extracellular spaces. The quasi-steady reaction-diffusion equation is assumed for the concentration $c(\mathbf{x}, t)$ of TAF in Ω_H and Ω_V

$$0 = \overline{D}_c \nabla^2 c - \overline{\beta}_D c - \overline{\beta}_U ce/\overline{e}_0 ,\tag{6.26}$$

where $\overline{D}_c$ is the diffusion constant, $\overline{\beta}_D$ is the rate of natural decay of TAF, $\overline{\beta}_U$ is the rate of uptake of TAF by endothelial cells (of density e), and $\overline{e}_0$ is the maximum density of endothelial cells in Ω. Here, as a simplifying step and to reduce unknowns, parameters in the last equation are assumed homogeneous, which is in general not valid. In particular, diffusion can be different inside the tumor than outside, as the diffusivity should depend upon parameters such as the cellular density of tumor and healthy tissues.

The concentration of TAF is constant at the necrotic interface. Modeling the release of TAF by tumor cells as they undergo necrosis,

$$c = \overline{c}_0 \text{ on } \Sigma_N .\tag{6.27}$$

No-flux boundary conditions are imposed on Σ_∞:

$$\zeta_\infty \cdot \nabla c = 0 ,\tag{6.28}$$

where ζ_∞ is the surface unit normal on Σ_∞.

A primary component of the ECM is fibronectin, a long binding molecule that does not diffuse. Endothelial cells produce, degrade, and attach to these molecules during their migration toward the tumor. The concentration of fibronectin $f(\mathbf{x}, t)$ obeys

$$\frac{\partial f}{\partial t} = \overline{\eta}_p \overline{f}_0 e/\overline{e}_0 - \overline{\eta}_U fe/\overline{e}_0 - \overline{\eta}_N \chi_{\Omega_N} f ,\tag{6.29}$$

where $\overline{\eta}_p$ is the rate of production of fibronectin by endothelial cells and $\overline{\eta}_U$ is the rate of degradation of fibronectin by endothelial cells. Degradation of fibronectin is modeled due to the presence of the necrotic core, where $\overline{\eta}_N$ is the rate of decay in the necrotic core. The initial condition for concentration of fibronectin is taken as $f(\mathbf{x}, 0) = \overline{f}_0$, where $\overline{f}_0$ is the fibronectin concentration in healthy tissue. χ_S is the characteristic function of the set S: $\chi_S(\mathbf{x}) = 1$ if $\mathbf{x} \in S$ and vanishes otherwise.

Endothelial cells are comparable in size to healthy and tumor cells. However, we assume that the former are few enough in number that the interaction of the former does not affect the calculation of the cell velocity $\mathbf{u}$. Indeed, the ratio of endothelial to tissue cells is of the order $1/50$ or $1/100$ [34]. On the other hand, the motion of healthy and tumor cells is an important consideration on the convection of endothelial cells. The density $e(\mathbf{x}, t)$ of endothelial cells (related to the probability to find the tip of a capillary at that location and time) obeys the convection-reaction-diffusion equation in Ω_H and Ω_V

$$\frac{\partial e}{\partial t} = \overline{D}_e \nabla^2 e - \nabla \cdot \left(\left(\frac{\chi_C}{1 + \alpha c / \overline{c}_0} \nabla c + \overline{\chi}_f \nabla f + \chi_{\mathbf{u}} \mathbf{u} \right) e \right)$$

$$-\overline{\rho}_D e + \overline{\rho}_p \frac{e(\overline{e}_0 - e)}{\overline{e}_0} \mathcal{H}(c - \overline{c}^*) \frac{(c - \overline{c}^*)}{\overline{c}_0} - \rho_N \chi_{\Omega_N} e , \tag{6.30}$$

where $\overline{D}_e$ is the diffusion constant, $\overline{\chi}_c$, $\overline{\chi}_f$ are chemotaxis and haptotaxis coefficients, respectively, and $\overline{\chi}_{\mathbf{u}}$ and α are dimensionless constants (herein, take $\chi_{\mathbf{u}} = 0.2$ and $\alpha = 0.1$). As assumed in [11], diffusion is dominated by convection. $\overline{c}^*$ is a concentration of TAF above which proliferation occurs. $\overline{\rho}_D$, $\overline{\rho}_p$, and $\overline{\rho}_N$ are rates of natural degradation, production, and necrosis of endothelial cells, respectively. The initial condition for e is

$$e(\mathbf{x}, 0) = \overline{e}_0 \sum_{i=1}^{m} \exp(-r_i^2 / s_e^2) , \tag{6.31}$$

where m is the number of initial capillary sprout-tips, r_i is the distance from the ith spout tip, and s_e is a distance measuring the spread of initial endothelial cell clusters. The boundary condition for $e(\mathbf{x}, t)$ is

$$\zeta_\infty \cdot (\overline{\mathbf{V}} e - \overline{D}_e \nabla e) = 0 \text{ on } \Sigma_\infty , \tag{6.32}$$

where ζ_∞ is the unit normal vector, and $\overline{\mathbf{V}}$ is the full convective velocity:

$$\overline{\mathbf{V}} = \frac{\overline{\chi}_C}{1 + \alpha c / \overline{c}_0} \nabla c + \overline{\chi}_f \nabla f + \chi_{\mathbf{u}} \mathbf{u} . \tag{6.33}$$

The model for motion of capillary sprout-tips is comprised of continuum and discrete components [11]. Equations (6.26), (6.29), and (6.30) constitute the continuum component. The discrete component is founded on the assumption that growth of the capillary is simply determined by the biased random migration (random walk) of a single endothelial cell at the sprout-tip. Given the time invariant spatial step size h_{reg}, and continuum fields $c(\mathbf{x}, t_0)$ and $f(\mathbf{x}, t_0)$, the model predicts the probabilities that at time $t_0 + \triangle t$ the single cell stays at $\mathbf{x}$ or moves to one of four nearest neighbor sites, $\mathbf{x} \pm h_{\text{reg}} \mathbf{e}_i$, where $\mathbf{e}_i$ are the canonical orthonormal basis vectors. These probabilities are calculated by finite differencing (6.30) following the method of [11]. The algorithm then updates the cell's position by a weighted random selection based on the five probabilities. Besides tip migration, the discrete-continuum scheme can predict capillary branching and anastomosis (fusion), and recently this framework has been used to include flow and the delivery of nutrients and drugs [140]. Unlike [11] or [140], we allow for the possibility that the entire capillary may be convected by the external cell velocity using the kinematic condition

$$\frac{d\mathbf{x}}{dt} = \mu_C \mathbf{u}, \tag{6.34}$$

where $\mathbf{x}$ is the position on the capillary and μ_C is to be interpreted as the mobility of the capillary (herein use the small value $\mu_C = 0.1$). This is a simplified model for the vasculature that treats all points on the vessels in the same way. In fact, as the network becomes more established in time the capillaries become harder to move, which is not accounted for here. Also, the precise characteristics of flow in the capillary network are not considered, except for accounting for the pressure effect on flow according to (6.18).

6.3.3 Results

The reaction-diffusion equations in the model outlined above are solved using an adaptive [53, 9] finite element/level set method in two spatial dimensions. We present a simulation using the combined growth and angiogenesis models. Complete model parameters are given in Fig. 6.9. The computational domain is $\Omega = (-40, 40) \times (-40, 40)$. Details of the simulation for nondimensional times $t = 0$ to 900 are displayed in Fig. 6.10 (only part of the domain is shown). The left column shows the current shape of the tumor interface (thick solid line), location of the necrotic rim (thin), and new capillaries (solid branching and looping lines) and contours of ECD (dashed). Plots of fibronectin concentration (FIB), nutrient concentration (N), pressure (P), endothelial cell density (ECD), and tumor angiogenic factor (TAF) concentration are also calculated; nutrient is shown in the right column. The tumor is initially centered at the origin with its interface given by

$$(x(\theta), y(\theta)) = (2 + 0.1\cos(2\theta))(\cos(\theta), \sin(\theta)), \tag{6.35}$$

where θ is the angle measured counterclockwise off the x-axis. The tumor is surrounded by six preselected capillary sprouts, which provide initial conditions for the free endothelial cell clusters. To accentuate the effect of angiogenesis, the transfer of nutrients from the uniform vasculature is assumed negligible in the near environment of the tumor ($v_p^{\mathrm{pre}} = 0$), and the nutrient is assumed to come only from the outside environment ($n = 1$ on Σ_∞) and from the neovasculature.

Microphysical Parameters for Malignant Glioma

Input parameters were selected based on the following considerations. In vivo, for malignant glioma (brain tumor), apoptosis is probably negligible ($\lambda_A = 0$)

Growth		Angiogenesis	
		$D_c = \bar{D}_c/(\bar{\beta}_D \mathcal{L}^2)$	2.5×10^3
$v_P^{ang} = \bar{v}_P^{ang}/\bar{v}_U$	2.5×10^{-2}	$\beta_U = \bar{\beta}_U/\bar{\beta}_D$	1.0
$v_P^{pre} = \bar{v}_P^{pre}/\bar{v}_U$	0	$\eta_P = \bar{\eta}_P/\bar{\lambda}_M$	2.5×10^{-3}
$n_C = \bar{n}_C/\bar{n}_\infty$	1.0	$\eta_U = \bar{\eta}_U/\bar{\lambda}_M$	5×10^{-3}
$n_N = \bar{n}_N/\bar{n}_\infty$	2.5×10^{-2}	$\eta_N = \bar{\eta}_N/\bar{\lambda}_M$	3×10^{-3}
$p_C^{ang} = \bar{p}_C^{ang}/\bar{p}_T$	1.0	$D_e = \bar{D}_e/(\bar{\lambda}_M \mathcal{L}^2)$	1.5×10^{-3}
$p_C^{pre} = \bar{p}_C^{pre}/\bar{p}_T$	0	$\chi_c = \frac{\bar{\chi}_c \bar{c}_0}{\lambda_M \mathcal{L}^2}$	2.0
$\lambda_A = \bar{\lambda}_A/\bar{\lambda}_M$	0	$\chi_f = \frac{\bar{\chi}_f \bar{f}_0}{\lambda_M \mathcal{L}^2}$	0.3
$\lambda_N = \bar{\lambda}_N/\bar{\lambda}_M$	0.25	$\rho_D = \bar{\rho}_D/\bar{\lambda}_M$	1.0×10^{-3}
$\gamma = \bar{\gamma}/(\bar{\lambda}_M \mathcal{L}^3/\bar{\mu})$	0.25	$\rho_P = \bar{\rho}_P/\bar{\lambda}_M$	1.0×10^{-2}
		$c^\star = \bar{c}^\star/\bar{c}_0$	0.1
		$\rho_N = \bar{\rho}_N/\bar{\lambda}_M$	1.0×10^{-2}

Fig. 6.9. Complete model parameters used in the full simulation, the results for which are displayed in Fig. 6.10. Reprinted with permission from *Bull. Math. Biol.*, Zheng et al. Vol. 67, p. 239, Copyright 2005 Springer. With kind permission of Springer Science and Business Media.

since mutated clones after the initial selection has occurred are typically characterized by suppression of the p53 pathway and enhanced proliferation [136], and even normal glial cells are immortal. From experiments [73] on the growth of glioblastoma cell lines (the most malignant and proliferative brain tumors) as multicellular millimeter-size spheroids in vitro, it was observed that typically the mitosis rate $\bar{\lambda}_M \approx 0.3$ day^{-1}, that the rate of volume loss in the necrotic core is comparable to or less than the rate of volume gain from mitosis, hence the choice $\lambda_N = 0.25$, and finally that minimum nutrient concentration for cell viability is a small fraction of outer uniform concentration in growth medium [73], hence the choice of a value for $n_N \ll 1$ (although the value of this parameter may be affected by the difficulty of reproducing the in vivo conditions in vitro). Dimensionless nutrient concentration in the blood is chosen as $n_C = 1$, i.e., in equilibrium with the concentration in the undisturbed tissue environment. Nutrient transfer rate v_p^{ang} is set after some experimentation to a value that provides a continuous supply of nutrient during the tumor's entire evolution, in order to reproduce in vivo growth and infiltration of neovascularized glioblastoma [136]. A value for the pressure is chosen as $p_C^{ang} = O(1)$ in the capillaries, which is in near equilibrium with interstitial pressure in glioma. By considering a characteristic diffusion constant for

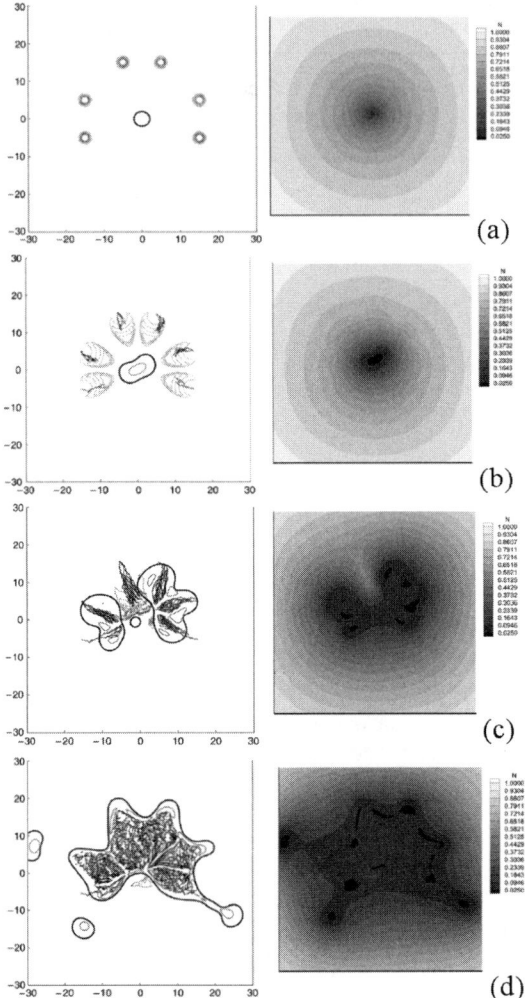

Fig. 6.10. Simulation of growth, neovascularization, and infiltration of the brain by a malignant glioma. Parameters are listed in Fig. 6.9. (a) Time $t = 0$; (b) Time $t = 200$; (c) Time $t = 400$ shows penetration into the tumor by the neovasculature and splitting of tumor into three fragments due to diffusional instability; (d) Time $t = 900$ shows that tumor fragments have co-opted the neovasculature, rejoined, and reached a nearly stationary state of centimeter size. Small clusters separate from the main tumor and migrate up nutrient concentration gradients. Reprinted with permission from *Bull. Math. Biol.*, Zheng et al. Vol. 67, pp. 240, 242, 244, 247, Copyright 2005 Springer. With kind permission of Springer Science and Business Media.

nutrient $\overline{D}_n \approx 10^{-5}$ cm$^2/s$ and a nutrient consumption rate $v_U \approx 1$ min^{-1} (the latter from the observation that brain cells run out of glucose and die on that time scale), a characteristic nutrient diffusion length $\mathcal{L} \approx 200 - 300$ μm is obtained. This is consistent with the observed thickness of the viable rim of cells in tumor spheroids in vitro [2, 73]. For the simulation illustrated in Fig. 6.10, the tumor grows to a size $\approx 40 \cdot \mathcal{L} \approx 8$ mm $- 1.2$ cm on a time scale $\approx 900\lambda_M^{-1} \approx 7$ years, which is in quite good agreement with the observed time of growth of high-grade malignant glioma (astrocytoma) to secondary glioblastoma [136]. The surface tension parameter was chosen at a value small enough that cell adhesive forces are weak and diffusional instability of the tumor shape occurs during growth as observed in the experiments [73]. Angiogenesis parameters were chosen to obtain continuous growth of neovasculature parallel to growth of the tumor as is observed clinically. The dimensionless diffusion constant of TAF was chosen to ensure a nonzero value of TAF concentration over the length scale of the tumor size. Rates characterizing fibronectin evolution were chosen to ensure an observable effect of haptotaxis (responsible for looping of the neocapillaries).

Diffusional Instability and Tissue Invasion

For the parameters given in Fig. 6.9 and an initial, noncircular shape (6.35), the tumor will experience unstable growth due to a diffusional instability [35] caused by the competition of growth of the tumor mass and surface tension (cell adhesive forces) that tends to influence this growth. Note that without angiogenesis, and with a circular initial shape, instabilities would grow only due to random numerical error or because of the nonradially symmetric nutrient distribution due to the use of a square computational domain. The instability is enhanced by the development of a necrotic core and its associated volume sink. The tumor forms bulbs and breaks up into fragments. Indeed, the beginning of instability can be seen at time $t = 200$ (Fig. 6.10b). The presence of the inhomogeneous nutrient field due to angiogenesis tends to further destabilize the tumor, because the tumor tends to co-opt the complexly shaped neovasculature in order to maximize nutrient transfer. Note that the resulting shape of the tumor is therefore stable to random noise or small perturbations because the patterns of growth of the tumor mass are mainly driven by the spatial distribution of the newly formed capillaries. By $t = 400$ the tumor breaks up into three parts, as fragments of the tumor "move." in opposite directions up the gradient of the nutrient concentration field (Fig. 6.10c). This net migration is due to the combination of cell death in low nutrient concentration and cell birth in high nutrient concentration. Note that in the simulations this migration is exaggerated because we use a simplified model (Darcy's law) for the mechanical response of the tissue.

At the same time the formation of necrosis leads to release of tumor angiogenic factors (TAFs) and thus triggers chemotaxis of endothelial cells and new capillary formation and migration towards the tumor from the preexisting blood vessels. At time $t = 400$ penetration of the capillaries into the tumor has occurred (Fig. 6.10b). It is assumed that the same model describes angiogenesis outside and inside the tumor, which implies that an ECM exists inside the tumor thus allowing chemotaxis and haptotaxis of endothelial cells to occur. This is probably a valid assumption for the case of malignant glioma, known to infiltrate through the brain ECM and co-exist there with healthy cells [136]. Note also that we assume infinitesimal thickness of capillaries and no mechanical interaction with the tissue (except for the small mobility μ_C). Thus here capillaries are line sources of nutrient. As the disjoint tumor fragments continue to grow, the tumor reconnects ($700 < t < 800$). Note also the small fragment in the middle ($t = 400$) later shrinks and disappears. By time $t = 900$ (Fig. 6.10d), the tumor has almost completely co-opted the neovasculature. It has been hypothesized that tissue invasion occurs in cycles. Within one cycle, angiogenesis occurs followed by tumor mass growth and co-option of the newly formed vessels. These cycles would repeat themselves. Here, one of these cycles is simulated. Further growth would require further vascularization. The complex tumor morphologies predicted in this simulation are ultimately due to the nonuniform distribution of nutrient sources following angiogenesis. The capability of simulating the coupled growth and angiogenesis processes leads to predictions of tumor morphologies that are more realistic than those predicted in previous investigations (Sect. 6.2).

By $t = 900$ two smaller tumor clusters have fragmented off because of diffusional instability and are migrating towards the computational boundary Σ_∞, where the nutrient level is highest (bottom of Fig. 6.10d), and a third will fragment off shortly. If the surface tension γ were larger, the tumor shape would remain compact, and fragmentation would not occur. Here low surface tension (and cell mobility) models weak adhesive forces that enable cell clusters to scatter and migrate and infiltrate through the extracellular matrix. In malignant glioma, weak cell adhesion is probably the effect of excitation of the FAK (focal adhesion kinase) pathways [148] that are triggered by overexpression of EGFR (epidermal growth factor receptor) and its numerous ligands on the tumor cell surfaces. EGFR signaling activates both MAPK proliferative pathways and FAK cell-scattering pathways [148]. In this simulation, fragment migration occurs in a manner similar to the migration of water droplets in ice in the presence of a temperature gradient [194] due to a melt-and-freeze mechanism. Proliferation occurs near the leading edge of the fragment, whereas necrosis occurs at the trailing edge, thus leading to a net migration of cells up the nutrient concentration levels (Fig. 6.11, left). This can be observed in the pressure field around the migrating fragments at time $t = 900$ (pressure (P) in Fig. 6.11, right). The pressure is higher at the leading edge, and lower at the trailing edge. In fact there is a mass sink at the trailing edge owing to the necrotic core. This provides insight into a possible mechanism for tissue invasion by tumor cell clusters [75], especially in brain tumors where the cancer cells are observed to powerfully infiltrate the brain's ECM. In addition there is migration due to gradients of adhesiveness, which is neglected in this model, but considered by [47]. Finally, here tumor cell apoptosis is neglected. However, if $\lambda_A > 0$, the same net migration is observed in the simulations without the presence of a necrotic core, in agreement with the infiltrative nature of low- and high-grade astrocytoma that do not exhibit necrosis [136].

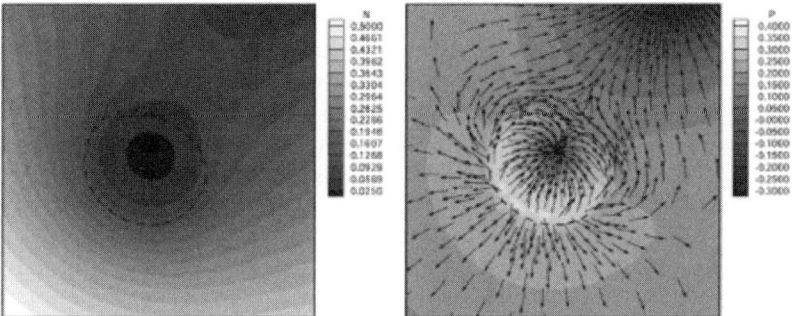

Fig. 6.11. Magnified view of the infiltrating tumor fragment in the bottom left of Fig. 6.10(d) ($t = 900$). **Left**: nutrient levels (N) and tumor fragment interface (dashed). **Right**: cell velocity (arrows) and interstitial pressure (P). A net migration of this fragment away from the main tumor body is the consequence of cell birth on the leading edge and death on the trailing edge due to the gradient of nutrient concentration. Note the high pressure in the proliferative leading edge, and the mass sink due to necrosis in the trailing edge. Reprinted with permission from *Bull. Math. Biol.*, Zheng et al. Vol. 67, p. 254, Copyright 2005 Springer. With kind permission of Springer Science and Business Media.

By multiplying the dimensionless tumor area at $t = 900$ by $\mathcal{L}^2$ with $\mathcal{L} = 300$ μm, and the dimensionless capillary length by $\mathcal{L}$, and then scaling the 2-D simulation to a 3-D tumor using an exponent $3/2$, one obtains a total predicted tumor volume ≈ 1 cm^3 and, by assuming an equivalent volume per cell of 1000 μm^3, a prediction of $\approx$ 1 billion tumor cells and a ratio of tumor-to-capillary cells ≈ 61, in good agreement with experimental observations [34].

Nutrient Transfer from the Neovasculature

The supply of nutrients is nonuniform and nonconstant in time in this model, owing to the extension of the capillaries to the tumor. This extension is a continuous feedback process because angiogenesis (i) occurs as a response to diminishing nutrient levels in the tumor and (ii) raises the nutrient supply in the tumor allowing for increased growth and increased nutrient demand. In addition there is a stabilizing effect of pressure in the nutrient transfer (6.18).

In the initial stages of neovascularization when the amount of nutrient coming from the new capillaries is low compared to that of other sources, the angiogenesis process is decoupled from growth, as in [11]. This is the case up to approximately time $t = 200$ (Fig. 6.10b). Note that the diffusional shape instability is not due to angiogenesis. After this point, the nutrient supply coming from the new capillaries is important for the growth of the tumor. By time $t = 400$ the capillaries penetrate the tumor. Splitting (branching) and looping (anastomosis) are also observed. In our implementation nutrients are transferred only from looped vessels, since these vessels can provide a more effective flow of blood. One can effectively control the density of looped vessels by adjusting the density of new capillaries through the splitting probability and the looping criteria through the minimum age for looping and the effective loop-receptive regions on the capillaries [11]. Subsequent to penetration, the tumor begins to co-opt the new capillaries. This process occurs because the tumor grows more near the (looped) capillaries. In this simulation (Fig. 6.10d), the tumor takes on the shape of the new vasculature, roughly. A recent hypothesis [136] for the infiltration of malignant glioma cells throughout the brain is that these cells co-opt and crawl around the preexisting brain vasculature. The behavior observed in the simulation seems to corroborate this hypothesis by providing an additional mechanism for infiltration.

In the present simulation, growth of the vasculature slows dramatically after about time $t = 400$ (and the capillaries are only advected by the growing tumor according to (6.34) thereafter). In the model, a minimum amount of ECD is required for the continued growth of the sprout tips. Here, the amount of endothelial cell proliferation is smaller than degradation and necrosis, and the amount of endothelial cells decreases. However, with sufficient proliferation, the neovascularization can even speed up, since the rate of capillary splitting generally depends on local levels of ECD [11]. Although only six activated sprout tips are included, one may also increase this number initially, or stochastically add more sites as the tumor grows, with activation probabilities depending upon the local TAF levels. In the simulation in Fig. 6.10, local levels of TAF generally increase along the radial direction as the tumor grows. Hence more active sprout tip sites are activated in time.

If suddenly the nutrient concentration became depleted, or the flow of nutrients were cut off ($n = 0$ everywhere in Ω) the tumor would shrink and vanish, owing to the death term λ_N in (6.21). If instead only the flow from the neovasculature were cut off, with the far field nutrient source in place ($n = 1$ on Σ_∞), the tumor would shrink to a diffusion-limited, stationary size. Additionally, the growth of the vascularized tumor depends vitally on the nutrient transfer rate ν_p^{ang}, the level of nutrient in the blood n_C, and the blood pressure in the new capillaries p_C^{ang}. Here we have taken the blood pressure to be $p_C^{\text{ang}} = 1$, i.e., equal to the characteristic pressure due to tumor cell mitosis. Because of the form of $b^{\text{ang}}(p)$, there is no nutrient transfer in an environment for which $p > 1$. This restricts growth by providing a stabilizing mechanism because the tumor must balance the rate of growth with the pressure level its growth causes. The result is that total pressure tends to be bounded away from p_C^{ang}. Increasing pressure in capillaries increases the rate of nutrient transfer, and hence the rate of growth. But again the pressure will be bounded away from p_C^{ang}. In vivo this pressure is responsible for the difficulties in delivering chemotherapeutic agents through the vasculature to tumor cells. The simulations in Figs. 6.10c and 6.10d reveal that inside the tumor the transfer from the vasculature nearly vanishes. As a result of these phenomena the tumor configuration at time $t = 900$ is nearly stationary; further growth will require an ongoing angiogenesis process. Finally note that the relatively small amount of necrosis in the last frame is an artifact of the model used, which implements a very sharp transition from live to necrotic cells at $n = n_N$. In reality, the transition is smoother and in the tumor body depicted in the last frame ($t = 900$) necrotic and nearly necrotic cells are mixed over a larger region.

6.3.4 Summary

The work presented here displays at least two new, important features vital for the development of a realistic virtual cancer simulator at the tumoral level. First, it successfully incorporates a realistic model of angiogenesis [11] with a continuum model for growth. Previous models for growth have only included constant vascularization [58] or a field variable representing spatially smooth vascularization [31]. In the model reviewed here, the capillary network extends due to direct interaction with the growing tumor, primarily through the TAF. At the same time, the tumor receives nutrient, by blood-to-tissue transfer from the extending capillary network. Second, this work is fully two dimensional, incorporating more realistic tumor evolution than can be realized in lower-dimensional (e.g., spherically symmetric, cylindrical, or 1-D) models of growth and angiogenesis. We used sophisticated numerical techniques to accomplish this: the level set method [153] for capturing complicated morphology and connectedness of the tumor interface, and finite element methods based on a fully adaptive unstructured mesh for accurately resolving multiple length scales at the lowest possible computational expense. Such efforts enable the simulator to model phenomena such as invasive fingering, tumor fragmentation, and healthy tissue capture. This work significantly extends that of Sect. 6.2, which used a simpler model for growth and vascularization and the boundary integral method for 2-D computation.

Our simulation results are supported by experimental data. In a parallel study [73], we used the grade IV glioma (glioblastoma multiforme) human cell line ACBT to culture spheroids in vitro over several weeks and observe their growth pattern as a function of nutrient (glucose) and growth factor (serum) variation. At high serum concentrations, spheroids were observed to grow to a diffusion-limited millimeter size and then become unstable and assume dimpled shapes as in our simulation. These sub-spheroidal structures may eventually break off from the main spheroid (as a "bubble" of cells or as spheroid fragments) or merge with neighboring structures to enlarge the over-all parental spheroid mass. This process can repeat itself on the sub-spheroid, leading to recursive sub-spheroidal growth as the main mechanism of spheroid morphogenesis. The stability of the sub-spheroidal components is dependent on the rate of cell proliferation and death, as controlled by access to nutrient and growth factors. Our simulations and these experiments indicate that diffusional shape instability may be a powerful tissue invasion mechanism, since for the same mitosis and death rates spherical tumors would remain of millimeter size and never become clinically relevant. The results indicate that diffusional instability allows clusters of tumor cells to invade and infiltrate the surrounding brain even without resorting to further genetic alterations that differentiate these cells from the bulk tumor by enhancing their mobility. Note that it has been observed that cancer cell migration is different from that of model cells. It has been shown that tumor cells migrate in cell clusters rather than as single cells [75]. Note also that in malignant glioma genotypes, heterogeneity in the mutations of the FAK pathways that regulate cell scattering and adhesion is rarely if ever observed [136], although this matter is still very unclear and caution should be used when drawing conclusions.

6.4 Solid Tumor Growth Using a Ghost Cell/Level Set Method[7]

6.4.1 Overview

In [134, 135] we extended tumor growth models considered by [58, 132, 211] and others, which reformulated classical models [89, 141, 3, 38, 39, 46] to include more detailed effects of the microenvironment. This was done by allowing variability in nutrient availability and the response to proliferation-induced mechanical pressure (which models hydrostatic stress) in the tissue surrounding the tumor. Using analysis and nonlinear numerical simulations, we explored the effects of the interaction between the genetic characteristics of the tumor and the tumor microenvironment on the resulting tumor progression and morphology. We found that the range of morphological responses can be placed in three categories that depend primarily upon the tumor microenvironment: tissue invasion via fragmentation due to a hypoxic microenvironment; fingering, invasive growth into nutrient-rich, biomechanically unresponsive tissue; and compact growth into nutrient-rich, biomechanically responsive tissue. The qualitative behavior of tumor morphologies was similar across a broad range of parameters that govern tumor genetic characteristics. These findings demonstrate the importance of the microenvironment on tumor growth and morphology and implications for therapy.

---

[7] This section includes an article published in *J. Theor. Biol.*, Vol. 245, Macklin and Lowengrub, pp. 677–704, Copyright Elsevier (2007), and portions reprinted from Macklin and Lowengrub (in press) [135].

Previously [131, 132, 133] we considered a level set-based extension of the tumor growth model by [58] (Sect. 6.2), where we developed new, highly accurate numerical techniques to solve the resulting system of partial differential equations in a moving domain. These methods are more accurate than those used in [211] (Sect. 6.3) and [96]. Using the new methods, we modeled tumor growth under a variety of conditions and investigated the role of necrosis in destabilizing the tumor morphology. We demonstrated that nonhomogeneous nutrient diffusion inside a tumor leads to heterogeneous growth patterns that, when interacting with cell-cell adhesion, cause sustained morphological instability during tumor growth, as well as repeated encapsulation of noncancerous tissue by a growing tumor. Building upon this earlier work, in [135] we developed an accurate ghost cell/level set technique for evolving interfaces whose normal velocity is given by normal derivatives of solutions to linear and nonlinear quasi-steady reaction-diffusion equations with curvature-dependent boundary conditions. The technique is capable of describing complex morphologies evolving in heterogeneous domains. The algorithm involves several new developments, including a new ghost cell technique for accurately discretizing jumps in the normal derivative without smearing jumps in the tangential derivative, a new adaptive solver for linear and nonlinear quasi-steady reaction-diffusion problems (NAGSI), an adaptive normal vector discretization for interfaces in close contact, and an accurate discrete approximation to the Heaviside function.

In our model, the region surrounding a tumor aggregates the effects of ECM and noncancerous cells, which are characterized by two nondimensional parameters that govern diffusional and biomechanical properties of the tissue. Fluids are assumed to move freely through interstitium and ECM, and thus these effects are currently neglected. External nutrient and pressure variations, in turn, affect tumor evolution. Due to the computational cost of 3-D simulations, we focus on 2-D tumor growth, although the model applies equally well in three dimensions. In [58] (Sect. 6.2), it was found that the baseline model predicts similar morphological behavior for 2-D and 3-D tumor growth. This has been borne out by recent 3-D simulations in [126], as seen in Sect. 6.2. Note that 2-D tumor growth may be well suited to study cancers that spread relatively thinly, such as melanoma.

We also investigated the internal structure of tumors, including volume fractions of necrotic and viable regions. We found that even during growth, the internal structure tends to stabilize due to apparent local equilibration of tumors as characteristic feature sizes and shapes emerge. Whereas tumor morphology depends primarily upon the microenvironment, internal structure is most strongly influenced by tumor genetic characteristics, including resistance to necrosis, the rate at which necrosis is degraded, and rate of apoptosis. These results are not obvious from examination of the model and underlying hypotheses alone. By hypothesis, the microenvironment, tumor genetics, and tumor morphology are all nonlinearly coupled. Tumor genetics determine biophysical properties like growth rates, which, in turn, are mediated by microenvironmental factors such as available nutrient supply. One would expect that tumor genetics have a greater impact on tumor morphology, and, indeed, [58] provides evidence that tumor genetics completely determine the morphological behavior when the microenvironment is not taken into account.

6.4.2 Governing Equations

We model an avascular tumor occupying volume $\Omega_T(t)$ with boundary $\partial\Omega$, denoted by Σ. The tumor is composed of a viable region Ω_V where nutrient (e.g., oxygen and glucose) levels are sufficient for tumor cell viability and a necrotic region Ω_N where tumor cells die due to low nutrient levels and are broken down. Note that $\Omega_T = \Omega_V \cup \Omega_N$. The growing tumor also interacts with the surrounding microenvironment in the host tissue; this region is denoted by Ω_H, which contains ECM and a mixture of noncancerous cells, fluid, and cellular debris. As observed in [58, 131, 132], a growing tumor may encapsulate regions of Ω_H, and so these regions may lack living noncancerous cells. Hereafter, we refer to Ω_H as noncancerous tissue, although the model applies equally well to the case in which Ω_H contains only ECM, fluid, and cellular debris.

Nutrient Transport

As defined in Sect. 6.3, we set capillary-to-tissue nutrient transfer function $\overline{T}_c = 0$ and use relative nutrient diffusivity D to control the level of nutrient in Ω_H: $\overline{D}_n = 1$ in Ω_T and $\overline{D}_n = D$ in Ω_H.

Cellular Velocity Field

Cells and ECM in host tissue Ω_H and viable tumor region Ω_V are affected by a variety of forces, each of which contributes to the cellular velocity field **u**. Proliferating tumor cells in Ω_V generate an internal (oncotic) mechanical pressure (hydrostatic stress) that also exerts force on surrounding noncancerous tissue in Ω_H. Tumor and noncancerous cells and ECM can respond to pressure variations by overcoming cell-cell and cell-ECM adhesion and moving within the scaffolding of collagen and fibroblast cells (i.e., ECM) that provides structure to host tissue. The ECM in Ω_H can deform in response to pressure. Following previous work, we assume constant cell density and model cellular motion within the ECM as incompressible fluid flow in a porous medium. The response of cells and ECM to pressure is governed by Darcy's law:

$$\mathbf{u} = -\mu_p \nabla P, \quad x \in \Omega_V \cup \Omega_H, \tag{6.36}$$

where the cellular mobility $\mu_p = \mu(\mathbf{x})$ measures the overall ability of tissue to respond to pressure. Note that μ_p also measures the permeability of tissue to tumor cells. See [7] and [42] for further motivation of this approach from a mixture modeling viewpoint. When tumor cells are hypoxic, cellular pathways that stimulate cell migration may be activated [94, 109, 125, 65, 165]. This may be modeled by increasing the mobility μ_p as nutrient level decreases or as a tactic response to nutrient gradients [77]. Here, we focus upon the effects of proliferative pressure only; effects of increased cellular mobility in response to hypoxia will be considered in future work. The outward normal velocity V of the tumor boundary Σ is given by

$$V = \mathbf{u} \cdot \mathbf{n} = -\mu_p \nabla P \cdot \mathbf{n}, \qquad (6.37)$$

where $\mathbf{n}$ is the outward unit normal vector along Σ.

Proliferation, Apoptosis, and Necrosis

In the viable region Ω_V, proliferation increases the number of tumor cells and thus the volume occupied by the viable region. Apoptosis decreases the total volume of Ω_V at a constant rate λ_A. We assume that cell birth and death are in balance in Ω_H, and so there is no change in volume in that region. (Note that if there are no cells in Ω_H, then there is no cell birth or death, and the assumption still holds.) In fact, poorly vascularized tumors are often hypoxic, leading to anaerobic glycolysis and acidosis [84, 85]. Noncancerous cells struggle survive in this condition, providing a relative survival advantage for tumor cells and a potential volume loss in Ω_H when cells are present.

As a computational convenience, we can achieve the correct volume loss by continuously extending the velocity $\mathbf{u}$ into Ω_N. We also assume that the normal velocity is continuous across the tumor boundary Σ, i.e., voids do not form between tumor and host tissue. Therefore, we choose our extension such that the normal velocity is continuous across the necrotic boundary, i.e., $[\mathbf{u} \cdot \mathbf{n}] = 0$ across Σ_N. Because the nutrient level determines Σ_N, the latter is not a material boundary and is not advected by the velocity field $\mathbf{u}$; the extension of the velocity field is used solely to yield the correct volume change in the tumor necrotic core. One means to attain this is to extend the pressure continuously into the necrotic core as well, by setting $\bar{\varepsilon} = 0$ in 6.22:

$$\mathbf{u} = -\mu_p \nabla P, \quad \mathbf{x} \in \Omega_N$$

$$[P] = 0, \quad \mathbf{x} \in \Sigma_N$$

$$[-\mu_p \nabla P \cdot \mathbf{n}] = 0, \quad \mathbf{x} \in \Sigma_N. \qquad (6.38)$$

The jump condition $[P] = 0$ across Σ_N models low cellular adhesion and is consistent with the increased cellular mobility observed in hypoxic cells [32, 43, 95, 164, 172, 165]. Note that (6.38) automatically satisfies $[\mathbf{u} \cdot \mathbf{n}] = 0$ on Σ_N.

Mechanical Pressure

We can obtain an equation for the mechanical pressure in $\Omega_T \cup \Omega_H$ by noting the pressure extension in Eq. (6.38):

$$\nabla \cdot (\mu_p \nabla P) = \begin{cases} 0 & \text{if } \mathbf{x} \in \Omega_H \\ bc - \lambda_A & \text{if } \mathbf{x} \in \Omega_V \\ -\lambda_N & \text{if } \mathbf{x} \in \Omega_N \end{cases} \tag{6.39}$$

By the continuity of the normal velocity across the tumor boundary, by Darcy's law (6.36) there is no jump in the normal derivative $\mu_p \nabla P \cdot \mathbf{n}$ across Σ. Following [58] and others, we model cell-cell adhesion forces in the tumor by introducing a Laplace–Young surface tension boundary condition. Therefore,

$$[P] = \gamma \kappa, \quad \mathbf{x} \in \Sigma \tag{6.40}$$

$$0 = [\mathbf{u} \cdot \mathbf{n}] = -[\mu_p \nabla P \cdot \mathbf{n}], \quad \mathbf{x} \in \Sigma, \tag{6.41}$$

where κ is the mean curvature and γ is a constant cell-cell adhesion parameter. Cellular proliferation and death are in balance outside of $\Omega_T \cup \Omega_H$. Therefore,

$$P \equiv P_\infty, \quad \mathbf{x} \in \partial(\Omega_T \cup \Omega_H) \tag{6.42}$$

on the far-field boundary.

Here we consider the special case of avascular growth in piecewise homogeneous tissue and take $\mu_p \equiv \mu$ in Ω_H and $\mu_p \equiv 1$ in Ω_T, where μ is a constant. Note that because μ is constant within the tumor (and across Σ_N), the pressure boundary conditions across Σ_N in (6.38) are automatically satisfied for any C^1 smooth solution P.

6.4.3 Results

We investigate the effects of the tumor microenvironment on the morphology and growth patterns of 2-D, avascular tumors growing into piecewise homogeneous tissues. Recall that D characterizes relative nutrient diffusivity, A is the amount of apoptosis, G measures tumor aggressiveness (proliferation compared to cellular adhesion), G_N characterizes rate of degradation of the necrotic tissue, and N is the threshold nutrient level for tumor cell viability. The viable rim size is determined by D, A, and N, while the necrotic core size is determined by G_N. In all simulations, we set the apoptosis parameter $A = 0$ because the tumors are assumed to ignore inhibitory signals for self destruction (apoptosis). We numerically compute the solutions using a computational mesh with $\triangle x = \triangle y = 0.08$. All tumors are simulated to a scaled nondimensional time of $T = Gt = \lambda_M t' = 20$, where t' is dimensional time. (The dimensional time is given by $t' = T/\lambda_M$.) Because $\lambda_M^{-1} \sim 1$ day, this nondimensional time allows us to compare tumors of varying simulated genotypes at fixed physical times (e.g., $T = 20 \approx 20$ days).

We characterize the effects of the modeled tumor microenvironment on growth by presenting a morphology diagram (Fig. 6.12). We simulate growth over a wide range of microenvironmental parameters (D and μ) with $G = 20$; $G_N = 1$, and $N = 0.35$, each with identical initial shape. Later, we shall consider the effect of G, G_N, and N. We let $D \in \{1, 50, 100, \infty\}$ and $\mu \in \{0.25, 1, 50, \infty\}$. When $D = \infty$, we set $\sigma \equiv 1$ in nonencapsulated regions of Ω_H and only solve the Poisson equation for σ in Ω_T and the encapsulated portions of Ω_H (with diffusion constant 1). Likewise, when $\mu = \infty$, we set $p \equiv 0$ in nonencapsulated regions of Ω_H and only solve the Poisson equation for p in Ω_T and the encapsulated portions of Ω_H (with mobility 1). In Fig. 6.12, we plot the shape of each tumor at time $T = 20.0$. In all figures, the black regions denote Ω_N where the tumor is necrotic, the gray regions show the viable tumor region Ω_V, and the white regions correspond to Ω_H, which consists of the ECM, noncancerous cells, and any other material outside of the tumor.

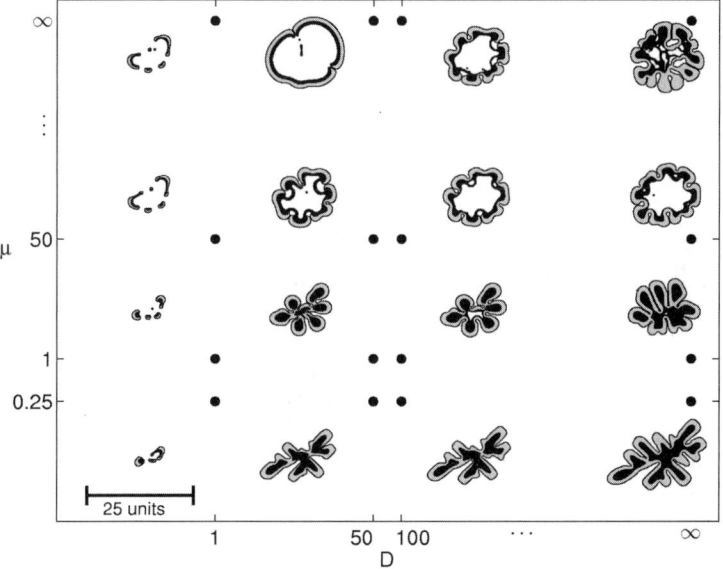

Fig. 6.12. Tumor morphological response to the microenvironment. External tissue nutrient diffusivity D increases from left to right, and the external tissue mobility μ increases from bottom to top. Three major morphologies are observed: fragmenting growth (left), invasive fingering (lower right), and compact/hollow (upper right). All tumors are plotted to the same scale, where the indicated length is $25L \approx 0 : 5$ cm. Necrosis in black, viable region in gray. Reprinted with permission from Macklin and Lowengrub, *J. Theor. Biol.* Vol. 245, p. 687 (2007). Copyright Elsevier.

On the horizontal axis, we vary the nutrient diffusivity of the surrounding tissue; as D increases from left to right, the simulated microenvironment varies from nutrient poor to nutrient rich. On the vertical axis, we vary the mobility of the surrounding material; as μ increases from bottom to top, the microenvironment ranges from low mobility to high mobility. The greater the mobility μ, the greater the ability of the external, noncancerous tissue to respond to the pressure generated by the growing tumor, and tumor cells are more able to penetrate the tissue. We observe three distinct tumor morphologies through this broad range of simulated tissue types. In the nutrient-poor regime on the left side of the diagram, tumors demonstrate fragmenting growth, characterized by the repeated breakup of the tumor in response to the low nutrient level. The nutrient-rich, low-mobility regime in the bottom right of the morphology diagram is characterized by fingering growth, where buds develop on the tumor boundary that invade the surrounding tissue, forming long, invasive fingers. The nutrient-rich, high-mobility regime in the top right of the diagram demonstrates compact/hollow growth, where the tumors tend to grow into spheroids and typically form abscesses filled with noncancerous tissue and fluid, similar to a necrotic core. These morphologies are similar to those observed experimentally in vitro (e.g., [73]).

We have found that the tumor morphologies in Fig. 6.12 are qualitatively similar when recomputed with different genetic characteristics (modeled by A, G, G_N, and N), although, as demonstrated in Sect. 6.4.3, large changes in the genetic parameter values can shift the morphology from one type to another. Therefore, a tumor's morphology depends primarily upon the characteristics of the microenvironment, as we shall see next.

Fragmenting Growth into Nutrient-Poor Microenvironments

Tumors growing into nutrient-poor microenvironments demonstrate repeated fragmentation through a wide range of mitosis rates (governed by the parameter G) and necrotic tissue degradation rates (G_N). Tumor fragmentation is observed in almost all cases, particularly for fast-proliferating, aggressive tumors with higher values of G. An increased aggressiveness (G) increases the rate of tumor fragmentation. Similarly, increasing the rate of necrotic tissue degradation (G_N) tends to destabilize the tumor, also leading to an increased rate of fragmentation. However, this effect is highly nonlinear: if G_N is large relative to G, then proliferation, necrosis, and cellular adhesion can balance to maintain spheroids and prevent further tumor fragmentation. Note that for sufficiently low levels of tumor aggressiveness (e.g., $G = 0.10$), tumor instability decreases until the steady state configuration is as tumor spheroids, as predicted in [58] for nonnecrotic tumors.

We found that the volume fractions of viable and necrotic tissue were largely independent of the tumor aggressiveness parameter G and the microenvironmental characteristics (D and μ) and were primarily functions of N and G_N. The occurrence of repeated tumor fragmentation is found to occur over a broad range of G and G_N. This demonstrates that in the nutrient-poor regime tumor morphology is largely determined by the characteristics of the surrounding microenvironment, while the genetic characteristics of the tumor (G, G_N, A, and N) determine the size and rate of evolution of the tumor. In addition, increasing the apoptosis rate A to positive values results in similar morphological behavior, only with more rapid tumor fragmentation and a greater number of fragments (results not shown).

The finding that tumor morphology in the nutrient-poor regime depends primarily upon the tumor microenvironment and not upon the tumor's genetic characteristics has important implications for cancer treatment. In anti-angiogenic therapy, drugs are supplied to prevent the neovascularization of the growing tumor and the surrounding tissue. The resulting nutrient-poor microenvironment may cause the tumors to fragment and invade nearby tissues, particularly in higher-mobility tissues. This can negate the positive effects of anti-angiogenic therapy and lead to recurrence and metastasis. This result is consistent with the findings of [54], who suggested that combining anti-angiogenic therapy with adhesion therapy may counteract the negative problems associated with tumor fragmentation in the nutrient-poor regime.

Invasive, Fingering Growth

In Fig. 6.13, we show the evolution of a tumor growing into a low-mobility, nutrient-rich tissue, where $D = 50$ and $\mu = 1$. As in the previous section, $G = 20$, $G_N = 1$, and $N = 0.35$. Because nutrient readily diffuses through the surrounding tissue Ω_H, the tumor is initially nonnecrotic, allowing for unchecked growth and the development of buds on the tumor periphery that protrude into the surrounding tissue (see time $T = 10$ in Fig. 6.13). Due to the cell-cell adhesion (modeled by the pressure jump in (6.40), the proliferation-induced mechanical pressure is greatest surrounding any protrusions of the tumor into the healthy tissue and approximately zero near flatter regions of the tumor boundary. Because the cellular mobility μ is low in the noncancerous tissue, the individual cells and the ECM cannot move to equilibrate the pressure. As a result, the cellular velocity field is mostly parallel to the buds, in spite of adequate nutrient levels between the growing buds. This makes it difficult for buds to merge, leading to the formation of long, invasive fingers (see $T = 30.0 - 50.0$ in Fig. 6.13). The net effect is highly invasive growth into the surrounding tissue.

Within the nutrient-rich, low-mobility tissue regime, we examined two levels of tissue mobility ($\mu \in \{0.25, 1\}$) and three nutrient diffusivities ($D \in \{50, 100, \infty\}$), for a total of six combinations of mobility and nutrient diffusivity. We found that the shape depended primarily upon the tissue mobility: the three lower-mobility tissue examples ($\mu = 0.25$) had an overall higher shape parameter than the higher-mobility tissue ($\mu = 1$), which reflects a higher degree of deformation. This trend is indeed observed in the morphologies along the $\mu = 0.25$ row of Fig. 6.12. This is because the lower the tissue

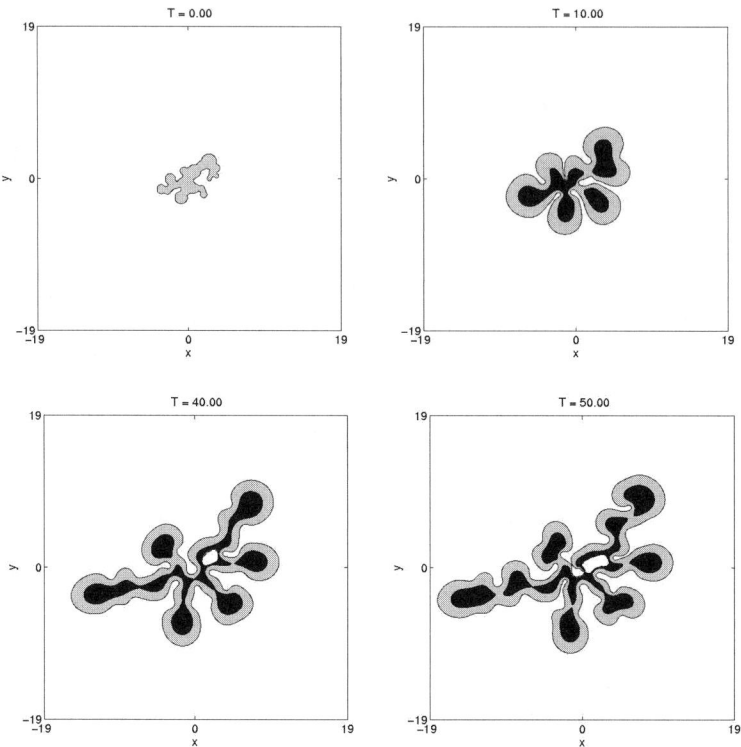

Fig. 6.13. Long-time simulation of invasive, fingering growth into nutrient-rich ($D = 50$), low-mobility ($\mu = 1$) tissue. $G = 20$; $G_N = 1$; $N = 0.35$, and $A = 0$. Necrosis in black, viable region in gray. Reprinted with permission from Macklin and Lowengrub, *J. Theor. Biol.* Vol. 245, p. 693 (2007). Copyright Elsevier.

mobility, the more difficult it is for cells in the healthy tissue to overcome the cell-cell and cell-ECM adhesion and move to equilibrate pressure variations, and the more difficult it is for the ECM to deform in response to the pressure, allowing for the formation of sharper corners and greater shape instabilities.

Overall, the larger deformation in the lower-mobility tissue simulations leads to overall larger perimeters in the low-mobility tissue cases than in the higher-mobility tissue cases. As a result of the increased surface area, the low-mobility tissue tumors had greater access to nutrient. This leads to a surprising result: the increased morphological instability from growing into lower-mobility tissues improves access to nutrient and leads to larger tumors, for each fixed nutrient diffusivity, the volume of the viable area of each tumor was larger for the lower-mobility tissue simulation ($\mu = 0.25$) than for the corresponding higher-mobility tissue example ($\mu = 1$). For all examples, interface length, relative to a circle with the same area, steadily rose as a function of time, which reflects the increasing shape instability as the tumors invade the surrounding tissue; this is characteristic of invasive, fingering growth. This has implications for therapies that target cell-cell and cell-ECM adhesiveness: if the therapy decreases the mobility in the surrounding microenvironment (by increasing the cell-cell or cell-ECM adhesiveness or rendering the ECM more rigid), then invasive, fingering growth into the surrounding tissue is likely. Likewise, a treatment that decreases the permeability of the host tissue to tumor cells may lead to an increase in tumor invasiveness.

The finger width is most strongly dependent upon the nutrient diffusivity D, and largely independent of the tissue mobility μ. As the nutrient diffusivity increases, nutrient is better able to diffuse between the growing fingers, allowing the nutrient to penetrate farther into the fingers. This allows the tumor to support thicker fingers. In all cases, the length scale tended toward a roughly fixed value, which demonstrates that each tissue can support a specific finger thickness.

In Fig. 6.14, we examine the effect of the tumor aggressiveness parameter G and the necrotic degradation parameter G_N on the invasive, fingering morphology. We fix $D = 50$, $\mu = 1$; $N = 0.35$, and take $0.1 \leq G_N \leq 10.0$ and $1 \leq G \leq 100$. For lower tumor aggressiveness values ($G = 1$) and $G_N \geq 1$, the fingering effect was significantly reduced, resulting in more stable, tubular-shaped tumors, an effect that has been observed in experiments [73]. These structures form because tumor cell proliferation (the numerator of G) and cell-cell adhesion (the denominator of G) are roughly in balance when $G = 1$. The competition between proliferation and adhesion smoothes but does not completely prevent shape instabilities, which may continue to grow. For sufficiently large values of G, the invasive fingering morphology was observed in all simulated tumors. For lower values of G_N (left column in Fig. 6.14), the low rate of degradation of the necrotic tumor tissue leads to the formation of very wide fingers; this morphology may be better described as a collection of spheroids. As G_N is increased, the necrotic core is degraded more quickly, leading to a decreased finger thickness, less stable morphology, and more aggressive tissue invasion. As G_N is increased toward $G_N = 10$ (right column in Fig. 6.14), the finger thickness is decreased to the point where the tumor periodically breaks into fragments and then reconnects, leading to the encapsulation of noncancerous tissue (white enclosed regions). This morphology, which we refer to as compact/hollow, is characterized by the presence of a large abscess containing a mixture of necrotic cells, fluid, ECM, and cellular debris, much like a necrotic core. In a long-time simulation of a tumor with the compact/hollow morphology, the effect of G_N on growth is seen to be non-monotonic: increasing G_N at first limits the size of the tumor by decreasing the thickness of the invasive fingers and limiting the overall spread of the tumor, but after a certain point, instability breaks the tumor and allows greater spread through the surrounding noncancerous tissue.

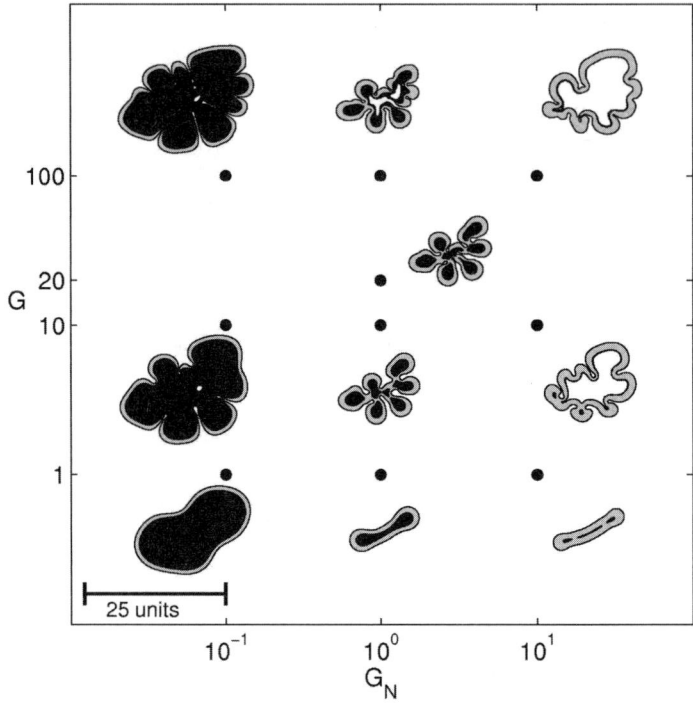

Fig. 6.14. Parameter study in G and G_N for invasive, fingering tumor growth into nutrient-rich, low-mobility tissue ($D = 50$, $\mu = 1$). The tumor aggressiveness parameter G increases from bottom to top, and the necrotic degradation parameter G_N increases from left to right. Necrosis in black, viable region in gray. Reprinted with permission from Macklin and Lowengrub, *J. Theor. Biol.* Vol. 245, p. 696 (2007). Copyright Elsevier.

Compact, Hollow Growth

We examine the effect of the tumor aggressiveness G and the necrotic degradation rate G_N on the compact tumor morphology. In these simulations, we fix $D = 50$, $\mu = \infty$, and $N = 0.35$. For lower values of G, the tumors remain in compact morphologies that fail to encapsulate noncancerous tissue, although shape instabilities may occur at long times. When $G = 1$, cell proliferation (numerator of G) and adhesion (denominator of G) are roughly in balance, which shrinks but does not completely prevent shape instabilities. For larger values of G, the cell proliferation rate outstrips cell-cell adhesion, resulting in folds in the outer tumor surface that encapsulate noncancerous tissue. For fixed values of G, we find that increasing the necrotic tissue degradation rate parameter G_N shrinks the necrotic volume fraction of the tumors. In the cases where noncancerous tissue has been encapsulated ($G > 1$), increasing G_N increases the size of the central tumor abscess. Lastly, as in the fragmenting and fingering cases, we find that varying N changes the tumor evolution quantitatively but not qualitatively. As N increases, the thickness of the viable rim decreases, the necrotic volume fraction increases, and morphological instability also increases.

Complex Tissue

We model growth in a complex, heterogeneous brain tissue as shown in the first frame in Fig. 6.15. We define B as the preexisting blood vessel density (as an indicator of bulk supply of nutrient to the vascularized tumor tissue). In the white region at the right side, $\mu = 0.0001$, $D = 0.0001$, and $B = 0$, which models a rigid material such as the skull. In the black regions, $\mu = 10$, $D = 1$, and $B = 0$, which models an incompressible fluid (cerebrospinal fluid). The light and dark gray regions model tissues of differing biomechanical properties (white and gray matter). In the light gray regions, $\mu = 1.5$, $D = 1$, and $B = 1$; in the dark gray regions, $\mu = 0.5$, $D = 1$, and $B = 1$. The tumor is denoted by a white thin boundary in the middle right of the frame. We smoothed μ, B, and D using a Gaussian filter with standard deviation $\sigma = 3 \triangle x = 0.3$ to satisfy smoothness requirements of the reaction-diffusion equations. We used (linear) extrapolation boundary conditions on the pressure along $x = 0$, $y = 0$, and $y = 50$ to simulate growth into a larger (not shown) tissue and set $p = 0$ along the rigid boundary at $x = 50$.

We simulated from $t = 0$ to $t = 60$. Using a 3.3 GHz Pentium 4 workstation and a C++ implementation, the 501×501 simulation required less than 24 hours to compute. Because the (mitosis) time scale ranges from approximately 18 to 36 hours for this problem, this corresponds to 45 to 90 days of growth. We plot the solution in $t = 10.0$ (approximately 10 days) increments in Fig. 6.15. In these plots, regions corresponding to viable tumor tissue (where $c > c_H$), hypoxic tumor tissue ($c_H \geq c > c_N$), and necrotic tumor cells ($c_N \geq c$) are shown. In hypoxic tissue, there is assumed to be no proliferation. In this simulation, the tumor grows rapidly until the nutrient level drops below $c_H = 0.30$, at which time a large portion of the tumor becomes hypoxic. The tumor continues to grow at a slower rate until the interior of the tumor becomes necrotic (see $t = 10.0$). This causes nonuniform volume loss within the tumor and contributes to morphological instability. Note that because the biomechanical responsiveness is continuous across the tumor boundary and the microenvironment has a moderate nutrient gradient, this simulation corresponds to the border between the invasive, fingering growth regime and the invasive, fragmenting growth regime that was investigated earlier.

However, additional effects can be seen that were not observed before. As the tumor grows out of the biomechanically permissive tissue (light gray; $\mu = 1.5$) and into the biomechanically resistant tissue (dark gray; $\mu = 0.5$), its rate of invasion into the tissue slows (see $t = 20.0$). This results in preferential

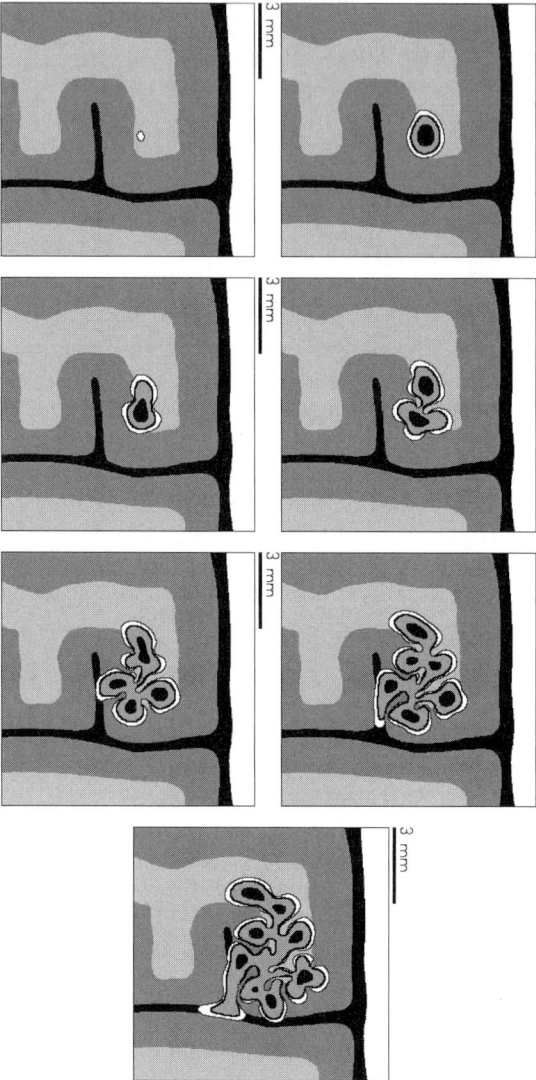

Fig. 6.15. Tumor simulation from $t = 0.0$ days (top left) to $t = 60.0$ days (bottom right) in 10 day increments. White band on the right of each frame models a rigid material such as the skull; black denotes an incompressible fluid (e.g., cerebrospinal fluid); light and dark gray regions represent tissues of differing biomechanical properties (e.g., white and gray matter). Tumor tissue is shown growing in the middle right with viable (outer layer, white), hypoxic (middle layer, gray), and necrotic (core, black) regions. Reprinted from Macklin and Lowengrub (in press) [135].

growth into the permissive (light gray) material, a trend which can be clearly seen from $t = 30.0$ onward. When the tumor grows through the resistive tissue (dark gray) and reaches the fluid (black) ($t = 40.0$), the tumor experiences a sudden drop in biomechanical resistance to growth. As a result, the tumor grows rapidly and preferentially in the $1/2$ mm fluid structures that separate the tissue ($t = 50.0 - 60.0$). Such growth patterns are not observed when simulating homogeneous tissues. Other observed differences are due to our new treatment of hypoxic (quiescent) tumor cells. Certain regions that had previously been classified as necrotic (in [131, 132, 133, 134]) are now treated as quiescent. As a result, tumor volume loss is reduced, and in particular, this may result in large hypoxic regions that have little or no viable rim. Had these regions been treated as necrotic, the invasive fingers would have been thinner, and the tumor may have fragmented. Therefore, the separate treatment of the hypoxic regions can have a significant impact on the details of the invasive morphology of the tumor.

6.4.4 Summary

In this work [134, 135] we developed a framework to investigate the interaction between avascular solid tumors and their microenvironment. In particular, we model perfusion of nutrient through a tumor and surrounding microenvironment, build-up of pressure in the tissue from proliferation of cancerous cells, cell-cell and cell-ECM adhesion, and loss of tumor volume due to necrosis. We observed three distinct morphologies: fragmenting, invasive/fingering, and compact/hollow growth. If the microenvironment is nutrient poor, tumors tend to break into small fragments and spread throughout the microenvironment, regardless of cellular mobility. Within this nutrient-poor growth regime, decreasing microenvironmental mobility (by increasing noncancerous cell-cell and cell-ECM adhesion or increasing ECM rigidity) decreases the extent of fragmentation and slows invasion into surrounding tissue, but does not completely prevent hypoxia-induced morphological instability. (Unstable tumor morphologies in the nutrient-poor regime have been observed in [10] and [54].) An invasive, fingering morphology was found in cases of growth into nutrient-rich, low-mobility microenvironments. Increasing nutrient perfusion does not prevent this invasive morphology, and the lower the microenvironmental mobility, the greater the degree of morphological instability and invasiveness. Tumors growing into nutrient-rich, high-mobility tissues develop compact/ hollow morphologies. A hallmark of this growth regime is formation and merger of buds on the tumor periphery, which leads to encapsulation of noncancerous regions and formation of a large abscess that qualitatively is similar to a necrotic core.

Since decreasing nutrient levels in the microenvironment tends to increase tumor fragmentation and invasion into the surrounding tissue, this may have to be taken into consideration during anti-angiogenic therapies, as it could lead to morphological instability in the form of fragmentation and invasion.

A number of experimental studies have recently shown that anti-angiogenic therapies may have this result [179, 176, 60, 172, 184, 121, 23]. Conversely, we found that increasing nutrient levels leads to greater morphological stability and increased tumor compactness, thereby rendering some tumors more resectable. These results support the contention [54] that treatments that seek to normalize tumor vasculature (by selectively "pruning" weak blood vessels with targeted anti-angiogenic therapy) may stabilize tumor morphology by providing increased access to nutrient. Since such treatments may also increase the accessibility to chemotherapeutic agents [104, 187], our results provide additional support for the use of targeted anti-angiogenic therapy as adjuvant to chemotherapy and resection.

As pointed out in [54], another approach to therapy is to use anti-invasive drugs such as Met inhibitors [29, 19, 145] or hepatocyte growth factor (HGF) antagonists [59, 143] in addition to anti-angiogenic therapies. Such therapies affect cell-cell and cell-ECM adhesive properties of the tumor. A recent experimental study on mouse models of malignant glioma shows that fragmentation can be prevented, and tumor satellites may be eliminated by a combined anti-angiogenic and anti-invasive therapy [23]. In the nutrient-poor growth regime, increasing cell-cell and cell-ECM adhesion of the microenvironment can help limit the rate of fragmentation and the extent of invasion. Decreasing permeability of the microenvironmental ECM to tumor cells by other means, such as making the ECM more dense, stiffer, and less able to support tumor cell movement, could also attain this effect.

Interestingly, the opposite approach is warranted in the nutrient-rich growth regime. In this case, decreasing cell-cell and cell-ECM adhesion in the microenvironment (while leaving tumor cells unaffected) or increasing the permeability of the microenvironment to tumor cells decreases invasive fingering. This could also be accomplished by increasing tumor cell-cell and cell-ECM adhesion or by decreasing the stiffness or density of the surrounding ECM, respectively. Such subtleties highlight the importance of considering tumor-microenvironment interactions when planning therapies that affect adhesive and mechanical properties of a tumor, its surrounding tissue, or both.

6.5 Vascularized 3-D Tumor Growth Using a Diffuse Interface Approach[8]

6.5.1 Overview

This section describes development of a model of Functional Collective Cell-Migration Units (FCCMU) [71] that describes the large-scale morphology and 3-D cell spatial arrangements during tumor growth and invasion. This includes

---

[8] This article was published in *NeuroImage*, Vol. 37, Frieboes et al., pp. S59–S70, Copyright 2007 Elsevier.

the application of mathematical and empirical methods to quantify the competition between cell substrate gradient-related pro-invasion phenomena and molecular forces that govern proliferation and taxis, and forces opposing invasion through cell adhesion. The latter, under normoxic conditions, often enforce compact non-infiltrative tumor morphology while local oxygen gradients promote invasion [189, 155, 184, 119, 159, 121, 23, 176, 172, 173, 60, 54, 73, 134]. Interactions between cellular proliferation and adhesion and other phenotypic properties may be reflected in both the surface characteristics, e.g., stability, of the tumor-host interface and the growth characteristics of tumors [58, 54, 73, 86, 134]. These characteristics give rise to various tumor morphologies and influence treatment outcomes. The model thus enables the deterministic linking of collective tumor cell motion on the balance between cellular properties and the microenvironment.

We assemble this 3-D multiscale computational model of cancer as a key step towards the transition from qualitative, empirical correlations of molecular biology, histopathology, and imaging to quantitative and predictive mathematical laws founded on the underlying biology. The model provides resolution at various tissue physical scales, including the microvasculature, and quantifies functional links of molecular factors to phenotype that currently for the most part can only be tentatively established through laboratory or clinical observation. This mathematical and computational approach allows observable properties of a tumor, e.g., its morphology, to be used to both understand the underlying cellular physiology and predict subsequent growth (or treatment outcome), providing a bridge between observable, morphologic properties of the tumor and its prognosis [55, 181].

6.5.2 Method Description

The FCCMU model is based on conservation laws (e.g., of mass and momentum) with conserved variables that describe the known determinants of glioma (e.g., cell density) and with parameters that characterize a specific glioma tissue. The conservation laws consist of well-established, biologically founded convection-reaction-diffusion equations that govern the densities of the tumor cell species, the diffusion of cytokines, and the concentration of vital nutrients. The model describes the cells' (collective) migratory response and interaction with the ECM and an evolving neovasculature. The collective tumor cell velocity depends on proliferation-driven mechanical pressure in the tissue, and chemotaxis and haptotaxis due to gradients of soluble cytokines and insoluble matrix macromolecules. The cell species velocity is obtained from a Darcy's law coarse-scale reformulation of the inertialess momentum equation, which is the instantaneous equilibrium among the following forces: pressure, resistance to motion (cell-adhesion), elastic forces, forces exchanged with the ECM leading to haptotaxis and chemotaxis, and other mechanical effects (see, e.g. [58, 211, 54, 73, 180, 126, 11, 10, 12, 50, 3, 24, 47, 78, 15, 132, 89, 38, 39, 5, 134, 6, 42, 49]). Cells produce proteases, which degrade the matrix locally, making room for cells to migrate. In the model, matrix degradation releases cytokines and growth promoters, thus having biological effects on tumor cells (see e.g., [47]). The model can account for cell-cell interactions (cell-cell adhesion and communications), high polarity, and strong pulling forces exchanged by cells and the ECM [77].

The FCCMU model is coupled nonlinearly to a hybrid continuum-discrete, lattice-free model of tumor-induced angiogenesis [160, 161]. The angiogenesis component describes proliferation and migration due to chemotaxis and haptotaxis of endothelial cells in response to tumor angiogenic factors (e.g., VEGF) and matrix macromolecules, respectively. The angiogenic factors are released by peri-necrotic tumor cells and host cells near the tumor-host interface [192, 185], which stimulate vascular endothelial cells of the brain vasculature to proliferate and begin to form vessels [106]. Anastomosed vessels may provide a source of nutrient in the tissue and may undergo spontaneous shutdown and regression during tumor growth [98]. We note that there are other related lattice-based models of tumor neovascularization (e.g., [190, 139]). Although tumor angiogenesis may occur via the formation of sprouts or intussusception [157], for simplicity here only the former process is incorporated in the model. Input parameter values to the model, e.g., cell proliferation and apoptosis, are estimated from in vitro cell lines and ex vivo patient data. The parameters governing the extent of neovascularization and nutrient supply due to blood flow are estimated in part from dynamic contrast-enhanced magnetic resonance imaging (DCE-MRI) observations in patients [151].

The model describes nutrient/oxygen delivery from the neovasculature (via convection and diffusion [45, 104, 105]) and cellular uptake, and nutrient, oxygen, and growth factor diffusion through the tumor tissue [35]. Oxygen/nutrient availability limits the fraction of cycling cells. Regions of tissue become hypoxic and then necrotic where nutrient/oxygen concentration falls below a threshold. The model describes evolution of local mass fractions of viable tumor species, and necrotic and host tissues. Cell mass exchange occurs due to mutations, mitosis, necrosis, and apoptosis. Lysis rates describe the disintegration of tumor cell mass and the radial effusion of fluid away from the necrotic regions. All rates are inverse times (unit time = 1 day). At any given time during tumor growth, the model outputs the computed values of all relevant variables at every location within the 3-D tumor tissue, e.g., the spatial distributions of oxygen, nutrients, and tumor cell species. The result is a description of the complex, multiscalar dynamics of in vivo 3-D tumors through avascular, neovascular, vascular growth, and invasion stages.

6.5.3 Multiscale Model

The minimal formulation of the FCCMU model is based on reaction-diffusion equations that govern a tumor cell density, an evolving neovasculature, a vital nutrient concentration, the ECM, and matrix degrading enzymes. Extensions to include more complex biophysics, e.g., multiple nutrients, growth inhibitors, and matrix remodeling, are straightforward.

In this approach, each constituent moves with its own velocity field; mass, momentum and energy equations are posed for each constituent. Through experimental comparisons and the inclusion of molecular-scale effects, we formulate functional relationships that close the FCCMU model. Generically, the reaction-diffusion equations take the form

$$\nu_t = -\nabla \cdot \mathbf{J} + \Gamma_+ - \Gamma_- , \tag{6.43}$$

where ν is the evolving variable, $\mathbf{J}$ is the flux, and Γ_+ and Γ_- are the sources and sinks. Letting $\nu = \rho_i$, σ, f, m, respectively be the tumor cell density of species i or the host density, the vital cell substrate concentration (e.g., oxygen), the (nondiffusible) matrix macromolecule (e.g., fibronectin [11, 10]), and matrix degrading enzyme, MDE (e.g., matrix metalloproteinases, urokinase plasminogen activators [12, 10, 50]) concentrations, we may take

$$\mathbf{J} = \begin{cases} \rho_i \mathbf{u}_i + \mathbf{J}_{\text{mechanics},i} & \text{if } \nu = \rho_i \\ \sigma \mathbf{u}_W - D_\sigma \nabla \sigma & \text{if } \nu = \sigma \\ 0 & \text{if } \nu = f \\ m \mathbf{u}_W - D_m \nabla m & \text{if } \nu = m \end{cases} \tag{6.44}$$

$$\Gamma_+ = \begin{cases} \rho_i \lambda_{\text{prolif},i} + \sum_j S_{ij}^+ & \text{if } \nu = \rho_i \\ \lambda_{\text{blood}} & \text{if } \nu = \sigma \\ \lambda_f & \text{if } \nu = f \\ \lambda_{\text{mde}} & \text{if } \nu = m \end{cases} \tag{6.45}$$

$$\Gamma_- = \begin{cases} \rho_i \lambda_{\text{death},i} + \sum_j S_{ij}^- & \text{if } \nu = \rho_i \\ \lambda_{\sigma,\text{uptake}} & \text{if } \nu = \sigma \\ \lambda_{f,\text{degrade}} & \text{if } \nu = f \\ \lambda_{\text{mde,degrade}} & \text{if } \nu = m \end{cases}, \tag{6.46}$$

where $\mathbf{u}_i$ is the cell velocity of species or host i, $\mathbf{u}_w$ is the velocity of water (i.e., assuming transport of chemical factors is primarily through the interstitial liquid), the D's are diffusion constants, and λ_{prolif}, λ_{death}, λ_{blood}, λ_{uptake}, λ_f, $\lambda_{f,\text{degrade}}$, λ_{mde}, and $\lambda_{\text{mde,degrade}}$ are the mitosis, apoptosis and necrosis, blood-tissue nutrient transfer and uptake and decay rates, respectively, for matrix molecules and MDE. An additional equation (not shown) is posed for the mass fraction of water. The flux $\mathbf{J}_{\mathrm{mechanics},i}$ accounts for the mechanical interactions among the different cell species. A major component of the FCCMU model is the development of the constitutive law for $\mathbf{J}_{\mathrm{mechanics},i}$. This is obtained from a variational approach from an energy formulation that accounts for the mechanical forces, e.g., cell-cell and cell-matrix adhesion, and elastic effects (residual stress). A feature of this approach is the incorporation of a novel continuum model of adhesion in this flux. Following the variational approach developed for diffuse interface models of multiphase flows and materials by Lowengrub and coworkers (e.g., [129, 123, 122, 111, 112, 202, 113]) and others (e.g., [83, 100, 11]) we introduce a continuum model of cell-cell and cell-matrix adhesion energy that can be written as an integral taken over the entire tumor/host domain $E_{\mathrm{adhesion},i} = \int f_i(\rho_1, \ldots, \rho_N) + \frac{1}{2} \sum_{j=1}^{N-1} \varepsilon_{i,j}^2 |\nabla \rho_j|^2 dx$. The first term is a bulk energy, which accounts for the degree of miscibility of cell and host species, as directed by experiments. The second term introduces cell-cell adhesion forces that generate a surface tension between the phases and further accounts for intermixing across a diffuse interface of thickness that roughly scales with $\varepsilon_{i,i}$. Typically, the cell-adhesion energy enforces phase separation of tumor and host tissues sharing a diffuse interface with thickness 1–100 μm. Under the assumption that tumor cells prefer to stay bonded with each other rather than being in any other configuration, that the cell density is roughly constant, and that there is only isotropic stress (pressure p), this reduces, in an asymptotic limit, to the "jump" boundary condition $[p] = \tau \kappa$ where τ measures the affinity and κ is the total curvature of the interface [201, 72]. This is akin to surface tension in multiphase flows and can also be used to describe tumor encapsulation by ECM fragments and is characteristic of collective cell migration [77].

A thermodynamically consistent constitutive law for the flux $\mathbf{J}_{\mathrm{mechanics},i}$ is obtained by taking the gradient of the variational derivative of the total energy: $\mathbf{J}_{\mathrm{mechanics},i} \propto \nabla(\delta E_{\mathrm{mechanics},i}/\delta \rho_i)$, where $E_{\mathrm{mechanics},i}$ is obtained by adding the contributions from each mechanism modeled, i.e., adhesion, elasticity, etc. The velocities $\mathbf{u}_i$ and $\mathbf{u}_w$ are determined from momentum equations. For example, following previous approaches (e.g., [58, 211, 54, 73, 126, 132, 134]) that are reformulations and generalizations of models in [89, 38, 39, 3, 24, 47] and neglecting viscoelastic effects, we take Darcy's law as a coarse-scale reformulation of the inertialess momentum equation, which is the instantaneous equilibrium among the following forces: pressure, resistance to motion, elastic forces, forces exchanged with the ECM leading to hapto- and chemotaxis and other mechanical effects within $E_{\mathrm{mechanics}}$ as discussed above. This leads to

$$\mathbf{u}_i = -M_i \nabla p + \gamma_i (\delta E_{\mathrm{mechanics},i}/\delta \rho_i) \nabla \rho_i + \chi_{f,i} \nabla f + \chi_{\sigma,i} \nabla \sigma \,, \qquad (6.47)$$

where p is the pressure (isotropic stress) and M, γ_i, χ_f, and χ_σ are the spatially inhomogeneous mobility, mechanotaxis, haptotaxis, and chemotaxis tensors that also take into account cell-matrix adhesion. The parameter M

depends on the extent of cell-to-cell and cell-to-ECM adhesion in bulk regions. Since a number of different parameters in the model describe various effects of cell-cell and cell-ECM adhesion it is expected that this model should have enough complexity to reproduce nontrivial and nonmonotonic dependences of migration on cell adhesion molecules (CAMs) [77]. Note that other models such as Stokes, viscoelastic, and nonlinear-elastic/plastic can be incorporated as required.

The FCCMU continuum-scale convection-reaction-diffusion equations are solved numerically using a novel adaptive finite-difference method [201, 72, 200]. This method features an adaptive, block-structured Cartesian mesh refinement algorithm (see, e.g., [26]), centered differences in space and an implicit time discretization for which there is no stability constraint on the space and time steps. The nonlinear equations at the implicit time level are solved efficiently using a multilevel, nonlinear multigrid method (see, e.g., [30]).

6.5.4 Tumor Vasculature

We model the physiology and evolution of glioma neovasculature in 3-D using a hybrid continuum-discrete, lattice-free model of tumor angiogenesis which is a refinement of earlier work [160, 161]. This was shown to create dendritic structures consistent with experimentally observed tumor capillaries [124, 188]. This random walk model generates vascular topology based on tumor angiogenic factors, e.g., VEGF [192], represented by a single continuum variable that reflects the excess of pro-angiogenic factors compared to inhibitory ones. Peri-necrotic tumor cells and host tissue cells close to the tumor boundary are assumed to be a source of angiogenic factors (e.g., VEGF). Endothelial cells near the sprout tips proliferate and their migration is described by chemotaxis and haptotaxis (e.g., motion up gradients of angiogenic factors and matrix proteins such as fibronectin). For simplicity, only leading endothelial cells are modeled and trailing cells passively follow. The vasculature architecture, i.e., interconnectedness and anastomoses, is captured via a set of rules, e.g., a leading endothelial cell has a fixed probability of branching at each time step while anastomosis occurs if a leading endothelial cell crosses a vessel trailing path. Glioma vessels are more tortuous than normal vessels [33]. This can be quantified by various means including a Sum of Angles Metric (SOAM) that sums total curvature along a space curve and normalizes by path length, indicating high frequency, low-amplitude sine waves or coils [33].

The tumor-induced vasculature does not initially conduct blood, as the vessels need to form loops first (anastomosis) [18]. As observed experimentally, the neovasculature model may also account for increasing vessel diameters and spontaneous shutdown and consecutive regression of initially functioning tumor vessel segments or whole microvascular areas [98]. Here, functional anastomosed vessels were assumed to provide a source of nutrient in the tissue proportionally to local pressure.

6.5.5 Calculation of Model Parameters

Previous measurements of growth and histopathology of in vitro ACBT (human glioblastoma multiforme) tumor spheroids [73], and of human glioma [22] were used to inform the parameters of the simulation presented herein. Briefly, higher-grade glioma mitosis and apoptosis rates were taken to be 1 day^{-1} and 0.32 day^{-1} respectively. The characteristic time scale was taken to be the inverse mitosis rate. The diffusion penetration length was measured to be 100 μm [58, 73], and is used herein as the characteristic unit of length. The necrosis threshold was taken to be $\sigma_N/\sigma_V = 0.5$, where σ_N is the nutrient concentration needed for viability and σ_V is the nutrient concentration in the far field. Mutation rates from low- to high-grade glioma were also estimated in previous work [22] but not utilized here. In previous work, a critical value of cell adhesion parameter was determined from shape stability analysis of experimental and simulated spheroids [73]: compact spherical morphologies exist only for sufficiently large adhesion, which is implemented via the parameter (after nondimensionalization) in (6.47). The above set of parameters provided the baseline for our simulations (the results show a simulation using a sub-critical value of the adhesion parameter). Simulations were performed using one fixed set of parameters as described above. Parameter sensitivity studies were performed where cell adhesion (γ_i) and cell chemotaxis ($\chi_{\sigma,i}$) parameters were varied to study their effect on the morphology of infiltrating collective-cell patterns (i.e., cell chains vs. strands vs. detached clusters [77]). Representative resulting morphologies are reported elsewhere and confirm that for relatively low cell adhesion morphologic instability occurs when nutrient heterogeneity is present, leading to the development of infiltrative cell protrusions [58, 73, 134, 22]. The shape features of these protrusions further depend on the relative strengths of cell proliferation and cell chemotaxis. A control was provided by simulations corresponding to relatively high cell adhesion, for which tumors grow spherically and morphologic instability does not occur.

6.5.6 Results

Fig. 6.16 shows a millimeter-sized glioblastoma during early stages of growth simulated using our 3-D multiscale model. The model predicts regions of viable cells, necrosis in inner tumor areas, and a tortuous neovasculature as observed in vivo [33]. Conducting vessels are capable of releasing nutrient. The rate of nutrient released may depend on their age and the solid pressure in the tissue. The vessels migrate towards the tumor/host interface since peri-necrotic tumor cells and host tissue cells close to the tumor boundary are assumed to produce angiogenic factors and other regulators. The tumor eventually coopts and engulfs the vessels. The tumor-induced vasculature does not initially conduct blood, as the vessels need to form loops first (anastomosis) [18], i.e., more mature vessels that have anastomosed conduct blood and may release nutrient. By hypothesizing the underlying mechanisms driving these phenomena, the model enables a quantitative analysis, e.g., a viable region thickness of about 100–200 μm and the extent of necrosis as seen in Fig. 6.16 are shown to be strongly dependent on diffusion gradients of oxygen/nutrient in the microenvironment and agree with previous experiments [93, 73]. Chaotic angiogenesis leads to heterogeneous perfusion in the tumor that then might be responsible for regression of parts of the vascular network and necrosis of tumor cells [44, 157], further enhancing variable tumor cell proliferation. By taking vessel maturation into account, the simulations correctly predict that as tumor size increases, inner vessels may regress or shut down, leading to nutrient depletion and resulting in the formation of a large necrotic core (data not shown), as observed in patients. For example, centimeter-sized human glioblastoma at later stages as seen through MRI in patients (e.g., [204]) is composed of viable cells delineating its boundary and surrounding extensive necrosis in its inner region.

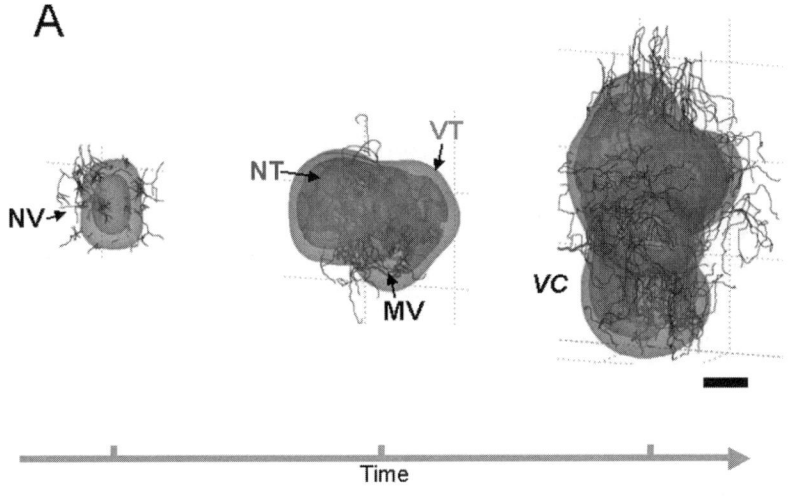

Fig. 6.16. Multiscale 3-D computer model predicts gross morphologic features of a growing glioblastoma. Viable (VT) and necrotic (NT) tissue regions, and vasculature (MV: mature blood-conducting vessels; NV: new nonconducting vessels) are shown. Time sequence (from left to right, over a period of 3 months) reveals that the morphology is affected by successive cycles of neovascularization, vasculature maturation, and vessel co-option (VC). Bar, 250 μm. Reprinted with permission from Frieboes et al., *NeuroImage*, Vol. 37, p. S63, (2007). Copyright Elsevier.

The multiscale model enables the prediction of tumor morphology by quantifying the spatial diffusion gradients of cell substrates maintained by heterogeneous cell proliferation and an abnormal, constantly evolving vasculature. Fig. 6.16 shows a simulated time sequence over the course of three months predicting that the glioblastoma grows with a thin layer of viable tissue on its periphery, displacing nearby tissue and internally generating necrosis. The morphology is directly influenced by angiogenesis, vasculature maturation, and vessel cooption [196, 18, 97]. The model predicts that the tumor boundary moves at a rate of about 50–100 μm per week, presenting a mass of diameter of about 5 cm in one year (data not shown). These results are supported by well-known clinical observations (e.g., [147]). As the tumor grows and engulfs vessels in its vicinity, the tumor may compress the vessels [154] and disrupt flow of nutrients, leading to further necrosis and even temporary mass and vascular regression [210, 98]. A growing tumor contends with increasing mechanical resistance from normal brain tissue, which has physical properties resembling a gel [152, 67]. Nevertheless, this resistance is insufficient to contain tumor growth, e.g., gliomas have been observed to displace cartilage [118]. Only hard bone (e.g., the skull) will be a physical barrier. The effect of such physical barriers on tumor morphology and growth can be incorporated in the multiscale model (see the methods in [71]).

6.5.7 Summary

We performed 3-D computer simulations of growing glioma and neovascular morphologies employing a multiscale mathematical model based on first principles and informed by experimental and clinical data, e.g., histopathology data transformed into model input parameters, and calibrated so that tumor morphology can be predicted beyond a purely empirical, observational approach [71]. The multiscale model predicts that glioma tissue structure and tumor invasiveness are significantly influenced by diffusion gradients in the microenvironment, as observed experimentally [176, 119, 121, 23, 73] and in human patients [22]. These gradients may have a strong effect on glioma morphology [54, 134], and are hypothesized in the model to reciprocally influence a growing tumor's continuously evolving vasculature in complex ways. The 3-D model facilitates this study by calculating the chemotactic and haptotactic response of the blood vessels at the cell scale and its cumulative effect at the tumor scale.

6.6 Conclusion

The mathematical models and simulation results reviewed in this chapter aim to develop theories and numerical analyses to study cancer as a system across physical scales linking tumor morphology with cellular and microenvironmental characteristics through experimentally tested functional relationships. The central hypothesis underlying this research is inspired by an engineering approach to tumor lesions as complex microstructured materials, where three-dimensional tissue architecture ("morphology" and dynamics are coupled in complex, nonlinear ways to cell phenotype, and this to molecular properties (e.g., genetics) and phenomena in the environment (e.g., hypoxia). These properties and phenomena act both as regulators of morphology and as determinants of invasion potential by controlling cell proliferation and migration mechanisms [77, 186, 197]. The importance of this close connection between tumor morphology and the underlying cellular/molecular scale is that it could allow observable properties of a tumor (e.g., morphology) to be used to understand the underlying cellular physiology and predict invasive behavior through mathematical modeling. Tumor morphology could also serve as a clinical prognostic factor because it may indicate the potential to respond to treatment; for instance, an indication of hypoxia could adversely affect oxygen-dependent treatment such as radiation therapy and some chemotherapies. This approach opens the possibility of using mathematical modeling to design novel therapeutic strategies in which the microenvironment and cellular factors are manipulated with the aim of both imposing compact morphology and reducing tumor invasion—an outcome that would benefit cancer therapy by improving local tumor control through surgery or radiation.

The models also strive to provide a more comprehensive understanding of the molecular and environmental bases of cellular diversity and adaptation by describing the complex interactions among tumor cells and their microenvironment [186, 197]. This approach is expected to improve current cancer modeling efforts because a multiscale approach model connects previous work focused on specific scales and specific processes (e.g., single cell motion) by performing 3-dimensional simulations of in vivo tumors. This methodology further allows the possibility to see beyond the current reductionist picture of invasion and migration [77, 110, 186, 197, 203, 116, 205, 63, 178, 74, 76, 52, 171], with the goal to enable prediction of disease progression and treatment response based on patient-specific tumor characteristics.

References

1. Abbott, R.G., Forrest, S., Pienta, K.J.: Simulating the hallmarks of cancer. Artif. Life, **12**, 617–634 (2006)
2. Acker, H.: Spheroids in Cancer Research: Methods and Perspectives. Springer-Verlag, Berlin and New York (1984)
3. Adam, J.: General aspects of modeling tumor growth and the immune response. In: Adam, J., Bellomo, N. (eds), A Survey of Models on Tumor Immune Systems Dynamics. Birkhauser, Boston, MA (1996)
4. Alarcón, T., Byrne, H.M., Maini, P.K.: A cellular automaton model for tumour growth in inhomogeneous environment. J. Theor. Biol., **225**, 257–274 (2003)
5. Ambrosi, D., Guana, F.: Stress-modulated growth. Math. Mech. Solids, **12**, 319–343 (2007)

6. Ambrosi, D., Mollica, F.: On the mechanics of a growing tumor. Int. J. Eng. Sci., **40**, 1297–1316 (2002)

7. Ambrosi, D., Preziosi, L.: On the closure of mass balance models for tumor growth. Math. Mod. Meth. Appl. Sci., **12**, 737–754 (2002)

8. Andersen, H., Mejlvang, J., Mahmood, S., Gromova, I., Gromov, P., Lukanidin, E., Kriajevska, M., Mellon, J.K., Tulchinsky, E.: Immediate and delayed effects of E-cadherin inhibition on gene regulation and cell motility in human epidermoid carcinoma cells. Mol. Cell. Biol., **25**, 9138–9150 (2005)

9. Anderson, A., Zheng, X., Cristini, V.: Adaptive unstructured volume remeshing-I: The method. J. Comput. Phys., **208**, 616–625 (2005)

10. Anderson, A.R.A.: A hybrid mathematical model of solid tumour invasion: the importance of cell adhesion. IMA Math. Appl. Med. Biol., **22**, 163–186 (2005)

11. Anderson, A.R.A., Chaplain, M.A.J.: Continuous and discrete mathematical models of tumor-induced angiogenesis. Bull. Math. Biol., **60**, 857–900 (1998)

12. Anderson, A.R.A. Chaplain, M.A.J., Newman, E.L., Steele, R.J.C., Thompson, A.M.: Mathematical modeling of tumour invasion and metastasis, J. Theor. Med., **2**, 129–154 (2000)

13. Anderson, A.R.A., Chaplain, M.A.J., Lowengrub, J.S., Macklin, P., McDougall, S.: Nonlinear simulation of tumour invasion and angiogenesis. Bull. Math. Biol., (in preparation)

14. Anderson, D.M., McFadden, G.B., Wheeler, A.A.: Diffuse interface methods in fluid mechanics. Ann. Rev. Fluid Mech., **30**, 139–165 (1998)

15. Araujo, R.P., McElwain, D.L.S.: A history of the study of solid tumor growth: the contribution of mathematical modeling. Bull. Math. Biol., **66**, 1039–1091 (2004)

16. Araujo, R.P., McElwain, D.L.S.: A linear-elastic model of anisotropic tumor growth. Eur. J. Appl. Math., **15**, 365–384 (2004)

17. Araujo, R.P., McElwain, D.L.S.: A mixture theory for the genesis of residual stresses in growing tissues II: solutions to the biphasic equations for a multicell spheroid. SIAM J. Appl. Math., **66**, 447–467 (2005)

18. Augustin, H.G.: Tubes, branches, and pillars: the many ways of forming a new vasculature. Circ. Research, **89**, 645–647 (2001)

19. Bardelli, A., Basile, M.L., Audero, E., Giordano, S., Wennström, S., Ménard, S., Comoglio, P.M., Ponzetto, C.: Concomitant activation of pathways downstream of Grb2 and PI 3-kinase is required for MET-mediated metastasis. Oncogene, **18**, 1139–1146 (1999)

20. Batchelor, G.: An Introduction to Fluid Dynamics. Cambridge University Press, Cambridge (1967)

21. Bauer, T.W., Liu, W.B., Fan, F., Camp, E.R., Yang, A., Somcio, R.J., Bucana, C.D., Callahan, J., Parry, G.C., Evans, D.B., Boyd, D.D., Mazar, A.P., Ellis, L.M.: Targeting of urokinase plasminogen activator receptor in human pancreatic carcinoma cells inhibits c-met- and insulin-like growth factor-1 receptor-mediated migration and invasion and orthotopic tumor growth in mice. Cancer Res., **65**, 7775–7781 (2005)

22. Bearer, E.L., Cristini, V.: Computational modeling identifies morphologic predictors of tumor invasion. Science, (in review)

23. Bello, L., Lucini, V., Costa, F., Pluderi, M., Giussani, C., Acerbi, F., Carrabba, G., Pannacci, M., Caronzolo, D., Grosso, S., Shinkaruk, S., Colleoni, F., Canron, X., Tomei, G., Deleris, G., Bikfalvi, A.: Combinatorial administration

of molecules that simultaneously inhibit angiogenesis and invasion leads to increased therapeutic efficacy in mouse models of malignant glioma. Clin. Cancer Res., **10**, 4527–4537 (2004)

24. Bellomo, N., Preziosi, L.: Modelling and mathematical problems related to tumor evolution and its interaction with the immune system. Math. Comput. Modelling, **32**, 413–452 (2000)

25. Bellomo, N., de Angelis, E., Preziosi, L.: Multiscale modelling and mathematical problems related to tumor evolution and medical therapy. J. Theor. Med., **5**, 111–136 (2003)

26. Berger, M., Colella, P.: Local adaptive mesh refinement for shock hydrodynamics. J. Comp. Phys., **82**, 64–84 (1989)

27. Bernsen, H.J.J.A., Van der Kogel, A.J.: Antiangiogenic therapy in brain tumor models. J. Neuro-oncology, **45**, 247–255 (1999)

28. Bloemendal, H.J., Logtenberg, T., Voest, E.E.: New strategies in anti-vascular cancer therapy. Euro. J. Clinical Investig., **29**, 802–809 (1999)

29. Boccaccio, C., Andò, M., Tamagnone, L., Bardelli, A., Michieli, P., Battistini, C., Comoglio, P.M.: Induction of epithelial tubules by growth factor HGF depends on the STAT pathway. Nature, **391**, 285–288 (1998)

30. Brandt, A.: Multi-level adaptive solutions to boundary-value problems, Math. Comput., **31**, 333–390 (1977)

31. Breward, C., Byrne, H., Lewis, C.: A multiphase model describing vascular tumour growth. Bull. Math. Biol., **65**, 609–640 (2003)

32. Brizel, D.M., Scully, S.P., Harrelson, J.M., Layfield, L.J., Bean, J.M., Prosnitz, L.R., Dewhirst, M.W.: Tumor oxygenation predicts for the likelihood of distant metastases in human soft tissue sarcoma. Cancer Res., **56**, 941–943 (1996)

33. Bullitt, E., Zeng, D., Gerig, G., Aylward, S., Joshi, S., Smith, J.K., Lin, W., Ewend, M.G.: Vessel tortuosity and brain tumor malignance: a blinded study. Acad. Radiol., **12**, 1232–1240 (2005)

34. Bussolino, F., Arese, M., Audero, E., Giraudo, E., Marchiò, S., Mitola, S., Primo, L., Serini, G.: Biological aspects of tumour angiogenesis. In: Cancer Modelling and Simulation. Chapman & Hall/CRC, London (2003)

35. Byrne, H.M.: The importance of intercellular adhesion in the development of carcinomas. IMA J. Math. Med. Biol., **14**, 305–323 (1997)

36. Byrne, H.M., Alarcón, T., Owen, M.R., Webb, S.D., Maini, P.K.: Modeling aspects of cancer dynamics: a review. Philos. Trans. R. Soc. A, **364**, 1563–1578 (2006)

37. Byrne, H.M., Chaplain, M.A.J.: Growth of nonnecrotic tumors in the presence and absence of inhibitors. Math. Biosci., **130**, 151–181 (1995)

38. Byrne, H.M., Chaplain, M.A.J.: Growth of necrotic tumors in the presence and absence of inhibitors. Math. Biosci., **135**, 187–216 (1996)

39. Byrne, H.M., Chaplain, M.A.J.: Modelling the role of cell-cell adhesion in the growth and development of carcinomas. Math. Comput. Modeling, **24**, 1–17 (1996)

40. Byrne, H.M., Chaplain, M.A.J.: Free boundary value problems associated with the growth and development of multicellular spheroids. Eur. J. Appl. Math., **8**, 639–658 (1997)

41. Byrne, H.M., Matthews, P.: Asymmetric growth of models of avascular solid tumors: exploiting symmetries. IMA J. Math. Appl. Med. Biol., **19**, 1–29 (2002)

42. Byrne, H., Preziosi, L.: Modelling solid tumour growth using the theory of mixtures. Math. Med. Biol., **20**, 341–366 (2003)

43. Cairns, R.A., Kalliomaki, T., Hill, R.P.: Acute (cyclic) hypoxia enhances spontaneous metastasis of KHT murine tumors. Cancer Res., **61**, 8903–8908 (2001)

44. Carmeliet, P., Jain, R.K.: Angiogenesis in cancer and other diseases. Nature, **407**, 249–257 (2000)

45. Chaplain, M.A.J.: Avascular growth, angiogenesis and vascular growth in solid tumours: the mathematic modelling of the stages of tumour development. Math. Comput. Modelling, **23**, 47–87 (1996)

46. Chaplain, M.A.J.: Pattern formation in cancer. In: Chaplain, M.A.J., Singh, G.D., MacLachlan, J.C. (eds), On Growth and Form: Spatio-Temporal Pattern Formation in Biology. Wiley Series in Mathematical and Computational Biology. Wiley, New York (2000)

47. Chaplain, M.A.J., Anderson, A.: Mathematical modelling of tissue invasion. In: Cancer Modelling and Simulation. Chapman & Hall/CRC, London (2003)

48. Chaplain, M.A.J., Ganesh, M., Graham, I.G.: Spatio-temporal pattern formation on spherical surfaces: numerical simulation and application to solid tumour growth. J. Math. Biol., **42**, 387–423 (2001)

49. Chaplain, M.A.J., Graziano, L., Preziosi, L.: Mathematical modelling of the loss of tissue compression responsiveness and its role in solid tumour development. Math. Med. Biol., **23**, 192–229 (2006)

50. Chaplain, M.A.J., Lolas, G.: Mathematical modeling of cancer cell invasion of tissue: the role of the urokinase plasminogen activation system. Math. Mod. Meth. Appl. Sci., **15**, 1685–1734 (2005)

51. Chaplain, M.A.J., Stuart, A.: A model mechanism for the chemotactic response of endothelial cells to tumor angiogenesis factor. IMA J. Math. Appl. Med. Biol., **10**, 149–168 (1993)

52. Condeelis, J., Singer, R.H., Segall, J.E.: The great escape: when cancer cells hijack the genes for chemotaxis and motility. Annu. Rev. Cell Dev. Biol., **21**, 695–718 (2005)

53. Cristini, V., Blawzdziewicz, J., Loewenberg, M.: An adaptive mesh algorithm for evolving surfaces: Simulations of drop breakup and coalescence, J. Comput. Phys., **168**, 445–463 (2001)

54. Cristini, V., Frieboes, H.B., Gatenby, R., Caserta, S., Ferrari, M., Sinek, J.: Morphological instability and cancer invasion. Clin. Cancer Res., **11**, 6772–6779 (2005)

55. Cristini, V., Gatenby, R., Lowengrub, J.: Multidisciplinary studies of tumor invasion and the role of the microenvironment. NIH 1R01CA127769-01. (2006)

56. Cristini, V., Li, X., Lowengrub, J., Wise, S.: Nonlinear simulations of solid tumor growth using a mixture model: Invasion and branching. J. Math. Biol., (in press)

57. Cristini, V., Lowengrub, J.: Three-dimensional crystal growth. I. Linear analysis and self-similar evolution. J. Crystal Growth, **240**, 267–276 (2002)

58. Cristini, V., Lowengrub, J.S., Nie, Q.: Nonlinear simulation of tumor growth. J. Math. Biol., **46**, 191–224 (2003)

59. Date, K., Matsumoto, K., Kuba, K., Shimura, H., Tanaka, M., Nakamura, T.: Inhibition of tumor growth and invasion by a four-kringle antagonist (HGF/NK4) for hepatocyte growth factor. Oncogene, **17**, 3045–3054 (1998)

60. DeJaeger, K., Kavanagh, M.C., Hill, R.: Relationship of hypoxia to metastatic ability in rodent tumors. Br. J. Cancer, **84**, 1280–1285 (2001)

61. Derycke, L., Van Marck, V., Depypere, H., Bracke, M.: Molecular targets of growth, differentiation, tissue integrity, and ectopic cell death in cancer cells. Cancer Biother. Radiopharm., **20**, 579–588 (2005)
62. Eble, J.A., Haier, J.: Integrins in cancer treatment. Curr. Cancer Drug Targets, **6**, 89–105 (2006)
63. Elvin, P., Garner, A.P.: Tumour invasion and metastasis: challenges facing drug discovery. Curr. Opin. Pharmacol., **5**, 374–381 (2005)
64. Enam, S.A., Rosenblum, M.L., Edvardsen, K.: Role of extracellular matrix in tumor invasion: migration of glioma cells along fibronectinpositive mesenchymal cell processes. Neurosurgery, **42**, 599–608 (1998)
65. Erler, J.T., Bennewith, K.L., Nicolau, M., Dornhoefer, N., Kong, C., Le, Q.-T., Chi, J.-T.A., Jeffrey, S.S., Siaccia, A.J.: Lysyl oxidase is essential for hypoxia-induced metastasis. Nature, **440**, 1222–1226 (2006)
66. Esteban, M.A., Maxwell, P.H.: HIF, a missing link between metabolism and cancer. Nature Med., **11**, 1047–1048 (2005)
67. Fallenstein, G.T., Hulce, V.D., Melvin, J.W.: Dynamic mechanical properties of human brain tissue. J. Biomechanics, **2**, 217–226 (1969)
68. Festjens, N., Vanden Berghe, T., Vandenabeele, P.: Necrosis, a well orchestrated form of cell demise: signalling cascades, important mediators and concomitant immune response. Biochim. Biophys. Acta, **1757**, 1371–1387 (2006)
69. Forsythe, J.A., Jiang, B.H., Iyer, N.V., Agani, F., Leung, S.W., Koos, R.D., Semenza, G.L.: Activation of vascular endothelial growth factor gene transcription by hypoxia-inducible factor 1. Mol. Cell. Bio., **16**, 4604–13 (1996)
70. Freyer, J.P.: Role of necrosis in regulating the growth saturation of multicellular spheroids. Cancer Res., **48**, 2432–2439 (1988)
71. Frieboes, H.B., Lowengrub, J.S., Wise, S., Zheng, X., Macklin, P., Bearer, E.L., Cristini, V.: Computer simulation of glioma growth and morphology. NeuroImage, **37**, S59–S70 (2007)
72. Frieboes, H.B., Wise, S.M., Lowengrub, J.S., Cristini, V.: Three dimensional multispecies nonlinear tumor growth-II: Investigation of tumor invasion. J. Theor. Biol., (in review)
73. Frieboes, H.B., Zheng, X., Sun, C.-H., Tromberg, B., Gatenby, R., Cristini, V.: An integrated computational/experimental model of tumor invasion. Cancer Res., **66**, 1597–1604 (2006)
74. Friedl, P.: Prespecification and plasticity: shifting mechanisms of cell migration. Curr. Opin. Cell Biol., **16**, 14–23 (2004)
75. Friedl, P., Brocker, E., Zanker, K.: Integrins, cell matrix interactions and cell migration strategies: fundamental differences in leukocytes and tumor cells. Cell Adhe. Commun., **6**, 225 (1998)
76. Friedl, P., Hegerfeldt, Y., Tilisch, M.: Collective cell migration in morphogenesis and cancer. Int. J. Dev. Biol., **48**, 441–449 (2004)
77. Friedl, P., Wolf, A.: Tumor cell invasion and migration: diversity and escape mechanisms. Nat. Rev. Cancer, **3**, 362–374 (2003)
78. Friedman, A.: A hierarchy of cancer models and their mathematical challenges. Discrete Cont. Dyn. Systems Ser. B, **4**, 147–159 (2004)
79. Friedman, A., Reitich, F.: Analysis of a mathematical model for the growth of tumors. J. Math. Biol., **38**, 262 (1999)
80. Friedman, A., Reitich, F.: On the existence of spatially patterned dormant malignancies in a model for the growth of non-necrotic vascular tumors. Math. Mod. Meth. Appl. Sci., **11**, 601–625 (2001)

81. Galaris, D., Barbouti, A., Korantzopoulos, P.: Oxidative stress in hepatic ischemia-reperfusion injury: the role of antioxidants and iron chelating compounds. Current Pharma. Design, **12**, 2875–2890 (2006)

82. Garber, K.: Energy boost: the Warburg effect returns in a new theory of cancer. J. Natl. Cancer Inst., **96**, 1805–1806 (2004)

83. Garcke, H., Nestler, B., Stinner, B.: A diffuse interface model for alloys with multiple components and phases, SIAM J. Appl. Math., **64**, 775–799 (2004)

84. Gatenby, R., Gawlinski, E.: A reaction-diffusion model of cancer invasion. Cancer Res., **56**, 5745 (1996)

85. Gatenby, R.A., Gawlinski, E.T.: The glycolytic phenotype in carcinogenesis and tumor invasion: insights through mathematical models. Cancer Res., **63**, 3847–3854 (2003)

86. Gatenby, R.A., Gawlinski, E.T., Gmitro, A.F., Kaylor, B., Gillies, R.J.: Acid-mediated tumor invasion: a multidisciplinary study. Cancer Res., **66**, 5216–5223 (2006)

87. Graeber, T.G., Osmanian, C., Jacks, T., Housman, D.E., Koch, C.J., Lowe, S.W., Giaccia, A.J.: Hypoxia-mediated selection of cells with diminished apoptotic potential in solid tumours. Nature, **379**, 88–91 (1996)

88. Greenspan, H.P.: Models for the growth of a solid tumor by diffusion. Stud. Appl. Math. LI, **4**, 317–340 (1972)

89. Greenspan, H.P.: On the growth and stability of cell cultures and solid tumors. J. Theor. Biol., **56**, 229–242 (1976)

90. Harris, A.L.: Hypoxia—a key regulatory factor in tumor growth. Nature Rev. Cancer **2**, 38–47 (2002)

91. Hashizume, H., Baluk, P., Morikawa, S., McLean, J.W., Thurston, G., Roberge, S., Jain, R.K., McDonald, D.M.: Openings between defective endothelial cells explain tumor vessel leakiness. American J. Pathology, **156**, 1363–80 (2000)

92. Hayot, C., Debeir, O., Van Ham, P., Van Damme, M., Kiss, R., Decaestecker, C.: Characterization of the activities of actin-affecting drugs on tumor cell migration. Toxicology Appl. Pharma., **211**, 30–40 (2006)

93. Helmlinger, G., Yuan, F., Dellian, M., Jain, R.K.: Interstitial pH and pO_2 gradients in solid tumors in vivo: high-resolution measurements reveal a lack of correlation. Nat. Med., **3**, 177–182 (1997)

94. Höckel, M., Schlenger, K., Aral, B., Mitze, M., Schaffer, U., Vaupel, P.: Association between tumor hypoxia and malignant progression in advanced cancer of the uterine cervix. Cancer Res., **56**, 4509–4515 (1996)

95. Höckel, M., Vaupel, P.: Tumor hypoxia: definitions and current clinical, biologic, and molecular aspects. J. Natl. Cancer Inst., **93**, 266–276 (2001)

96. Hogea, C.S., Murray, B.T., Sethian, J.A.: Simulating complex tumor dynamics from avascular to vascular growth using a general level-set method. J. Math. Biol., **53**, 86–134 (2006)

97. Holash, J., Maisonpierre, P.C., Compton, D., Boland, P., Alexander, C.R., Zagzag, D., Yancopoulos, G.D., Wiegand, S.J.: Vessel cooption, regression, and growth in tumors mediated by angiopoietins and VEGF. Science, **284**, 1994–1998 (1999)

98. Holash, J., Wiegand, S.J., Yancopoulos, G.D.: New model of tumor angiogenesis: dynamic balance between vessel regression and growth mediated by angiopoietins and VEGF. Oncogene, **18**, 5356–5362 (1999)

99. Huang, Q., Shen, H.M., Ong, C.N.: Emodin inhibits tumor cell migration through suppression of the phosphatidylinositol 3-kinase-Cdc42/Rac1 pathway. Cell. Mol. Life Sci., **62**, 1167–1175 (2005)

100. Jacqmin, D.: Calculation of two-phase Navier-Stokes flows using phase-field modeling. J. Comput. Phys., **155**, 96–127 (1999)

101. Jain, R.K.: Determinants of tumor blood flow: a review. Cancer Res., **48**, 2641–2658 (1988)

102. Jain, R.K.: Physiological Barriers to Delivery of Monoclonal Antibodies and Other Macromolecules in Tumors. Cancer Res. (Suppl.), **50**, 814s-819s (1990)

103. Jain, R.K: Delivery of molecular and cellular medicine to solid tumors. J. Control. Release, **53**, 49–67 (1998)

104. Jain, R.K.: Normalizing tumor vasculature with anti-angiogenic therapy: a new paradigm for combination therapy. Nat. Med., **7**, 987–989 (2001)

105. Jain, R.K.: Delivery of molecular medicine to solid tumors: lessons from in vivo imaging of gene expression and function. J. Control. Release, **74**, 7–25 (2001)

106. Jain, R.K.: Molecular regulation of vessel maturation. Nature Med., **9**, 685–693 (2003)

107. Jones, A.F., Byrne, H.M., Gibson, J.S., Dold, J.W.: A mathematical model of the stress induced during avascular tumor growth. J. Math. Biol., **40**, 473–499 (2000)

108. Kansal, A.A., Torquato, S., Harsh IV, G.R., Chiocca, E.A., Deisboeck, T.S.: Simulated brain tumor growth dynamics using a 3-D cellular automaton. J. Theor. Biol., **203**, 367–382 (2000)

109. Kaur, B., Khwaja, F.W., Severson, E.A., Matheny, S.L., Brat, D.J., VanMeir, E.G.: Hypoxia and the hypoxia-inducible-factor pathway in glioma growth and angiogenesis. Neuro-oncol., **7**, 134–153 (2005)

110. Keller, P.J., Pampaloni, F., Stelzer, E.H.K.: Life sciences require the third dimension. Curr. Op. Cell Biol., **18**, 117–124 (2006)

111. Kim, J.S., Kang, K., Lowengrub, J.S.: Conservative multigrid methods for Cahn-Hilliard fluids. J. Comp. Phys., **193**, 511–543 (2004)

112. Kim, J.S., Kang, K., Lowengrub, J.S.: Conservative multigrid methods for ternary Cahn-Hilliard systems. Comm. Math. Sci., **12**, 53–77 (2004)

113. Kim, J.S., Lowengrub, J.S.: Phase field modeling and simulation of three-phase flows. Int. Free Bound., **7**, 435 (2005)

114. Kloner, R.A., Jennings, R.B.: Consequences of brief ischemia: stunning, preconditioning, and their clinical implications: part 1. Circulation, **104**, 2981–2989 (2001)

115. Konopleva, M., Zhao, S.R., Hu, W., Jiang, S.W., Snell, V., Weidner, D., Jackson, C.E., Zhang, X., Champlin, R., Estey, E., Reed, J.C., Andreeff, M.: The anti-apoptotic genes Bcl-X-L and Bcl-2 are over-expressed and contribute to chemoresistance of non-proliferating leukaemic cells. Br. J. Haematol., **118**, 521–534 (2002)

116. Kopfstein, L., Christofori, G.: Metastasis: cell-autonomous mechanisms versus contributions by the tumor microenvironment. Cell. Mol. Life Sci., **63**, 449–468 (2006)

117. Kuiper, R.A.J., Schellens, J.H.M., Blijham, G.H., Beijnen, J.H., Voest, E.E.: Clinical research on antiangiogenic therapy. Pharmacol Res., **37**, 1–16 (1998)

118. Kumar, M., Krishnan, G., Arumainanthan, U., Singh, K.: Endoscopic excision of a nasal glioma. The Internet Journal of Otorhinolaryngology, **2** (2003)

119. Kunkel, P., Ulbricht, U., Bohlen, P., Brockmann, M.A., Fillbrandt, R., Stavrou, D., Westphal, M., Lamszus, K.: Inhibition of glioma angiogenesis and growth in vivo by systemic treatment with a monoclonal antibody against vascular endothelial growth factor receptor-2. Cancer Res., **61**, 6624–6628 (2001)

120. Lah, T.T., Alonso, M.B.D., Van Noorden, C.J.F.: Antiprotease therapy in cancer: hot or not? Exp. Op. Biol. Ther., **6**, 257–279 (2006)

121. Lamszus, K., Kunkel, P., Westphal, M.: Invasion as limitation to anti-angiogenic glioma therapy. Acta Neurochir. Suppl., **88**, 169–177 (2003)

122. Lee, H., Lowengrub, J.S., Goodman, J.: Modeling pinchoff and reconnection in a Hele-Shaw cell I. The models and their calibration, Phys. Fluids, **14**, 492–513 (2002)

123. Leo, P.H., Lowengrub, J.S., Jou, H.-J.: A diffuse interface model for elastically stressed solids. Acta Metall., **46**, 2113–2130 (1998)

124. Less, J.R., Skalak, T.C., Sevick, E.M., Jain, R.K.: Microvascular architecture in a mammary carcinoma: branching patterns and vessel dimensions. Cancer Res., **51**, 265–273 (1991)

125. Lester, R.D., Jo, M., Campana, W.M., Gonias, S.L.: Erythropoietin promotes MCF-7 breast cancer cell migration by an ERK/mitogenactivated protein kinase-dependent pathway and is primarily responsible for the increase in migration observed in hypoxia. J. Biol. Chem., **280**, 39273–39277 (2005)

126. Li, X., Cristini, V., Nie, Q., Lowengrub, J.S.: Nonlinear three dimensional simulation of solid tumor growth. Disc. Cont. Dyn. Sys. B, **7**, 581–604 (2007)

127. Lockett, J., Yin, S.P., Li, X.H., Meng, Y.H., Sheng, S.J.: Tumor suppressive maspin and epithelial homeostasis. J. Cell. Biochem., **97**, 651–660 (2006)

128. Lowengrub, J.S., Macklin, P.: A centimeter-scale nonlinear model of tumor growth in complex, heterogeneous tissues. J. Math. Biol., (in preparation)

129. Lowengrub, J.S., Truskinovsky, L.: Quasi-incompressible Cahn-Hilliard fluids and topological transitions. Proc. R. Soc. London A, **454**, 2617–2654 (1998)

130. Lubarda, V., Hoger, A.: On the mechanics of solids with a growing mass. Int. J. Solids Structures, **39**, 4627 (2002)

131. Macklin, P.: Numerical simulation of tumor growth and chemotherapy. MS thesis, University of Minnesota, Minnesota (2003)

132. Macklin, P., Lowengrub, J.S.: Evolving interfaces via gradients of geometry-dependent interior Poisson problems: application to tumor growth. J. Comput. Phys., **203**, 191–220 (2005)

133. Macklin, P., Lowengrub, J.: An improved geometry-aware curvature discretization for level-set methods: application to tumor growth, J. Comput. Phys., **215**, 392–401 (2006)

134. Macklin, P., Lowengrub, J.: Nonlinear simulation of the effect of microenvironment on tumor growth. J. Theor. Biol., **245**, 677–704 (2007)

135. Macklin, P., Lowengrub, J.: A new ghost cell/level set method for moving boundary problems: application to tumor growth. J. Scientific Comp., (in press) doi:10.1007/S10915-008-9190-Z

136. Maher, E., Furnari, F., Bachoo, R., Rowitch, D., Louis, D., Cavenee, W., De-Pinho, R.: Malignant glioma: genetics and biology of a grave matter. Genes Dev., **15**, 1311 (2001)

137. Mallett, D.G., de Pillis, L.G.: A cellular automata model of tumorimmune system interactions. J. Theor. Biol., **239**, 334–350 (2006)

138. Mansury, Y., Kimura, M., Lobo, J., Deisboeck, T.S.: Emerging patterns in tumor systems: simulating the dynamics of multicellular clusters with an agent-based spatial agglomeration model. J. Theor. Biol., **219**, 343–370 (2002)
139. McDougall, S.R., Anderson, A.R.A., Chaplain, M.A.J.: Mathematical modeling of dynamic adaptive tumour-induced angiogenesis: clinical applications and therapeutic targeting strategies. J. Theor. Biol., **241**, 564–589 (2006)
140. McDougall, S.R., Anderson, A.R.A., Chaplain, M.A.J., Sherratt, J.: Mathematical modelling of flow through vascular networks: implications for tumour-induced angiogenesis and chemotherapy strategies. Bull. Math. Biol., **64**, 673–702 (2002)
141. McElwain, D.L.S., Morris, L.E.: Apoptosis as a volume loss mechanism in mathematical models of solid tumor growth. Math. Biosci., **39**, 147–157 (1978)
142. McLean, G.W., Carragher, N.O., Avizienyte, E., Evans, J., Brunton, V.G., Frame, M.C.: The role of focal-adhesion kinase in cancer. A new therapeutic opportunity. Nat. Rev. Cancer, **5**, 505–515 (2005)
143. Michieli, P., Basilico, C., Pennacchietti, S., Maffè, A., Tamagnone, L., Giordano, S., Bardelli, A., Comoglio, P.M.: Mutant Met mediated transformation is ligand-dependent and can be inhibited by HGF antagonists. Oncogene, **18**, 5221–5231 (1999)
144. Montesano, R., Matsumoto, K., Nakamura, T., Orci, L.: Identification of a fibroblast-derived epithelial morphogen as hepatocyte growth factor. Cell, **67**, 901–908 (1991)
145. Morotti, A., Mila, S., Accornero, P., Tagliabue, E., Ponzetto, C.: K252a inhibits the oncogenic properties of Met, the HGF receptor. Oncogene, **21**, 4885–4893 (2002)
146. Mueller-Klieser, W.: Multicellular spheroids: a review on cellular aggregates in cancer research. J. Cancer Res. Clin. Oncol., **113**, 101–122 (1987)
147. Naganuma, H., Kimurat, R., Sasaki, A., Fukamachi, A., Nukui, H., Tasaka, K.: Complete remission of recurrent glioblastoma multiforme following local infusions of lymphokine activated killer cells. Acta Neurochir., **99**, 157–160 (1989)
148. Natarajan, M., Hecker, T.P., Gladson, C.L.: Fak signaling in anaplastic astrocytoma and glioblastoma tumors. Cancer J., **9**, 126–133 (2003)
149. Netti, P.A., Baxter, L.T., Boucher, Y., Skalak, R., Jain, R.K.: Time dependent behavior of interstitial fluid pressure in solid tumors: implications for drug delivery. Cancer Res., **55**, 5451–5458 (1995)
150. Nor, J.E., Christensen, J., Liu, J., Peters, M., Mooney, D.J., Strieter, R.M., Polverini, P.J.: Up-regulation of Bcl-2 in microvascular endothelial cells enhances intratumoral angiogenesis and accelerates tumor growth. Cancer Res., **61**, 2183–2188 (2001)
151. O'Connor, J.P.B., Jackson, A., Parker, G.J.M., Jayson, G.C.: DCE-MRI biomarkers in the clinical evaluation of antiangiogenic and vascular disrupting agents. Br. J. Cancer, **96**, 189–195 (2007)
152. Ommaya, A.K.: Mechanical properties of tissues of the nervous system. J. Biomechanics, **1**, 127–138 (1968).
153. Osher, S., Sethian, J.: Fronts propagating with curvature-dependent speed: algorithms based on Hamilton-Jacobi formulation. J. Comput. Phys., **79**, 12 (1988)
154. Padera, T.P., Stoll, B.R., Tooredman, J.B., Capen, D., di Tomaso, E., Jain, R.: Cancer cells compress intratumour vessels. Nature, **427**, 695 (2004)

155. Page, D.L., Anderson, T.J., Sakamoto, G: In: Diagnostic Histopathology of the Breast, Churchill Livingstone, Edinburgh, Scotland, 193–235 (1987)

156. Paku, S., Paweletz, N.: First step of tumor-related angiogenesis. Lab. Invest., **65**, 334–346 (1991)

157. Patan, S., Tanda, S., Roberge, S., Jones, R.C., Jain, R.K., Munn, L.L.: Vascular morphogenesis and remodeling in a human tumor xenograft: blood vessel formation and growth after ovariectomy and tumor implantation. Circ. Research, **89**, 732–739 (2001)

158. Paweletz, N., Knierim, M.: Tumor-related angiogenesis. Crit. Rev. Oncol. Hematol., **9**, 197–242 (1989)

159. Pennacchietti, S., Michieli, P., Galluzzo, M., Giordano, S., Comoglio, P.: Hypoxia promotes invasive growth by transcriptional activation of the met protooncogene. Cancer Cell, **3**, 347–361 (2003)

160. Plank, M.J., Sleeman, B.D.: A reinforced random walk model of tumour angiogenesis and anti-angiogenic strategies. Math. Med. Biol., **20**, 135–181 (2003)

161. Plank, M.J., Sleeman, B.D.: Lattice and non-lattice models of tumour angiogenesis. Bull. Math. Biol., **66**, 1785-1819 (2004)

162. Please, C.P., Pettet, G., McElwain, D.L.S.: A new approach to modeling the formation of necrotic regions in tumors. Appl. Math. Lett., **11**, 89–94 (1998)

163. Polette, M., Gilles, C., de Bentzmann, S., Gruenert, D., Tournier, J.M., Birembaut, P.: Association of fibroblastoid features with the invasive phenotype in human bronchial cancer cell lines. Clin. Exp. Metastasis, **16**, 105–112 (1998)

164. Postovit, L.M., Adams, M.A., Lash, G.E., Heaton, J.P., Graham, C.H.: Oxygen-mediated regulation of tumor cell invasiveness. Involvement of a nitric oxide signaling pathway. J. Biol. Chem., **277**, 35730-35737 (2002)

165. Pouysségur, J., Dayan, F., Mazure, N.M.: Hypoxia signalling in cancer and approaches to enforce tumour regression. Nature, **441**, 437–443 (2006)

166. Putz, E., Witter, K., Offner, S., Stosiek, P., Zippelius, A., Johnson, J., Zahn, R., Riethmüller, G., Pantel, K.: Phenotypic characteristics of cell lines derived from disseminated cancer cells in bone marrow of patients with solid epithelial tumors: establishment of working models for human micrometastases. Cancer Res., **59**, 241–248 (1999)

167. Quaranta, V., Weaver, A.M., Cummings, P.T., Anderson, A.R.A.: Mathematical modeling of cancer: the future of prognosis and treatment. Clin. Chim. Acta, **357**, 173–179 (2005)

168. Ramakrishnan, S.: Department of Pharmacology, University of Minnesota. Personal communication (2003)

169. Ramanathan, A., Wang, C., Schreiber, S.L.: Perturbational profiling of a cell-line model of tumorigenesis by using metabolic measurements. Proc. Natl Acad. Sci., **102**, 5992–5997 (2005)

170. Ravandi, F., Estrov, Z.: Eradication of leukemia stem cells as a new goal of therapy in leukemia. Clin. Cancer Res., **12**, 340–344 (2006)

171. Ridley, A.J., Schwartz, M.A., Burridge, K., Firtel, R.A., Ginsberg, M.H., Borisy, G., Parsons, J.T., Horwitz, A.R.: Cell migration: integrating signals from front to back. Science, **302**, 1704–1709 (2003)

172. Rofstad, E., Halsør, E.: Hypoxia-associated spontaneous pulmonary metastasis in human melanoma xenographs: involvement of microvascular hotspots induced in hypoxic foci by interleukin. Br. J. Cancer, **86**, 301–308 (2002)

173. Rofstad, E., Rasmussen, H., Galappathi, K., Mathiesen, B., Nilsen, K., Graff, B.A.: Hypoxia promotes lymph node metastasis in human melanoma xenografts by up-regulating the urokinase-type plasminogen activator receptor. Cancer Res., **62**, 1847–1853 (2002)
174. Rohzin, J., Sameni, M., Ziegler, G., Sloane, B.F.: Pericellular pH affects distribution and secretion of cathepsin B in malignant cells. Cancer Res., **54**, 6517-6525 (1994)
175. Roose, T., Netti, P.A., Munn, L.L., Boucher, Y., Jain, R.: Solid stress generated by spheroid growth estimated using a linear poroelastic model. Microvasc. Res., **66**, 204–212 (2003)
176. Rubenstein, J.L., Kim, J., Ozawa, T., Zhang, K., Westphal, M., Deen, D.F., Shuman, M.A.: Anti-VEGF antibody treatment of glioblastoma prolongs survival but results in increased vascular cooption. Neoplasia, **2**, 306–314 (2000)
177. Saad, Y., Schultz, M.H.: GMRES: a generalized minimal residual algorithm for solving nonsymmetric linear systems, SIAM J. Sci. Stat. Comput. **7**, 856–869 (1986)
178. Sahai, E.: Mechanisms of cancer cell invasion. Curr. Opin. Genet. Dev., **15**, 87–96 (2005)
179. Sakamoto, G.: Infiltrating carcinoma: major histological types. In: Page, D.L., Anderson, T.J. (eds), Diagnostic Histopathology of the Breast. Churchill-Livingstone, London, UK (1987)
180. Sanga, S., Sinek, J.P., Frieboes, H.B., Fruehauf, J.P., Cristini, V.: Mathematical modeling of cancer progression and response to chemotherapy. Expert. Rev. Anticancer Ther., **6**, 1361–1376 (2006)
181. Sanga, S., Frieboes, H.B., Zheng, X., Bearer, E.L., Cristini V.: Predictive oncology: a review of multidisciplinary, multiscale in silico modeling linking phenotype, morphology and growth. NeuroImage., **37**, S120–S134 (2007)
182. Sanson, B.C., Delsanto, P.P., Magnano, M., Scalerandi, M.: Effects of anatomical constraints on tumor growth. Phys. Rev. E, **64**, 21903ff (2002)
183. Schmeichel, K.L., Weaver, V.M., Bissel, M.J.: Structural cues from the tissue microenvironment are essential determinants of the human mammary epithelial cell phenotype. J. Mammary Gland Biol. Neoplasia, **3**, 201–213 (1998)
184. Seftor, E.A., Meltzer, P.S., Kirshmann, D.A., Pe'er, J., Maniotis, A.J., Trent, J.M., Folberg, R., Hendrix, M.J.: Molecular determinants of human uveal melanoma invasion and metastasis. Clin. Exp. Metastasis, **19**, 233–246 (2002)
185. Shweiki, D., Itin, A., Soffer, D., Keshet, E.: Vascular endothelial growth factor induced by hypoxia may mediate hypoxia-initiated angiogenesis. Nature, **359**, 843–845 (1992)
186. Sierra, A.: Metastases and their microenvironments: linking pathogenesis and therapy. Drug Resistance Updates, **8**, 247–257 (2005)
187. Sinek, J., Frieboes, H., Zheng, X., Cristini, V.: Two-dimensional chemotherapy simulations demonstrate fundamental transport and tumor response limitations involving nanoparticles. Biomed. Microdev., **6**, 197–309 (2004)
188. Skinner, S.A.: Microvascular architecture of experimental colon tumors in the rat. Cancer Res., **50**, 2411–2417 (1990)
189. Steeg, P.S.: Angiogenesis inhibitors: motivators of metastasis? Nature Med., **9**, 822–823 (2003)
190. Sun S., Wheeler, M.F., Obeyesekere, M., Patrick Jr., C.: Multiscale angiogenesis modeling using mixed finite element methods, Multiscale Model. Simul., **4**, 1137–1167 (2005)

191. Sutherland, R.M.: Cell and environment interactions in tumor microregions: the multicell spheroid model. Science, **240**, 177–184 (1988)

192. Takano, S., Yoshii, Y., Kondo, S., Suzuki, H., Maruno, T., Shirai, S., Nose, T.: Concentration of vascular endothelial growth factor in the serum and tumor tissue of brain tumor patients. Cancer Res., **56**, 2185–2190 (1996)

193. Tester, A.M., Ruangpani, N., Anderso, R.L., Thompson, E.W.: MMP-9 secretion and MMP-2 activation distinguish invasive and metastatic sublines of a mouse mammary carcinoma system showing epithelial-mesenchymal transition traits. Clin. Exp. Metastasis, **18**, 553–560 (2000)

194. Tiller, W. Migration of a liquid zone through a solid. Part 3. J. Appl. Phys., **36**, 261 (1965)

195. Truskey, G., Yuan, F., Katz, D.: Transport Phenomena in Biological Systems. Pearson Prentice-Hall, Upper Saddle River, NJ (2004)

196. Vajkoczy, P., Farhadi, M., Gaumann, A., Heidenreich, R., Erber, R., Wunder, A., Tonn, J.C., Menger, M.D., Breier, G.: Microtumor growth initiates angiogenic sprouting with simultaneous expression of VEGF, VEGF receptor-2, and angiopoietin-2. J. Clin. Invest., **109**, 777–785 (2002)

197. van Kempen, L.C.L.T., Ruiter, D.J., van Muijen, G.N.P., Coussens, L.M.: The tumor microenvironment: a critical determinant of neoplastic evolution. Eur. J. Cell. Biol., **82**, 539–548 (2003)

198. Vaupel, P., Haugland, H.K., Nicklee, T., Morrison, A.J., Hedley, D.W.: Hypoxia-inducible factor-1 alpha is an intrinsic marker for hypoxia in cervical cancer xenografts. Cancer Res., **61**, 7394–7398 (2001)

199. Vaupel, P., Kallinowski, F., Okunieff, P.: Blood flow, oxygen and nutrient supply, and metabolic microenvironment of human tumours: a review. Cancer Res., **49**, 6449–6465 (1989)

200. Wise, S.M., Kim, J., Lowengrub, J.: Solving the regularized, strongly anisotropic Cahn-Hilliard equation by an adaptive nonlinear multigrid method. J. Comput. Phys., **226**, 414–446 (2007)

201. Wise, S.M., Lowengrub, J.S., Frieboes, H.B., Cristini, V.: Three dimensional multispecies nonlinear tumor growth-I: Model and numerical method. J. Theor. Biol., (in press)

202. Wise, S.M., Lowengrub, J.S., Kim, J.S., Johnson, W.C.: Efficient phase-field simulation of quantum dot formation in a strained heteroepitaxial film. Superlattices and Microstructures, **36**, 293–304 (2004)

203. Wolf, K., Friedl, P.: Molecular mechanisms of cancer cell invasion and plasticity. Br. J. Dermatology, **154**, 11–15 (2006)

204. Wurzel, M., Schaller, C., Simon, M., Deutsch, A.: Cancer cell invasion of brain tissue: guided by a prepattern? J. Theor. Medicine, **6**, 21–31 (2005)

205. Yamaguchi, H., Wyckoff, J., Condeelis, J.: Cell migration in tumors. Curr. Op. Cell Biol., **17**, 559–564 (2005)

206. Yin, S.P., Lockett, J., Meng, Y.H., Biliran, H., Blouse, G.E., Li, X.H., Reddy, N., Zhao, Z.M., Lin, X.L., Anagli, J., Cher, M.L., Sheng, S.J.: Maspin retards cell detachment via a novel interaction with the urokinase-type plasminogen activator/urokinase-type plasminogen activator receptor system. Cancer Res., **66**, 4173–4181 (2006)

207. Young, S.D., Hill, R.P.: Effects of reoxygenation of cells from hypoxic regions of solid tumors: anticancer drug sensitivity and metastatic potential. J. Natl. Cancer Inst., **82**, 338–339 (1990)

208. Young, S.D., Marshall, R.S., Hill, R.P.: Hypoxia induces DNA overreplication and enhances metastatic potential of murine tumor cells. Proc. Natl. Acad. Sci. USA, textbf85, 9533–9537 (1988)
209. Yu, J., Rak, J., Coomber, B., Hicklin, D., Kerbel, R.: Effect of p53 status on tumor response to antiangiogenic therapy. Science, **295**, 1526–1528 (2002)
210. Zagzag, D., Amirnovin, R., Greco, M.A., Yee, H., Holash, J., Wiegand, S.J., Zabski, S., Yancopoulos, G.D., Grumet, M.: Vascular apoptosis and involution in gliomas precede neovascularization: a novel concept for glioma growth and angiogenesis. Lab Invest., **80**, 837–849 (2000)
211. Zheng, X., Wise, S.M., Cristini, V.: Nonlinear simulation of tumor necrosis, neo-vascularization and tissue invasion via an adaptive finite element/level set method. Bull. Math. Biol., **67**, 211–259 (2005)

7

Tumour Cords and Their Response to Anticancer Agents

Alessandro Bertuzzi,[1] Antonio Fasano,[2] Alberto Gandolfi,[1]
and Carmela Sinisgalli[1]

[1] Istituto di Analisi dei Sistemi ed Informatica "A. Ruberti" - CNR,
   Viale Manzoni 30, 00185 Roma, Italy
   `bertuzzi@iasi.cnr.it` `gandolfi@iasi.cnr.it` `sinisgalli@iasi.cnr.it`
[2] Dipartimento di Matematica "U. Dini", Università di Firenze,
   Viale Morgagni 67/A, 50134 Firenze, Italy
   `fasano@math.unifi.it`

7.1 Introduction

7.1.1 Modelling Cords and Spheroids

Blood vessels in vascularized tumours are in general irregular and chaotically oriented. However, more ordered structures have been observed, mainly in experimental tumours, where tumour cells proliferating around a blood vessel give rise to approximately axisymmetric aggregates called *tumour cords* [36, 29, 33]. Tumour cords generally differ from each other in size and orientation and, depending on their stage of development and on the way they are organized in space, may or may not be surrounded by a necrotic region. In the presence of necrosis, the mean thickness of a cord is 60–130 μm in different tumours, with a mean radius of central vessels of 10–40 μm. Fig. 7.1 shows a schematic cross section of a system of cords in the absence of necrosis (panel A) or separated by a connected necrotic region (panel B). We have assumed in this figure that blood vessels are parallel, identical, and regularly spaced, as in the Krogh model of microcirculation [32]. The assumption of a Krogh-like vasculature allows us to formulate a highly idealized model of a vascular tumour.

The main difficulty in the experimental study of tumour cords is that they cannot be grown *in vitro*. This explains why much more attention, also by mathematicians, has been devoted to what are called multicellular tumour spheroids, i.e. approximately spherical aggregates of tumour cells which can be easily grown *in vitro* under well-controlled conditions (see the review [34] for the experimental issues, and [17, 3] for the mathematical modelling).

From the modelling point of view, the fact that cords receive nutrients from the central blood vessel offers some advantages. For instance, the zone

N. Bellomo et al. (eds.), *Selected Topics in Cancer Modeling*,
DOI: 10.1007/978-0-8176-4713-1_7, © Springer Science+Business Media, LLC 2008

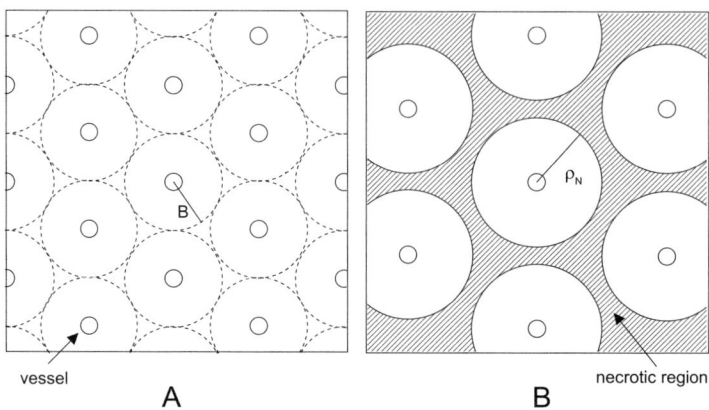

Fig. 7.1. Scheme of an array of tumour cords. Panel A: vessels close enough to provide nutrient supply to all surrounding cells. Panel B: the increased distance among vessels causes peripheral necrosis. Symbols are explained in Section 7.2.

of more intense proliferation can be identified as the innermost region, with a progressive weakening of activity toward the periphery, possibly reaching a region of complete necrosis. For avascular tumour nodules receiving nutrients from the surroundings the situation is obviously reversed, but there is no general agreement on how deep in the tumour the cells proliferate. In some models, proliferation is assumed to be allowed only for cells situated in a thin peripheral rim, or even just at the surface of the tumour. This question is particularly important when dealing with the geometrical instability of the tumour (see [26]), that from a slightly perturbed spherical shape may eventually produce finger-like structures. Besides [16], the formation of fractal structures is described in [25] on the basis of a discrete model. We may have an idea of how delicate the issue of the surface proliferative activity is by observing that there are models that concentrate the whole activity on the tumour surface, and assume opposite views about the relative importance of the growth-favouring nutrient concentration and the growth-inhibiting pressure (both higher in tips in a nonspherical shape). Compare for instance the models in [1] and [16], both able to generate complicated shapes by means of different mechanisms.

If we concentrate on modelling the evolution of just one cord in the interior of a more or less regular cohort, the chosen element confines with other similar elements. Thus we do not deal with the problem of how the active surface of a tumour interacts with the surrounding tissue in the body. This subject, however, is receiving growing attention. For instance, it has been suggested that as a by-product of glucose metabolism an acidic environment can be created.

The corresponding pH level can be lethal to the adjacent normal tissue, while tolerated by the tumour cells [35]. Another advantage in modelling cords is that the cell velocity is known at the inner boundary: cells adhering to the central blood vessel have zero velocity. This information is of great help in integrating the differential equation for the cell velocity (see Section 7.2.2). On the contrary, in spheroids carrying a necrotic core there is no point where the velocity of live cells is known a priori, and information must be retrieved by describing the dynamics of the necrotic core.

That said, there are also questions that turn out to be more complicated in tumour cords than in spheroids. The most evident one is about the geometry. While approximating the spheroid with a sphere is an obvious choice in the framework of the continuum approach, attributing a circular cylindrical shape to a cord is certainly questionable for the reasons already mentioned. Moreover, the concentration of nutrients and the blood pressure change along the cord and restrictions on their relative variations must be imposed. We will briefly discuss this point in Section 7.2.3. The reward of cylindrical symmetry is however remarkable, because this assumption allows us to bypass the mechanical problem of the cell-cell and cell-liquid interactions (if we confine ourselves to these two constituents) that determine the cell motion.

A disadvantage of the cylindrical *vs.* the spherical geometry is the higher dimensionality of the dynamics of extracellular fluid, which permeates the whole tumour. The role of the fluid is essential, because it provides the material for the growth of dividing cells. In a sphere we may suppose that the fluid velocity, as well as the cell velocity, is purely radial (we obviously refer to average quantities). In cylindrical tumour cords, it is still reasonable to take a radial velocity field for the cells in a stage in which expansion in the direction of the blood vessel has been completed. On the contrary, the fluid, which comes from the central blood vessel and crosses the whole cord, must eventually leave the cylinder formed by the cord and the peripheral necrosis from the two bases, thus acquiring a velocity with a longitudinal component.

Another difficulty, which is present in modelling tumour cords and is common to the modelling of all vascular tumours, is the possibility that internal stresses grow so large as to produce the collapse of blood vessels, cutting out the nutrient supply. Predicting this event obviously requires the computation of the stress at the blood vessel wall. Studies in this direction have been performed in [15, 2] on the basis of suitable constitutive laws for the mechanical behaviour of the tumour. So far such an analysis has not been performed for tumour cords. Not including the stresses in the model is a strong limitation, not only concerning the blood vessel collapse, but also for the inhibitory action that compression may have on cell proliferation. Such an effect has been considered by some authors [18, 20], mainly in the context of models that consider cells and extracellular liquid as two interacting fluids. Radial compression, however, could also be the cumulative result of the traction exerted on the expanding cell layers. We believe that this aspect should receive adequate attention in the future.

Despite all differences between spheroids and tumour cords, they share many features and what is obtained in one context should not be ignored in the other. One of the most interesting aspects emphasized in modelling tumour cords is that their evolution is constantly accompanied by the presence of *unilateral constraints*, as will be illustrated later. These constraints should also be accounted for in the evolution of the live cells-necrosis interface in spheroids subjected to treatment.

One last general remark about the modelling of tumour cords, applicable also to spheroids, is about the justification of adopting the continuum approach. This choice may look rather questionable, since a typical cord thickness is of the order of 4–7 cellular diameters (as in many cases is the viable rim in spheroids), thus pointing in favour of a discrete approach. One should not forget, however, that the typical length of a cord is about 30 cellular diameters, so that the number of cells in a cord is of the order of 10^3. We may take advantage of this fact by selecting the representative elementary volume in the form of a thin cylindrical shell, which, despite its small thickness, intersects a sufficiently large number of cells. Thus, basic quantities such as the local volume fraction occupied by cells acquire a physical relevance.

7.1.2 Modelling Treatments

Coming to treatments, we enter a huge subject because there are many different techniques, each presenting peculiar difficulties for mathematical modelling. The ultimate target of the models should be the optimization of the treatment. Let us briefly introduce some of them, restricting our discussion to treatments whose effects can be more directly investigated by means of tumour cord modelling.

Chemotherapy. A mathematical model should take into account the way the drug is transported within the tumour and delivered to the cells, the way the drug is taken up and possibly released after cell death, and the modality of the cytotoxic action exerted. Relatively small molecules are mainly transported by diffusion, while advection by extracellular liquid may have an important role for molecules of larger molecular weight. Also, the interaction with the cell membrane may decide whether the drug permeates the whole tumour volume or is selectively concentrated in the extracellular liquid. In vascular tumours, the intricacy of the vessel network may be an obstacle to the drug delivery because of the inefficient blood flow [31].

Radiation. The short duration of the delivery of a single radiation dose is usually translated into the model by updating the initial conditions. The difficulty here consists in describing the kinds of damage suffered by the cells, taking into account their damage repair ability, and phenomena, such as reoxygenation, that influence the cell population radiosensitivity. Optimizing the intensity and frequency of radiation doses is obviously of great importance, trying not only to maximize the effect on the tumour, but at the same time to keep the damage to the normal tissues at an acceptable level. Models have been proposed for the spatially homogeneous case and only very recently for tumour cords.

Antibodies. Antibodies target specific receptors on the tumour cells. They can be charged with toxins or radionuclides. Advection may be important in their transport. We will return to this subject later in the chapter.

Viruses. Specific viruses able to infect tumour cells, replicate inside them and cause cell lysis, are deployed in the tumour. Some mathematical models have been proposed [40, 27]. Other therapeutic applications under study use viruses as vectors for gene therapy. Due to the size of viruses, diffusion looks negligible but even advection is scarcely efficient, so that transmission takes place mainly by direct infection of neighbouring cells.

In this chapter we shortly review the model for the evolution of tumour cords developed in [7, 8, 9, 10], as well as the attempts of modelling the response to drugs and radiation, and the transport of antibodies able to bind to tumour cell surface antigens [11, 12, 13].

7.2 The Basic Model for the Evolution of Tumour Cords

A first model of tumour cords was proposed in [5], including the age structure of the cell population, and mathematical aspects of this approach were investigated in [39, 23]. This model was sketched in the review paper [24]. Age structure is essential in many cases, e.g. when studying the distribution of a proliferation marker taken up at a specific phase of the cell cycle [6], but for other purposes age effects can be averaged out. The model described in the following does not include age structure, whereas it includes the diffusion and consumption of the nutrient, and the flow of interstitial fluid, and it predicts the evolution caused by treatments.

7.2.1 Structure of the Cord: Cell and Fluid Dynamics

Fig. 7.2 depicts the idealized geometry of a tumour cord surrounded by necrosis. Let r_0 denote the blood vessel radius and ρ_N denote the cord radius. In the domain $r_0 < r < \rho_N$, the cell population may be subdivided into proliferating (P), quiescent (Q), and apoptotic cells, all surrounded by extracellular liquid. Such constituents are supposed to have the same mass density, and the corresponding local volume fractions ν_P, ν_Q, ν_A, ν_E add up to one. The surface $r = \rho_N$ is the interface with the necrotic region, $\rho_N < r < B$. Assuming the cord to be inside an array of parallel and regularly spaced cords, the outer boundary B prevents any mass exchange with the neighbouring cords. Although we will mainly deal with the case of cords surrounded by necrosis, we may also consider the case in which the necrotic region is absent (Fig. 7.1A). In such a case, B is the cord radius. The longitudinal coordinate z varies in the interval $[-H, +H]$. The liquid, which enters the system at $r = r_0$, leaves from the bases $z = \pm H$.

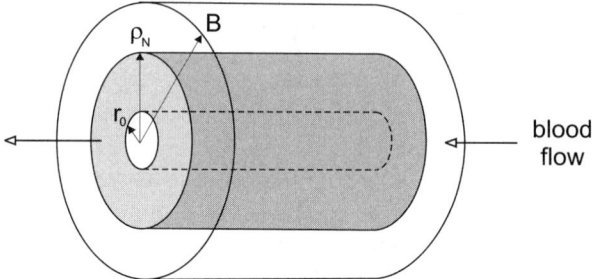

Fig. 7.2. Geometry of the tumour cord (symbols explained in the text).

We assume that cells form a porous medium of *constant* porosity (that is, ν_E is constant) and, irrespectively of their state, they move with the radial velocity $\mathbf{u} = (u(r,t), 0)$. The porosity is thus independent of the stress the cells are experiencing (we also will neglect the possible influence of the stress on the proliferation rate). The assumption that the cord can always be viewed as a packed arrangement of cells, possibly including dead and already degrading cells, limits the applicability of the model to cases in which the cellular component maintains some adhesion and is not severely reduced as a consequence of treatment. Therefore, the model could be significantly improved by including the computation of the stress and the possible degradation of the structure.

The velocity $\mathbf{v}$ of the fluid relative to the cells in the live cord is given by Darcy's law

$$\nu_E(\mathbf{v} - \mathbf{u}) = -\kappa \nabla \tilde{p}, \tag{7.1}$$

where κ is the hydraulic conductivity and $\tilde{p}$ is the pressure of the liquid. Dealing with (7.1) in our case is not simple, in view of the fact that the dynamics of the fluid in the cord is coupled with the dynamics of the fluid in the necrotic region. The rigorous way to proceed would be to take the divergence of both sides in (7.1) and use the information on $\nabla \cdot \mathbf{v}$, $\nabla \cdot \mathbf{u}$ derived from mass balance, thus obtaining an elliptic equation for $\tilde{p}$ to be associated with complicated interface conditions. We choose instead an approximate description that retains the most relevant information, that is the total fluid flow across each cylindrical section. This procedure amounts to considering the longitudinal average of the radial component of $\mathbf{v}$. Performing the longitudinal average of $\nabla \cdot \mathbf{v}$, where $\mathbf{v} = (v_r, v_z)$, and setting

$$v(r,t) = \frac{1}{2H} \int_{-H}^{H} v_r(r, z, t)\, dz,$$

one gets

$$\frac{1}{r}\frac{\partial}{\partial r}(rv) + \frac{1}{2H}[v_z(r, H, t) - v_z(r, -H, t)].$$

The second term expresses the outflow rate from $z = \pm H$, which has to be specified in some way. Our choice is to introduce the longitudinal average of the pressure,

$$p(r,t) = \frac{1}{2H} \int_{-H}^{H} \tilde{p}(r,z,t)\,dz\,,$$

and to assume that the outflow rate is proportional to the difference $p-p_\infty$. The constant p_∞ is identifiable as a "far field" pressure, namely the pressure in the lymphatic vessels. Thus, the quantities utilized in our model are $v(r,t)$, $p(r,t)$. We remark that the difficulties we have emphasized are peculiar to the cord geometry. The averaging procedure is not required in the case of a spheroid.

7.2.2 Mass Balance and Oxygen Dynamics

We are now ready to write down the mass balance equations for the various cell subpopulations

$$\frac{\partial \nu_P}{\partial t} + \frac{1}{r}\frac{\partial}{\partial r}(ru\nu_P) = \chi\nu_P + \gamma\nu_Q - \lambda\nu_P - \mu_P\nu_P\,, \tag{7.2}$$

$$\frac{\partial \nu_Q}{\partial t} + \frac{1}{r}\frac{\partial}{\partial r}(ru\nu_Q) = -\gamma\nu_Q + \lambda\nu_P - \mu_Q\nu_Q\,, \tag{7.3}$$

$$\frac{\partial \nu_A}{\partial t} + \frac{1}{r}\frac{\partial}{\partial r}(ru\nu_A) = \mu_P\nu_P + \mu_Q\nu_Q - \mu_A\nu_A\,, \tag{7.4}$$

and for the liquid

$$\nu_E \nabla \cdot \mathbf{v} = \mu_A\nu_A - \chi\nu_P\,. \tag{7.5}$$

In the above equations, χ is the proliferation rate, γ and λ are the rates of the transition Q→P and, respectively, P→Q, μ_P and μ_Q are death rates, and μ_A is the volume loss rate of dead cells. The coefficients γ and λ are increasing and, respectively, decreasing functions of the oxygen concentration $\sigma(r,t)$; the coefficients μ_P, μ_Q rather than spontaneous death represent the action of a cytotoxic agent, or can be associated to the damage produced by radiation. Thus, the knowledge of μ_P, μ_Q relies on the determination of other quantities, whose evolution should also be modelled.

Summing (7.2)–(7.4) (remember that $\nu_P+\nu_Q+\nu_A = \nu^\star$ is constant) produces a simple differential equation for u:

$$\frac{1}{r}\frac{\partial}{\partial r}(ru) = \frac{1}{\nu^\star}(\chi\nu_P - \mu_A\nu_A)\,.$$

Adding also (7.5), we get

$$\nabla \cdot (\nu_E \mathbf{v} + (1 - \nu_E)\mathbf{u}) = 0\,, \tag{7.6}$$

which expresses global incompressibility. Taking the longitudinal average of (7.6) as we have described above, we find

$$\frac{1}{r}\frac{\partial}{\partial r}(rv) = -\frac{1}{\nu_E}\left(\chi\nu_P - \mu_A\nu_A + \frac{\zeta_{out}}{H}(p - p_\infty)\right)\,,$$

where the coefficient ζ_{out}, possibly dependent on r, measures the drainage efficiency from the cord ends. Going back to Darcy's law (7.1), we can now derive its averaged form as

$$\nu_E(v - u) = -\kappa \frac{\partial p}{\partial r},$$

which in our scheme is used to obtain the pressure:

$$p(r, t) = p_0(t) - \frac{\nu_E}{\kappa} \int_{r_0}^{r} [v(r', t) - u(r', t)] \, dr', \qquad (7.7)$$

where the new unknown $p_0(t) = \lim_{r \to r_0^+} p(r, t)$ appears.

We consider the oxygen as the critical "nutrient," although other substances are important for cell energy metabolism, see for instance [19] and the recent paper [38] where oxygen, glucose, and lactate concur in determining the level of ATP in the cell. The high permeability of cell membrane to oxygen allows us to disregard the difference between extracellular and intracellular concentration. Due to the high diffusivity of oxygen, the quasi-steady diffusion-consumption equation

$$\Delta \sigma = f_P(\sigma)\nu_P + f_Q(\sigma)\nu_Q \qquad (7.8)$$

is assumed to be valid, where the functions f_P, f_Q that are related to oxygen consumption are of Michaelis–Menten type. We assume that all cells die if σ falls to a threshold value σ_N.

Before modelling the necrotic region, let us write down the boundary conditions for the equations written so far.

7.2.3 Boundary and Initial Conditions

As we said, at the vessel wall we may impose

$$u(r_0, t) = 0.$$

This condition guarantees that $r = r_0$ is a characteristic for (7.2)–(7.4), so that the quantities ν_P, ν_Q, ν_A do not have to be prescribed there.

Concerning the oxygen, we have

$$\sigma(r_0, t) = \sigma_b,$$

where σ_b is the oxygen concentration in blood, taken constant.

For the liquid exchange between blood and tumour tissue, a simple condition is the following:

$$\nu_E v(r_0, t) = \zeta_{in}(p_b - p_0(t)),$$

where p_b is the (constant) blood pressure, p_0 is the unknown introduced in (7.7), and ζ_{in} is a coefficient expressing the exchange efficiency. We recall here that the assumption that σ_b and p_b are both constant is an approximation because of the occurrence of two competing phenomena. Since oxygen is continuously transferred to the cord, its concentration in blood tends to decrease along the vessel in the direction of blood flow. In order to make the concentration as uniform as possible it is necessary that blood flow is sufficiently rapid, which however requires a high pressure drop. The vessel radius and the size of the cord are crucial in determining whether or not a compromise can be reached. On the basis of perfusion data, it has been checked that for cords of average size the two assumptions may be accepted [9].

Considering the interface $r = \rho_N$, a first condition is the continuity of the averaged pressure:

$$p(\rho_N, t) = p_N(t),$$

where p_N is unknown.

The most delicate conditions are concerned with the oxygen dynamics, because here we find two possible regimens:

(s1) cells enter the necrotic region, that is

$$u(\rho_N(t), t) > \dot{\rho}_N(t), \tag{7.9}$$

which means that σ has reached the necrosis threshold

$$\sigma(\rho_N(t), t) = \sigma_N; \tag{7.10}$$

(s2) cells do not enter the necrotic region, that is

$$u(\rho_N(t), t) = \dot{\rho}_N(t), \tag{7.11}$$

while σ is free to rise above σ_N

$$\sigma(\rho_N(t), t) \geq \sigma_N. \tag{7.12}$$

In both cases, according to the quasi-steady diffusion assumption, we impose

$$\left. \frac{\partial \sigma}{\partial r} \right|_{r = \rho_N(t)} = 0.$$

Thus, the motion of the interface takes place under two unilateral constraints. Note that (7.10) actually defines $\rho_N(t)$. Typically the switch from (7.9)–(7.10) to (7.11)–(7.12) occurs when cells are killed by a treatment that reduces oxygen consumption and pushes the interface outwards. The interface velocity cannot, however, exceed the cell velocity, since no living cell can be produced from the necrotic material. The converse switch is instead typical of the tumour regrowth, which, under the conditions (7.11)–(7.12) would tend to force

σ below σ_N. Simulations performed in [7] show clearly the essential role of these constraints in the evolution of the cord.

In the absence of necrosis, we have to prescribe for σ the no-flux conditions at $r = B(t)$. This boundary is now a material surface, and we have $\dot{B} = u(B(t), t)$. Concerning the pressure p, we cannot assign its value at $r = B$. Instead we will have there $\partial p/\partial r\big|_{r=B(t)} = 0$.

Prescribing initial conditions is not as simple as it may look. For instance, when one wants to investigate the effects of treatments it makes sense in many cases to start from the steady state (the steady state problem includes the equations for the necrotic region, still to be written). Finding the equilibrium solution is itself a highly nontrivial problem. All such issues have been discussed in detail [8, 9].

7.2.4 The Necrotic Region

We recall that the necrotic region occupies the domain $\rho_N(t) < r < B(t)$, $-H < z < H$. The way the forces exerted at $r = B$ enter the evolution of the system depends on the composition of the necrotic region, which contains a fraction of solid material (dead cells retaining some structural integrity) and a fraction of liquid. We have two possible regimes: (n1) the solid is packed in a sufficiently dense way to withstand the external action; (n2) the surrounding medium acts directly on the liquid. We take the simplifying assumption that both the pressure and the local volume fraction of dead cells are space independent.

The total volume of the necrotic region is

$$V_N = 2H\pi(B^2 - \rho_N^2) \tag{7.13}$$

and it splits into the sum $V_N^c + V_N^l$ of the solid and of the liquid volume. The evolution of the latter quantities, disregarding the loss of dead cells through $z = \pm H$, is ruled by mass balance:

$$\dot{V}_N^c = 4H\pi\rho_N(1 - \nu_E)[u(\rho_N, t) - \dot{\rho}_N] - \mu_N V_N^c, \tag{7.14}$$

$$\dot{V}_N^l = 4H\pi\rho_N\nu_E[v(\rho_N, t) - \dot{\rho}_N] + \mu_N V_N^c - q_{out}(t), \tag{7.15}$$

where μ_N is the rate of conversion of solid to liquid (remember also that $u - \dot{\rho}_N \geq 0$ which implies $V_N^c > 0$), and q_{out} is proportional to the difference $(p_N - p_\infty)$ and to the area of the cross section $\pi(B^2 - \rho_N^2)$, with the weight V_N^l/V_N, i.e. the liquid volume fraction. Thus

$$q_{out} = 2\zeta_{out}^N \frac{V_N^l}{V_N}\pi(B^2 - \rho_N^2)(p_N - p_\infty), \tag{7.16}$$

where the coefficient ζ_{out}^N is comparable to ζ_{out}/ν_E.

The complement to one of V_N^l/V_N, that is V_N^c/V_N, is subject to the constraint

$$\frac{V_N^c}{V_N} \leq \nu_N^\star , \qquad (7.17)$$

with the equality corresponding to regime (n1). Thus, in regime (n1), imposing $\dot{V}_N^c = \nu_N^\star \dot{V}_N$ in (7.14) yields a differential equation for B^2:

$$\frac{d}{dt}(B^2 - \rho_N^2) = 2\frac{1 - \nu_E}{\nu_N^\star}\rho_N\big(u(\rho_N, t) - \dot{\rho}_N\big) - \mu_N(B^2 - \rho_N^2) . \qquad (7.18)$$

By setting $\dot{V}_N^l = (1 - \nu_N^\star)\dot{V}_N$ and $V_N^c = \nu_N^\star V_N$ in (7.15) gives an expression for q_{out}, which defines p_N via (7.16).

So far we have ignored the stress, but during regime (n1) p_N is required not to exceed the stress that the surrounding material is able to exert on the system. Such a stress may be considered a function of the overall size of the cohort of cords, that is, a function of B. Let $\Psi(B)$ denote such a function, increasing with B. Thus, the following constraint has to be satisfied during regime (n1):

$$p_N < \Psi(B) . \qquad (7.19)$$

Violating the constraint (7.19) marks the transition to regime (n2), in which the condition $V_N^c = \nu_N^\star V_N$ is replaced by the condition

$$p_N = \Psi(B) , \qquad (7.20)$$

and (7.17) as a strict inequality is present as a new constraint. Now (7.14) can be integrated, providing V_N^c as a functional of ρ_N and u, while the combination of (7.13), (7.15), (7.16), (7.20) leads to the differential equation for B replacing (7.18). This picture of the necrotic region is the one proposed in [10].

In the formation of a spheroidal tumour the early stage of the necrotic core will be under the regime (n1). The same is true for the first appearance of a necrotic zone around the cord. However, predicting in a more precise way the transition to the other regime would require a definition of the age of the outer rim of the necrotic region around the viable core (or of the inner core in the case of the spheroid), abandoning the simple model of the homogeneous mixture.

We conclude this section by recalling that the well-posedness of the model was investigated in [8, 9], including the analysis of the steady state in the case of an untreated tumour. Needless to say, the presence of constraints in the dynamical case produces serious mathematical difficulties.

7.3 Response of Cords to Treatments

The model illustrated in the previous section has been applied to study the response of cords to various types of treatment. Here we comment the work done in this direction. Although the results give several interesting clues on the effects of treatments, we must say that they are far from being conclusive. One of the reasons is that the model used, despite the many details it contains, does not give a full description of the tumour.

7.3.1 Treatments by Drugs

Already in [7], where the model was first presented in a version not including the dynamics of the fluid, the effect of a cytotoxic drug was considered. That model was only applicable to drugs whose transport mechanism is mainly diffusive. We estimated that advective transport is indeed negligible if diffusivity is not less than 5×10^{-8} cm^2/s, a condition satisfied by many anticancer drugs. Moreover the drug was assumed to diffuse the same way in the liquid and in the cells. The cell death rate was taken as a given function of the drug concentration c. Of course the diffusion equation for c contains a sink term, expressing drug uptake and consumption by the cells, which vanishes in the necrotic region. The value of c was prescribed at the blood vessel wall as a function of time, following drug administration, while zero flux was prescribed at the boundary $r = B(t)$.

The effect of cell killing on the evolution of the cord, including the distribution of pressure and the change experienced by the necrotic zone, was investigated (in the context of the full model illustrated in Section 7.2) in [10]. However, instead of examining the dynamics of the drug, the death rates μ_P, μ_Q were chosen as a combination of space independent functions decaying exponentially with time, so as to reproduce the *expected* effect of the delivery of a bolus dose. Namely, we chose [10, 11]

$$\mu_P(t) = \frac{m_P}{\tau_1 - \tau_2}(e^{-t/\tau_1} - e^{-t/\tau_2}),$$

$$\mu_Q(t) = \frac{m_Q}{\tau_1 - \tau_2}(e^{-t/\tau_1} - e^{-t/\tau_2}),$$

where τ_1 is related to drug removal and τ_2 to the drug distribution in the body compartments.

This shortcut made the simulation simpler, and allowed us to reach some significant qualitative conclusions. For instance it was pointed out that cell killing alone is not enough to produce a marked reduction of the overall size of the tumour, but it must be accompanied by an effective drainage of the liquid (meaning a sufficiently high value of the coefficients ζ_{out}, ζ_{out}^N of the model). Fig. 7.3 shows an example of the time evolution of the cord in the case of a cycle-specific drug, that is, a drug affecting mainly the proliferating cells ($m_P > m_Q$). Panel A reports the ratio between the total volume (per unit cord length) of viable cells and its value at $t = 0$, describing the dynamics of the viable cell population following the treatment. The reduction of the number of viable cells lowers oxygen consumption and thus causes reoxygenation of the cord as shown by the time course of mean oxygen concentration (panel B). The increase in oxygen concentration induces a recruitment of quiescent cells into proliferation, as seen in panel A, so that a transient phase in which the proliferating fraction is higher than the initial one may occur. The radius ρ_N shows an initial shrinkage followed by a regrowth leading to the steady state (panel C). Very soon after the rise of drug concentration the interface

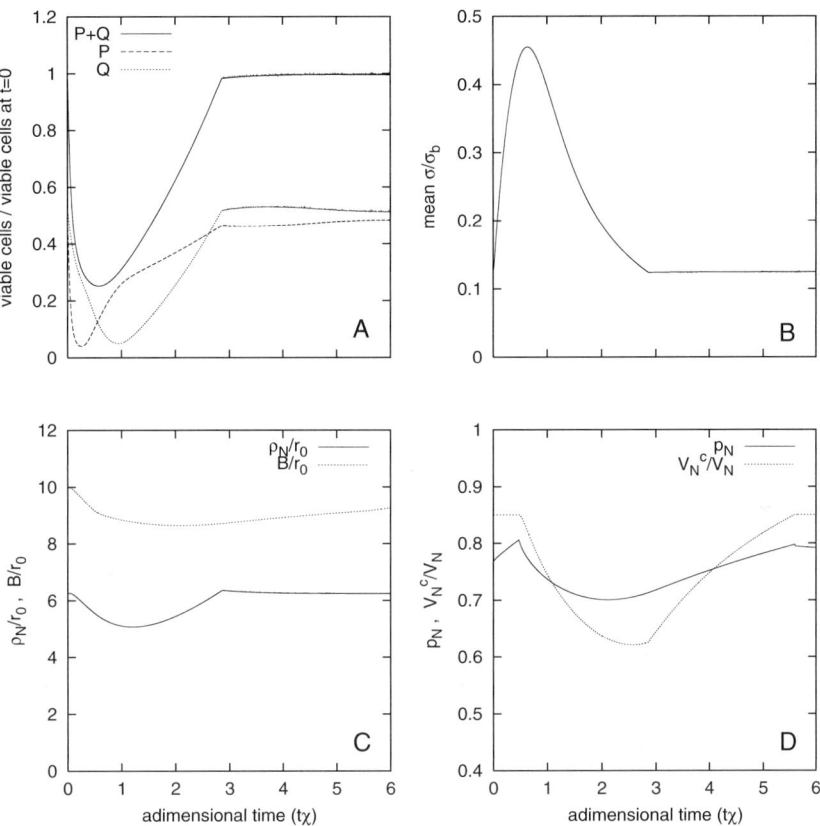

Fig. 7.3. Panel A: time course of the viable cell subpopulations after a single-dose treatment; P proliferating cells, Q quiescent cells. Panel B: mean oxygen concentration. Panel C: cord radius ρ_N and outer boundary B. Panel D: pressure and cell fraction in the necrotic region. Parameters as in [24] with $m_P/m_Q = 5$.

$r = \rho_N$ becomes a material surface (see Section 7.2.3). The slope discontinuity that occurs later marks the switching of the interface from the material to the nonmaterial nature. In the same panel, the time course of the boundary B is plotted. Panel D shows the time evolution of the pressure p_N and of the cellular fraction in the necrotic region. In the initial state the constraint (7.17) is satisfied with the equality sign and the pressure is less than $\Psi(B)$. Due to the enhanced influx of liquid caused by cell death, p_N increases reaching $\Psi(B)$. At this point the regime changes, p_N is given by $\Psi(B)$, and the cellular fraction goes below $\nu_N^\star$. During the cord regrowth, the influx of liquid decreases and the system switches again to the regime characterized by a cellular fraction equal to $\nu_N^\star$. It was found that the time evolution of the average interstitial pressure in the viable cord closely follows the pressure in the necrotic region because of the high value of Darcy's conductivity.

This numerical experiment opened the way to the mathematical investigation of another question of great interest: what is the effect of splitting a dose of drug? We have considered the case of splitting the dose into two equal boluses spaced by a time interval T, and found the splitting advantageous if the sensitivity of the cell population to the drug significantly increases when the oxygen level increases [11]. A comparison between the single dose and the split dose was made by using the survival ratio defined as

$$ \text{SR} = \frac{\min(\text{viable cell volume})_2}{\min(\text{viable cell volume})_1} , \tag{7.21} $$

where the subscripts 1,2 refer to the single and to the split dose, respectively.

A crucial role is played by the ratio m_P/m_Q. To understand how dose splitting can enhance the cell killing, one should go back to equations (7.2)–(7.3), in which the coefficients γ, λ regulating the transitions $P \rightleftarrows Q$ are monotonically dependent (in opposite ways) on the oxygen concentration σ. As shown by Fig. 7.3B, when the first half-dose kills a certain fraction of cells, oxygen concentration increases favouring the transition of the surviving Q cells to the P-state. Then, if the ratio m_P/m_Q is large, the "upgraded" cells will have a much greater chance to be killed by the application of the second half-dose. This phenomenon is called *resensitization*. Fig. 7.4, left panel, shows the behaviour of SR as a function of the inter-fraction interval, when using different values for m_P, m_Q. Of course, taking $m_P/m_Q = 1$ eliminates resensitization completely, while a ratio $m_P/m_Q = 5$ shows a marked effect of the dose splitting procedure. The figure also shows the existence of an optimal choice of the splitting time, corresponding to the time in which the ratio between P and Q cells is maximal. These results are obviously qualitative, but they strongly suggest the promotion of experimental research in this direction.

Dose splitting is an interesting topic also in the context of radiation therapy [14], as we will see in the following section.

7.3.2 Response to Impulsive Irradiation

A spatially uniform model

Radiation can produce cell damages which may later lead to cell death either by a direct action or as a consequence of a misrepair process. In order to understand and to model the latter mechanism, suppose that the DNA double strand is broken by radiation at one point. This damage has a certain probability of being repaired, thus allowing the cell to survive. However, along with the repair consisting in joining the two segments of the same DNA molecule, there can also be "cross-repairs" in which two segments originally belonging to different strands are joined, giving rise to two misrepaired strands. The outcome of such mixing may, or may not, be lethal for the cell. Each DNA double strand has a specific point, known as its centromere, acting as a pivotal center during mitosis. Now, the "cross-repair" can produce two chromosomes

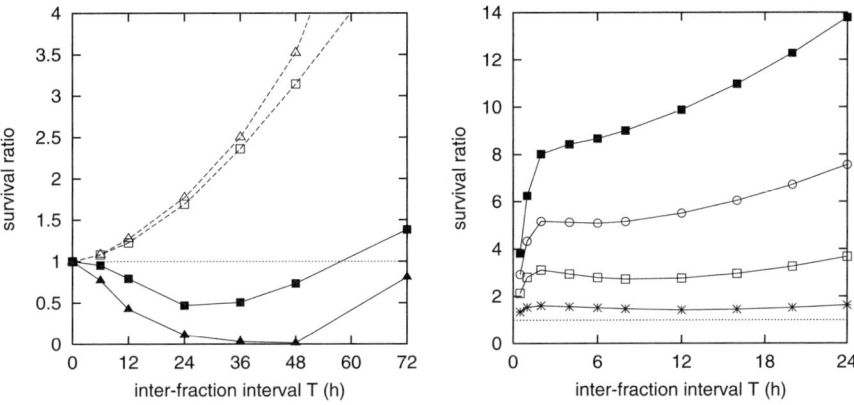

Fig. 7.4. Survival ratio as a function of the time interval between the two fractions. Left panel: SR for split-dose drug delivery. Closed symbols: $m_P/m_Q = 5$; $m_P = 4$ for each fraction (squares), $m_P = 8$ (triangles). Open symbols: $m_P/m_Q = 1$; $m_P = 2$ (squares), $m_P = 4$ (triangles). Other parameter values given in [11]. Right panel: SR for split-dose radiation delivery. Effect of the intervessel distance on the survival ratio. Closed squares, $B(0) = 80\,\mu m$; open circles, $B(0) = 90\,\mu m$; open squares, $B(0) = 100\,\mu m$; stars, cord surrounded by necrosis ($\rho_N = 124.75\,\mu m$). Other parameter values given in [13].

with one centromere each, or one with two centromeres and one with no centromere. The occurrence of the latter kind of misrepair produces cells unable to replicate and destined to death. Lethally damaged cells are called "clonogenically dead." Other types of lethal misrepairs can be accounted for in the direct action.

A simple spatially homogeneous differential model describing the repair-misrepair process was proposed in [22, 30] and can be written as

$$\frac{dN}{dt} = -[\alpha\dot{D} + \frac{1}{2}kU^2]N\,, \tag{7.22}$$

$$\frac{dU}{dt} = \delta\dot{D} - \omega U - 2kU^2\,, \tag{7.23}$$

where N is the number of viable cells, $\dot{D}$ the radiation dose rate, and U the mean number of DNA double strand breaks (DSBs) per cell. The term ωU represents the rate of correct repairs, the term kU^2 is the rate of binary cross-repairs, which on one hand eliminate two DSBs each, and on the other have a probability $1/2$ of ending up with a lethal damage. Direct lethal action of radiation is represented by the term $-\alpha\dot{D}$, whereas $\delta\dot{D}$ is the rate of DSB production per cell. Cells carrying DSBs are counted in N as long as they do not become lethally damaged.

The duration of pulse irradiation is usually so short that the direct action of radiation and the DSB production can be described simply by setting the initial conditions for N and for U:

$$N(0^+) = N(0^-)\,e^{-\alpha D}$$

$$U(0^+) = U(0^-) + \delta D, \qquad U(0^-) = 0,$$

where D is the radiation dose. The solution of (7.22)–(7.23) with the above initial conditions provides, in the limit $t \to \infty$, the surviving fraction $S = N(\infty)/N(0^-)$:

$$\ln S = -\alpha D + \frac{\omega}{8k}\left[\ln\left(1 + \frac{2k\delta D}{\omega}\right) - \frac{2k\delta D}{\omega}\right].$$

For $2k\delta D/\omega \ll 1$, which corresponds to neglecting the quadratic term in (7.23), we obtain

$$S = \exp\left[-\alpha D - \frac{k(\delta D)^2}{4\omega}\right]. \tag{7.24}$$

Defining $\beta = k\delta^2/(4\omega)$, we recognize in (7.24) what is called the linear-quadratic (LQ) model previously proposed on empirical bases [37].

When the dose D is split into two fractions $D/2$, given with an interval T, (7.22)–(7.23) still allow us to evaluate the surviving fraction (after the second dose). For simplicity we just report the new value of S in the case $k\delta D/\omega \ll 1$:

$$S_{\text{split}} = \exp\left[-\alpha D - \beta\frac{1 + e^{-\omega T}}{2}D^2\right]. \tag{7.25}$$

Clearly

$$\frac{S_{\text{split}}}{S} = \exp\left[\beta\frac{1 - e^{-\omega T}}{2}D^2\right] > 1, \tag{7.26}$$

showing that, according to this theory, splitting the dose is never advantageous in terms of cell killing. We can also see that by splitting D into hD and $(1 - h)D$, the factor $(1 + e^{-\omega T})/2$ in (7.25) is replaced with $2h(h-1)(1-e^{-\omega T})+1$, showing that the above ratio is maximum for $h = 1/2$.

However, the analysis sketched above ignores the dynamics of the tumour and, in particular, the possible reoxygenation of the tumour following the first dose as experimentally observed [21]. It must be stressed that the parameters α, δ are increasing functions of the oxygen concentration [41].

Effects of radiation on a tumour cord

In [13] we studied the dose splitting effect on the basis of the following tumour cord model:

$$\frac{\partial \nu_P}{\partial t} + \frac{1}{r}\frac{\partial}{\partial r}(ru\nu_P) = \chi\nu_P + \gamma\nu_Q - \lambda\nu_P - m_P(r,t)\nu_P, \tag{7.27}$$

$$\frac{\partial \nu_Q}{\partial t} + \frac{1}{r}\frac{\partial}{\partial r}(ru\nu_Q) = -\gamma\nu_Q + \lambda\nu_P - m_Q(r,t)\nu_Q, \tag{7.28}$$

$$\frac{\partial \nu^\dagger}{\partial t} + \frac{1}{r}\frac{\partial}{\partial r}(ru\nu^\dagger) = m_P(r,t)\nu_P + m_Q(r,t)\nu_Q - \mu\nu^\dagger, \tag{7.29}$$

$$\frac{\partial \nu_A}{\partial t} + \frac{1}{r}\frac{\partial}{\partial r}(ru\nu_A) = \mu\nu^\dagger - \mu_A\nu_A, \tag{7.30}$$

where ν_P, ν_Q, and ν_A have the same meaning as in the basic model of Section 7.2, and $\nu^\dagger$ is the volume fraction of lethally damaged cells. The rates m_P and m_Q represent the effect of the misrepair process that induces lethal damage, and μ is the death rate of lethally damaged cells.

In view of (7.22)–(7.23) for the kinetics of DSB repair/misrepair, for the rates m_P and m_Q we assume

$$m_P(r,t) = \frac{1}{2}kX_P^2(r,t), \quad m_Q(r,t) = \frac{1}{2}kX_Q^2(r,t), \tag{7.31}$$

where $X_P(r,t)$ and $X_Q(r,t)$ denote the mean number of DSBs in an "equivalent" P cell and, respectively, Q cell at the position r at time t. These quantities, as derived in [13], satisfy the following equations:

$$\frac{\partial X_P}{\partial t} + u\frac{\partial X_P}{\partial r} = -\omega X_P - 2kX_P^2, \tag{7.32}$$

$$\frac{\partial X_Q}{\partial t} + u\frac{\partial X_Q}{\partial r} = -\omega X_Q - 2kX_Q^2. \tag{7.33}$$

The assumption that all cellular volume fractions in (7.27)–(7.30) sum up to a constant $\nu^\star$ yields the equation for the common cellular velocity u, as seen in Section 7.2. The dynamics of the interstitial liquid is here of less importance and is disregarded.

If a sequence of impulsive irradiation is given with dose D_k at time t_k, $k = 1, 2, \ldots$, $t_1 = 0$, we have the following conditions:

$$\nu_i(r, t_k^+) = \nu_i(r, t_k^-)\exp[-\alpha_i(\sigma(r, t_k^-))D_k], \quad i = P, Q,$$
$$\nu^\dagger(r, t_k^+) = \nu^\dagger(r, t_k^-) + \sum\nolimits_{i=P,Q}\left(\nu_i(r, t_k^-) - \nu_i(r, t_k^+)\right),$$
$$X_i(r, t_k^+) = X_i(r, t_k^-) + \delta_i(\sigma(r, t_k^-))D_k, \quad i = P, Q,$$

that define the initial data for the differential system (7.27)–(7.33) by setting $\nu_i(r, 0^-) = \nu_{i0}(r)$, $\nu^\dagger(r, 0^-) = 0$, $X_i(r, 0^-) = 0$, $i = P, Q$, and the data update at the subsequent delivery times. We have allowed the sensitivity parameters α_i, δ_i to depend on the oxygen concentration according to experimental evidence [41]. Oxygen concentration satisfies the free boundary problem described in Section 7.2, in which in (7.8) the absorption term due to the population $\nu^\dagger$ must be added.

The model was simulated [13] under different conditions to elucidate the influence of reoxygenation on the split-dose response compared with the response to the undivided dose. Fig. 7.4, right panel, shows the pattern of the survival ratio defined by (7.21) for three different values of the radius B at $t = 0$ in the absence of necrosis (i.e., for different intervessel distances, see Fig. 7.1A). In addition, the response of a cord surrounded by necrosis is also shown. When B increases, the whole SR curve is lowered and reaches a minimum in the case of necrosis. This is explained by considering that the mean oxygen concentration decreases as B increases and therefore the average β value decreases. Smaller β values, according to the LQ model, are expected to produce smaller SR values (see (7.26)). Moreover, if the cord radius is small, the reoxygenation induces only a small increase in radiosensitivity because the initial mean oxygen concentration is high, with σ falling in the saturating portion of the $\alpha(\sigma)$ and $\delta(\sigma)$ curves. At the higher values of B, the SR curve shows an appreciable relative minimum due to the reoxygenation of the cell population that makes the second dose more effective. The initial rising branch of the curve corresponds to the repair process, whose duration is proportional to $1/\omega$. The increase for large T is due to the regrowth of surviving cells between the two doses.

On the basis of the results shown in Fig. 7.4, we can conclude that the enhancing effect of reoxygenation on cell killing, which was emphasized for drug treatments, is present here too, although it is not strong enough to reduce the survival ratio below unity. This apparently negative situation can however prove advantageous since the increase of the survival ratio upon splitting may be higher for the normal tissue than for the tumour [13]. Therefore repeated treatments with fractionated doses may lead to a more selective destruction of the tumour mass.

7.3.3 Transport of Monoclonal Antibodies

Specific antibodies may bind to antigens on the tumour cell membrane. This property can be exploited to deliver a killing agent to the targeted cell (a toxin or a radionuclide [4]). In some cases antibodies can directly exert a cytotoxic action. As a preliminary analysis to the study of tumour therapies based on the use of antibodies, in the paper [12] we have examined the problem of their transport through a cord that has reached a steady state, without considering any cytotoxic action. The scheme that follows may be the basis for a further study.

We consider monoclonal IgG antibodies with two equivalent binding sites. The antigens are uniformly distributed on the cell membrane and are monovalent. Thus the antibodies can be found in three states: (i) free in the extracellular liquid with concentration c, (ii) monovalently bound with surface concentration $\hat{b}_1$, (iii) bivalently bound with surface concentration $\hat{b}_2$. All concentrations are supposed to be independent of the longitudinal coordinate z. We schematize antigens as receptors with surface concentration $\hat{S}$, and we denote by $\eta^\star$ the ratio of total cellular surface per unit volume to extracellular volume fraction. Consistent with the assumption that the volume fraction occupied by cells in the cord is constant, $\eta^\star$ is a known constant. The formation of bonds is a reversible process, and the formation of double bonds is taken as a sequential process. We introduce the following rate constants: $2k_a$ for the formation of the first bond, k'_a for the formation of the second bond, and k_d for the dissociation of a bond.

That said, after performing the longitudinal mean, the dynamics of the antibodies in the cord is described by the following system [12]:

$$\frac{\partial c}{\partial t} - \frac{D}{r}\frac{\partial}{\partial r}(r\frac{\partial c}{\partial r}) + fv(r)\frac{\partial c}{\partial r} = f\chi\frac{\nu_P(r)}{1 - \nu^\star}c - 2k_a\eta^\star c\hat{s} + k_d\eta^\star\hat{b}_1 \, , \quad (7.34)$$

$$\frac{\partial\hat{b}_1}{\partial t} + u(r)\frac{\partial\hat{b}_1}{\partial r} = -\chi\frac{\nu_P(r)}{\nu^\star}\hat{b}_1 + 2k_a c\hat{s} - k_d\hat{b}_1 - k_a'\hat{s}\hat{b}_1 + 2k_d\hat{b}_2 \, , \quad (7.35)$$

$$\frac{\partial\hat{b}_2}{\partial t} + u(r)\frac{\partial\hat{b}_2}{\partial r} = -\chi\frac{\nu_P(r)}{\nu^\star}\hat{b}_2 + k_a'\hat{s}\hat{b}_1 - 2k_d\hat{b}_2 \, , \quad (7.36)$$

with

$$\hat{s} = \hat{S} - \hat{b}_1 - 2\hat{b}_2 \, .$$

Here, u, v, and ν_P are functions of the radial distance only because the cord is at the steady state. The velocities u, v and the size of the cord are provided by the solution of the steady state version of the model in Section 7.2 (with $\mu_P = \mu_Q = 0$, $\nu_A = 0$). In equation (7.34) we have considered that the transport of antibodies takes place through diffusion (with diffusivity D) and advection (with retardation factor $f < 1$).

For the flux of antibodies at the blood vessel wall, once the concentration of antibodies in blood $c_b(t)$ is prescribed, we assume the expression

$$-D\frac{\partial c}{\partial r}\Big|_{r=r_0} + fv(r_0)c(r_0,t) = \frac{P}{\nu_E}(c_b(t) - c(r_0,t))\frac{\text{Pe}}{e^{\text{Pe}}-1} + v(r_0)(1 - \sigma_f)c_b(t) \, ,$$

with Pe (Peclet number) given by $\text{Pe} = \nu_E v(r_0)(1 - \sigma_f)/P$, where P is the permeability of the vessel wall, and σ_f is the filtration reflection coefficient. No condition is required for $\hat{b}_1$, $\hat{b}_2$ at $r = r_0$, since $u(r_0) = 0$. At $t = 0$ all the unknown concentrations are taken to be zero. The second boundary condition for c requires the description of the antibody transport in the necrotic region.

In the necrotic region, little is known about the interaction of antibodies with degrading cells. Here we suppose that the antigens are retained on the surface of dead cells and are destroyed after cell degradation. Concerning the antibodies bound to cells entering the necrotic region, we suppose that upon cell degradation either (i) antibodies are lost, or (ii) antibodies are set free. Of course these are opposite options describing two extreme situations. They are supposed to provide bounds to the real behaviour which will be somehow in between. Whatever model is chosen, we have to write the evolution equations for c, $\hat{b}_1$, $\hat{b}_2$ and this requires the knowledge of the fields $u(r)$, $v(r)$ also in the necrotic region. A derivation of these quantities is provided in [12], and it is not reported here for the sake of brevity. In that paper, the same approach as in Section 7.2.4 has been followed to determine the outer boundary $r = B$ and the necrotic pressure p_N.

Once we have determined the global equilibrium solution for the cord plus the necrotic region, it is possible to write the evolution equations for c, $\hat{b}_1$, $\hat{b}_2$ in the necrotic region, which in case (i) take the form

$$\frac{\partial c}{\partial t} - \frac{D}{r}\frac{\partial}{\partial r}\left(r\frac{\partial c}{\partial r}\right) + fv(r)\frac{\partial c}{\partial r}$$
$$= -f\mu_N\frac{\nu_N}{1-\nu_N}c - 2k_a\eta_N c\hat{s} + k_d\eta_N\hat{b}_1, \quad (7.37)$$

$$\frac{\partial\hat{b}_1}{\partial t} + u(r)\frac{\partial\hat{b}_1}{\partial r} = 2k_a c\hat{s} - k_d\hat{b}_1 - k'_a\hat{s}\hat{b}_1 + 2k_d\hat{b}_2, \quad (7.38)$$

$$\frac{\partial\hat{b}_2}{\partial t} + u(r)\frac{\partial\hat{b}_2}{\partial r} = k'_a\hat{s}\hat{b}_1 - 2k_d\hat{b}_2, \quad (7.39)$$

where $\nu_N = V_N^c/V_N$ is the volume fraction of dead cells and η_N is the ratio of the cellular surface per unit volume in the necrotic region to the extracellular volume fraction $1 - \nu_N$. In case (ii), the term $\mu_N\eta_N(\hat{b}_1 + \hat{b}_2)$ must be added to the right-hand side of (7.37).

The conditions at the necrotic interface $r = \rho_N$ are: the continuity of c; the continuity of the flux of antibodies which, in view of the mass flux continuity, and supposing that the factor f is also continuous, takes the form

$$(1 - \nu_N)\frac{\partial c}{\partial r}\bigg|_{r=\rho_N^+} = (1 - \nu^\star)\frac{\partial c}{\partial r}\bigg|_{r=\rho_N^-};$$

and the continuity of $\hat{b}_1$, $\hat{b}_2$. Finally we have no flux at the outer boundary B:

$$\frac{\partial c}{\partial r}\bigg|_{r=B} = 0.$$

Numerical simulations have been performed for the input data given by

$$c_b(t) = c_{b0}\left(me^{-t/\tau_1} + (1 - m)e^{-t/\tau_2}\right),$$

with values of m, τ_1, and τ_2 as in [28], and are illustrated in Fig. 7.5. This figure shows the evolution of free and bound antibody for different values of the parameters $k_a = k'_a$ and k_d. As expected, the affinity parameter $K = k_a/k_d$ plays an important role: for $K = 50$ (left panel) antibodies are mainly present in the doubly bound state while, for $K = 2$ (right panel), $\hat{b}_1$ and $\hat{b}_2$ are much closer to each other. In the simulated cases the concentration of free antibodies decays very strongly with the radial distance: this is a clinically interesting information, since it says that the injected antibodies basically do not leave the cord, thus causing no harm to the surrounding tissue. Moreover, we observe that the high binding to cell surface antigens results in a "barrier" to antibody penetration generating a more heterogeneous antibody distribution due to the preferential binding in the inner region of the cord. A comparison between the options (i) and (ii) showed that the fate of antibodies after cell degradation is not particularly important apart from cases in which both the degradation rate of dead cells and the binding affinity are large.

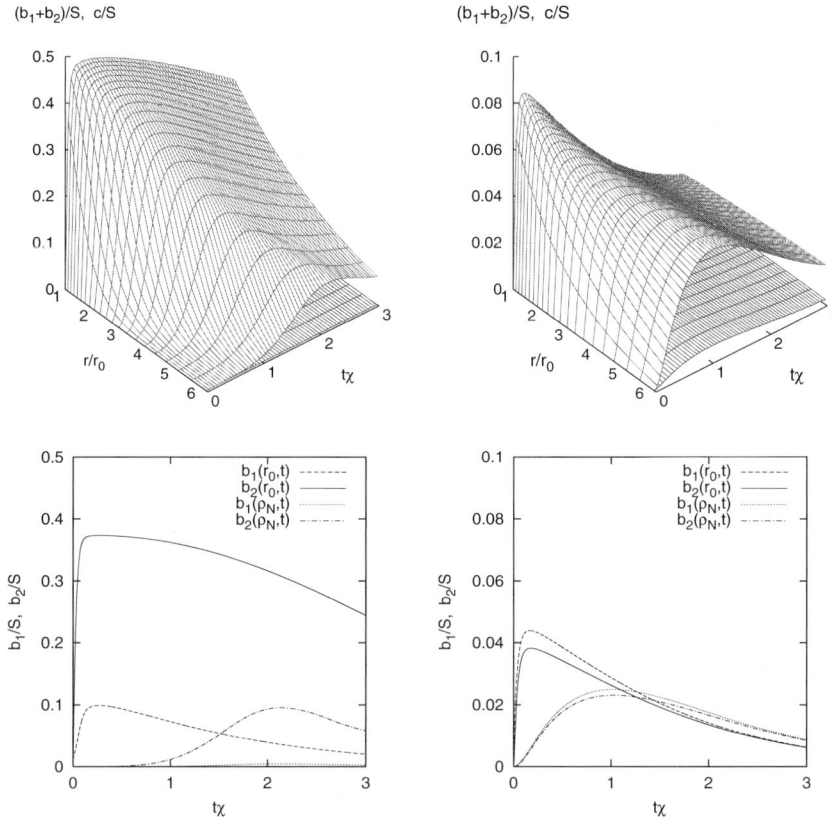

Fig. 7.5. Upper panels: distribution of bound and free antibodies (in both panels the lower surface represents free antibodies). The concentrations reported are normalized. Lower panels: time course of b_1 and b_2 at $r = r_0$ and $r = \rho_N$. Left panels: $k_a = k_a' = 1000$, $k_d = 20$; right panels: $k_a = k_a' = 100$, $k_d = 50$ (nondimensional units). Other parameters given in [12].

7.4 Conclusions

With reference to an array of tumour cords, taken as a paradigm of a vascular tumour, we have reviewed some models describing the action of treatments. Three classes of treatments have been considered: chemotherapy, radiotherapy, and treatments using antibodies. We have tried to emphasize both the clinical interest of the results obtained and the limitations accompanying the corresponding mathematical models, which are necessarily formulated on a selection of the many processes accompanying tumour evolution. We also tried to provide sufficient motivations for the choices at the basis of the illustrated approaches. The final goal was to reach conclusions of some practical relevance by means of numerical simulations in which the various parameters involved have been taken from the experimental literature.

The theories presented contain some concepts that should always be taken into account when dealing with tumour cords or spheroids. At the same time other aspects have been ignored, like the analysis and influence of stresses, whose role can be important. The reason is, on one hand, to limit the complexity of the models, which nevertheless is still remarkable, and on the other the lack of a convincingly complete constitutive law for the cell-liquid mixture. The very same idea of adopting a two-component scheme cannot be completely satisfactory, although it may be reasonably acceptable for tumour cords that do not seem to develop a substantial extracellular matrix. Because of the importance of the subject and the intrinsic complexity of tumours, we believe that when attempting to formulate a mathematical model, particularly in the critical field of treatments, one should explicitly declare its limits of applicability.

That said, we can also affirm that the results we have illustrated have implications of practical interest. This refers in particular to the conclusions about the effectiveness of splitting the dose in chemotherapy and the different scenario that is offered when one poses the same question for radiation treatments. The description of how monoclonal antibodies are absorbed in a cord also appears to be of practical relevance. Model predictions, although substantially qualitative, appear sufficiently precise to suggest experimental work aimed at their confirmation.

References

1. Anderson, A.R.: A hybrid mathematical model of solid tumour invasion: the importance of cell adhesion. Math. Med. Biol., **22**, 163–86 (2005).
2. Araujo, R.P., McElwain, D.L.S.: New insights into vascular collapse and growth dynamics in solid tumors. J. Theor. Biol., **228**, 335–46 (2004).
3. Araujo, R.P., McElwain, D.L.S.: A history of the study of solid tumour growth: the contribution of mathematical modelling. Bull. Math. Biol., **66**, 1039–91 (2004).
4. Berinstein, N.L.: Biological therapy of cancer. In: Tannock, I.F., Hill, R.P. (eds) The Basic Science of Oncology. McGraw-Hill, New York, pp. 420–42 (1998).
5. Bertuzzi, A., Gandolfi, A.: Cell kinetics in a tumour cord. J. Theor. Biol., **204**, 587–99 (2000).
6. Bertuzzi, A., Fasano, A., Gandolfi, A., Marangi, D.: Cell kinetics in tumour cords studied by a model with variable cell cycle length. Math. Biosci., **177/178**, 103–25 (2002).
7. Bertuzzi, A., d'Onofrio, A., Fasano, A., Gandolfi, A.: Regression and regrowth of tumour cords following single-dose anticancer treatment. Bull. Math. Biol., **65**, 903–31 (2003).
8. Bertuzzi, A., Fasano, A., Gandolfi, A.: A free boundary problem with unilateral constraints describing the evolution of a tumour cord under the influence of cell killing agents. SIAM J. Math. Anal., **36**, 882–915 (2004).

9. Bertuzzi, A., Fasano, A., Gandolfi, A.: A mathematical model for tumor cords incorporating the flow of interstitial fluid. Math. Mod. Meth. Appl. Sci., **15**, 1735–77 (2005).

10. Bertuzzi, A., Fasano, A., Gandolfi, A., Sinisgalli, S.: Interstitial pressure and extracellular fluid motion in tumor cords. Math. Biosci. Engng., **2**, 445–60 (2005).

11. Bertuzzi, A., Fasano, A., Gandolfi, A., Sinisgalli, C.: Cell resensitization after delivery of a cycle-specific anticancer drug and effect of dose splitting: learning from tumour cords. J. Theor. Biol., **244**, 388–99 (2007).

12. Bertuzzi, A., Fasano, A., Gandolfi, A., Sinisgalli, C.: The transport of specific monoclonal antibodies in tumour cords. In: Aletti, G., Burger, M., Micheletti, A., Morale, D. (eds) Math Everywhere: Deterministic and Stochastic Modelling in Biomedicine, Economics and Industry. Springer-Verlag, Berlin and Heidelberg, pp. 151–64 (2007).

13. Bertuzzi, A., Fasano, A., Gandolfi, A., Sinisgalli, C.: Reoxygenation and split-dose response to radiation in tumours with Krogh-like vasculature. Bull. Math. Biol., in press. DOI 10.1007/s11538-007-9287-9 (2008).

14. Brenner, D.J., Hlatky, L.R., Hahnfeldt, P.J., Hall, E.J., Sachs, R.K.: A convenient extension of the linear-quadratic model to include redistribution and reoxygenation. Int. J. Radiat. Oncol. Biol. Phys., **32**, 379–90 (1995).

15. Breward, C.J.W., Byrne, H.M., Lewis, C.E.: A multiphase model describing vascular tumour growth. Bull. Math. Biol., **65**, 609–40 (2003).

16. Bru, A., Albertos, S., Luis Subiza, J., Garcia-Asenjo, J.L., Bru, I.: The universal dynamics of tumor growth. Biophys. J., **85**, 2948–61 (2003).

17. Byrne, H.M.: Modelling avascular tumour growth. In: Preziosi, L. (ed) Cancer Modelling and Simulation. Chapman & Hall/CRC, Boca Raton, pp. 75–120 (2003).

18. Byrne, H.M., Preziosi, L.: Modelling solid tumour growth using the theory of mixtures. Math. Med. Biol., **20**, 341–66 (2003).

19. Casciari, J.J., Sotirchos, S.V., Sutherland, R.M.: Mathematical modelling of microenvironment and growth in EMT6/Ro multicellular tumour spheroids. Cell. Prolif., **25**, 1–22 (1992).

20. Chaplain, M.A., Graziano, L., Preziosi, L.: Mathematical modelling of the loss of tissue compression responsiveness and its role in solid tumour development. Math. Med. Biol., **23**, 197–229 (2006).

21. Crokart N., Jordan, B.F., Baudelet, C., Ansiaux, R., Sonveaux, P., Grégoire, V., Beghein, N., DeWever, J., Bouzin, C., Feron, O., Gallez, B.: Early reoxygenation in tumors after irradiation: determining factors and consequences for radiotherapy regimens using daily multiple fractions. Int. J. Radiat. Oncol. Biol. Phys., **63**, 901–10 (2005).

22. Curtis, S.B.: Lethal and potentially lethal lesions induced by radiation-a unified repair model. Radiat. Res., **106**, 252–70 (1986).

23. Dyson, J., Villella-Bressan, R., Webb, G.F.: The evolution of a tumor cord cell population. Comm. Pure Appl. Anal., **3**, 331–52 (2004).

24. Fasano, A., Bertuzzi, A., Gandolfi, A.: Mathematical modelling of tumour growth and treatment. In: Quarteroni, A., Formaggia, L., Veneziani, A. (eds) Complex Systems in Biomedicine. Springer-Verlag Italia, Milano, pp. 71–108 (2006).

25. Ferreira Junior, S.C., Matrins, M.L., Vilela, M.J.: The reaction diffusion model for the growth of avascular tumors. Phys. Rev. E, **65**, 1–8 (2002).

26. Friedman, A., Reitich, F.: Analysis of a mathematical model for the growth of tumors. J. Math. Biol., **38**, 262–84 (1999).

27. Friedman, A., Tao, Y.: Analysis of a model of a virus that replicates selectively in tumor cells. J. Math. Biol., **47**, 391–423 (2003).

28. Fujimori, K., Covell, D.G., Fletcher, J.E., Weinstein, J.N.: Modeling analysis of the global and microscopic distribution of immunoglobulin G, $F(ab')_2$, and Fab in tumors. Cancer Res., **49**, 5656–63 (1989).

29. Hirst, D.G., Denekamp, J.: Tumour cell proliferation in relation to the vasculature. Cell Tissue Kinet., **12**, 31–42 (1979).

30. Hlatky, L.R., Hahnfeldt, P., Sachs, R.K.: Influence of time-dependent stochastic heterogeneity on the radiation response of a cell population. Math. Biosci., **122**, 201–20 (1994).

31. Jain, R.K.: Normalization of tumor vasculature: an emerging concept in antiangiogenic therapy. Science, **307**, 58–62 (2005).

32. Krogh, A.: The number and distribution of capillaries in muscles with calculations of the oxygen pressure head necessary to supply the tissue. J. Physiol., **52**, 409–15 (1919).

33. Moore, J.V., Hasleton, P.S., Buckley, C.H.: Tumour cords in 52 human bronchial and cervical squamous cell carcinomas: inferences for their cellular kinetics and radiobiology. Br. J. Cancer, **51**, 407–13 (1985).

34. Mueller-Klieser, W.: Multicellular spheroids: A review on cellular aggregates in cancer research. J. Cancer Res. Clin. Oncol., **113**, 101–22 (1987).

35. Smallbone, K., Gavaghan, D.J., Gatenby, R.A., Maini, P.K.: The role of acidity in solid tumour growth and invasion. J. Theor. Biol., **235**, 476–84 (2005).

36. Tannock, I.F.: The relation between cell proliferation and the vascular system in a transplanted mouse mammary tumour. Br. J. Cancer, **22**, 258–73 (1968).

37. Thames, H.D.: An 'incomplete-repair' model for survival after fractionated and continuous irradiations. Int. J. Radiat. Biol., **47**, 319–39 (1985).

38. Venkatasubramanian, R., Henson, M.A., Forbes, N.S.: Incorporating energy metabolism into a growth model of multicellular tumor spheroids. J. Theor. Biol., **242**, 440–53 (2006).

39. Webb, G.F.: The steady state of a tumor cord cell population. J. Evolut. Equat., **2**, 425–38 (2002).

40. Wein, L.M., Wu, J.T., Kirn, D.H.: Validation and analysis of a mathematical model of a replication-competent oncolytic virus for cancer treatment: implications for virus design and delivery. Cancer Res., **63**, 1317–24 (2003).

41. Wouters, B.G., Brown, J.M.: Cells at intermediate oxygen levels can be more important than the "hypoxic fraction" in determining tumor response to fractionated radiotherapy. Radiat. Res., **147**, 541–50 (1997).

8

Modeling Diffusely Invading Brain Tumors: An Individualized Approach to Quantifying Glioma Evolution and Response to Therapy

Russell Rockne, Ellsworth C. Alvord Jr., Mindy Szeto, Stanley Gu, Gargi Chakraborty, Kristin R. Swanson

Department of Pathology, University of Washington, 1959 NE Pacific St., Box 357470, Seattle, WA 98195, USA
rockne@u.washington.edu, swanson@amath.washington.edu

8.1 Introduction

Gliomas are highly aggressive primary brain tumors that extensively invade the surrounding normal tissue prior to the onset of symptoms. They are classified from low to high grade (I–IV) malignancy depending on specific histological characteristics [24]. High-grade gliomas (most commonly glioblastoma multiforme, WHO grade IV) are distinguished by necrosis and are the most common type of gliomas found in adults, as well as the most rapidly growing and the most invasive. Patients with glioblastomas (GBM) have a 100% fatality rate and a median survival time of 10–12 months after diagnosis and treatment, with very few patients surviving beyond three years [2]. This combination of high degree of invasiveness and the inability of current medical imaging technology to capture the full extent of invasion creates an ideal situation for the development of a mathematical model that can shed light on the extent of invasion and the possibility of improving treatments.

The present mathematical model characterizes glioma growth and invasion in terms of only two dominant parameters: net rates of diffusion/motility (D) and proliferation (ρ) [36]. Using data collected from as few as two pre-treatment observations on standard clinical magnetic resonance imaging (MRI) scanners, these parameters can be computed for individual patients *in vivo* and in real time [21], [36], [37], [44]. Full 3-dimensional simulations can then be performed to provide a metric for the extent of significant invasion beyond the clinically imageable tumor boundary. The model specifically describes the behavior of untreated tumor growth and has been extended to include surgical resections of various extents, chemotherapeutic drug delivery [42], and simulation and quantification of the response to external radiation therapy [45] such that individuals can serve as their own controls against variations in treatment schedule and protocol (reviewed in [21]). These math-

N. Bellomo et al. (eds.), *Selected Topics in Cancer Modeling*,
DOI: 10.1007/978-0-8176-4713-1_8, © Springer Science+Business Media, LLC 2008

ematical models offer a unique and individualized approach to quantifying—
and even predicting—tumor evolution and response to therapy utilizing parameters obtained only from current routine medical imaging techniques [9],
[20].

8.2 Growth Dynamics of Gliomas *in Vivo*

As early as the mid-1900s, experimental and human studies demonstrated
that cancer cells divide at a relatively constant rate, though this rate can vary
greatly depending on the type of cancer. One of the first studies, performed by
Collins et al. [12] on X-ray visualizations of metastases in the lungs, established
a constant volume-doubling growth rate that is in accordance with a simple
exponential law. Their conclusion was the spark for the proposal of many
now classical theoretical models for cancer cell proliferation, with the growth
rate taken to be exponential, gompertzian, or logistic without regard to the
spatial distribution of tumor cells within the patient, as extensively reviewed
by Araujo and McElwain [5].

None of these was able to properly describe the characteristically dynamic
invasiveness of glioma growth. In the early 1990s, Murray [29] took advantage
of the fact that gliomas rarely metastasize outside of the brain [1] to simplify
the classical definition of cancer as cells proliferating and invading locally
(with the ability to metastasize distantly eliminated since gliomas practically
never metastasize) to produce a conservation-diffusion equation, written in
word form as

$$\begin{matrix} \text{rate of change} \\ \text{in glioma cell density} \end{matrix} = \begin{matrix} \text{net diffusion} \\ \text{of glioma cells} \end{matrix} + \begin{matrix} \text{net proliferation} \\ \text{of glioma cells} \end{matrix} .$$

By assuming that the diffusion of glioma cells is gradient driven according to
Fick's law, Murray re-stated the equation mathematically as follows:

$$\frac{\partial c}{\partial t} = \nabla \cdot (D \nabla c) + \rho c. \tag{8.1}$$

Here $c = c(\boldsymbol{x}, t)$ denotes the tumor concentration at time t and spatial location
$\boldsymbol{x}$, D is the diffusion coefficient representing the net motility of tumor cells in
units $\text{cm}^2 \text{day}^{-1}$, and ρ is the net proliferation rate in units day^{-1}. Boundary
conditions are imposed to prevent cells from leaving the finite space domain,
with a point-source initial condition of concentration $c_0 = c(\boldsymbol{x}, 0)$.

8.2.1 The CT Era

Analysis by Tracqui et al. [46] of computerized tomographic (CT) scans monitoring the growth of a recurrent malignant astrocytoma gave rise to the first
approximations of model parameters D and ρ ($D = 0.0013 \text{ cm}^2 \text{day}^{-1}$, $\rho =$

0.012/day) [46]. Woodward et al. [50] speculated that these values may be about average for all high-grade gliomas and about 10 times that of low-grade gliomas.

Initial investigation of the model assumed two-dimensional tumor growth in homogeneous tissue bounded by the ventricles and skull and relied on data derived from CT observations. Simulated tumors used crude estimates of 1.5 cm and 3 cm tumor radii at diagnosis and death, respectively, derived from the small amount of data available at the time [13]. Woodward et al. [50] included resection in the simulations by setting the tumor concentration to zero within the resection bed. These preliminary results showed good agreement with published data on duration of survival following gross total resection or biopsy. The model predicted the observed difference of only 7 weeks even though 115 patients were not sufficient to provide statistical significance in the clinical study.

8.2.2 The MRI Era

Despite the relative inexpense and wide availability of CT, magnetic resonance imaging (MRI) rapidly became the gold standard for imaging brain tumors in the 1980s. With the improved resolution and anatomical accuracy provided by MRI in mind, Swanson [36] extended the model to 3-dimensional heterogeneous brain tissue with grey and white matter anatomically accurate to 1 mm^3, taking advantage of the BrainWeb anatomical atlas [10], [11], [36].

MR scans utilized in the present model derive from three sequences: T1- or T2-weighted, and fluid-attenuated inversion recovery (FLAIR). T1-weighted MRIs show the overall structure of the brain, with abnormalities frequently visualized by a leaky blood-brain barrier (BBB) revealed as enhancement by intravenously injected gadolinium (T1Gd). In the normal brain, there is no penetration of the BBB, but in malignant tumors, where the BBB is broken due to the immature and malformed blood vessels in the tumor mass, gadolinium leaks into the surrounding tissue. Regions of contrast enhancement on T1Gd MRI reveal the bulk mass of the tumor but not the peripherally invading isolated tumor cells, which are at such low concentrations that the BBB, though permeable enough to allow water to pass into the tissue as edema, is not sufficiently permeable to allow penetration of gadolinium [9], [20].

T2-weighted (T2) and FLAIR modalities reveal increased water concentration or edema (extra-vascular interstitial fluid), which has been shown to also contain isolated tumor cells at low but significant concentrations [14], [23]. These regions do not enhance on T1Gd, but their visualization on T2-weighted and FLAIR MRI sequences allows us to assume tumor invasion at a much lower threshold than that of T1Gd, since the T1Gd abnormality is almost always encompassed by the T2 abnormality (Fig. 8.1).

Thus, with T1Gd and T2/FLAIR sequences, MRIs reveal several regions of interest: central necrosis, "edge of solid tumor," and some estimate of the peripheral extent of the invading tumor cells.

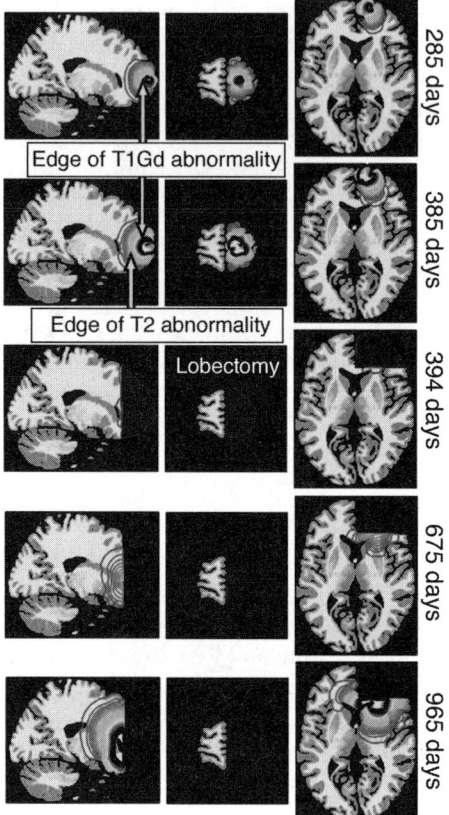

Fig. 8.1. Snapshots of sagittal, coronal, and axial virtual MRIs using the BrainWeb virtual brain from a full 3-dimensional simulation of the recurrence of a "favorable" glioblastoma (unusually small, 1 cm in diameter, and unusually far forward in frontal polar cortex) following extensive resection of most of the frontal lobe. Thick black contours represent the edge of the gadolinium-enhanced T1-weighted MRI (T1Gd) signal. Glioma cell concentration gradient decreases from dark to light.

8.2.3 The MRI-Detectable Edge as a Traveling Wave

An essential and characteristic property of the model includes Fisher's approximation, which states that for spherically symmetric growth, the expansion of the MRI-detectable edge of the tumor resembles a traveling wave (though an actual traveling wave only develops for the 1-dimensional case) and asymptotically approaches a constant velocity $v = 2\sqrt{D\rho}$, or $D = v^2/4\rho$ [16], [29], [38]. Two MRIs without intervening treatment are necessary for the measurement of v. This asymptotic approximation is valid only for large time, but this is well within the time frame of MRI-observable tumor growth.

The first evidence of the validity of Fisher's approximation as applied to gliomas came from Swanson *et al.* [37], [44], who observed one untreated high-grade glioma with constant radial velocity of 12 mm/year. Further confirmation came from the analysis of 27 low-grade gliomas (LGGs, WHO grade II) followed for up to 15 years with serial T2-weighted MRIs [28]: each maintained a constant velocity, the average having a radial velocity of approximately 2 mm/year. This six-fold difference between the low-grade and high-grade patient population was consistent with the prediction of a 10-fold difference by Woodward et al. [50].

A recent addition to this part of the story is due by Pallud et al. [30], who showed that the duration of survival correlates inversely with the velocity of radial expansion. We suspect that contrast enhancement develops somewhat earlier, indicating "progression" to a higher grade of glioma with its implication of a rather short survival thereafter. With this in mind, we have constructed a simple table in which size and velocity predict the duration of survival of individual patients [3] (Table 8.1).

Table 8.1. Model-predicted survival of a patient with an LGG of known size (mm diameter) and velocity (mm diameter/year).

Model-Predicted Survival Time (years)

Velocity	Size at Diagnosis			
	20	40	60	80
1.5	58	45	31	18
2.5	35	27	19	11
3.5	25	19	13	7.7
4.5	19	15	10	6
5.5	16	12	8.5	5
7.0	12.4	9.6	6.7	4
11.0	7.9	6	4.3	2.5

8.2.4 Individualization of Contrast-Enhancing Gliomas

For high-grade gliomas, which generally show contrast enhancement on T1Gd MRI, discovery by Swanson of a formula for the ratio D/ρ, calculable from a single pair of T1Gd and T2 MRI sequences, provided a second equation in the two unknowns, D and ρ, allowing explicit definition of these two parameters in individual patients [21], [37], [44].

Tumor volumes visualized by MRIs are computed using a semi-automated segmentation software developed by Swanson *et al.* The sum of the series of segmented 2-dimensional areas produces a gross tumor volume (GTV), which is then translated to a radius by assuming the volume to be spherical: $v = 4/3\pi r^3$. This supposition is consistent with the detectable edge of the tumor acting as a spherically symmetric traveling wave via Fisher's approximation [16]. Tumor volume is taken as the average of two measurements made by independent observers. Intra-observer variation in tumor segmentation with the semi-automated technique is equal to that of completely manual delineation at approximately 20% of volume, well within published and acceptable ranges [48], [49], translating to a 6–7% variation in radius and therefore a maximum of -6 to $+14\%$ variation in velocity. This methodology suffices to provide net radial velocity and a unique set of parameters (D,ρ) for individual patients. Fig. 8.2 illustrates this on a 3-cycle log-log graph. The shaded area corresponds to our experience with contrast-enhancing gliomas generally falling between 10 and 200 mm/yr in velocity and 2 and 20 mm^2 for D/ρ [42]. LGGs have velocities averaging 2 mm/yr [28], but ranging up to 20 mm/yr [30]; however, we cannot calculate both D and ρ for these noncontrast-enhancing cases.

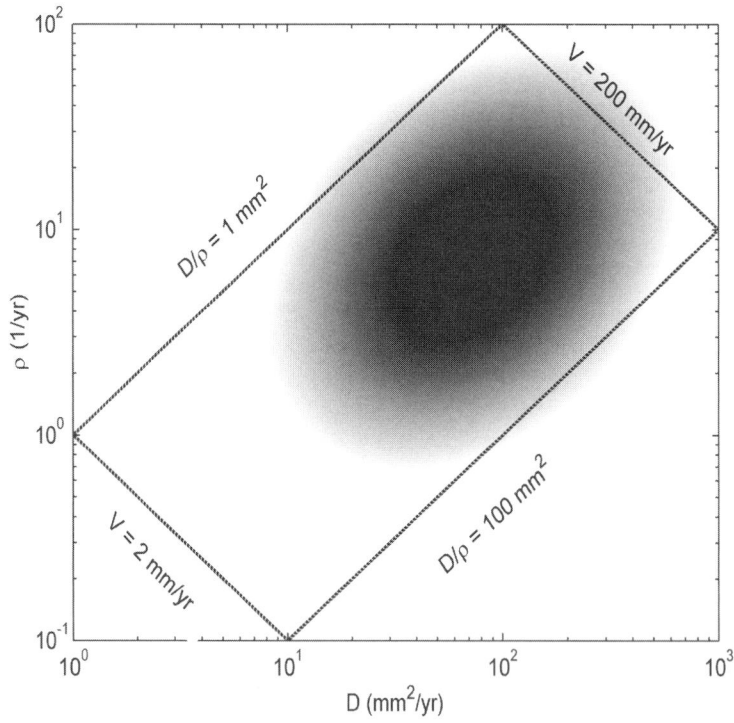

Fig. 8.2. This 3-cycle log-log graph of D vs. ρ has an overlay of velocity vs. D/ρ and encompasses the ranges of values seen in LGGs and HGGs.

8.3 Tissue Heterogeneity: Grey and White Matter

Gross and microscopic patterns of growth have suggested that glioma cells tend to migrate along white matter tracts in the brain and, indeed, *in vitro* experiments have shown that cells exhibit greater motility in white matter than in grey [18]. Swanson [36] reformulated the model in order to more accurately reflect the spatial limitation of cellular proliferation and inherent heterogeneity in the brain by introducing k, the carrying capacity of the tissue, and by allowing the diffusion coefficient D to depend on the tissue environment, changing D to $D(\boldsymbol{x})$:

$$\frac{\partial c}{\partial t} = \nabla \cdot (D(\boldsymbol{x})\nabla c) + \rho c \left(1 - \frac{c}{k}\right), \qquad (8.2)$$

where $D(\boldsymbol{x}) = D_g$ for $\boldsymbol{x}$ in grey matter and $D(\boldsymbol{x}) = D_w$ for $\boldsymbol{x}$ in white matter and k is taken to be approximately 10^8 cells/cm^3. Simulations of virtual tumor growth were achieved using the BrainWeb atlas [10] (Fig. 8.1). Initial studies assumed a ratio of $D_w/D_g = 5$, but a wide range is expected. We have extended this isotropic model of glioma cellular diffusion to also consider anisotropic migration by defining D as a tensor ($D = \mathsf{D}$) using diffusion tensor imaging (DTI) [22].

8.4 Modeling Glioma Response to Therapy

In clinical practice, an algorithmic approach to glioma treatment includes an MRI followed by surgical resection (and accompanying second MRI if the operation is under neuro-navigational guidance), external beam X-ray therapy (XRT) concurrent with and followed by chemotherapy, with MRIs conducted at various times during treatment as prescribed by the physician. Serial observations of gliomas prior to and during treatment afford an opportunity to quantitatively model response to therapy, and then to develop predictions as to the efficacy of treatments, which are arguably the most important goals of cancer modeling as a whole.

8.4.1 Surgical Resection

Practically all gliomas are treated with surgical resection of some extent. The diffuse extent of glioma invasion in the brain produces a difficult environment for complete surgical removal. Depending on the tumor's location in the brain, the extent of resection (EOR) can be classified into one of three categories by the operating surgeon supported by post-operative scans: biopsy (Bx), sub-total resection (STR), or gross total resection (GTR). Although intuition suggests that surgery of any extent should hinder disease progression and thus perhaps extend survival, the clinical evidence is at best ambiguous. In general,

Bx and STR show only a little more difference and, indeed, GTR shows little difference over the combination of Bx and STR. Of course, these groups of patients have been considered statistically homogeneous only on the basis of histologic similarity. Almost certainly the failure to find differences relates to the poor correlation between histologic appearances and the actual values of D and ρ. Perhaps the best study was published by Lacroix et al. [27] but there were no controls. By creating virtual controls matched for size, D and ρ, we have been able to show that part of the difference can be accounted for by operating on the best patients (i.e., those with the smallest amounts of tumor) and part by the GTR itself [32].

From a modeling viewpoint, resection can be approximated by setting the tumor concentration in the resection bed to zero and continuing the simulation (Fig. 8.1) [36].

8.4.2 Chemotherapy

First implemented in the early 1970s with the introduction of nitrosoureas, chemotherapeutic options appear to be the most promising treatments for high-grade gliomas if the drug can penetrate the normal BBB and reach the peripherally diffusing cells as well as the bulk tumor with its leaky BBB. However, published clinical trials exploring the role of chemotherapy highlight disappointing results, and a significant positive impact on survival time has not been observed [17]. Nevertheless, some form of chemotherapy is generally administered throughout the clinical course depending on the patient's ability to withstand the toxic side effects.

Swanson *et al.* demonstrated that the extent of glioma invasion may be unaffected by chemotherapy due to continued tumor cell motility, even though the total number of cells may be decreasing due to the treatment's cytotoxic nature [40], [39]. As invaded cells remain occult and under the threshold of MRI detection, diffuse tumor recurrence is practically certain upon conclusion of a chemotherapy cycle. This suggests that treatment response cannot be reliably measured by T1Gd images alone: expansion of T2 and restriction of T1Gd radii suggest that peripheral invasion is continuing even though the bulk tumor may be controlled.

8.4.3 Radiation Therapy

Radiation therapy is routinely used as a treatment for gliomas because of its precision, minimal invasiveness, and ability to circumvent the BBB. External beam radiation therapy (XRT) relies on linear energy transfer (LET) to produce arrest of growth and death of the tumor cells. Highly energized particles are emitted from a radioactive source that ionizes the atoms which constitute the DNA, causing single strand breaks (SSBs) and double strand breaks (DSBs). These DNA injuries make the cell unable to reproduce itself during the next mitotic phase since transcription is impossible.

Assessing response to XRT in gliomas has historically focused on visible changes in GTV as measured on MRI [7], [8]. With only a single pre-treatment MRI little can be said quantitatively. However, with two pre-treatment MRIs to measure D and ρ, and a third, post-XRT, we are able to model an analogous virtual glioma's response to XRT for comparisons with the actual response as seen by serial MRIs. Of course, MRIs do not necessarily perfectly track the response of gliomas to therapy—there are temporal delays as well as alternative biological mechanisms at play when interpreting imaging. Therefore, it is important to note that these model interpretations are restricted by the limited nature of the MRIs themselves in accurately characterizing the lesion. Alternatively, clinical imaging is used routinely to assess treatment effects on the basis that the imaging is providing some, albeit limited, insight.

Using the classic linear-quadratic model for radiation efficacy [6], [19], [33], and *in vivo* radiation dose distributions as reference, we extended the fundamental glioma model to include the spatio-temporal effects of radiation therapy [31], [45]. This is approached via a death term as follows:

$$
\underbrace{\frac{\partial c}{\partial t}}_{\substack{\text{rate of change} \\ \text{of glioma cell} \\ \text{concentration}}} = \underbrace{\nabla \cdot (D(\boldsymbol{x})\nabla c)}_{\substack{\text{net dispersal} \\ \text{of glioma cells}}} + \underbrace{\rho c \left(1 - \frac{c}{k}\right)}_{\substack{\text{net proliferation} \\ \text{of glioma cells}}} - \underbrace{R(\alpha, d(\boldsymbol{x}, t))c}_{\substack{\text{loss due} \\ \text{to therapy}}}. \quad (8.3)
$$

Here, the fractionated dose is defined in both space and time $d = d(\boldsymbol{x}, t)$ by a 3-dimensional dose mapping system, similar to those used by radiation oncologists.

The form of the loss term utilizes the linear-quadratic model for radiation efficacy which relates the cell survival probability S with the biologically effective dose (BED) as follows:

$$
S\left(\alpha, d(\boldsymbol{x}, t)\right) = e^{-\alpha BED}, BED = \alpha n \left(d + \frac{d^2}{\alpha/\beta}\right), \quad (8.4)
$$

where d is the per-fraction dose and n the number of fractions [15], [19], [33], [35], [43]. Typically, α is considered a constant proportional to the number of repairable SSBs and β with DSBs. The ratio α/β represents tissue response, with $\alpha/\beta = 3Gy$ for normal, early responding tissue and $\alpha/\beta = 10Gy$ for later responding, cancerous tissue [19]. With the ratio α/β fixed at $10Gy$, and n and d determined by the treatment schedule, the strong dependence on the single parameter $\alpha(/Gy)$ is made clear. Large α implies low resistance (i.e., high sensitivity) to therapy, whereas small α implies high resistance (i.e., low sensitivity) as seen in Fig. 8.3. We therefore regard α as our primary radiation sensitivity parameter, and our loss term $R(\alpha, d(\boldsymbol{x}, t))$ takes the form

$$
R(\alpha, d(\boldsymbol{x}, t)) = \begin{cases} 0, & \text{for } t \notin \text{therapy} \\ 1 - S(\alpha, d(\boldsymbol{x}, t)), & \text{for } t \in \text{therapy}. \end{cases} \quad (8.5)
$$

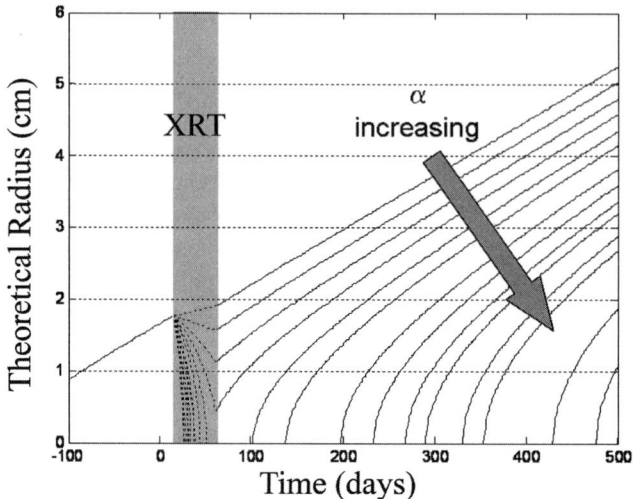

Fig. 8.3. Simulations of a virtual glioma with a specific velocity determined by the first two MRIs pre-treatment and with increasing degrees of radiosensitivity (α) following a standard dose of XRT.

Although our model allows for any imaginable treatment schedule or dose distribution, the current standard radiation treatment protocol at the University of Washington Medical Center is as follows: 7 weeks of treatment, using a 5 days on, 2 days off schedule (to allow for weekends) delivering 1.8Gy to the T2 region plus a 2.5 cm margin for 28 days, followed by 1.8Gy to the T1Gd region plus a 2 cm margin for the remaining 6 days, yielding 61.2Gy total maximum dose to the tumor bed.

Based on volumetric measurements to calculate tumor radii, a unique value for the radiation sensitivity parameter α is defined by the third MRI (i.e., the post-XRT/MRI). Because $S(\alpha, d(\boldsymbol{x}, t))$ is a one-to-one function in α, we are assured a unique correspondence between α and response. A study of 13 glioblastoma multiforme patients [43] reveals a strong correlation between ρ and α, confirming intuition that faster-growing tumors respond more to treatment since they will be more often in the mitotic phase of the cell cycle which is more susceptible to radiation damage. This result may also provide a metric for predicting the response (expected changes in imaging) for each patient to radiotherapy. We suspect that each tumor has an inherent radiosensitivity that can not only be measured after treatment but also be predicted before treatment.

8.5 Improvements in Medical Imaging and Tumor Evolution

While MRI (T1Gd and T2) allows anatomical analysis of gliomas, other imaging modalities can shed light on the functional and evolutionary dynamics of gliomas [4], [25], [26], [34], [47]. Functional imaging, such as positron emission tomography (PET), allows visualization of radio-labeled tracers to monitor biochemical activity. Usually, more activity is associated with tumor cells. A quite different biochemical mechanism of interest with regard to tumor morphology is hypoxia, a state of low oxygenation, which constitutes a harsh tumor micro-environment and has been implicated in inducing formation of blood vessels and resistance to therapy. 18F-Fluoromisonidazole (FMISO) labeled PET allows visualization of hypoxia. FMISO, delivered intravenously, crosses the BBB and migrates into cells. However, once inside a hypoxic cell, this tracer does not leave during the time scale of the imaging procedure, providing an easily viewable hyper-intensity associated with hypoxic regions. Interestingly, we have found a substantial correlation between the relative hypoxia of a glioma and the aggressiveness of the lesion defined by D and ρ [43]. Thus, the mathematical model (D, ρ) provides a language to translate between clinical anatomical imaging (MRI) and a functional characteristic of the tumor, hypoxia, visualized on FMISO-PET.

To further elucidate the connection between imaging with FMISO-PET and T1Gd and T2 MRI, we have extended the mathematical modeling framework to consider the biological connection between angiogenesis and hypoxia. As tumor cells proliferate, crowding of the cells occurs and the native vasculature cannot supply enough nutrients. The hypoxic cells secrete tumor angiogenic factors (TAFs) that stimulate angiogenesis, the formation of new blood vessels, in the surrounding region to increase blood flow to the area. If tumor cell proliferation is not too high, this angiogenesis would return hypoxic regions to their original normoxic state. However, in the case of high-grade gliomas, the rate of tumor growth (proliferation) exceeds that of nutrient resupply by angiogenesis, resulting in irreversible necrosis of some regions and the further increase of hypoxic regions. This chain of events is known as the angiogenic cascade and is the basis for an extension to our model. Interestingly, we have found that simulations of this model accurately recreate the key characteristics of all grades of gliomas by simply varying the net rates of invasion (D) and proliferation (ρ) [21].

8.6 Conclusion

A new bio-mathematical formulation of the behavior of gliomas, based only on the classical definition of cancer as cells proliferating and invading locally (with the capacity to metastasize distantly being an unnecessary mathematical complication since gliomas practically never metastasize), begins with two unmeasurable concepts, net rates of proliferation (ρ) and diffusion (D). These can be calculated, however, from measurements on routinely available clinical MRIs and lead to the ability to monitor the effects of any treatments and to predict the effects of surgical resections of any extent and the degree of sensitivity to X-ray irradiation. Although the behavior of the most malignant and most common glioma, glioblastoma, has been emphasized, the model is applicable to any histologic type and grade of glioma. For those gliomas that do not show contrast enhancement, serial MRIs define at least the velocity of radial expansion (which is approximately linear with time). Together with the size at any particular time the velocity predicts the time to "progression" to high grade (with the development of contrast enhancement) and the duration of survival. For those gliomas that show contrast enhancement, the degree of invisible invasiveness can also be estimated, providing additional information which should be useful in planning surgical, radiological, and chemical therapies. Ultimately, the individual patient parameters D and ρ also provide unique insight into the biochemistry of each tumor (e.g., hypoxia), further suggesting the clinical applications of this spatially complex Fisher's model for growth and invasion of gliomas *in vivo*.

Acknowledgments

KRS gratefully acknowledges the support of the following foundations and institutions: the James S. McDonnell Foundation, the Charles A. Dana Foundation, NIH - NCI grants P01-CA42405, P30-CA15704, S10-RR17229, the University of Washington Academic Pathology Fund, the Shaw Professorship, and the Mary Gates Endowment.

References

1. Alvord E.C. Jr.: Why do gliomas not metastasize. Arch. Neurol., **33**, 73–75 (1976)
2. Alvord E.C. Jr., Shaw C.M.: Neoplasms affecting the nervous system in the elderly. In: Duckett S (ed), The Pathology of the Aging Human Nervous System. Lea & Febiger, Philadelphia (1991)
3. Alvord E.C. Jr., Swanson K.R.: Using mathematical modeling to predict survival of low-grade gliomas. Ann. Neurol., **61**, 496; author reply 496–497 (2007)
4. Anderson H., Price P.: What does positron emission tomography offer oncology? Euro. J. Cancer., **26**, 2028–2035 (2000)
5. Araujo R.P., McElwain D.L.: A history of the study of solid tumour growth: the contribution of mathematical modelling. Bull. Math. Biol., **66**, 1039–1091 (2004)
6. B. Jones R.G.D.: Cell loss factors and the linear-quadratic model. Rad. Onc., **37**, 136–139 (1995)

7. Barker F.G. II, Prados M.D., Chang S.M., et al.: Radiation response and survival time in patients with glioblastoma multiforme. J. Neurosurg., **84**, 442–448 (1996)

8. Bloor R., Templeton A.W., Quick R.S.: Radiation therapy in the treatment of intracranial tumors. Am J. Roentgenol. Radium Ther. Nucl. Med., **87**, 463–472 (1962)

9. Brown M.A., Semelka R.C.: MRI: Basic Principles and Applications ed. 2. Wiley-Liss Inc., New York (1999)

10. Cocosco C.A., Kollokian V., et al.: Brainweb: online interface to a 3D simulated brain database. Neuroimage., **5**, 425 (1997)

11. Collins D.L., Zijdenbos A.P., Kollokian V., et al.: Design and construction of a realistic digital brain phantom. IEEE T. Med. Imaging., **17**, 463–468 (1998)

12. Collins V.P., Loeffler R.K., Tivey H.: Observations on growth rates of human tumors. Am. J. Roentgenol. Radium. Ther. Nucl. Med., **76**, 988–1000 (1956)

13. Concannon J.P., Kramer S., Berry R.: The extent of intracranial gliomata at autopsy and its relationship to techniques used in radiation therapy of brain tumors. Am. J. Roentgenol. Radium. Ther. Nucl. Med., **84**, 99–107 (1960)

14. Dalrymple S.J., Parisi J.E., Roche P.C., et al.: Changes in proliferating cell nuclear antigen expression in glioblastoma multiforme cells along a stereotactic biopsy trajectory. Neurosurg., **35**, 1036–1044; discussion 1044–1045 (1994)

15. Enderling H., Anderson A.R., Chaplain M.A., et al.: Mathematical modelling of radiotherapy strategies for early breast cancer. J. Theor. Biol., **241**, 158–171 (2006)

16. Fisher R.A.: The wave of advance of advantageous genes. Ann. Eugenics., Vol. 7 (1937)

17. Galanis E., Buckner J.: Chemotherapy for high-grade gliomas. Brit. J. Cancer, **82**, 1371–1380 (2000)

18. Giese A., Westphal M.: Glioma invasion in the central nervous system. Neurosurg., **39**, 235–250; discussion 250-252 (1996)

19. Hall E.: Radiobiology for the Radiologist, ed. 4. J.B. Lippincott Company, Philadelphia (1994)

20. Hammoud M.A., Sawaya R., Shi W., et al.: Prognostic significance of preoperative MRI scans in glioblastoma multiforme. J. Neuroonc., **27**, 65–73 (1996)

21. Harpold H., Alvord E.C. Jr., Swanson K.R.: The evolution of mathematical modeling of glioma proliferation and invasion. J. Neuropathol. Exp. Neurol., **66**, 1–9 (2007)

22. Jbabdi S., Mandonnet E., Duffau H., et al.: Simulation of anisotropic growth of low-grade gliomas using diffusion tensor imaging. Magn. Reson. Med., **54**, 616–624 (2005)

23. Kelly P.J.: Computed tomography and histologic limits in glial neoplasms: tumor types and selection for volumetric resection. Surg. Neurol., **39**, 458–465 (1993)

24. Kleihues P., Louis D.N., Scheithauer B.W., et al.: The WHO classification of tumors of the nervous system. J. Neuropathol. Exp. Neurol., **61**, 215–225; discussion 226-229 (2002)

25. Koh W.J., Griffin T.W., Rasey J.S., et al.: Positron emission tomography. A new tool for characterization of malignant disease and selection of therapy. Acta. Oncol., **33**, 323–327 (1994)

26. Koh W.J., Rasey J.S., Evans M.L., et al.: Imaging of hypoxia in human tumors with [F-18]fluoromisonidazole. Int. J. Rad. Oncol. Biol. Phys., **22**, 199–212 (1992)

27. Lacroix M., Abi-Said D., Fourney D.R., et al.: A multivariate analysis of 416 patients with glioblastoma multiforme: prognosis, extent of resection, and survival. J. Neurosurg., **95**, 190–198 (2001)

28. Mandonnet E., Delattre J.Y., Tanguy M.L., et al.: Continuous growth of mean tumor diameter in a subset of grade II gliomas. Ann. Neurol., **53**, 524–528 (2003)

29. Murray J.D.: Mathematical Biology II. Spatial Models and Biological Applications. ed. 3. Vol. 2. Springer-Verlag, New York (2003)

30. Pallud J., Mandonnet E., Duffau H., et al.: Prognostic value of initial magnetic resonance imaging growth rates for World Health Organization grade II gliomas. Ann. Neurol., **60**, 380–383 (2006)

31. Rockne R., Alvord E.C. Jr., Rockhill J.K.: A mathematical model for brain tumor response to radiation therapy, J. Math. Biol. (2008), *in press*

32. Swanson K.R., Rostomily R.C., Alvord E.C. Jr.: A mathematical modeling tool for predicting survival of individual patients following resection of glioblastoma. Brit. J. Cancer, **98**, 113–119 (2008)

33. Sachs R.K., Hlatky L.R., Hahnfeldt P.: Simple ODE models of tumor growth and anti-angiogenic or radiation treatment. Math. Comp. Mod., **33**, 1297–1305 (2001)

34. Spence A.M., Mankoff D.A., Muzi M.: Positron emission tomography imaging of brain tumors. Neuroimag. Clin. N. Am., **13**, 717–739 (2003)

35. Stamatakos G.S., Antipas V.P., Uzunoglu N.K., et al.: A four-dimensional computer simulation model of the in vivo response to radiotherapy of glioblastoma multiforme: studies on the effect of clonogenic cell density. Brit. J. Rad., **79**, 389–400 (2006)

36. Swanson K.R.: Mathematical modeling of the growth and control of tumors. PhD Thesis, University of Washington, Seattle, Washington (1999)

37. Swanson K.R., Alvord E.C. Jr. (eds): A biomathematical and pathological analysis of an untreated glioblastoma. NeuroPath. Annual Meeting. Helsinki, Finland. (2002)

38. Swanson K.R., Alvord E.C. Jr.: Serial imaging observations and postmortem examination of an untreated glioblastoma: A traveling wave of glioma growth and invasion. Neuro-Oncol., **4**, 340 (2002)

39. Swanson K.R., Alvord E.C. Jr., Murray J.: Virtual brain tumours (gliomas) enhance the reality of medical imaging and highlight inadequacies of current therapy. Brit. J. Cancer., **86**, 14–18 (2002)

40. Swanson K.R., Alvord E.C. Jr., Murray J.: Dynamics of a model for brain tumors reveals a small window for therapeutic intervention. Disc. Con. Dyn. Sys.-Series. B., **4**, 289–295 (2004)

41. Swanson K.R., Alvord E.C. Jr., Murray J.D.: A quantitative model for differential motility of gliomas in grey and white matter. Cell. Prolif., **33**, 317–329 (2000)

42. Swanson K.R., Alvord E.C. Jr., Murray J.D.: Quantifying efficacy of chemotherapy of brain tumors with homogeneous and heterogeneous drug delivery. Acta. Biotheoretica, **50**, 223–237 (2002)

43. Swanson K.R., Chakraborty G., Rockne R., et al.: A mathematical model for glioma growth and invasion links biological aggressiveness assessed by MRI with hypxoia assessed by FMISO-PET. 53rd Annual Meeting of the Soc. Nuc. Med., 48–115 (2007)

44. Swanson K.R., Murray J.D., Alvord E.C. Jr.: Combining radiological observations with a three-dimensional model to predict behavior of brain tumors in real patients. SIAM Life Sci. Imag. Sci. Conference. Boston, MA. (2002)
45. Swanson K.R., Rockne R., Rockhill J.K., et al.: Mathematical modeling of radiotherapy in individual glioma patients: quantifying and predicting response to radiation therapy. AACR Annual Meeting. Los Angeles, CA. (2007)
46. Tracqui P., Cruywagen G.C., Woodward D.E., et al.: A mathematical model of glioma growth: the effect of chemotherapy on spatio-temporal growth. Cell. Prolif., **28**, 17–31 (1995)
47. Valk P.E., Mathis C.A., Prados M.D., et al.: Hypoxia in human gliomas: demonstration by PET with fluorine-18-fluoromisonidazole. J. Nucl. Med., **33**, 2133–2137 (1992)
48. Vos M.J., Uitdehaag B.M.J., Barkhof F., et al.: Interobserver variability in the radiological assessment of response to chemotherapy in glioma. Neurology **60**, 826–830 (2003)
49. Weltens C., Menten J., Feron M., et al.: Interobserver variations in gross tumor volume delineation of brain tumors on computed tomography and impact of magnetic resonance imaging. Radiother Oncol., **60**, 49–59 (2001)
50. Woodward D.E., Cook J., Tracqui P., et al.: A mathematical model of glioma growth: the effect of extent of surgical resection. Cell. Prolif., **29**, 269–288 (1996)

9

Multiphase Models of Tumour Growth

Sergey Astanin and Luigi Preziosi

Dipartimento di Matematica, Politecnico di Torino,
Corso Duca degli Abruzzi 24, 10129 Torino, Italy
{sergey.astanin, luigi.preziosi}@polito.it

9.1 Introduction

Mixture theory has been applied to describe the mechanics of biological tissues since the 1960s. Most of the work was focused on the behaviour of articular cartilages [HHLM89, KLM90, LHM90, MHL84, MKLA80, ML79, MRS90], but applications can be found to many soft tissues, e.g., brain [Nic85, SCZM06], heart mechanics [SS86, TIZB84, YTC94], subcutaneous layer [OVCG87], and flow through arteries [Jay83, Ken79, KT87].

In the last few years mixture theory has also been applied with success to tumour growth. Examples of applications can be found in [BBL02, BBL03, BKMP03, BP04, CGP06, FBK$^+$03, FBM$^+$03, FK03] while [AP02, AM05, GP07] are review papers on this approach and on the mechanical aspects related to tumour growth. Here, we shall deduce a general multiphase modelling framework for a few essential constituents (cells, extracellular matrix, and extracellular liquid with the solutes dissolved in it). We shall also show how to take into account several subpopulations of the cells, and several components of the extracellular matrix (ECM).

There are three basic hypotheses that allow us to obtain a manageable model even when more constituents are involved. The first hypothesis is an assumption that the components of the ECM form such an intricate network that they all move together so that the same deformation and velocity describe their evolution. The second one consists in assuming that the pressure gradient and the interaction forces involving the liquid are much smaller than the others, e.g., the adhesion force between cells and ECM. The third one consists in assuming that cells mechanically respond to the compression coming from the surrounding cells in the same way independently of the cell type.

All the steps of the modelling procedure are explained in detail, special attention being paid to the meaning of all the different terms involved in the model. Some examples are given to clarify how to model them. Specifically, in Section 9.2 we deal with mass balance equations, and in Section 9.3 with force balance equations. Section 9.4 is in large part devoted to the description of

N. Bellomo et al. (eds.), *Selected Topics in Cancer Modeling*,
DOI: 10.1007/978-0-8176-4713-1_9, © Springer Science+Business Media, LLC 2008

the interaction between the cells and the ECM. In Section 9.5 we address the issue of how to deduce a proper constitutive model for the stress, though the reader is referred to more specific literature for further details [AP02, AP08, AM05, GP07]. Finally, in the last sections, the general model is specialized to describe tumour growth in an immutable ECM (rigid, non-remodelling), including the mechanical interaction with the host tissue, the growth in a rigid remodelling ECM with the aim of showing the formation of fibrosis, and the growth of a vascularized tumour, with a particular focus on how to relate cell metabolism to growth terms.

9.2 Mass Balance

Soft tissues are mainly made of cells and ECM. The porous material that this ensemble forms is wet by an extracellular liquid full of chemicals: nutrients, growth factors, chemotactic factors, and so on (see Fig. 9.1a).

Of course, the typical size of cells and ECM composed of aggregated proteins is much bigger than that of dissolved proteins. So, one can assume that the space occupied by the latter is negligible and one can treat them as part of the extracellular liquid.

For all the constituents of the mixture we define their volume ratios as follows. Given a point in the mixture consider a sequence of spheres with the centres at the point (Fig. 9.1b). Measuring the ratio of the volume of a given constituent inside the sphere to the volume of the sphere one may observe the dependency shown in Fig. 9.1c. For small sample volumes the ratio is likely to oscillate due to microscopic inhomogeneity. Macroscopic inhomogeneities may affect the ratio for large sample volumes. However, for sample volumes in between, at scales larger than the cell size and smaller than typical tissue scale, it is nearly constant and allows us to define a quantity called volume ratio of the constituent.

Let us denote by $\phi \in [0, 1]$ and $m \in [0, 1]$ the volume ratios occupied by cells and by the ECM respectively. The mixture is *saturated* if the rest of the space is filled by extracellular liquid $\ell \in [0, 1]$, i.e.,

$$\phi + m + \ell = 1 \,. \tag{9.1}$$

In some models the upper constraint on the volume ratio is replaced by a constant value $\overline{\phi} < 1$, possibly space dependent, allowing for some fixed portion of space to be occupied by other constituents not considered in the mixture, e.g., vessels or a general stroma. In this case the saturation constraint is replaced by

$$\phi + m + \ell = \overline{\phi} \,, \tag{9.2}$$

with all volume ratios in $[0, \overline{\phi}]$.

If $\overline{\phi}$ is space independent, it is possible to rescale the variables as $\tilde{\phi} := \phi/\overline{\phi}$, $\tilde{m} := m/\overline{m}$, $\tilde{l} := l/\overline{l}$ to have $\tilde{\phi} + \tilde{m} + \tilde{l} = 1$.

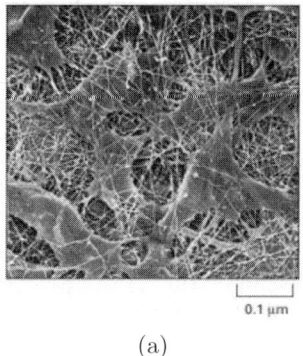

(a)

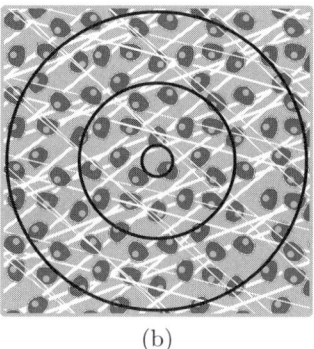

(b)

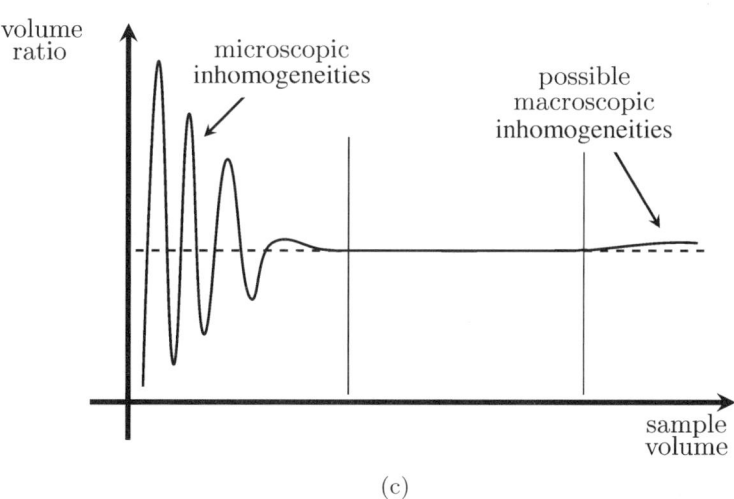

(c)

Fig. 9.1. (a) Tissue with fibroblasts and ECM. Three sample volumes are shown as black circles in (b), ECM in white, cells in darker tint, the rest is extracellular liquid. (c) Volume ratio of the constituent as a function of sample volume size.

In order to define the mass balance equations for the different constituents consider a general volume $\mathcal{V}$ fixed in space with boundary $\partial\mathcal{V}$. To be specific we shall focus on the cellular constituent of the tissue. If ρ is the density within the cells, the mass of the constituent in $\mathcal{V}$

$$\int_{\mathcal{V}} \rho\phi \, dV$$

can change due to:

1. Flux caused by the motion of the constituent through the boundary $\partial\mathcal{V}$

$$-\int_{\partial\mathcal{V}} \rho\phi\mathbf{v}_\phi \cdot \mathbf{n} \, d\Sigma \,,$$

   where $\mathbf{v}_\phi$ is the cell velocity and $\mathbf{n}$ is an external normal to the boundary $\partial\mathcal{V}$;

2. Growth or death of cells

$$\int_{\mathcal{V}} \rho\Gamma_\phi \, dV \,,$$

   where Γ_ϕ is the exchange rate or growth/death rate for the cellular mass.

One then has

$$\frac{d}{dt}\int_{\mathcal{V}} \rho\phi \, dV = -\int_{\partial\mathcal{V}} \rho\phi\mathbf{v}_\phi \cdot \mathbf{n} \, d\Sigma + \int_{\mathcal{V}} \rho\Gamma_\phi \, dV \,.$$

Using Gauss's theorem, one can write

$$\int_{\mathcal{V}} \left[\frac{\partial}{\partial t}(\rho\phi) + \nabla \cdot (\rho\phi\mathbf{v}_\phi) - \rho\Gamma_\phi \right] dV = 0 \,,$$

and, if the integrands are smooth, because of the arbitrariness of the volume of integration $\mathcal{V}$,

$$\frac{\partial}{\partial t}(\rho\phi) + \nabla \cdot (\rho\phi\mathbf{v}_\phi) = \rho\Gamma_\phi \,, \tag{9.3}$$

where ρ can be taken constant and equal to the density of water.

Generalizing the procedure for all the variables mentioned above one can write the mass balance equations

$$\frac{\partial\phi}{\partial t} + \nabla \cdot (\phi\mathbf{v}_\phi) = \Gamma_\phi \,,$$

$$\frac{\partial m}{\partial t} + \nabla \cdot (m\mathbf{v}_m) = \Gamma_m \,, \tag{9.4}$$

$$\frac{\partial\ell}{\partial t} + \nabla \cdot (\ell\mathbf{v}_\ell) = \Gamma_\ell \,.$$

If the mixture is *closed* so that mass exchange occurs only between the constituents taken into consideration, then

$$\Gamma_\phi + \Gamma_m + \Gamma_\ell = 0 \,, \tag{9.5}$$

where for the sake of simplicity we assumed that all constituents of the tissue have equal density ρ, the density of the extracellular liquid.

In other cases, when external mass sources/sinks are introduced to describe outflow/inflow processes related, for example, to a homogenized vascular or lymphatic structure, the condition (9.5) might be dropped. This approach is, for instance, used in [FBK$^+$03, FBM$^+$03, FK03]. However, also in this case one needs to ensure that the solution never violates the positivity of the volume ratios and the geometrical constraint (9.1) or (9.2) during the evolution.

According to the details needed to describe the phenomenon of interest, it may be necessary to distinguish different cell populations, e.g., tumour cells, endothelial cells, epithelial cells, fibroblasts, macrophages, and lymphocytes, or to distinguish different clones within the same population characterized by relevant differences in their behaviour, or to distinguish the cells according to their phase in the cell cycle, e.g., G_0, G_1, G_2.

If this is the case, the first equation in (9.4) must be split in I equations, one for each of the I subpopulations:

$$\frac{\partial \phi_i}{\partial t} + \nabla \cdot (\phi_i \mathbf{v}_{\phi_i}) = \Gamma_{\phi_i} \,, \qquad i = 1, \dots, I \,, \tag{9.6}$$

where ϕ_i is the volume ratio of the subpopulation i, $\mathbf{v}_i$ is its velocity, and Γ_{ϕ_i} is its mass exchange rate. Of course,

$$\sum_{i=1}^{I} \phi_i = \phi \,, \qquad \sum_{i=1}^{I} \phi_i \mathbf{v}_{\phi_i} = \phi \mathbf{v}_\phi \,, \qquad \sum_{i=1}^{I} \Gamma_{\phi_i} = \Gamma_\phi \,, \tag{9.7}$$

and therefore summing all (9.6) over i gives back the first equation in (9.4).

Similarly, because of the different mechanical behaviour and chemical properties, it might be necessary to distinguish the different components of the ECM, e.g., collagen, elastin, fibronectin, vitronectin, and proteoglycans. One then has

$$\frac{\partial m_j}{\partial t} + \nabla \cdot (m_j \mathbf{v}_m) = \Gamma_{m_j} \,, \qquad j = 1, \dots, J \,, \tag{9.8}$$

where m_j is the volume ratio of the jth component and Γ_{m_j} is its remodelling rate. We explicitly notice that in (9.8) the ECM velocity is taken to be the same for all ECM components, which means describing them as an intricate network of fibres that have to move all together. This is called a *constrained submixture assumption*. As before,

$$\sum_{j=1}^{J} m_j = m \,, \qquad \sum_{j=1}^{J} \Gamma_{m_j} = \Gamma_m \,, \tag{9.9}$$

and summing (9.8) over j gives the second equation in (9.4).

Other fundamental factors influencing tumour evolution are the various proteins and chemicals that govern the growth and the behaviour of the cells. One can treat them as solutes dispersed in the extracellular liquid, transported and diffusing with it. Their concentrations are the quantities of interest from the modelling point of view.

For simplicity, consider some chemical and denote by c_α its concentration per unit volume within the constituent α of the mixture, where for instance α might be ϕ, ℓ, or m. However, the concentration c_α has to be related to the volume ratio occupied by the constituent in which it is present, so that finally the relevant entities for an overall balance over the whole mixture are the *reduced* (or *weighted*) *concentrations*, e.g., $C_\ell = \ell c_\ell$.

To be specific consider the diffusion in the liquid constituent. In order to compute its balance we have to consider the motion of the fluid, the diffusive flux, the absorption of the liquid in which the chemical is dissolved, and the absorption of the chemical without absorption of the liquid, e.g., by osmosis.

One then has the following integral balance equation:

$$\frac{d}{dt}\int_V \ell c_\ell\, dV = -\int_{\partial V} \ell c_\ell \mathbf{v}_\ell\cdot\mathbf{n}\, d\Sigma - \int_{\partial V} \ell \mathbf{j}_\ell\cdot\mathbf{n}\, d\Sigma + \int_V \Gamma_\ell c_\ell\, dV + \int_V G_c\, dV\,, \quad (9.10)$$

where $\mathbf{j}_\ell$ is the diffusive flux inside liquid and Γ_c is the chemical exchange rate (rate of production/uptake). Taking for instance Γ_ℓ negative, the term $\int_V \Gamma_\ell c_\ell\, dV$ reflects adoption of the chemical by other constituents of the mixture by means of capturing the liquid.

Therefore, the following reaction-convection-diffusion equation can be deduced:

$$\frac{\partial}{\partial t}(\ell c_\ell) + \nabla\cdot(\ell c_\ell \mathbf{v}_\ell) = -\nabla\cdot(\ell \mathbf{j}_\ell) + G_c + \Gamma_\ell c_\ell\,. \quad (9.11)$$

This equation can be written in terms of $C_\ell = \ell c_\ell$, but Fick's law states that the diffusive flux can be assumed to be proportional to the concentration gradient in the liquid, that is

$$\mathbf{j}_\ell = -\mathbf{D}_\ell \nabla c_\ell = -\mathbf{D}_\ell \nabla \frac{C_\ell}{\ell}\,, \quad (9.12)$$

where $\mathbf{D}_\ell = \mathbf{D}_\ell(\phi_\ell)$ is the effective diffusion tensor in the liquid which accounts for diffusion of the chemical in the liquid due to Brownian motion as well as for molecule dispersion due to the porous structure of the mixture (see [BB90]). Hence, one has

$$\frac{\partial C_\ell}{\partial t} + \nabla\cdot(C_\ell \mathbf{v}_\ell) = \nabla\cdot\left(\ell \mathbf{D}_\ell \nabla \frac{C_\ell}{\ell}\right) + G_c + \Gamma_\ell \frac{C_\ell}{\ell}\,. \quad (9.13)$$

On the other hand, using the mass balance equation for the liquid (9.4)$_3$, Eq. (9.11) simplifies to

$$\ell \left(\frac{\partial c_\ell}{\partial t} + \mathbf{v}_\ell \cdot \nabla c_\ell \right) = \nabla \cdot (\ell \mathbf{D}_\ell \nabla c_\ell) + G_c \,. \tag{9.14}$$

Similar equations can be written for the concentration of chemicals in the other constituents. However, if exchange of the chemical between the constituents is so fast that one might assume that concentration of the chemical is the same for all the constituents:

$$c = c_\ell = c_\phi = c_m,$$

then the summation gives

$$\frac{\partial c}{\partial t} + \mathbf{v}_c \cdot \nabla c = \nabla \cdot (\mathbf{D} \nabla c) + G \,, \tag{9.15}$$

where $\mathbf{D}$ is an effective diffusivity tensor in the mixture, G contains production/source terms and degradation/uptake terms relative to the entire mixture, and $\mathbf{v}_c = \phi \mathbf{v}_\phi + \ell \mathbf{v}_\ell + m \mathbf{v}_m$ is the composite velocity. Actually, the related convective term can be neglected in most applications, so that one can write

$$\frac{\partial c}{\partial t} = \nabla \cdot (\mathbf{D} \nabla c) + G \,. \tag{9.16}$$

The procedure above can be generalized to all soluble molecules which are considered relevant to tumour development.

9.3 Force Balance

Several methods have been used to close the system of mass balance equations introduced in the previous section (the reader is referred to [AP02] for a critical review on this aspect). We focus here on the use of momentum balance equations, which we start writing in integral form for a generic constituent for pedagogical reasons to clarify the origin of all terms appearing in the equations.

Focusing again on the cellular constituent of the tissue, the variation of momentum of the constituent in the fixed volume $\mathcal{V}$

$$\int_\mathcal{V} \rho \phi \mathbf{v}_\phi \, dV$$

is due to

1. Momentum flux caused by the motion of the cells through the boundary $\partial \mathcal{V}$

$$-\int_{\partial \mathcal{V}} \rho \phi \mathbf{v}_\phi (\mathbf{v}_\phi \cdot \mathbf{n}) \, d\Sigma \,;$$

2. Contact forces within the constituent acting through the boundary $\partial \mathcal{V}$, which are codirected with **n**, therefore yielding

$$\int_{\partial \mathcal{V}} \widetilde{\mathbf{T}}_\phi^T \mathbf{n} \, d\Sigma \,,$$

where $\widetilde{\mathbf{T}}_\phi$ is called the partial stress;

3. Contact forces due to the interaction with the other constituents within the domain through the interface separating the constituents, say the cell membrane wet by the extracellular liquid or in contact with the extracellular matrix through the adhesion sites

$$\int_{\mathcal{V}} \widetilde{\mathbf{m}}_\phi \, dV \,,$$

where $\widetilde{\mathbf{m}}_\phi$ is called the interaction force;

4. Momentum supply related to phase changes

$$\int_{\mathcal{V}} \rho \Gamma_\phi \mathbf{v}_\phi \, dV \,,$$

e.g., fluid absorbed by a growing cell, ECM production or degradation;

5. Body forces

$$\int_{\mathcal{V}} \rho \phi \mathbf{b} \, dv \,,$$

e.g., chemotaxis or haptotaxis can be modelled in this way, though they actually involve the activation of subcellular mechanisms rather than an external action.

One then has

$$\frac{d}{dt} \int_{\mathcal{V}} \rho \phi \mathbf{v}_\phi \, dV = \int_{\partial \mathcal{V}} \left[-\rho \phi \mathbf{v}_\phi (\mathbf{v}_\phi \cdot \mathbf{n}) + \widetilde{\mathbf{T}}_\phi^T \mathbf{n} \right] d\Sigma + \int_{\mathcal{V}} (\rho \phi \mathbf{b} + \widetilde{\mathbf{m}}_\phi + \rho \Gamma_\phi \mathbf{v}_\phi) \, dV \,. \tag{9.17}$$

So using Gauss's theorem we can write

$$\int_{\mathcal{V}} \left[\frac{\partial}{\partial t} (\rho \phi \mathbf{v}_\phi) + \nabla \cdot (\rho \phi \mathbf{v}_\phi \otimes \mathbf{v}_\phi) - \nabla \cdot \widetilde{\mathbf{T}}_\phi - \rho \phi \mathbf{b} - \widetilde{\mathbf{m}}_\phi - \rho \Gamma_\phi \mathbf{v}_\phi \right] dV = 0 \,. \tag{9.18}$$

This holds for any volume of integration $\mathcal{V}$. So, if the integrand is smooth, one can write the following local form of the momentum balance for the solid constituent in conservative form:

$$\frac{\partial}{\partial t} (\rho \phi \mathbf{v}_\phi) + \nabla \cdot (\rho \phi \mathbf{v}_\phi \otimes \mathbf{v}_\phi) = \nabla \cdot \widetilde{\mathbf{T}}_\phi + \rho \phi \mathbf{b} + \widetilde{\mathbf{m}}_\phi + \rho \Gamma_\phi \mathbf{v}_\phi \,. \tag{9.19}$$

Actually using the mass balance equation $(9.4)_1$, Eq. (9.19) can be simplified as

$$\rho\phi\left(\frac{\partial\mathbf{v}_\phi}{\partial t} + \mathbf{v}_\phi\cdot\nabla\mathbf{v}_\phi\right) = \nabla\cdot\widetilde{\mathbf{T}}_\phi + \rho\phi\mathbf{b} + \widetilde{\mathbf{m}}_\phi\,, \qquad (9.20)$$

where the inertial term on the left-hand side can usually be neglected when describing biological growth phenomena.

If a saturation condition like (9.1) is assumed, then the constitutive equations for the partial stresses and for the interaction forces are characterized by the presence of a Lagrange multiplier classically identified with the interstitial pressure of the extracellular liquid [Bow76, RT95]. Without going into technical details, this is related to the fact that in checking the validity of the second principle of thermodynamics, one is considering only those processes satisfying the saturation constraint. The presence of a constraint implies the need of introducing a Lagrange multiplier in the Clausius–Duhem inequality, so that it is considered for any process such that the saturation constraint holds.

A similar reasoning is usually applied in fluid dynamics where enforcing incompressibility implies that one is studying only flows satisfying such a constraint and for this class of processes the second principle of thermodynamics should hold. The consequence is that in the constitutive equation for the fluid, the isotropic part of the stress tensor cannot be determined constitutively but is a reaction that adjusts so that the incompressibility constraint is satisfied.

In the case of the saturated mixture, for instance, it can be proved [Bow76, RT95] that

$$\widetilde{\mathbf{T}}_\phi = -\phi P\mathbf{I} + \phi\mathbf{T}_\phi\,, \qquad \widetilde{\mathbf{m}}_\phi = P\nabla\phi + \mathbf{m}_\phi\,, \qquad (9.21)$$

where $\mathbf{T}_\phi$ is called the excess stress and $\mathbf{m}_\phi$ the excess interaction force.

One then has

$$-\phi\nabla P + \nabla\cdot(\phi\mathbf{T}_\phi) + \mathbf{m}_\phi + \rho\phi\mathbf{b} = \mathbf{0}\,. \qquad (9.22)$$

Proceeding in a similar way for the other constituents and specifying, if needed, the different force balance equations for the cellular components one can write

$$-\phi_i\nabla P + \nabla\cdot(\phi_i\mathbf{T}_{\phi_i}) + \mathbf{m}_{\phi_i} + \rho\phi_i\mathbf{b}_i = \mathbf{0}\,,$$

$$-m\nabla P + \nabla\cdot(m\mathbf{T}_m) + \mathbf{m}_m = \mathbf{0}\,, \qquad (9.23)$$

$$-\ell\nabla P + \mathbf{m}_\ell = \mathbf{0}\,,$$

where the excess stress tensor for the extracellular liquid is assumed to be negligible, as is usually assumed in the theory of deformable porous media to obtain Darcy's law-like behaviour, and the body forces are dropped in the equations for the ECM and for the liquid.

We observe explicitly that, even if several ECM components must be specified, the constrained submixture hypothesis allows us to write a single force balance equation to determine the common velocity $\mathbf{v}_m$. Of course, all the ECM components will contribute to the constitutive equation for the stress tensor according to their relative proportion.

9.4 Interaction Forces

If the mixture is closed, one may demonstrate that in mixture theory the sum of interaction forces and of the momentum transfers due to mass exchange is zero [Bow76, RT95]. However, the contribution due to mass exchange is negligible with respect to that due to the interaction forces [PF01], compatible with the fact that inertial terms are negligible. Hence, one can say that the interaction forces sum to zero, as might be expected since they act as internal forces among the constituents of the whole mixture.

We reinforce this concept of internal forces by assuming that if the constituent β exerts an interaction force $\mathbf{m}_{\alpha\beta}$ on the constituent α, in turn the constituent α will exert on β an equal and opposite force, i.e., $\mathbf{m}_{\alpha\beta} = -\mathbf{m}_{\beta\alpha}$, being aware of the fact that this equality is an approximation, for instance, for the presence of exchanges of mass.

We distinguish among the interaction forces those involving the extracellular liquid, because they can be treated as drag forces. The others might require a better understanding of the adhesion mechanisms.

Compatible with Darcy's law, the interaction forces of all the constituents with the liquid can be taken to be proportional to the velocity difference between the liquid and the other constituents through invertible matrices $\mathbf{M}_i$, and $\mathbf{M}_m$, so that

$$\begin{aligned}
\mathbf{m}_{\ell\phi_i} &= -\mathbf{M}_i(\mathbf{v}_\ell - \mathbf{v}_{\phi_i})\,, \\
\mathbf{m}_{\ell m} &= -\mathbf{M}_m(\mathbf{v}_\ell - \mathbf{v}_m)\,.
\end{aligned} \qquad (9.24)$$

Therefore, in the last equation of (9.23), $\mathbf{m}_\ell = \mathbf{m}_{\ell m} + \sum_i \mathbf{m}_{\ell\phi_i}$, and one then has

$$\mathbf{M}_m(\mathbf{v}_\ell - \mathbf{v}_m) + \sum_{i=1}^I \mathbf{M}_i(\mathbf{v}_\ell - \mathbf{v}_{\phi_i}) = -\ell\nabla P\,, \qquad (9.25)$$

or

$$\mathbf{v}_\ell = \mathbf{M}^{-1}\left(\mathbf{M}_m\mathbf{v}_m + \sum_{i=1}^I \mathbf{M}_i\mathbf{v}_{\phi_i} - \ell\nabla P\right)\,, \qquad (9.26)$$

where $\mathbf{M} = \mathbf{M}_m + \sum_i \mathbf{M}_i$, which explicitly gives the liquid velocity in terms of the other velocities and of the pressure gradient.

Furthermore, summing the mass balance equations (9.4) one has for a closed mixture

$$\nabla \cdot \left(\ell \mathbf{v}_\ell + m \mathbf{v}_m + \sum_{i=1}^{I} \phi_i \mathbf{v}_{\phi_i} \right) = 0 \,, \tag{9.27}$$

which, substituting the velocity of the liquid, reduces to

$$\nabla \cdot (\ell^2 \mathbf{M}^{-1} \nabla P) = \nabla \cdot \Big[\sum_{i=1}^{I} (\phi_i \mathbf{I} + \ell \mathbf{M}^{-1} \mathbf{M}_i) \mathbf{v}_{\phi_i}$$
$$+ (m \mathbf{I} + \ell \mathbf{M}^{-1} \mathbf{M}_m) \mathbf{v}_m \Big] \,. \tag{9.28}$$

It is now useful to distinguish between two contributions in the momentum equations for cells and the ECM:

- Contributions due to the interactions with the extracellular liquid and to the pressure gradient;
- Contributions related to the interaction between cells and between cells and the ECM.

In many cases the former contribution is less important and can be dropped. Then the momentum equations can be simplified into

$$\nabla \cdot (\phi_i \mathbf{T}_{\phi_i}) + \sum_{\substack{j=1 \\ j \neq i}}^{I} \mathbf{m}_{ij} + \mathbf{m}_{im} = \mathbf{0} \,, \qquad i = 1, \dots, I \,,$$
$$\nabla \cdot (m \mathbf{T}_m) - \sum_{i=1}^{I} \mathbf{m}_{im} = \mathbf{0} \,. \tag{9.29}$$

Under these hypotheses Eq. (9.29) does not depend on the interstitial pressure or on the liquid velocity. Therefore, the equations of (9.29) can in principle be solved without solving (9.27) and (9.28). Integration of (9.27) and (9.28) is only required if we want to describe the evolution of either the interstitial pressure or the liquid velocity. They are obtained in cascade after integrating the equations (9.29) above.

Regarding the behaviour of the cell population, we can assume as a first approximation that they respond to the compression of other cells independently of their type, i.e.,

$$\mathbf{T}_{\phi_i} = \mathbf{T}_\phi \,. \tag{9.30}$$

An additional requirement is that the sum of the equations for the cell constituents yields

$$\nabla \cdot (\phi \mathbf{T}_\phi) + \sum_{i=1}^{I} \mathbf{m}_{im} = \mathbf{0} \,. \tag{9.31}$$

This can be achieved assuming that the cells belonging to the ith population press those of the jth population with a force proportional to $\nabla \cdot (\phi_i \mathbf{T}_\phi)$, and at the same time are pressed by the latter with a force proportional to $\nabla \cdot (\phi_j \mathbf{T}_\phi)$. In view of an integral balance law, these contributions need to be multiplied by the volume ratio of the population they act upon, with reference to the overall cellular component of the mixture ϕ. This suggests that the net interaction force $\mathbf{m}_{ij}$ might take the following form:

$$\mathbf{m}_{ij} = \frac{\phi_i}{\phi} \nabla \cdot (\phi_j \mathbf{T}_\phi) - \frac{\phi_j}{\phi} \nabla \cdot (\phi_i \mathbf{T}_\phi) , \qquad (9.32)$$

so that the momentum equations for the cell populations $(9.29)_1$ specialize as

$$\frac{\phi_i}{\phi} \nabla \cdot (\phi \mathbf{T}_\phi) + \mathbf{m}_{im} = \mathbf{0} , \qquad i = 1, \ldots, I , \qquad (9.33)$$

which sum up to the force balance equation for the submixture of cells (9.31).

We observe that summing all Eqs. (9.33) and $(9.29)_2$ gives the force balance equation for the tissue

$$\nabla \cdot (\phi \mathbf{T}_\phi + m \mathbf{T}_m) = \mathbf{0} , \qquad (9.34)$$

with the pressure gradient term and the interaction forces with the liquid neglected, compatibly with the assumptions done before writing Eqs. (9.29).

Let us focus now more specifically on the interaction between cells and the ECM which of course depends on both the volume ratios of the ECM constituents and of the cells, and therefore also on the available portion of space ℓ occupied by the liquid.

Though as a first approximation one can still assume the interaction terms to be proportional to the velocity differences as done when the liquid phase was involved, i.e.,

$$\mathbf{m}_{im} = -\mathbf{M}_{im}(\mathbf{v}_i - \mathbf{v}_m) , \qquad (9.35)$$

a better description of the attachment/detachment mechanisms between cells and the ECM would be desirable.

An alternative form for the interaction terms is proposed in [PT08] on the basis of the experiments performed by Baumgartner et al. [BHN+00], Canetta et al. [CDLV05], and Sun et al. [SGH+05] who measured the adhesive strength of a cell attached to a microsphere linked to the tip of an atomic force microscopy cantilever. The microsphere was assumed to present proper adhesion molecules on its surface in order to check the specific interaction of the cell adhesion molecule with those on the tip of the cantilever.

After putting the microsphere in contact with the cell, the cantilever is pulled away at a constant speed (in the range 0.2–4 μm/sec). If there is no adhesion between the microsphere and the cell, the force measured presents no stretching when the microsphere is taken away from the cell. This is experimentally obtained, for instance, by the addition of an antibody attaching to the external domain of the adhesion molecule, or by interfering with the links between the adhesion molecules and the cell cytoskeleton.

On the other hand, adhesion gives rise to the measurement of a stretching force and a characteristic jump indicating the rupture of an adhesive bond. Therefore, these bonds have a limited strength quantified to be in the range 35–55 pN each by Baumgartner et al. [BHN+00].

A similar result was also obtained by Sun et al. [SGH+05] who did not functionalize the microsphere and allowed a longer resting period on the cell surface, ranging from 2 to 30 seconds. Again, pulling away the cantilever at a constant speed in the range 3–5 μm/sec caused the rupture of one or more adhesive bonds. They used different cell types (Chinese hamster ovary cells, endothelial cells, and human brain tumour cells), all showing an adhesive strength of a single bond slightly below 30 pN. Coating the bead with poly-L-lysine or collagen did not lead to significant changes in the measurement.

On the other hand, big differences were observed interfering with the adhesion mechanism either by capping the external domain of the adhesion molecule with a proper antibody [BHN+00], or by disrupting the actin cytoskeleton [SGH+05], or by eliminating the link between adhesion molecules and the cytoskeleton [CDLV05].

It is not trivial to quantitatively transfer this measurement done at a molecular scale to a constitutive law at a tissue scale. However, we can say that this phenomenological description suggests that if cells are not pulled strongly enough to detach from the ECM, they remain attached to it. If they detach the force in excess can be assumed to be proportional to the velocity difference, as suggested by viscoplasticity theory.

This translates into the following constitutive assumption:

$$\mathbf{v}_i = \mathbf{v}_m , \qquad \text{if} \quad |\mathbf{m}_{im}| \le \sigma_{im} ,$$

$$(|\mathbf{m}_{im}| - \sigma_{im}) \frac{\mathbf{m}_{im}}{|\mathbf{m}_{im}|} = \alpha_{im}(\mathbf{v}_m - \mathbf{v}_i) , \qquad \text{if} \quad |\mathbf{m}_{im}| > \sigma_{im} . \tag{9.36}$$

The coefficient σ_{im} can be compared to a friction force and as such it is expected to depend on the adhesion mechanisms and on the volume ratio of the actors, the cells and the ECM. Proportionality between velocity and the force is a starting assumption made in absence of more precise experimental data.

From (9.33)

$$\mathbf{m}_{im} = -\frac{\phi_i}{\phi} \nabla \cdot (\phi \mathbf{T}_\phi) ,$$

and therefore Eq. (9.36) can be rewritten as

$$\mathbf{v}_i - \mathbf{v}_m = K_{im} \left(\frac{\phi_i}{\phi} - \frac{\sigma_{im}}{|\nabla \cdot (\phi \mathbf{T}_\phi)|} \right)_+ \nabla \cdot (\phi \mathbf{T}_\phi) , \tag{9.37}$$

where $(\cdot)_+$ stands for the positive part in the parentheses and $K_{im} = \alpha_{im}^{-1}$ is called in this chapter the motility coefficient of the ith cell population. This behaviour is presented in Fig. 9.2. Equation (9.37) replaces Eq. (9.33) and has to be solved jointly with Eq. (9.29)$_2$ or (9.34).

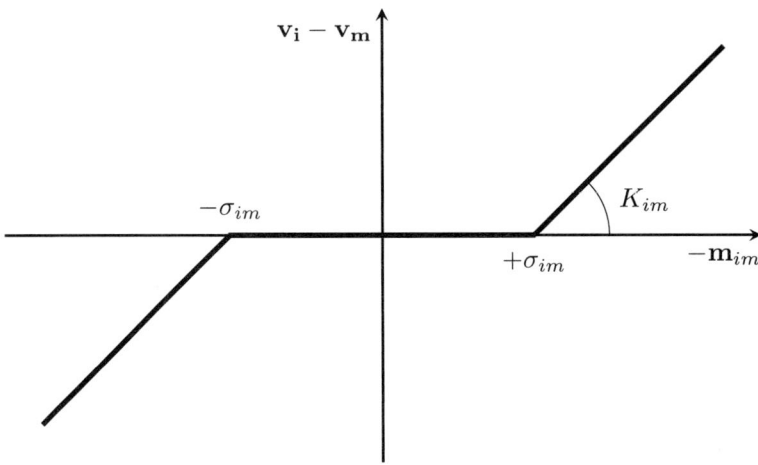

Fig. 9.2. Viscoplastic cell-ECM interaction.

To better understand the meaning of the constitutive equations above we can make some calculations for $|\mathbf{m}_{im}| > \sigma_{im}$. Taking the modulus of Eq. (9.36), one has

$$\alpha_{im}|\mathbf{v}_m - \mathbf{v}_i| = |\mathbf{m}_{im}| - \sigma_{im} .$$

Replacing $|\mathbf{m}_{im}|$ in the same equation, it can be rewritten as

$$\alpha_{im}|\mathbf{v}_i - \mathbf{v}_m|\frac{\mathbf{m}_{im}}{\sigma_{im} + \alpha_{im}|\mathbf{v}_i - \mathbf{v}_m|} = \alpha_{im}(\mathbf{v}_m - \mathbf{v}_i) ,$$

or

$$\mathbf{m}_{im} = \sigma_{im}\frac{\mathbf{v}_m - \mathbf{v}_i}{|\mathbf{v}_m - \mathbf{v}_i|} + \alpha_{im}(\mathbf{v}_m - \mathbf{v}_i) ,$$

which allows us to distinguish in $\mathbf{m}_{im}$ a static contribution in the direction of the relative motion (the first term) from a drag contribution proportional to the velocity difference. Of course, a viscous drag force is recovered in the limit $\sigma_{im} = 0$. As already mentioned the friction force σ_{im} strongly depends on the concentration of ECM. For instance, increasing the concentration of ECM leads to an increase in activated adhesion sites and therefore to a stronger friction threshold. In addition, it is known that there is an optimal concentration of the ECM favouring motility, because the content of the ECM cannot become too small; otherwise the lack of substratum would lead to a decrease in cell motility. Then the observation that cells hardly move when there is little or too much ECM can be translated as σ_{im} increasing for small and "large" m, thus, effectively, prohibiting cellular motion.

9.5 Stress Tensors

The momentum equations discussed in the previous sections need to be accompanied by the constitutive equations describing the response of the cells and ECM component to stress.

The basic questions are: How does the tumour behave? Is it a liquid or a solid? How should we summarize in a macroscopic constitutive equation cell adhesion properties? Should we take viscous or viscoelastic effects into account? What about plastic or viscoplastic deformations? Does a multicellular spheroid possess surface tension?

These questions are not at all trivial and there is no definitive answer yet, especially because of the lack of experiments. In fact, from the experimental point of view it is very difficult to perform mechanical tests on living matter, and in particular on ensembles of cells. In this respect Winters et al. [WSF05] performed a wonderful and very promising experiment consisting in a uniaxial compression test. More precisely, multicellular spheroids with radii in the range 0.15–0.7 mm were positioned between two plates immersed in a physiological liquid. The lower plate was raised and the force acting on the upper plate was measured using a Cahn electrobalance. Two different compressions were performed for each multicellular spheroid in order to check whether an elastic model or a liquid model with surface tension was more proper to describe the mechanical response. In the latter case the measured surface tension should be independent of the deformation. In the former case it would not and their ratio should be close to the ratio of the measured force. Of course, as stated in the paper, only measurements in which surface tension is independent of the applied force and size can be used to calculate for each cell line the value of surface tension. In most cases they concluded that the multicellular spheroid behaves like a liquid. However, in other cases they found that the behaviour was elastic (see Table 9.1). They argue that this might be explained with a production of ECM by the cells in the multicellular spheroid.

Table 9.1. Force ratio and deduced surface tension measurement for different cell lines (data from [WSF05]).

Cell line	Surface tension (dynes/cm±SEM)	ratio	force ratio	material
U-87MG	6.9 ± 0.4 and 7.1 ± 0.3	1.0	1.6	liquid
U-118MG	16.3 ± 0.3 and 17.2 ± 0.5	1.1	1.5	liquid
LN-229 TE/C	10.3 ± 0.3 and 10.0 ± 0.4	1.0	1.5	liquid
LN-229 TE	8.2 ± 0.9 and 12.4 ± 0.9	1.6	1.6	elastic

Unfortunately, uniaxial tests cannot exclude that what they are measuring is actually the yield stress that must be imposed before rupturing the adhesion sites among molecules. It would be interesting to perform shear tests. This would establish with no doubt what class of material we should look at to obtain a good constitutive equation to describe tumour growth.

Some results in this direction are obtained by Iordan and Verdier [Iord08]. They put in a plate-and-plate rheometer a cell suspension at different concentrations, proving the existence of a yield stress at higher concentrations (say, greater than 40%, i.e., $\phi > 0.4$).

Another theoretical difficulty comes when one wants to describe tumours as solids, because they are growing, remodelling, and re-organizing while deforming. This brings us to two difficulties that need to be properly addressed if we want to describe tumours as solid masses:

- defining a reference configuration with respect to which we can measure deformations;
- defining a proper Lagrangian coordinate system.

More precisely, following the ideas presented in [HR02, RHR03] (see also [MPR07]), one needs to describe how the natural configuration evolves in time due to growth and internal re-organization. Ambrosi and Mollica [AM02, AM04] use a purely elastic one-component model to evaluate residual stress formation in a growing multicellular spheroid. This approach was developed in [AP08] working in a multiphase framework and also taking internal re-organization and ECM deformation into account. This gave rise to an elasto-viscoplastic description for the cell population and a compressive elastic description for the ECM.

We refrain from discussing in detail this type of constitutive model, because it is too lengthy to fit in this chapter. We suggest that our readers refer to the works mentioned above for further details on this topic.

We also refrain from dealing with viscoelastic constitutive models for a different reason. In fact, although viscoelastic characteristics are important in describing the mechanical behaviour of tissues, they are less important in describing growth. This is due to the fact that the characteristic times of the mechanical response of biological materials are of the order of tens of seconds (see for instance, Forgacs et al. [FFSS98]), and therefore much less than the characteristic times of cell duplication (a day). Therefore, the effect of viscoelasticity fades away quite quickly with respect to the time the material requires to grow, leaving only a viscous heritage [PJ87, Pre89].

In most of the multiphase models of tumour growth deduced in the literature the tumour is modelled as a fluid. This approach, in fact, circumvents the difficulties mentioned above, mainly for two related reasons:

- the stress depends on the volume ratios and on the rate of deformations;
- it is possible to use an Eulerian approach.

Of course, tissues are not liquid and as stated above even ensembles of cells are unlikely to behave as a liquid. However, in this modelling approach the "cellular liquid" is contained in a solid structure of the ECM, so the material as a whole would look like a viscoelastic solid.

The easiest constitutive equation for the ensemble of cells consists in assuming that they behave as an elastic fluid, i.e.,

$$\mathbf{T}_\phi = -\Sigma\mathbf{I}\,,$$

where Σ is taken positive in compression. The use of this constitutive equation would result in a multicellular spheroid that in the absence of an ECM is not able to sustain shear.

In this case one can substitute (9.37) in the mass balance equations to obtain the following model:

$$
\begin{cases}
\dfrac{\partial \phi_i}{\partial t} + \nabla \cdot (\phi_i \mathbf{v}_m) + \nabla \cdot \left[\phi_i K_{im} \left(\dfrac{\phi_i}{\phi} - \dfrac{\sigma_{im}}{|\nabla(\phi\Sigma)|}\right)_+ \nabla(\phi\Sigma)\right] + \Gamma_{\phi_i}\,, \\[3mm]
\dfrac{\partial m_j}{\partial t} + \nabla \cdot (m_j \mathbf{v}_m) = \Gamma_{m_j}\,, \\[3mm]
\nabla \cdot (m\mathbf{T}_m) - \nabla(\phi\Sigma) = \mathbf{0}\,,
\end{cases}
$$

$$(9.38)$$

for $i = 1,\ldots,I$ and $j = 1,\ldots,J$.

A possible extension is to consider a viscous behaviour as in [BP04, FBK$^+$03, FBM$^+$03, FK03]

$$\hat{\mathbf{T}}_T = (-\Sigma + \lambda\nabla \cdot \mathbf{v}_\phi)\mathbf{I} + 2\mu\mathbf{D}\,, \qquad (9.39)$$

where $\mathbf{D} = (\nabla\mathbf{v}_\phi + \nabla\mathbf{v}_\phi^T)/2$ is the rate of strain tensor. This constitutive equation has the advantage to confer more stability to the growing mass.

9.6 Tumour Growth in a Rigid ECM

Regarding applications we start with the easiest case, when the ECM is rigid and does not change. The reader must be aware that an immediate consequence of this hypothesis would be that from the macroscopic point of view the tissue would behave like a rigid porous medium, with cells and water moving inside a rigid scaffold. Any stress acting on the bulk tissue would be sustained by the ECM, and cells in the core of the tissue would experience no stress deriving directly from the external actions.

From the mathematical point of view, this means that the stress tensor $\mathbf{T}_m$ acts as a (tensor) Lagrangian multiplier to satisfy the constraint $\mathbf{v}_m = \mathbf{0}$.

As an example, we apply the modelling approach above to the growth of a tumour in a host enviroment using only two cell populations, tumour cells with volume ratio ϕ_t and host cells with volume ratio ϕ_n initially occupying different domains $\Omega_t(t = 0)$ and $\Omega \setminus \Omega_t(t = 0)$.

The interface $\partial\Omega_t(t)$ between tumour and environment is a material surface moving with the common velocity of the cells

$$\mathbf{n} \cdot \frac{d\mathbf{x}_t}{dt} = \mathbf{n} \cdot \mathbf{v}_t = \mathbf{n} \cdot \mathbf{v}_n \,, \qquad \text{on} \quad \partial\Omega_t(t) \,. \tag{9.40}$$

It can be shown that the two cell populations stay segregated at all times. Taking into account that the interface conditions are enforced through continuity of stress and velocity, and treating, for simplicity, the ensemble of cells as elastic fluids, we have the following free boundary problem:

$$\begin{cases} \dfrac{\partial\phi_t}{\partial t} + \nabla \cdot (\phi_t \mathbf{v}_{\phi_t}) = \Gamma_{\phi_t} \,, & \text{in } \Omega_t \,, \\[2ex] \mathbf{v}_t = -K_{tm} \left(1 - \dfrac{\sigma_{tm}}{|\nabla(\phi_t \Sigma)|}\right)_{+} \nabla(\phi_t \Sigma) \,, & \text{in } \Omega_t \,, \\[2ex] \dfrac{\partial\phi_n}{\partial t} + \nabla \cdot (\phi_n \mathbf{v}_{\phi_n}) = \Gamma_{\phi_n} \,, & \text{in } \Omega - \Omega_t \,, \\[2ex] \mathbf{v}_n = -K_{nm} \left(1 - \dfrac{\sigma_{nm}}{|\nabla(\phi_n \Sigma)|}\right)_{+} \nabla(\phi_n \Sigma) \,, & \text{in } \Omega - \Omega_t \,, \\[2ex] \mathbf{v}_t \cdot \mathbf{n} = \mathbf{v}_n \cdot \mathbf{n} \,, & \text{on } \partial\Omega_t \,, \\[2ex] \phi_t \Sigma(\phi_t) = \phi_n \Sigma(\phi_n) \,, & \text{on } \partial\Omega_t \,. \end{cases} \tag{9.41}$$

Since the cell populations stay segregated, it is possible to introduce only one variable for the volume ratio of cells: ϕ, and assume that ϕ is the volume ratio of tumour cells ϕ_t in Ω_t and the volume ratio of normal host cells ϕ_n in $\Omega \setminus \Omega_t$:

$$\phi = \begin{cases} \phi_t, & \text{in } \Omega_t \,, \\ \phi_n, & \text{in } \Omega \setminus \Omega_t \,. \end{cases}$$

We can rewrite the main equation as

$$\frac{\partial\phi}{\partial t} = \nabla \left[\phi K_m \left(1 - \frac{\sigma_m}{|\nabla(\phi\Sigma)|}\right)_{+} \nabla(\phi\Sigma)\right] + \Gamma \,, \tag{9.42}$$

where, for instance, $K_m = K_{tm}$ in Ω_t and $K_m = K_{nm}$ in $\Omega \setminus \Omega_t$. In this formulation it is natural to use level set methods with the interface dividing the domains moving according to (9.40).

In [CGP06] $K_{tm} = K_{nm} = K_m$, $\sigma_{tm} = \sigma_{nm} = 0$, and $\Sigma = \Sigma(\psi)$ with $\psi = \phi_t + \phi_n + m$. In addition, the growth terms are modelled on the basis of the observation that when cells live in a crowded environment they sense the presence of other cells through the activation of mechanotransduction pathways. This phenomenon is called contact inhibition of growth and is one of the fundamental phenomena in controlling cell concentration. In the model this means that mitosis stops when the volume ratio (or the compression) overcomes a given threshold.

The behaviour of the cells in terms of growth and motion then crucially depends on how they feel the presence of other cells and how they translate the mechanical cues. What Chaplain et al. [CGP06] showed that if, for instance, for some reason, e.g., a fault in the mechanotransduction pathway, there is a misperception of the compression state of the local tissue and then of the subsequent stress which is exerted on a cell, then this degeneration can cause a clonal advantage on the surrounding cells leading to the replacement and the invasion of the healthy tissue with the formation of hyperplasia and therefore tumour lesions.

From the mathematical point of view the phenomenological description above can be formalized by saying that the threshold value for tumour cells to overcome the restriction point and commit themselves to divide is slightly larger than the physiological one. Actually, it may even tend to infinity, meaning that the cells are completely insensitive to compression and continue replicating independently of the compression level.

We shall then consider the following growth terms:

$$\Gamma_i = [\gamma_i H_\sigma(\psi - \psi_i) - \delta_i(\psi)]\phi_i, \qquad i = n, t, \tag{9.43}$$

where $\psi = \phi_n + \phi_t + m$. We assume that what makes the difference between a normal and a tumour cell is expressed in the growth term and in its dependence on the stress level.

Of course, cellular mechanotransduction is not the only cause of formation of hyperplasia and tumours. In fact, chemical factors operate to regulate the reproduction rates so that the growth terms crucially depend on the presence of growth promoting factors, growth inhibitory factors, and of course nutrients.

However, here we shall only focus on the possible role of stress on tumour invasion and therefore assume that all the constituents required to sustain growth and mitosis are abundant in the extracellular liquid.

In (9.43) $H_\sigma(\psi - \psi_i)$ is a mollifier of the step function, which is at least continuous, is constantly equal to 1 for ψ smaller than the threshold value ψ_i, and vanishes for $\psi > \psi_i + \sigma$. According to the discussion above, the threshold values ψ_n and ψ_t are such that $\psi_n < \psi_t$. For the following discussion it is useful to observe that a balance between cell growth and death occurs when $\gamma_i H_\sigma(\psi - \psi_i) = \delta_i(\psi)$, or, in the case in which δ_i is considered constant as in the following simulations,

$$\psi = \psi_i + H_\sigma^{-1}\left(\frac{\delta_i}{\gamma_i}\right). \tag{9.44}$$

The simulation in Fig. 9.3 shows how some tumour cells originating from the surface of a bone diffuse in the surrounding tissue. Initially, the interface

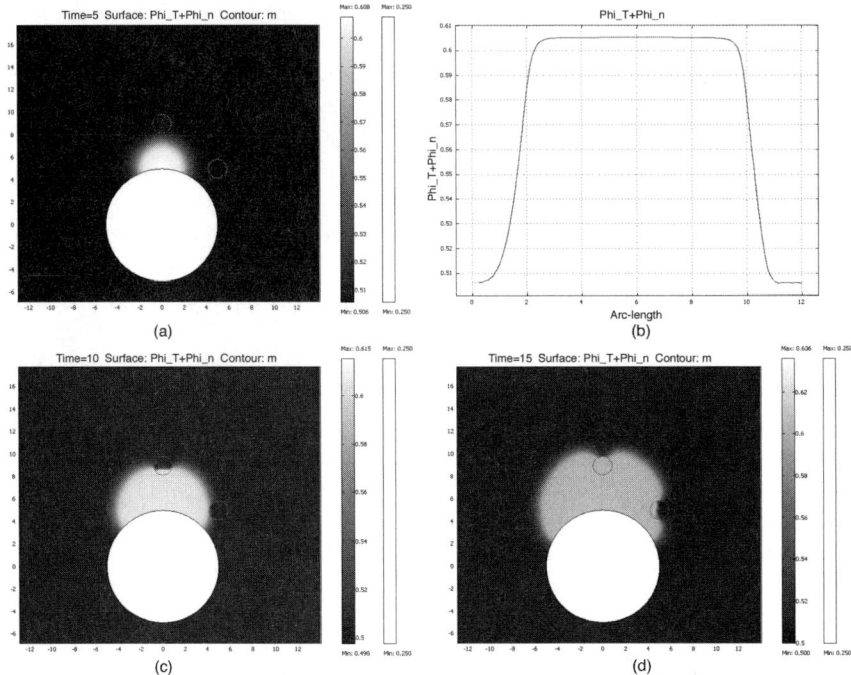

Fig. 9.3. Growth of a tumour in a heterogeneous tissue surrounding a bone. Denser ECM is found near the points (0,10) and (5,5). (a), (c), and (d) give the cell volume ratio $\phi_t + \phi_n$ at the dimensionless times 5, 10, and 15. (b) gives the cell volume at the section of the tumour along $y = 6$ for $x \in [-6, 6]$ and $t = 5$.

dividing the tumour from the host tissue is nearly circular. Far away from the tumour mass the volume ratio occupied by the cells is that given in (9.44) with $\psi_n = 0.5$, while in the core of the tumour it is that corresponding to $\psi_n = 0.6$. Near the surface it is possible to observe a compression of the host tissue as put in evidence by a cross section ($y = 0.6$) in Fig. 9.3b, showing the cell volume ratio. The interface between the two is located near the level $\phi_t + \phi_n = 0.6$. However, growth is not occurring in a homogeneous tissue. In fact, while in most of the domain the volume ratio occupied by the ECM is 0.2, there are two regions centered at (0,10) and (5,5) with a higher volume ratio increasing up to 0.3. The presence of these heterogeneities breaks the symmetry of the tumour, as already evident in Fig. 9.3b. Figs. 9.3c,d show how the presence of more ECM slows down tumour invasion.

9.7 Tumour Growth in a Remodelling ECM

With little effort we can adjust the model to take ECM remodelling into account. This is essential to describe the formation of fibrotic tissues and therefore of stiffer stroma.

So we additionally consider

- the volume ratio m occupied by the extracellular matrix;
- the concentration c of matrix degrading enzymes (MDEs).

The numerous constituents of the ECM are produced in a stress-dependent way by the cells and are degraded by MDEs [CM97, Mat92, PWB$^+$97, SSHC96].

Hence the remodelling process can be described by adding an equation for m:

$$\frac{\partial m}{\partial t} = \mu_n(\Sigma)\phi_n + \mu_t(\Sigma)\phi_t - \nu cm \,, \tag{9.45}$$

where μ_n and μ_t are the ECM production rates respectively by normal and tumour cells and ν is the degradation coefficient due to the action of MDEs.

Active MDEs are produced (or activated) by the cells, diffuse throughout the tissue, and undergo some decay (either passive or active). So one has to introduce the following reaction-diffusion equation governing the evolution of MDE concentration:

$$\frac{\partial c}{\partial t} = \kappa \nabla^2 c + \pi_n(\Sigma)\phi_n + \pi_t(\Sigma)\phi_t - \frac{c}{\tau} \,, \tag{9.46}$$

where π_n and π_t are the MDE production rates respectively by normal and tumour cells and τ is its half-life.

In (9.45) it is important that the production coefficients of ECM by normal and tumour cells be different in order to describe the formation of fibrosis characterizing many tumours. Also the functions π_n and π_t describe the production levels of active MDEs by normal and tumour cells, respectively. They may be different and certainly depend on the compression level. As proved in [CGP06] they also can be the cause of the formation of fibrotic tissues.

Thus the complete system of equations with matrix remodelling effects taken into account is

$$\begin{cases} \dfrac{\partial \phi_n}{\partial t} = \nabla \cdot [\phi_n K_m \nabla(\phi_n \Sigma(\psi))] + \gamma_n H_\sigma(\psi - \psi_n)\phi_n - \delta_n(\psi)\phi_n \,, \\[2mm] \dfrac{\partial \phi_t}{\partial t} = \nabla \cdot [\phi_t K_m \nabla(\phi_t \Sigma(\psi))] + \gamma_t H_\sigma(\psi - \psi_t)\phi_t - \delta_t(\psi)\phi_t \,, \\[2mm] \dfrac{\partial m}{\partial t} = \mu_n(\Sigma)\phi_n + \mu_t(\Sigma)\phi_t - \nu cm \,, \\[2mm] \dfrac{\partial c}{\partial t} = \kappa \nabla^2 c + \pi_n(\Sigma)\phi_n + \pi_t(\Sigma)\phi_t - \dfrac{c}{\tau} \,. \end{cases} \tag{9.47}$$

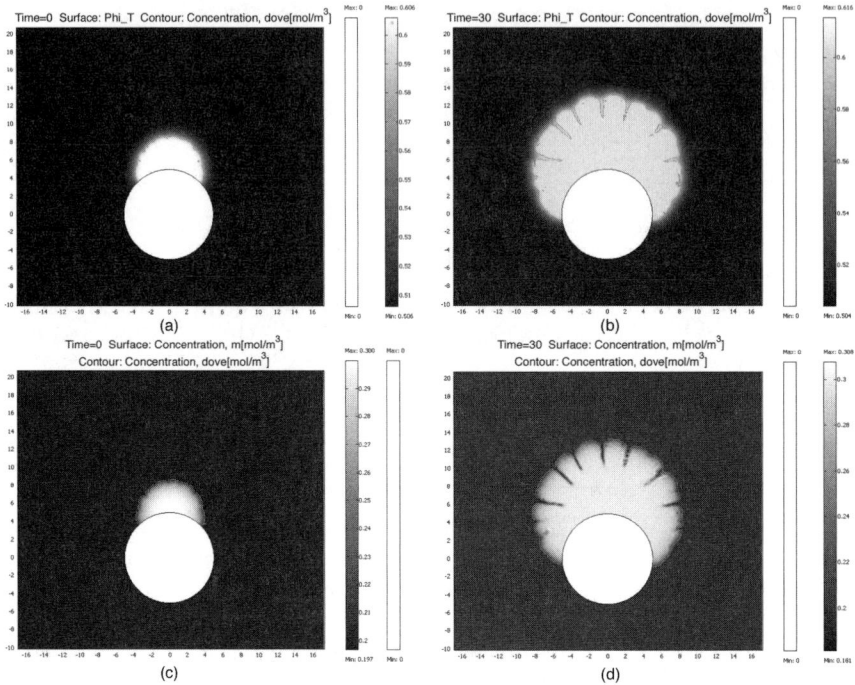

Fig. 9.4. Growth of the fibrosis in a homogeneous tissue surrounding a bone. Cell volume ratio $\phi_t + \phi_n$ at the dimensionless times 30 and 60 is given in (a) and (b). ECM volume ratio is given in (c) and (d). The line delimits the tumour from the host tissue.

One of the by-products of this model is the description of the formation of fibrotic tissues and of tissues stiffer than normal so that they may be sometimes felt with a self-test. This is the aim of the simulation shown in Fig. 9.4. The situation is similar to the previous one. However, now the ECM is initially distributed homogeneously with $m = 0.2$. On the other hand, while proliferating tumour cells will produce the same amount of MDE as the host cells, they will produce more ECM than normal. This causes the formation of a tumour characterized by an amount of ECM with a volume ratio close to $m = 0.3$. From the mechanical point of view this increase in the percentage of ECM would lead to an increase of almost one order of magnitude in tissue stiffness.

9.8 Vascularized Tumour Growth

The general model can be modified to describe vascular tumour growth. To start, consider the most simple configuration: a vessel and tumour tissue in the direct vicinity of the vessel. As a vessel is a natural source of oxygen and nutrients the region near the vessel is beneficial for tumour growth. On the contrary, regions very distant from the vessel are likely to be prohibitive for the tumour.

This configuration may lead to the formation of a tumour along the vessel that we shall call a *tumour cord*.

Let us consider a two-dimensional domain Ω where tumour occupies the region Ω_t, and the rest of the domain $\Omega_h = \Omega \setminus \Omega_t$ is occupied by the normal host tissue (Fig. 9.5).

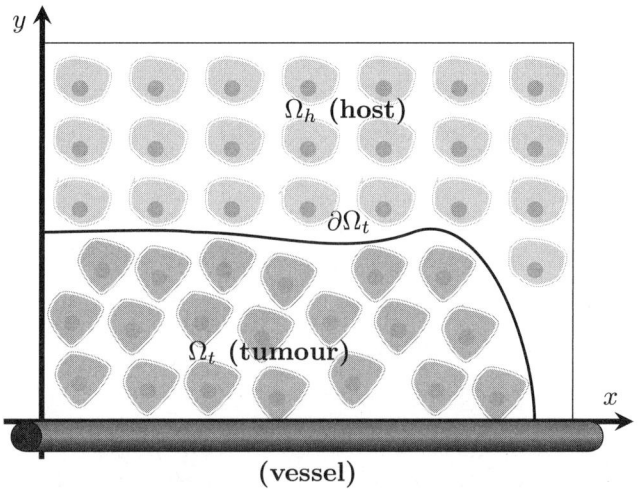

Fig. 9.5. Tumour cord region Ω_t and region of host tissue Ω_h. Blood vessel is positioned along the x-axis ($\partial\Omega_{south}$).

We assume that there is a blood vessel which coincides with some of the boundaries. In particular we shall consider the case when there is a vessel along the x-axis.

The basic model is given in Eq. (9.41). However, for simplicity, we shall neglect any viscoplastic effects, effectively substituting $\sigma_{im} = 0$, $i = t, n$.

The model should be accompanied by the selection of an appropriate growth term. One might expect that any growth process within the tissue is closely related to cell metabolism and energy balance. Thus we need to introduce equations governing the distribution and consumption of various nutrients, like Eq. (9.15).

The type of the tumour metabolism assumed shall define which nutrients are of the most interest and should be included in the model.

For example, let us consider glucose catabolism. In normal conditions its fission produces approximately 32 molecules of ATP per molecule of glucose [NC02] and requires 6 molecules of oxygen. However incomplete glucose oxydation is also possible in hypoxic condition. In this case there are only 2 molecules of ATP produced per molecule of glucose, and the by-product in this case is lactic acid (Fig. 9.6).

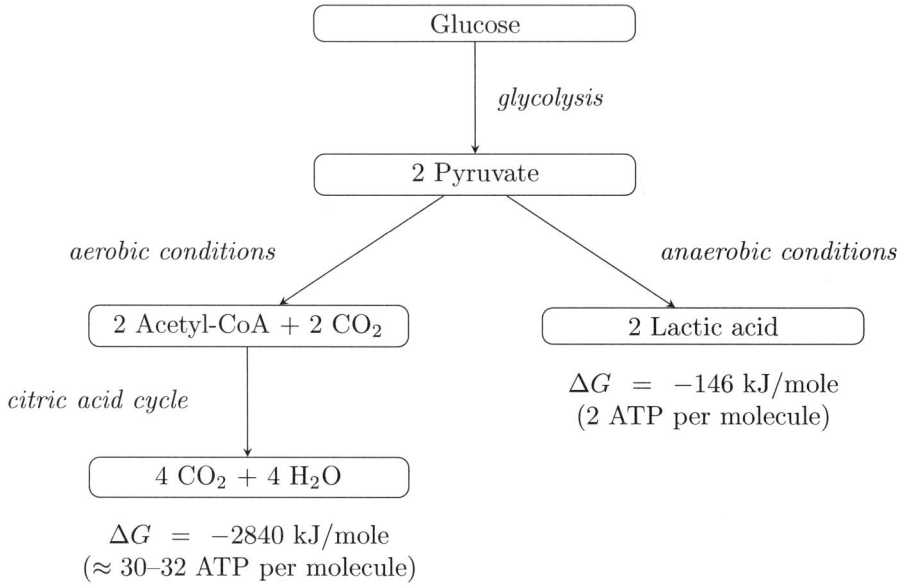

Fig. 9.6. Glucose catabolic pathways (based on [NC02]). Anaerobic pathway is less energy efficient and in addition it acidifies the microenvironment, but many tumours rely on this type of metabolism.

While the anaerobic pathway is less energy efficient, it proved to give an evolutionary advantage to tumours as they tend to develop and heavily rely on their ability for a glycolysis-oriented metabolism [SGG$^+$07, GG07, GGG$^+$06].

Thus the proper description of the metabolism is essential for obtaining a model valid for a wide range of tumours. In the most simple case one may assume that the tumour has not yet developed an ability for anaerobic metabolism. In this case one may show that it is only the concentration of oxygen that is important within the model.

Let c be the concentration of oxygen, and let its distribution be governed by the reaction-diffusion equation

$$\frac{\partial c}{\partial t} = D\Delta c + G(c, \phi),$$

where G is the oxygen consumption term:

$$G(c, \phi) = \begin{cases} \alpha\phi f(\phi)c, & \text{in } \Omega_t \\ 0, & \text{in } \Omega_h, \end{cases}$$

We assume that consumption of the host tissue is negligible with respect to growing tumour tissue. The rate of oxygen uptake is described by α. Function $f(\phi)$ characterizes intensity of metabolic processes: we expect that cells stop proliferating (and consuming) at maximum packing density ϕ_*.

Then we may define a growth/death term of the cellular phase in the tumour subdomain as

$$\Gamma = \gamma\phi(f(\phi)c - \theta)_+ - \epsilon\phi(\theta - f(\phi)c)_+,$$

where γ and ϵ are growth and death rates respectively, θ is the minimal life maintenance cost per cell, and $(\cdot)_+$ denotes the positive part of $(\cdot)$. More details on how this form of the growth term is obtained can be found in [AT08].

For the host subdomain Ω_h we assume

$$\Gamma \equiv 0.$$

Let both tissues have identical mechanical properties, and have the same stress-free packing density ϕ_0; then Σ may be chosen as

$$\Sigma(\phi) = \phi - \phi_0.$$

Initially both tissues are in a stress-free condition:

$$\phi(x, y, 0) = \phi_0. \tag{9.48}$$

We distinguish three kinds of exterior boundaries:

- a boundary coinciding with a blood vessel,
- a remote boundary,
- a symmetry axis.

For the vascular boundary we assume that the cells do not penetrate into the vessel, and the oxygen supply is always sufficient to maintain its constant concentration c_{in}:

$$\frac{\partial\phi\Sigma(\phi)}{\partial\mathbf{n}}(x, y, t) = 0, \quad c(x, y, t) = c_{in}, \quad \text{for } (x, y) \text{ at vascular boundaries,} \tag{9.49}$$

where $\mathbf{n}$ is an external normal of Ω.

We assume that remote boundaries stay undisturbed by the growth and there is zero flux of oxygen through those boundaries:

$$\phi(x, y, t) = \phi_0, \quad \frac{\partial c}{\partial\mathbf{n}}(x, y, t) = 0, \quad \text{for } (x, y) \text{ at remote boundaries.} \tag{9.50}$$

And for a symmetry axis we use

$$\frac{\partial\phi\Sigma(\phi)}{\partial\mathbf{n}}(x, y, t) = 0, \quad \frac{\partial c}{\partial\mathbf{n}}(x, y, t) = 0, \quad \text{for } (x, y) \text{ at an axis of symmetry.} \tag{9.51}$$

In the configuration shown in Fig. 9.5 there are five boundaries: the four exterior boundaries of model domain Ω, and $\partial\Omega_{th}$, the boundary between Ω_t and Ω_h, or the tumour-host interface.

We consider the right and the top boundaries to be remote, the bottom boundary to coincide with the vessel, and the left boundary to be a symmetry axis.

For the tumour-host interface $\partial\Omega_{th}$ we assume continuity of stress (this implies continuity of ϕ). For mass preservation reasons the velocity of the interface should be

$$\mathbf{v}_{\partial\Omega_{th}} \cdot \mathbf{n} = -K_m \nabla(\phi\Sigma(\phi)) \cdot \mathbf{n},$$

where $K_m = K_{tm} = K_{nm}$.

A typical cord growth in single-vessel configuration is shown in Fig. 9.7. The initial cord size was 0.2, and the values of the other parameters are $\gamma = 1$, $\epsilon = 0.8$, $\alpha = 200$, $K_m = 0.01$, $\theta = 0.15$. The stress-free density was $\phi_0 = 0.75$, $f(\phi) = 1 - \phi$, $D = 1$, $c_{in} = 1$.

The source code used for computer simulations using the model is freely available at http://code.google.com/p/cord/.

One may observe that the growth of the tumour region is highly anisotropic with the preferred direction of the vessel. The cord reaches and maintains the same radius along all the cord except the very tip. The packing density profile of the late stages suggests that it is at the tip of the cord where proliferation of the tumour is most intensive. In contrast, in the region of the steady radius, there is a hypoxic region near the outer rim of the cord, where cell death is observed in the simulation.

In general the behaviour of the tumour observed in the simulation confirms a well-known observation that there exists a certain distance from the vessels above which the tumour may not go unless it develops the ability to utilize anaerobic metabolism.

9.9 Final Remarks and Open Problems

The general modelling framework illustrated in this chapter has been developed on the basis of the following observations.

- Tumour cells duplicate in a tissue characterized by the presence of other host cells, a deformable ECM made of many constituents and of extracellular liquid. If we want to model tumour growth from the macroscopic viewpoint, this induces the need to use a multiphase mathematical model with several constituents.
- Also due to the action of tumour cells themselves, the environment changes considerably during the evolution which in turn influences the behaviour of the cells.

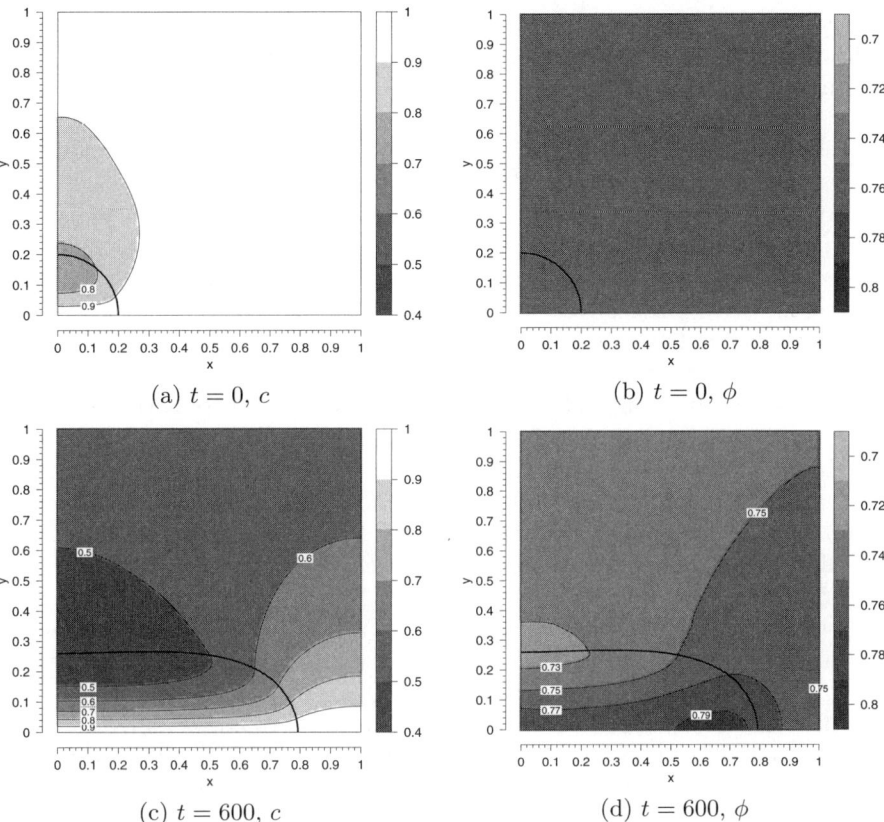

Fig. 9.7. Cord growth. Thick line lines shows position of the tumour-host interface $\partial\Omega_{th}$. (a) and (c) show oxygen concentration. (b) and (d) show packing density profile.

- Cells are bound to the ECM through adhesion molecules, mainly integrins, that have a limited strength. In a similar way cells are also attached to other cells through other adhesion molecules, mainly cadherins, that also have a limited strength. On the basis of these experimental evidences it is proposed that there exists a threshold condition below which the ensemble of cells sticks to the ECM and moves with it. Above the threshold cells gradually detach to move with respect to the ECM.

The model presented here can be specialized in several different ways, e.g., specifying the cell populations (endothelial cells, epithelial cells, fibroblasts, macrophages, lymphocytes), or including the different phases of the cell cycle, i.e., G_0, G_1, G_2, in view of the application of the model to the study of possible treatments, or distinguishing different tumour clones characterized by relevant differences in their behaviour, e.g., cells with normal and abnormal expression of the tumour suppressor gene, p53, and hormone sensitive and insensitive cells.

In this respect, one of the breakthroughs in modelling tumour growth consists in including what happens inside the cells and therefore in developing multiscale models which take into account the cascades of events regulating the behaviour of cells.

Another interesting problem which has not been studied yet is the growth of tumours in a mechanically heterogeneous environment, which includes network structures like blood vasculature, airways, and lymphatic system, the interaction with physical barriers like bones and cartilages, and the pressure on the surrounding tissues. This would allow us to understand vessel collapse due to tumour growth, capsule formation and degradation, cell compartmentalization due to strong inhomogeneities of the ECM distribution, or tissue invasion related to changes in the adhesion mechanisms.

However, research in this direction still needs a characterization of the mechanical behaviour of growing tissues and their environment, in order to evaluate the importance of nonlinear effects, to quantify viscoelastic and plastic effects, and to identify the proper constitutive equation.

So, in developing all the generalizations above, one has to keep in mind the objective difficulties in obtaining specific measurements from experiments. For instance, characterizing the behaviour of a growing and remodelling tissue from the mechanical viewpoint is not easy. Quantifying the dependence of the production rates of ECM and MDEs from the level of stress and/or strain is not easy and data are not available yet, though the effects were put in evidence many years ago and related therapies have been applied in clinical practice, e.g., application of traction in bone healing and orthodoncy. For this reason, in our opinion, the development of mathematical models and of experiments have to run along parallel paths, stimulating and cross-fertilizing each other.

Acknowledgments

Partially supported by the European Community, through the Marie Curie Research Training Network Project HPRN-CT-2004-503661: Modelling, Mathematical Methods and Computer Simulation of Tumour Growth and Therapy and by the Italian Ministry for University and Research, through a PRIN project on Modelli matematici di crescita e vascolarizzazione di tumori e tessuti biologici.

References

[AM02]   Ambrosi, D., Mollica, F.: On the mechanics of a growing tumor. Int. J. Engng. Sci., **40**, 1297–1316 (2002)

[AM04]   Ambrosi, D., Mollica, F.: The role of stress in the growth of a multicell spheroid. J. Math. Biol., **48**, 477–499 (2004)

[AM05]   Araujo, R., McElwain, D.: A mixture theory for the genesis of residual stresses in growing tissues, I: A general formulation. SIAM J. Appl. Math., **65**, 1261–1284 (2005)

[AP02]   Ambrosi, D., Preziosi, L.: On the closure of mass balance models for tumor growth. Math. Mod. Meth. Appl. Sci., **12**, 737–754 (2002)

[AP08]   Ambrosi, D., Preziosi, L.: Tumors as elasto-viscoplastic growing bodies. Biomechanics and Modeling in Mechanobiology (2008), submitted

[AT08]   Astanin, S., Tosin, A.: Mathematical model of tumour cord growth along the source of nutrient. Math. Mod. Nat. Phen. (2008), in press

[BB90]   Bear, J., Bachmat, Y.: Introduction to Modeling of Transport Phenomena in Porous Media. Kluwer Academic Publishers, Dordrecht (1990)

[BBL02]   Breward, C., Byrne, H.: Lewis, C., The role of cell-cell interactions in a two-phase model for avascular tumor growth. J. Math. Biol., **45**, 125–152 (2002)

[BBL03]   Breward, C., Byrne, H., Lewis, C.: A multiphase model describing vascular tumor growth. Bull. Math. Biol., **65**, 609–640 (2003)

[BHN+00] Baumgartner, W., Hinterdorfer, P., Ness, W., Raab, A., Vestweber, D., Schindler, H., Drenckhahn, D.: Cadherin interaction probed by atomic force microscopy. Proc. Nat. Acad. Sci. USA, **97**, 4005–4010 (2000)

[BKMP03] Byrne, H., King, J., McElwain, D., Preziosi, L.: A two-phase model of solid tumor growth. Appl. Math. Letters, **16**, 567–573 (2003)

[Bow76]   Bowen, R.M.: The theory of mixtures. In: A. Eringen (ed.) Continuum Physics, vol. 3, Academic Press, New York (1976)

[BP04]   Byrne, H., Preziosi, L.: Modeling solid tumor growth using the theory of mixtures. Math. Med. Biol., **20**, 341–366 (2004)

[CDLV05] Canetta, E., Duperray, A., Leyrat, A., Verdier, C.: Measuring cell viscoelastic properties using a force-spectrometer: Influence of the protein-cytoplasm interactions. Biorheology, **42**, 298–303 (2005)

[CGP06]   Chaplain, M., Graziano, L., Preziosi, L.: Mathematical modelling of the loss of tissue compression responsiveness and its role in solid tumour development. Math. Med. Biol., **23**, 197–229 (2006)

[CM97]   Chambers, A., Matrisian, L.: Changing views of the role of matrix metalloproteinases in metastasis. J. Natl. Cancer Inst., **89**, 1260–1270 (1997)

[FBK+03] Franks, S., Byrne, H., King, J., Underwood, J., Lewis, C.: Modelling the early growth of ductal carcinoma in situ of the breast. J. Math. Biol., **47**, 424–452 (2003)

[FBM+03] Franks, S., Byrne, H., Mudhar, H., Underwood, J., Lewis, C.: Mathematical modelling of comedo ductal carcinoma in situ of the breast. Math. Med. Biol., **20**, 277–308 (2003)

[FFSS98] Forgacs, G., Foty, R., Shafrir, Y., Steinberg, M.: Viscoelastic properties of living embryonic tissues: A quantitative study. Biophys. J., **74**, 2227–2234 (1998)

[FK03]   Franks, S., King, J.: Interactions between a uniformly proliferating tumor and its surroundings. Uniform material properties. Math. Med. Biol., **20**, 47–89 (2003)

[GG07]   Gillies, R., Gatenby, R.: Hypoxia and adaptive landscapes in the evolution of carcinogenesis. Cancer Metastasis Rev. (2007), e-publication

[GGG+06]   Gatenby, R., Gawlinski, E., Gmitro, A., Kaylor, B., Gillies, R.: Acid-mediated tumour invasion: A multidisciplinary study. Cancer Res., **66**, 5216–5223 (2006)

[GP07]   Graziano, L., Preziosi, L.: Mechanics in tumour growth. In: F. Mollica, L. Preziosi, K. Rajagopal (eds.) Modeling of Biological Materials, 267–328, Birkhäuser, Boston, MA (2007)

[HHLM89]   Hou, J., Holmes, M., Lai, W., Mow, V.: Boundary conditions at the cartilage-synovial fluid interface for joint lubrication and theoretical verifications. J. Biomech. Engng., **111**, 78–87 (1989)

[HR02]   Humphrey, J., Rajagopal, K.: A constrained mixture model for growth and remodeling of soft tissues. Math. Mod. Meth. Appl. Sci., **12**, 407–430 (2002)

[Iord08]   Iordan, A., Duperray, A., Verdier, C.: Fractal approach to the rheology of concentrated cell suspension. Phys. Rev. E, **77**, 011911 (2008)

[Jay83]   Jayaraman, G.: Water transport in the arterial wall. A theoretical study. J. Biomech., **16**, 833–840 (1983)

[Ken79]   Kenion, D.: A mathematical model of water flux through aortic tissue. Bull. Math. Biol., **41**, 79–90 (1979)

[KLM90]   Kwan, M., Lai, W., Mow, V.: A finite deformation theory of cartilage and other soft hydrated connective tissues: Part I – Equilibrium results. J. Biomech., **23**, 145–155 (1990)

[KT87]   Klanchar, M., Tarbell, J.: Modeling water flow through arterial tissue. Bull. Math. Biol., **49**, 651–669 (1987)

[LHM90]   Lai, W., Hou, J., Mow, V.: A triphasic theory for the swelling properties of hydrated charged soft biological tissues. In: Biomechanics of Diarthroidal Joints, vol. 1, 283–312, Springer, New York (1990)

[Mat92]   Matrisian, L.: The matrix-degrading metalloproteinases. Bioessays, **14**, 455–463 (1992)

[MHL84]   Mow, V., Holmes, M., Lai, W.: Fluid transport and mechanical problems of articular cartilage: A review. J. Biomech., **17**, 377–394 (1984)

[MKLA80]   Mow, V., Kuei, S., Lai, W., Armstrong, C.: Biphasic creep and stress relaxation of articular cartilage: Theory and experiment. J. Biomech. Engng., **102**, 73–84 (1980)

[ML79]   Mow, V., Lai, W.: Mechanics of animal joints. Ann. Rev. Fluid Mech., **11**, 247–288 (1979)

[MPR07]   Mollica, F., Preziosi, L., Rajagopal, K.: Modelling of Biological Materials. Birkhäuser, Boston, MA (2007)

[MRS90]   Mow, V., Ratcliffe, A., Savio, L.Y: (eds.) Biomechanics of Diarthroidal Joints. Springer-Verlag, New York (1990)

[NC02]   Nelson, D., Cox, M.: I principi di biochimica di Lehninger. Zanichelli (2002), translated by M. Averna, E. Melloni, A. Sdraffa

[Nic85]   Nicholson, C.: Diffusion from an injected volume of a substance in brain tissue with arbitrary volume fraction and tortuosity. Brain Res., **333**, 325–329 (1985)

[OVCG87]   Oomens, C., Van Campen, D., Grootenboer, H.: A mixture approach to the mechanics of skin. J. Biomech., **20**, 877–885 (1987)

[Pre89]   Preziosi, L.: On an invariance property of the solution to Stokes first problem for viscoelastic fluids. J. Non-Newtonian Fluid Mech., **33**, 225-228 (1989)

[PF01]   Preziosi, L., Farina, A.: On Darcy's law for growing porous media. Int.
           J. Nonlinear Mech., **37**, 485–491 (2001)
[PJ87]   Preziosi, L., Joseph, D.: Stokes' first problem for viscoelastic fluids. J.
           Non-Newtonian Fluid Mech., **25**, 239–259 (1987)
[PT08]   Preziosi, L., Tosin, A.: Multiphase modeling of tumor growth and ex-
           tracellular matrix interaction: Mathematical tools and applications. J.
           Math. Biol. (2008), in press
[PWB+97]   Parson, S., Watson, S., Brown, P., Collins, H., Steele, R.: Matrix met-
           alloproteinases. Brit. J. Surg., **84**, 160–166 (1997)
[RHR03]   Rao, I., Humphrey, J., Rajagopal, K.: Biological growth and remod-
           eling: A uniaxial example with possible application to tendons and
           ligaments. Comp. Mod Engr. Sci., **4**, 439–455 (2003)
[RT95]   Rajagopal, K., Tao, L.: Mechanics of Mixtures. World Scientific, Sin-
           gapore (1995)
[SCZM06]   Sarntinoranont, M., Chen, X., Zhao, J., Mareci, T.: Computational
           model of interstitial transport in the spinal cord using diffusion tensor
           imaging. Ann. Biomed. Eng., **34**, 1304–1321 (2006)
[SGG+07]   Smallbone, K., Gatenby, R., Gillies, R., Maini, P., Gavaghan, D.:
           Metabolic changes during carcinogenesis: Potential impact on inva-
           siveness. J. Theor. Biol., **244**, 703–713 (2007)
[SGH+05]   Sun, M., Graham, J., Hegedus, B., Marga, F., Zhang, Y., Forgacs, G.,
           Grandbois, M.: Multiple membrane tethers probed by atomic force
           microscopy. Biophys. J., **89**, 4320–4329 (2005)
[SS86]   Sorek, S., Sideman, S.: A porous medium approach for modelling heart
           mechanics. Part 1: Theory. Math. Biosci., **81**, 1–14 (1986)
[SSHC96]   Stetler-Stevenson, W., Hewitt, R., Corcoran, M.: Matrix metallo–
           proteinases and tumour invasion: From correlation to causality to the
           clinic. Cancer Biol., **7**, 147–154 (1996)
[TIZB84]   Tsaturyan, A., Izacov, V., Zhelamsky, S., Bykov, B.: Extracellular fluid
           filtration as the reason for the viscoelastic behaviour of the passive
           myocardium. J. Biomech., **17**, 749–755 (1984)
[WSF05]   Winters, B., Shepard, S., Foty, R.: Biophysical measurement of brain
           tumor cohesion. Int. J. Cancer, **114**, 371–379 (2005)
[YTC94]   Yang, M., Taber, L., Clark, E.: A nonlinear poroelastic model for the
           trabecular embryonic heart. J. Biomech. Engng., **116**, 213–223 (1994)

10

The Lymphatic Vascular System in Lymphangiogenesis, Invasion and Metastasis: A Mathematical Approach

Michael S. Pepper[1] and Georgios Lolas[2]

[1] Department of Immunology, Faculty of Health Sciences, University of Pretoria, and Netcare Institute of Cellular and Molecular Medicine,
Lifestyle Management Park, 223 Clifton Avenue, 0157 Lyttleton, South Africa
mpepper@doctors.netcare.co.za
[2] Technological and Educational Institute of Athens, Department of Mathematics, Ag. Spyridonos, 12210 Aigaleo, Athens, Greece
georgioslolas@hotmail.com

10.1 Introduction

Cancer growth involves many interrelated processes with varying spatio-temporal scales. There are two distinct phases of solid tumor growth: avascular and vascular. During the early avascular phase, solid tumors remain confined to the tissue in which they arise [1]. For an avascular tumor to grow, it needs a supply of nutrients, delivered by the blood. The tumor therefore secretes growth factors which induce the formation of new blood vessels from preexisting vasculature and directs them toward the tumor. The process by which vascularization occurs is called *angiogenesis* ([9], [16], [17], [18]). Cells of a vascularized tumor have the possibility to invade and destroy the surrounding tissues and, by exploiting the blood or the lymphatic systems, establish new colonies, a process called *metastasis* [19].

Metastasis is the most significant turning point in cancer. There are four major routes of neoplastic dissemination: (1) local invasion; (2) direct seeding of body cavities; (3) hematogenous spread; and (4) lymphatic spread, initially to regional lymph nodes and later to distant sites [50].

Targeting angiogenesis, namely, interrupting blood supply, is one of the strategies for blocking tumor growth and dissemination. A similar, although far less well-studied, process is referred to as *lymphangiogenesis* ([50], [56]). The lymphatic system comprises a vascular network of one-way, blind-ending, thin-walled capillaries leading into larger vessels, collecting vessels, lymph nodes, trunks, and ducts that transport lymph and cells from body tissues back to the circulatory system ([26], [46], [45]). Lymph is a protein-rich interstitial fluid drained from peripheral extracellular spaces, composed of inter-

N. Bellomo et al. (eds.), *Selected Topics in Cancer Modeling*,
DOI: 10.1007/978-0-8176-4713-1_10, © Springer Science+Business Media, LLC 2008

stitial fluid components, metabolites, and plasma proteins extravasated from blood capillaries, and cells from the immune system ([50], [27], [59]).

Over the past few years a major impetus in lymphangiogenesis research has come from the discovery of specific markers that could accurately differentiate blood endothelial cells (BECs) from lymphatic endothelial cells (LECs) ([50], [2], [22], [49]). These factors include VEGFR-3, a receptor for VEGFs -C and -D, well-defined lymphangiogenic factors [23]. VEGFR-3 is mainly restricted to LECs although it is expressed by blood vascular endothelium during early development ([74], [48], [25]). Other reliable lymphatic markers are LYVE-1 (lymphatic vessel endothelial hyaluronan receptor-1), podoplanin and Prox1 ([21], [20]).

Additionally, several forms of VEGF-C and VEGF-D are generated by proteolytic processing. Proteolytic processing increases their binding affinity to VEGFR-2 and VEGFR-3, cell surface receptors that are predominantly expressed on blood and lymphatic vascular endothelia, respectively [42]. Thus, proteolytically processed VEGF-C and VEGF-D have a dual role since they are able to induce both angiogenesis and lymphangiogenesis (see Fig. 10.1). VEGF-C also stimulates the migration of BECs and induces vascular permeability and endothelial cell proliferation, but is less effective than VEGF at equimolar concentrations [60].

Tumor angiogenesis and lymphangiogenesis provide new vessels that malignant cells can use to escape the confines of the primary tumor [29]. However, existing vessels also provide a mechanism of escape, and therefore the relative importance of preexisting versus new vessels is still to be determined [61]. Various studies have shown that angiogenesis is important for solid tumor growth and also in hematogenous metastasis [10]. In contrast, the role of lymphatic vessels and the relevance of lymphangiogenesis to tumor pathology is less clear. Until recently only limited information concerning the molecular mechanisms and pathways involved in tumor lymphangiogenesis and tumor lymphatic invasion had been obtained ([27], [50], [69], [70], [22]).

Unlike the blood vascular network, the lymphatic network does not provide nutrients to cells. It is, however, more conductive to tumor invasion and metastasis [54]. The lymphatic system is optimally suited for the entry and transport of cells (e.g., immune cells), and it also seems to have many advantages over the blood circulation as a pathway for tumor cell dissemination [46]. Even the smallest initial lymphatics are larger than blood capillaries. In comparison to blood vessels, lymphatic vessels have thinner walls and a poorly developed basement membrane, devoid of pericytes. Additionally, lymphatic vessel endothelium lacks tight junctions. LECs are equipped with overlapping junctions, which function as mechanical flap valves ([71], [26]). Anchoring filaments and collagen anchor the LECs into the surrounding connective tissue ([57]). Following an increase in interstitial fluid pressure, the anchoring filaments become stretched, thereby widening the lymphatic lumen. The LECs, which under normal conditions overlap, then move apart, effectively opening intercellular channels to allow fluid and macromolecules access to the

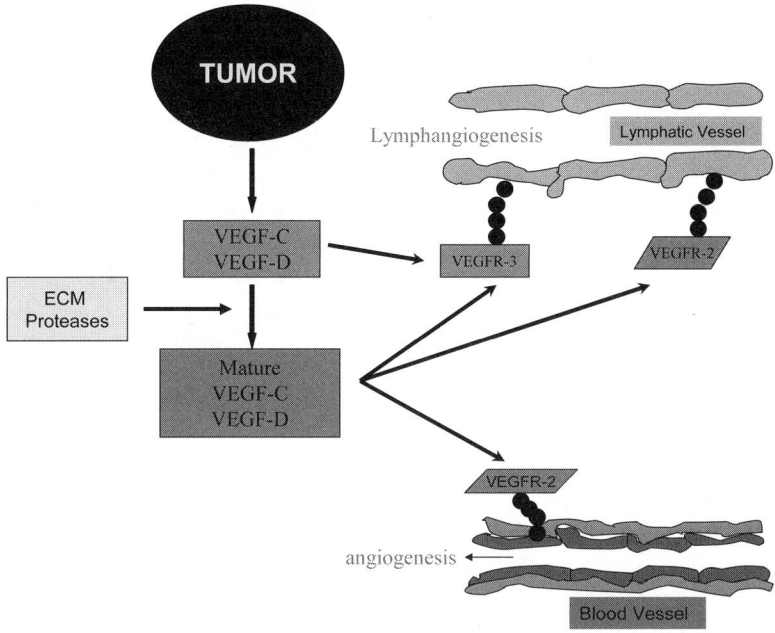

Fig. 10.1. The different effects that tumor-secreted VEGF-C and VEGF-D have on blood angiogenesis versus lymphangiogenesis are dependent on their protelytic processing by extracellular matrix proteases.

lymphatic lumen [71]. It has been speculated that this may contribute to the greater permeability of the lymphatic vessels. Flow velocities inside the lymphatic system are orders of magnitude lower than those observed in the blood system. Additionally, lymph composition is nearly identical to that of the interstitial fluid and in this regard is able to promote the viability of invading tumor cells ([50], [55]).

In contrast, the bloodstream is a highly aggressive medium for neoplastic cells due to serum toxicity, high shear stresses and mechanical deformation. Moreover, blood vessels have a more robust structure with a well-defined basement membrane and supporting cells [26]. As a consequence, hematogenous metastasis is a low-efficiency phenomenon, where a significant number of the neoplastic cells within bloodstream routes are quiescent or in apoptosis. Thus, altogether, the lymphatic system provides a much better environment than the blood vasculature for both the survival and metastatic efficiency of disseminating tumor cells. In addition, metastatic cells may reach the bloodstream via lymphatic-venous shunts, high endothelial venules inside lymph nodes or by lymphatic drainage into the thoracic duct ([50], [69]).

Until recently, nearly all investigations (both mathematical and biological) of metastatic mechanisms such as intravasation, survival, and extravasation, have focused on tumor cell behavior in the bloodstream ([33], [11], [12], [3], [47], [30], [32], [31]). However, from what has been presented above, there is an urgent need to understand the way in which tumor cells interact with lymphatics and the mechanism of lymphatic metastasis.

As mentioned above, until recently the lack of specific lymphatic markers and identified lymphangiogenic growth factors and their receptors has hampered progress in this field. Several recent studies have demonstrated that it is possible to culture pure populations of LECs, and that they are largely dependent on the activation of vascular endothelial growth factor receptor-3 (VEGFR-3) by one of its cytokine ligands, VEGF-C or VEGF-D ([28], [37], [65], [66], [68], [63]).

10.2 A Mathematical Model

In this section we present a mathematical model of lymphangiogenesis. The model consists of a coupled system of eight partial differential equations (PDEs) describing the evolution in time and space of the following key physical variables: tumor cell density (denoted by c); LEC density (denoted by e); extracellular matrix protein density (ECM) (denoted by m); urokinase plasminogen activator concentration (uPA) secreted by LECs (denoted by u_e), and by cancer cells (denoted by u_c); plasmin concentration activated by LECs (denoted by p_e), and by cancer cells (denoted by p_c); and vascular endothelial growth factor-C concentration (VEGF-C) (denoted by f). In the following we first give the model equations together with the employed initial and boundary conditions. Following that, we comment in more detail on some of the terms in the model equations.

$$
\frac{\partial c}{\partial t} = \underbrace{\nabla \cdot (D_c \nabla c)}_{dispersion} - \underbrace{\nabla \cdot (\zeta_c\, c\nabla u_c + \psi_c\, c\nabla p_c)}_{chemotaxis} - \underbrace{\nabla \cdot (\xi_c\, c\nabla m)}_{haptotaxis}
$$

$$
+ \underbrace{\mu_{11}\, c\,(1-c)}_{proliferation},
$$

$$
\frac{\partial e}{\partial t} = \underbrace{\nabla \cdot (D_e \nabla e)}_{dispersion} - \underbrace{\nabla \cdot (\chi_e e\, \nabla f + \zeta_e e\, \nabla u_e + \psi_e e\, \nabla p_e)}_{chemotaxis}
$$

$$
- \underbrace{\nabla \cdot (\xi_e e\, \nabla m)}_{haptotaxis} + \underbrace{\mu_{21}\, e\,(1-e) + \mu_{22}\, e f + \mu_{23}\, p_c f\, e}_{proliferation},
$$

$$
\frac{\partial m}{\partial t} = \underbrace{-\delta_{31}\, p_e\, m - \delta_{32}\, p_c\, m}_{proteolysis} + \underbrace{\mu_{31}\, m\,(1-m)}_{reestablishment},
$$

$$\tag{10.1}$$

$$\frac{\partial f}{\partial t} = \underbrace{D_f \nabla^2 f}_{diffusion} + \underbrace{\underbrace{\alpha_{41} c}_{secreted} + \underbrace{\alpha_{42} p_c f c}_{mature\,form} + \underbrace{\alpha_{43} p_c m f}_{mature\,form}}_{production}$$

$$- \underbrace{\underbrace{\beta_{41} e f}_{} - \underbrace{\beta_{42} p_c e f}_{}}_{neutralization} - \underbrace{\beta_{43} f}_{natural\,decay} \quad,$$

$$\frac{\partial u_e}{\partial t} = \underbrace{D_{u_e} \nabla^2 u_e}_{dispersion} + \underbrace{\alpha_{51} e + \alpha_{52} e f + \alpha_{53} p_c f e}_{production} - \underbrace{\beta_{51} e u_e}_{neutralization}$$

$$- \underbrace{\beta_{52} (p_e m + p_c m) u_e}_{inhibition} - \underbrace{\beta_{53} u_e}_{natural\,decay} \quad,$$

$$\frac{\partial u_c}{\partial t} = \underbrace{D_{u_c} \nabla^2 u_c}_{dispersion} + \underbrace{\alpha_{61} c}_{production} - \underbrace{\beta_{61} c u_c}_{neutralization} - \underbrace{\beta_{62} (p_c m + p_e m) u_c}_{inhibition}$$

$$- \underbrace{\beta_{63} u_c}_{natural\,decay} \quad,$$

$$\frac{\partial p_e}{\partial t} = \underbrace{D_{p_e} \nabla^2 p_e}_{diffusion} + \underbrace{\alpha_{71} e u_e}_{production} - \underbrace{\beta_{71} p_e}_{natural\,decay} \quad,$$

$$\frac{\partial p_c}{\partial t} = \underbrace{D_{p_c} \nabla^2 p_c}_{diffusion} + \underbrace{\alpha_{81} c u_c}_{production} - \underbrace{\beta_{81} p_c}_{natural\,decay} \quad.$$

These model equations coincide with those given in [35]. The non-dimensional system was obtained by rescaling distance with the maximum distance of the lymphatic vessels to the cancer cells at a typical stage of lymphangiogenesis $L := 0.1$–0.5 cm [10], time with $\tau = \frac{L^2}{D}$, where $D := 10^{-6}$ cm^2 s^{-1} [8] is a representative chemical diffusion coefficient, and with the dependent variables $e, c, m, f, u_c, u_e, p_c, p_e$ with appropriate reference cancer and lymphatic endothelial cell density e_o, c_o and reference concentration values $m_o, f_o, u_{c_o}, u_{e_o}, p_{c_o}, p_{e_o}$ in the nanomolar range, 1 nM $= 10^{-9}$ mol/l.

System (10.1) must be closed by appropriate initial and boundary conditions for each of the dependent variables. As for the initial conditions for system (10.1), we assume that initially (i) there is a cluster of LECs already present and a cluster of cancer cells that have penetrated just a short distance into the ECM; (ii) the concentrations of VEGF-C, cancer cell secreted urokinase, and cancer cell activated plasmin are proportional to the initial tumor density; and finally (iii) LEC-secreted urokinase as well as LEC-activated plasmin have not yet been secreted and activated, respectively. Specifically, the initial conditions for system (10.1) are taken to be

$$c(x,0) = \exp(\frac{-x^2}{\epsilon}), \ x \in [0,1] \text{ and } \epsilon > 0,$$

$$e(x,0) = \exp(\frac{-(x-1)^2}{\epsilon}), \ x \in [0,1] \text{ and } \epsilon > 0,$$

$$m(x,0) = 1 - \frac{1}{2} \exp(\frac{-x^2}{\epsilon}) - \frac{1}{2} \exp(\frac{-(x-1)^2}{\epsilon}), \ x \in [0,1] \text{ and } \epsilon > 0,$$

$$f(x,0) = \frac{1}{10} \exp(\frac{-x^2}{\epsilon}), \ x \in [0,1] \text{ and } \epsilon > 0,$$

(10.2)

$$u_e(x,0) = 0, \ x \in [0,1],$$

$$u_c(x,0) = \frac{1}{20} \exp(\frac{-x^2}{\epsilon}), \ x \in [0,1] \text{ and } \epsilon > 0,$$

$$p_e(x,0) = 0, \ x \in [0,1],$$

$$p_c(x,0) = \frac{1}{20} \exp(\frac{-x^2}{\epsilon}), \ x \in [0,1] \text{ and } \epsilon > 0,$$

where throughout this chapter we have taken $\epsilon = 0.01$.

We assume that cancer cells, LECs, uPA, plasmin and VEGF-C remain within the domain of tissue under consideration and therefore zero-flux boundary conditions are imposed. For the ECM density no boundary conditions can be prescribed.

We now give a description of the fundamental biological interactions that are known to occur during lymphangiogenesis and are presented in the model. A full description may be found in [35].

(a) Cancer Cells. It is well known that prognosis in cancer patients is primarily dependent on the ability of the tumor to invade and metastasize. A crucial component of these processes is the dissolution of the ECM by tumor cell-associated proteases. In addition, invasive cells *in vivo* adhere to surrounding ECM molecules via specific receptors such as integrins and produce and secrete uPA as well as activate other proteases such as matrix metalloproteinases (MMPs) ([4], [5], [58]).

A major protease system responsible for ECM degradation is the plasminogen activation (PA) system which generates the potent serine protease plasmin ([34], [13], [64]). uPA is an extracellular protease. Cells including macrophages, endothelial cells and tumor cells secrete its enzymatically inactive pro-uPA into the extracellular space. pro-uPA is activated by plasmin to its active form uPA. The binding of uPA to the cancer cell membrane-anchored urokinase receptor (uPAR) accelerates plasminogen activation and, hence, generates plasmin, a serine protease capable of digesting directly or indirectly, most basement membrane and ECM proteins. Plasmin itself is a broadly acting enzyme that not only catalyzes the breakdown of many of the known ECM and basement membrane molecules, such as vitronectin, fibrin, laminin and collagens, but also may activate metalloproteinases. Thus, the unrestrained generation of plasmin from plasminogen by the action of uPA is potentially hazardous to cells, since this destroys their mechanical and chemical scaffold required for adhesion and migration.

ECM degradation allows the cells to move into the spaces thereby created, and also sets up tissue gradients, which the cells then exploit to move forward ([38], [39], [40], [72], [6], [7]). Movement up concentration gradients of ECM has been reported as a mechanism enabling movement through tissues by a variety of cell types. Tumor cell motility toward high concentrations/densities of substratum-bound insolubilized components is termed *haptotaxis*.

Another cause of tumor cell motility is *chemotaxis* whereby tumor cells undergo migration in the direction of a gradient of a soluble attractant [72]. Tumors secrete a number of diffusible chemical substances such as uPA into the surrounding tissues and ECM to which cancer cells respond chemotactically ([4], [5]).

We assume that there is a change in cell number density due to dispersion: cells disperse from higher to lower densities in a random motion with diffusion coefficient D_c. The flux arising from this random motion is

$$\mathbf{J_{random}} = -D_c \nabla c .$$

We shall choose D_c to be constant.

The second important term that quantifies the change in cell number density is that of the directional flow of cells due to spatial gradients of environmental stimuli, such as those stimulating chemotactic or haptotactic responses mentioned above. To incorporate these responses into our mathematical model we take the cancer cell flux (due to gradients) to be

$$\mathbf{J_{flux}} = \mathbf{J_{chemo}} + \mathbf{J_{hapto}} ,$$

where

$$\mathbf{J_{chem}} = \zeta_c\, c \nabla u_c + \psi_c\, c \nabla p_c, \quad \mathbf{J_{hapt}} = \xi_c\, c \nabla m ,$$

ζ_c and ψ_c are the chemotactic coefficients and ξ_c is the haptotactic coefficient; these coefficients are positive, and for simplicity we assume that they are constant.

Regarding the proliferation of cancer cells, we assume that this satisfies a logistic growth law. Hence the resulting PDE for cancer cell motion is

$$\frac{\partial c}{\partial t} = \underbrace{\nabla \cdot (D_c \nabla c)}_{dispersion} - \underbrace{\nabla \cdot (\zeta_c\, c \nabla u_c + \psi_c\, c \nabla p_c)}_{chemotaxis} - \underbrace{\nabla \cdot (\xi_c\, c \nabla m)}_{haptotaxis}$$

$$+ \underbrace{\mu_{11}\, c\, (1 - c)}_{proliferation} ,$$

(10.3)

where μ_{11} is the proliferation rate of the cancer cells.

(b) Lymphatic Endothelial Cells. LECs in the neighboring lymphatic vessels secrete matrix degrading enzymes in response to cancer cell secreted lymphangiogenic stimulus (*e.g.* VEGF-C). The dominating factors governing LEC migration are random motion, chemotaxis due to VEGF-C secreted by the cancer cells ([44], [36]), uPA and plasmin as well as haptotaxis due to VN or other ECM proteins [64]. Besides migration, LEC mitosis is also included in the model in the form of a logistic type growth $e\,(1-e)$. Moreover, LEC proliferation is also increased by unproteolytically and proteolytically processed VEGF-C at a rate proportional to $e\,f$ and $e\,p_c\,f$ respectively since it has been shown experimentally ([27], [46], [44]) that proteolytically and unproteolytically processed VEGF-C can lead to the proliferation and enlargement of peritumoral and intratumoral lymphatic vessels. The above considerations lead to the following equation for lymphatic endothelial cells:

$$\frac{\partial e}{\partial t} = \underbrace{\nabla \cdot (D_e \nabla e)}_{dispersion} - \underbrace{\nabla \cdot (\chi_e e\,\nabla f + \zeta_e e\,\nabla u_e + \psi_e e\,\nabla p_e)}_{chemotaxis}$$

$$\underbrace{- \nabla \cdot (\xi_e e\,\nabla m)}_{haptotaxis} + \underbrace{\mu_{21}\,e\,(1-e) + \mu_{22}\,e f + \mu_{23}\,p_c f\,e}_{proliferation}\,,$$

(10.4)

where D_e is a diffusion coefficient, χ_e, ζ_e, ψ_e and ξ_e are the chemotactic and haptotactic coefficients, respectively, while μ_{21}, μ_{22}, μ_{23} are proliferation coefficients. We assume that D_e, χ_e, ζ_e, ψ_e, ξ_e, μ_{21}, μ_{22} and μ_{23} are positive constants.

(c) Extracellular Matrix. It is known that the ECM does not diffuse and therefore we omit any diffusion term (or other "migration" terms) from its model equation. However, the ECM is not "static" in the sense that it is continually produced and remodelled. Furthermore, based on the experimental evidence ([4], [5]) that uPA activates plasminogen to its cell-surface associated form plasmin, which in turn catalyzes the breakdown of VN as well as other ECM proteins, we model the fact that plasmin degrades VN upon contact at a (degradation) rate $\delta_{31}\,p_e m$, $\delta_{32}\,p_c m$ to represent the rates of degradation due to plasmin generation that is regulated by the lymphatic endothelial and cancer cells, respectively.

Moreover, we suggest that ECM components reestablish or remodel in a logistic manner similar to that described above for cancer cell proliferation. Using a logistic growth with rate constant μ_{31} to describe ECM renewal, and taking $\delta_{31}\,p_e m$, $\delta_{32}\,p_c m$ to represent the rates of degradation due to plasmin regulated by lymphatic endothelial and cancer cells, respectively, we have the following equation for the ECM:

$$\frac{\partial m}{\partial t} = \underbrace{-\delta_{31}\, p_e\, m \,-\, \delta_{32}\, p_c\, m}_{proteolysis} \,+\, \underbrace{\mu_{31}\, m\,(1-m)}_{reestablishment} \;.$$ (10.5)

(d) Vascular Endothelial Growth Factor-C (VEGF-C). VEGF-C with concentration $f(x,t)$ is released rapidly by the solid tumor and diffuses into the surrounding tissue ([23], [24]). As stated already in the Introduction, both VEGF-C and VEGF-D stimulate lymphangiogenesis in tissues as well as in tumors by activating LEC surface tyrosine kinase receptors VEGFR-3 and VEGFR-2. For simplicity we shall focus our attention only on VEGF-C.

Proteolytic cleavage removes the propeptide forms of tumor secreted VEGF-C to generate mature forms that bind LEC surface receptors such as VEGFR-3 (or VEGFR-2) with much greater affinity than the full-length cancer-cell secreted VEGF-C (VEGF-D) forms [24]. In fact, McColl [41] reported that the serine protease plasmin cleaved both cancer secreted VEGF-C and VEGF-D propeptides and thereby generated a mature form exhibiting greatly enhanced binding and cross linking of VEGFR-2 and VEGFR-3 in comparison to full-length secreted VEGF-C and VEGF-D ($\alpha_{42}p_c cf$). Additionally, regarding the process of angiogenesis it has been demonstrated by Oh [43] and Pepper [53] that the process of ECM degradation by plasmin leads to the release and cleavage of matrix-bound latent cytokines, such as VEGF. Therefore, we assume that tumor-activated plasmin can also release and cleave matrix-bound VEGF-C during the process of tumor ECM proteolysis ($\alpha_{43}p_c mf$).

We shall therefore assume that cancer cell regulated plasmin proteolytically cleaves tumor secreted and ECM-bound VEGF-C to generate its mature VEGF-C form.

We also assume that VEGF-C undergoes some form of decay, either natural ($\beta_{43}f$) or proportional to the neutralization of proteolytically and unproteolytically processed VEGF-C by its binding to the LEC surface receptor VEGFR-3 ($\beta_{41}\, f\, e$, $\beta_{42}p_c\, f\, e$). Summarizing, we have

$$\frac{\partial f}{\partial t} = \underbrace{D_f\,\nabla^2 f}_{diffusion} \,+\, \underbrace{\underbrace{\alpha_{41}\, c}_{secreted} \,+\, \underbrace{\alpha_{42}\, p_c\, c f}_{mature\, form} \,+\, \underbrace{\alpha_{43}\, p_c\, m f}_{mature\, form}}_{production} \,-\, \underbrace{\beta_{41}\, e\, f \,-\, \beta_{42}\, p_c\, e\, f}_{neutralization}$$

(10.6)

$$-\, \underbrace{\beta_{43}\, f}_{natural\, decay} \;.$$

(e) uPA in Lymphatic Endothelial Cells. Pepper ([51], [52]) demonstrated that angiogenic cytokines such as bFGF and VEGF increase uPA and uPAR expression in bovine lymphatic endothelial (BLE) cells in a manner very similar to that described for endothelial cells derived from the blood vascular system.

In a more recent paper, Tille [73] showed that this effect (*i.e.* regulation of the plasminogen activation system) is mediated by the binding of VEGF-C to its receptors. Although other proteolytic systems may be involved, we have used the PA-plasmin system in our model.

Therefore, factors influencing the LEC regulated uPA concentration are assumed to be diffusion, uPA production and uPA neutralization and decay. During its secretion by the LECs ($\alpha_{51} e$) uPA diffuses throughout the ECM, with constant diffusion coefficient D_{u_e}, while uPA production is also enhanced by the binding of proteolytically and unproteolytically cleaved VEGF-C to the LEC surface receptor VEGFR-3, and this is represented by terms $\alpha_{52} e f$ and $\alpha_{53} p_c e f$. Moreover, urokinase is decreased by natural decay ($\beta_{53} u_e$), by its neutralization via its binding to the LEC surface receptor uPAR ($\beta_{51} u_e e$), and indirectly via its inhibition by PAI-1 that is activated by the process of plasmin degrading the ECM ($\beta_{52} (p_e m + p_c m) u_e$). The equation governing the evolution of uPA concentration is therefore given by

$$
\frac{\partial u_e}{\partial t} = \underbrace{D_{u_e} \nabla^2 u_e}_{dispersion} + \underbrace{\alpha_{51} e + \alpha_{52} e f + \alpha_{53} p_c f e}_{production} - \underbrace{\beta_{51} e u_e}_{neutralization}
$$

$$
- \underbrace{\beta_{52} (p_e m + p_c m) u_e}_{inhibition} - \underbrace{\beta_{53} u_e}_{natural\,decay} \quad .
$$

(10.7)

(f) uPA by the Cancer Cells. Cancers possess the ability to actively invade peritumoral local tissue. Mimicking the proteolysis of the extracellular space by LECs, cancer cells also secrete urokinase plasminogen activator ($\alpha_{61} c$) which diffuses throughout the peritumoral extracellular space, with constant diffusion coefficient D_{u_c} ([4], [5]). Additionally, cancer cell secreted uPA undergoes some form of decay either natural ($\beta_{63} u_c$), or in proportion to its neutralization by its binding to the cancer cell surface receptor (uPAR) ($\beta_{61} u_c c$). Cancer cell secreted uPA concentration is decreased even further by its inhibition by PAI-1 which in turn is activated by cancer and LEC regulated plasmin degradation of peritumoral tissue ($\beta_{62} (p_c m + p_e m) u_c$). Under the aforementioned assumptions the equation governing cancer cell secreted uPA concentration is given by

$$
\frac{\partial u_c}{\partial t} = \underbrace{D_{u_c} \nabla^2 u_c}_{dispersion} + \underbrace{\alpha_{61} c}_{production} - \underbrace{\beta_{61} c u_c}_{neutralization} - \underbrace{\beta_{62} (p_c m + p_e m) u_c}_{inhibition}
$$

(10.8)

$$
+ \underbrace{\beta_{63} u_c}_{natural\,decay} \quad .
$$

(g) Plasmin by the Lymphatic Endothelial Cells. In examining the spatio-temporal evolution of plasmin concentration, we assume that it also diffuses. Furthermore, we assume that the binding of LEC secreted uPA to its LEC surface receptor (uPAR) provides the LEC with potential proteolytic activity via activation of plasminogen, and thus enhances the rate of plasmin formation ($\alpha_{71} u_e e$) ([4], [5]). Finally, the term ($\beta_{72} p_c$) models the deactivation of plasmin either by natural decay or by the action of the plasmin inhibitor α_2-antiplasmin. Hence we have

$$\frac{\partial p_e}{\partial t} = \underbrace{D_{p_e} \nabla^2 p_e}_{diffusion} + \underbrace{\alpha_{71} e\, u_e}_{production} - \underbrace{\beta_{71} p_e}_{natural\, decay} \quad . \tag{10.9}$$

(h) Plasmin by the Cancer Cells. Plasmin regulation by cancer cells is assumed to diffuse with a constant diffusion coefficient D_{p_c}, and to be produced through the binding of cancer cell secreted uPA to its cancer cell surface receptor uPAR ($\alpha_{81} c\, u_c$). Additionally, cancer cell generated plasmin undergoes some form of natural decay ($\beta_{82} p_c$). Hence we have

$$\frac{\partial p_c}{\partial t} = \underbrace{D_{p_c} \nabla^2 p_c}_{diffusion} + \underbrace{\alpha_{81} c\, u_c}_{production} - \underbrace{\beta_{81} p_c}_{natural\, decay} \quad . \tag{10.10}$$

The lymphangiogenesis model that was first presented by [35] and is also analyzed here shares common features with the angiogenesis models presented by Chaplain and co-workers and Levine and co-workers ([11], [12], [3], [30], [32], [31]). However, there are also some significant differences.

Angiogenesis results in tumor growth, but the models developed so far do not incorporate this feature. In contrast, the lymphatic system does not directly provide nutrients to tumor cells, lymphangiogenesis is not essential for tumor growth and therefore there is less of a need to incorporate tumor growth into the lymphangiogenesis model.

The continuum models of both angiogenesis and lymphangiogenesis can only describe the corresponding vasculatures in terms of the concentration of endothelial and lymphatic endothelial cells. However, blood vasculature is a closed system and thus angiogenesis requires an account of anastomosis whereas the lymphatic system is a unidirectional system, and anastomoses less frequently.

Unlike VEGF in angiogenesis, VEGF-C in both angiogenesis and lymphangiogenesis does not appear to be regulated by hypoxia but rather by numerous pro-inflammatory cytokines (*e.g.* interleukin) ([14], [60]).

Lymphatic vessels remain intact at least for up to 6 months and in many mice for up to one year, while new capillary blood vessels in the cornea usually begin to regress about two weeks after growth factors have become depleted [10]. For this reason we shall carry out subsequent calculations for several weeks.

10.3 Numerical Results

In this section we show numerical results for model (10.1) in one space dimension together with the initial conditions and zero-flux conditions given in Section 10.2 using the NAG library subroutine D03PCF. Routine D03PCF is a method of lines (MOL) discretization for parabolic PDEs in one space variable using standard central finite differences for the discretization in space and backward differentiation formulas for the time stepping. Typically we take 1501 spatial points in $[0, 1]$ while the accuracy in the time integration is 1.0×10^{-5}.

In the simulations of Figs. 10.2–10.4, we consider a default set of parameters which are given by: $D_e = 1.05 \times 10^{-4}$, $D_c = 9.75 \times 10^{-5}$, $D_f = 5 \times 10^{-3}$, $D_{u_e} = 1.75 \times 10^{-3}$, $D_{u_c} = 1.75 \times 10^{-3}$, $D_{p_e} = 1.12 \times 10^{-3}$, $D_{p_c} = 1.12 \times 10^{-3}$, $\chi_e = 3.05 \times 10^{-2}$, $\xi_e = 9.5 \times 10^{-3}$, $\zeta_e = 8.75 \times 10^{-3}$, $\psi_e = 5.7510^{-3}$, $\xi_c = 3.5 \times 10^{-3}$, $\zeta_c = 7.85 \times 10^{-3}$, $\psi_c = 6.85 \times 10^{-3}$, $\delta_{31} = 3.25$, $\delta_{32} = 0.25$, $\alpha_{41} = 0.15$, $\alpha_{42} = 0.4$, $\alpha_{43} = 0.015$, $\alpha_{51} = 0.015$, $\alpha_{52} = 0.05$, $\alpha_{53} = 0.35$, $\alpha_{61} = 0.25$, $\alpha_{71} = 2.075$, $\alpha_{81} = 2.915$, $\beta_{41} = 0.05$, $\beta_{42} = 0.35$, $\beta_{43} = 0.25$, $\beta_{51} = 3.35$, $\beta_{52} = 0.105$, $\beta_{53} = 0.35$, $\beta_{61} = 3.315$, $\beta_{62} = 0.125$, $\beta_{63} = 0.475$, $\beta_{71} = 0.785$, $\beta_{81} = 0.55$, $\mu_{11} = 0.1335$, $\mu_{21} = 0.1135$, $\mu_{22} = 0.05$, $\mu_{23} = 0.035$, $\mu_{31} = 0.0535$.

In Fig. 10.2, at $t = 5$ (~ 14 hours), we note that large clusters of both the lymphatic endothelial and the cancer cells have migrated a short distance into the extracellular space; cancer cells secrete uPA and VEGF-C while they activate plasmin in order to degrade the peritumoral space. By $t = 15$ (~ 2 days), a large custer of LECs has already been formed at the leading edge and migrates chemotactically mainly in response to cancer cells secreted VEGF-C.

As time evolves, at $t = 24$ (≈ 3 days) in Fig. 10.3, two large clusters of LEC have formed at the leading and the rear edge of the lymphatic network. By $t = 35$ (≈ 4 days), the leading edge of the LEC is already in the inter- and peri-tumoral space and there is increased proliferation of the leading clusters of LEC due to increased amounts of VEGF-C present. By $t = 50$ (≈ 5.7 days), two different clusters of cancer cells have been formed as a consequence of cancer cell proliferation. By $t = 90$ (≈ 10.5 days), a lymphatic endothelial cell network has been established in the whole intra- and peri-tumoral space.

As time evolves, at $t = 160$ (≈ 18.5 days) in Fig. 10.4, several clusters of lymphatic endothelial and cancer cells have formed. The spatial heterogeneity of cancer and lymphatic endothelial cells is still evident by $t = 250$ (≈ 29 days) as a result of the dynamic activity of the interactions between lymphatic growth factors, proteases, ECM, cancer cells and LECs ([15], [67]).

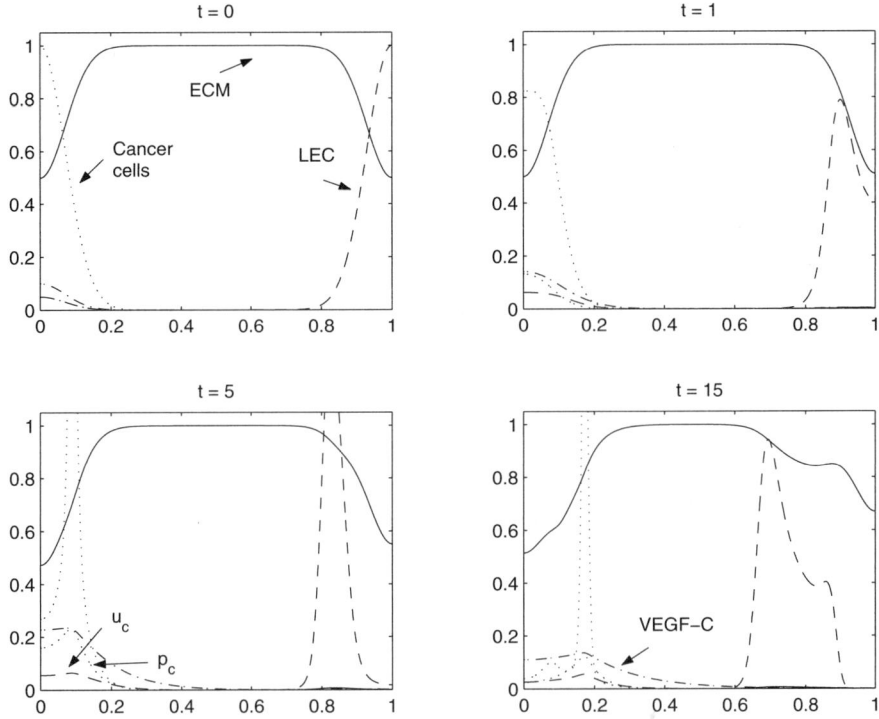

Fig. 10.2. Sequence of profiles showing the evolution of the tumor cell density $c(x,t)$ (dotted black line), the LEC density $e(x,t)$ (dashed black line), the ECM density $m(x,t)$ (solid black line), the VEGF-C concentration $f(x,t)$ (dot-dashed black line), the cancer cells secreted uPA concentration $u_c(x,t)$ (dashed black line), the cancer cells activated plasmin $p_c(x,t)$ (dotted black line), the LEC secreted uPA concentration $u_e(x,t)$ (dot-dashed black line) and LEC activated plasmin concentration $p_e(x,t)$ (solid black line).

Our model can be used to simulate the effects of anti-lymphangiogenic drugs on the progress of tumor lymphangiogenesis and tumor invasion into the lymphatic system. We shall demonstrate this with one example.

It has been suggested that the secretion of VEGF-C by cancer cells, as well as its proteolytic cleavage by cancer cell activated plamsin, is a special candidate for anti-lymphangiogenic strategies. In order to reduce the chemotactic effect of VEGF-C at the parental lymphatic vessel, we may inject a soluble form of the LEC receptor-3 (VEGFR-3) into the peritumoral space. We model this by setting $\beta_{43} = 5.0$.

The forced decay of naturally secreted VEGF-C would also result in a decrease in VEGF-C binding to LEC receptors, in both cancer cells and LECs. We model this by taking $\beta_{41} = 0.025$, $\beta_{42} = 0.175$, $\alpha_{52} = 0.025$, $\alpha_{53} = 0.175$. The forced reduction of VEGF-C will also affect the effect that proteolytically

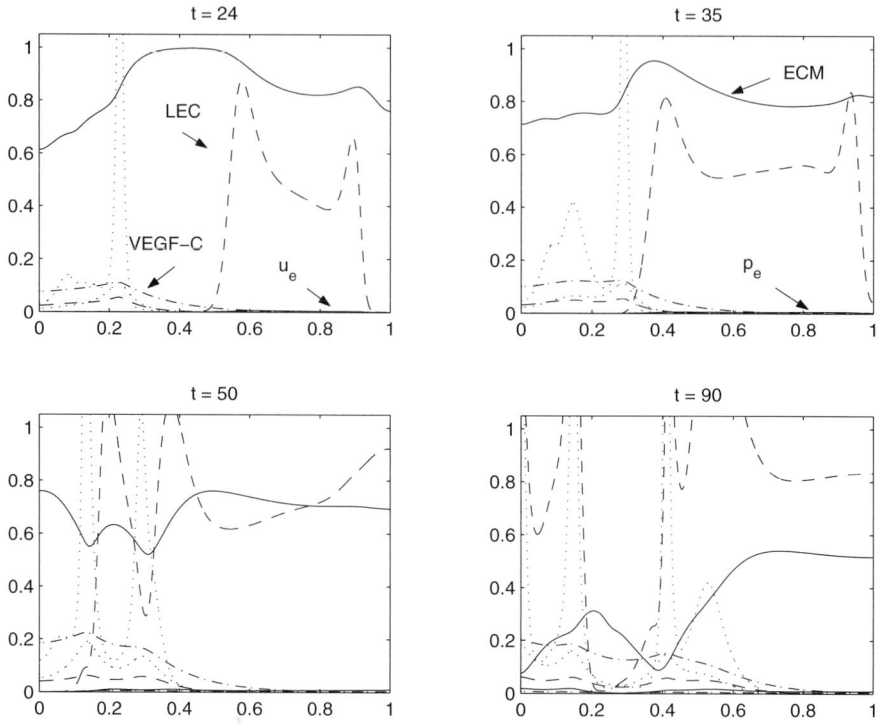

Fig. 10.3. Further sequence of profiles subsequent to Fig. 10.2, with the same notation.

and unproteolytically processed VEGF-C has in LEC proliferation, and we therefore chose $\mu_{22} = 0.025$, $\mu_{23} = 0.175$.

It has been shown that the proteolytic cleavage of VEGF-C and VEGF-D increases their binding affinity to LEC VEGFRs. Therefore, by blocking cancer and lymphatic endothelial cell secreted uPA using soluble forms of the plasminogen activator inhibitor-1 (PAI-1), we can reduce plasmin formation and subsequently matrix degradation as well. We incorporate the above effects by setting $\beta_{53} = 6.7$, $\beta_{63} = 9.5$, $\beta_{71} = 15.7$, $\beta_{81} = 11.0$.

Reducing uPA and plasmin formation will result in a reduction of their binding constants to their respective ligands. We model this by setting $\beta_{52} = 1.675$, $\beta_{62} = 1.675$, $\alpha_{71} = 0.2075$, $\alpha_{81} = 0.2915$.

Fig. 10.5 shows the result of the above changes in the model parameters resulting from the injection of soluble forms of VEGFR-3 and PAI-1. Comparing Fig. 10.5 with Figs. 10.2–10.4 we see, for example, that in Fig. 10.3, at $t = 35$ (~ 4 days) the LECs have already migrated through more than half of the domain, while in Fig. 10.5 they have migrated appreciably less; at

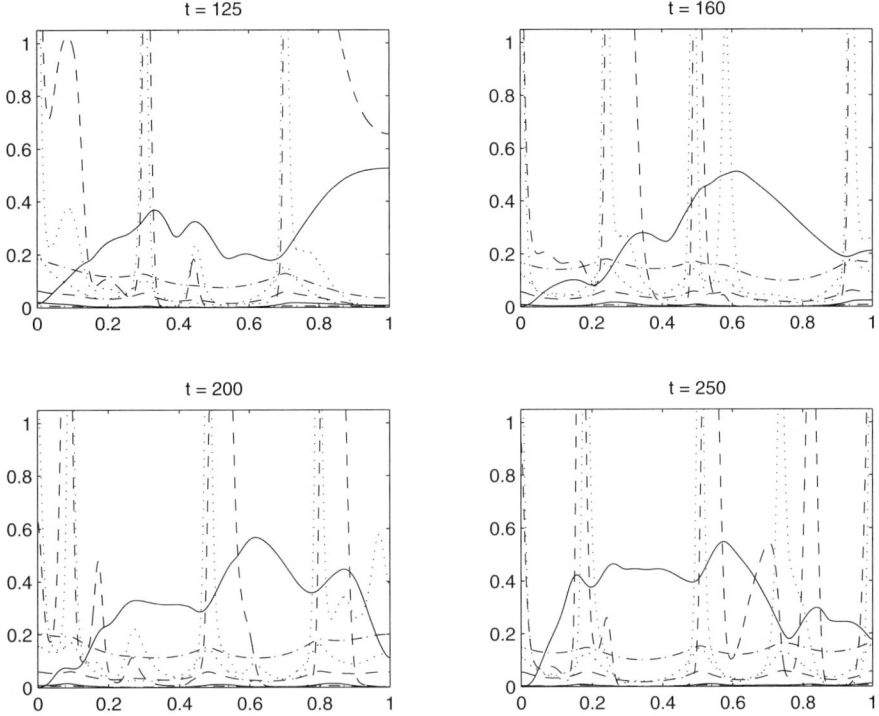

Fig. 10.4. Sequence of profiles subsequent to Fig. 10.2, with the same notation.

$t = 90$ (~ 10 days) in Fig. 10.3 the profile of LECs is highly heterogeneous, whereas in Fig. 10.5 their profile is approximately Gaussian.

10.4 Conclusions

In this chapter we have formulated and developed a continuum model of tumor lymphangiogenesis based on recent experimental results. The model consists of eight PDEs for the densities of tumor and lymphatic endothelial cells, the concentrations of ECM macromolecules, the concentrations of vascular endothelial growth factor and the concentrations of urokinase plasminogen activator and plasmin secreted and activated respectively by both tumor and lymphatic endothelial cells.

A key biological focus of the model is lymphangiogenesis and invasion of tissue. The lymphatic system plays an important role in tumor invasion and metastasis. Recent experimental evidence has established a connection between the tumor and lymphangiogenesis in its vicinity. For this reason it is important to develop a mathematical model for the growth of lymphatic

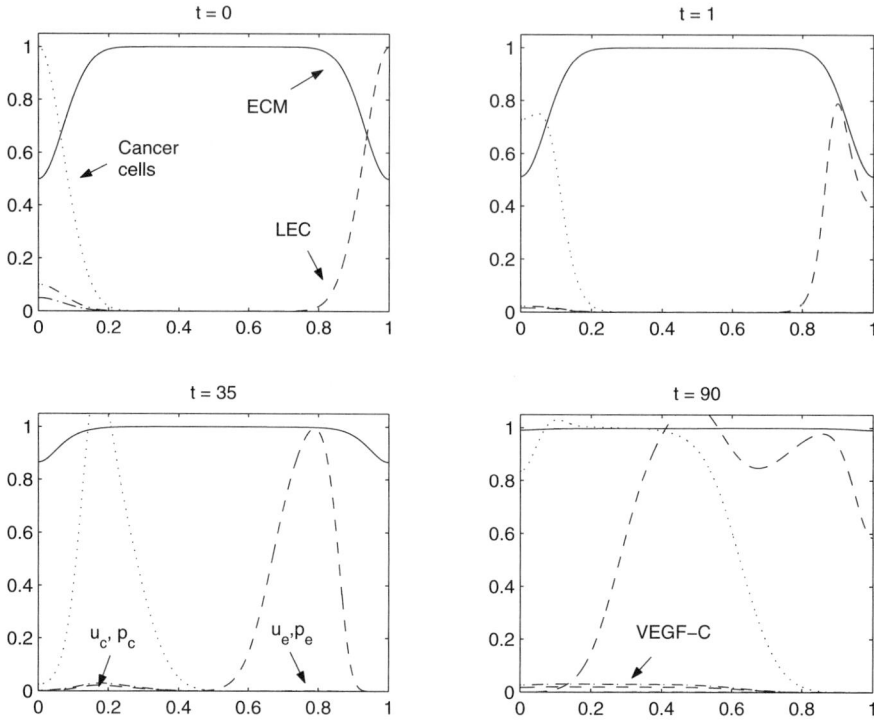

Fig. 10.5. Sequence of profiles showing the evolution of the same densities and concentrations as in Figs. 10.2–10.4, with the change of parameters resulting from anti-lymphangiogenic potential drugs mentioned above.

vessels caused by tumor secreted lymphatic growth factors. Since it is difficult to account directly for the growth of new vessels, we have taken the approach of viewing the lymphatic system as a density of LECs. A very important role in the model is attributed to tumor-activated plasmin. Tumor-activated plasmin not only proteolytically cleaves tumor secreted VEGF-C and therefore produces its mature form which binds with high affinity to the lymphatic specific endothelial cell surface receptor VEGFR-3, but it can also, via its role as an ECM degrading protease release matrix-bound inactive VEGF-C.

Although there is no *in vivo* evidence regarding the activation of urokinase plasminogen activator secreted by the LECs as well as plasmin activation by them as a result of tumor secreted VEGF-C, we take our model one step further, assuming that the plasminogen activation system behaves in the same way that has been experimentally established for endothelial cells.

We have simulated our model in the one-dimensional case and have shown that, ("dynamic") spatio-temporal heterogeneity does clearly develop within

20 days with very sharp levels of densities of LECs in several locations. Thus the model produces what may be viewed as a network of lymphatic vessels.

In our model, we have worked on the basis that lymphangiogenesis is occurring in and around tumors. We do however recognize that many tumors utilize preexisting lymphatics as a means to disseminate tumor cells. In this case, VEGF-C may also be important in that it may alter the function of preexisting endothelial cells (for example by altering endothelial to tumor cell adhesion or by producing chemokines), as may the role of uPA and plasmin in activating VEGF-C. In other words, our model may also be indirectly applicable to preexisting lymphatics in the absence of lymphangiogenesis.

Tumors are heterogeneous in the fact that they consist of subpopulations of neoplastic cells with different metastatic, migration, and invasion potential relative to the newly formed lymphatic vessels. Our simulation captures this tumor heterogeneity: mimicking lymphatic endothelial heterogeneity, we observe proliferative cancer cells near the LECs already within 20 days. Thus although lymphangiogenesis is essentially a two- (*in vitro*) or three-dimensional (*in vivo*) process, our one-dimensional results already successfully uncover the complex dynamics following tumor lymphangiogenesis.

In terms of future work and model development, we note that the model considered in this paper has some limitations. Future work will deal with this and we now comment on these limitations briefly. The model presented here does not take into consideration any competition for space. Cancer cells, ECM and LECs all take up space and compete with each other for it. In a future model we will therefore consider taxis terms which prevent overcrowding, and also have the (cancer and lymphatic endothelial) cell proliferation and ECM remodelling terms obey spatial restrictions.

Other effects of the lymphatic vascular system and its relation to lymphangiogenesis, invasion and metastasis which are observed biologically will also be considered for inclusion in the model. One example would be to incorporate the role of the plasminogen activator inhibitor-1 (PAI-1), α_2-antiplasmin and tumor-associated macrophages into the model. Recently, Schoppmann [62] identified tumor-associated macrophages (TAMs) producing VEGF-C and VEGF-D while they also expressed VEGFR-3. These macrophages could play a novel role in peritumoral lymphangiogenesis and subsequent tumor cell dissemination in human cancer. Co-expression of VEGF-C, VEGF-D and their receptor by the same cell provide an autocrine regulatory system within the peritumoral stroma and a potential stimulus for peritumoral lymphangiogenesis.

Finally, we show how lymphatic invasion and spatio-temporal heterogeneity can be slowed down by injecting VEGFR-3 into the peritumoral space or increasing PAI-1 and α_2-antiplasmin. Thus this model can be used as a tool for examining the effect of potential anti-cancer drugs.

References

1. Alberts, B., Bray, D., Lewis, J., Raff, M., Roberts, K., and Watson, J.D.: Molecular Biology of the Cell, Garland Publishing, New York (1994).
2. Alitalo, K., and Carmeliet, P.: Molecular mechanisms of lymphangiogenesis in health and disease, *Cancer Cell*, **1**, 219–227 (2002).
3. Anderson, A.R.A., and Chaplain, M.A.J.: Continuous and discrete mathematical models of tumor induced angiogenesis, *Bulletin of Mathematical Biology*, **60**, 857–899 (1998).
4. Andreasen, P.A., Kjøller, L., Christensen, L. and Duffy, M.J.: The urokinase-type plasminogen activator system in cancer metastasis: A review, *International Journal of Cancer*, **72**, 1–22 (1997).
5. Andreasen, P.A., Egelund, R., and Petersen, H.H.: The plasminogen activation system in tumor growth, invasion, and metastasis, *Cellular and Molecular Life Sciences*, **57**, 25–40 (2000).
6. Aznavoorian, S., Stracke, M.L., Krutzsch, H., Schiffmann, E., and Liotta, L.A.: Signal transduction for chemotaxis and haptotaxis by matrix molecules in tumor cells, *Journal of Cell Biology*, **110**, 1427–1438 (1990).
7. Aznavoorian, S., Stracke, M.L., Persons, J., McClanahan, J., and Liotta, L.A.: Integrin $\alpha_v\beta_3$ mediates chemotactic and haptotactic motility in human melanoma cells through different signaling pathways, *Journal of Biological Chemistry*, **271**, 3247–3254 (1996).
8. Bray, D.: *Cell Movements from Molecules to Motility*, Garland Publishing, New York (2000).
9. Carmeliet, P., and Jain, R.K.: Angiogenesis in cancer and other diseases, *Nature*, **407**, 249–257 (2000)
10. Chang, L., Kaipainen, A., and Folkman, J.: Lymphangiogenesis new mechanisms, *Annals New York Academy of Sciences*, **979**, 111–119 (2002).
11. Chaplain, M.A.J.: Avascular growth, angiogenesis and vascular growth in solid tumours: The mathematical modelling of the stages of tumour development, *Mathematical and Computer Modelling*, **23**, 47–87 (1996).
12. Chaplain, M.A.J.: Mathematical modelling of angiogenesis, *Journal of Neuro-Oncology*, **50**, 37–51 (2000).
13. Chaplain, M.A.J., and Lolas, G.: Mathematical modelling of cancer cell invasion of tissue: The role of the urokinase plasminogen activation system, *Mathematical Models and Methods in Applied Sciences*, **15** (11), 1685–1734 (2005).
14. Enholm, B., Paavonen, K., Ristimäki, A., Kumar, V., Gunji, Y., Klefstrom, J., Kivinen, L., Laiho, M., Olofsson, B., Joukov, V., Eriksson, U., and Alitalo, K.: Comparison of VEGF, VEGF-B, VEGF-C and Ang-1 mRNA regulation by serum, growth factors, oncoproteins and hypoxia, *Oncogene*, **14**, 2475–2483 (1997).
15. Fidler, I.J.: Tumor heterogeneity and the biology of cancer invasion and metastasis, *Cancer Research*, **38**, 2651–2660 (1978).
16. Folkman, J.: Tumor angiogenesis: Therapeutic implications, *New England Journal of Medicine*, **285**, 1182–1186 (1971).
17. Folkman, J.: The vascularization of tumors, *Scientific American*, **234**, 58–73 (1976).
18. Folkman, J.: Tumor angiogenesis, In: *Cancer Medicine,* Bast, R.C., Kufe, D.W., Pollock, R.E., Weichselbaum, R.R., Holland, J.F., Frei, E., and Gansler, T.S., editors, Decker, Ontario, Canada, 132–152 (2000).

19. Hanahan, D., and Weinberg, R.A.: The hallmarks of cancer, *Cell*, **100**, 57–70 (2000).

20. Hong, Y.-H., and Detmar, M.: Prox1, master regulator of the lymphatic vasculature phenotype, *Cell & Tissue Research*, **314**, 85–92 (2003).

21. Jackson, D.G., Prevo, R., Clasper, S., and Banerji, S.: LYVE-1, the lymphatic system and tumor lymphangiogenesis, *TRENDS in Immunology*, **22**, 317–321 (2001).

22. Ji, R-C.: Lymphatic endothelial cells, tumor lymphangiogenesis and metastasis: New insights into intratumoral and peritumoral lymphatics, *Cancer Metastasis Reviews*, **25**, 677–694 (2006).

23. Joukov, V., Pajusola, K., Kaipainen, A., Chilov, D., Lahtinen, I., Kukk, E., Saksela, O., Kalkkinen, N., and Alitalo, K.: A novel vascular endothelial growth factor, VEGF-C, is a ligand for the Flt4 (VEGFR-3) and KDR (VEGFR-2) receptor tyrosine kinases, *The EMBO Journal*, **15**, 1751 (1996).

24. Joukov, V., Sorsa, T., Kumar, V., Jeltsch, M., Claesson-Welsh, L., Cao, Y., Saksela, O., Kalkkinen, N., and Alitalo, K.: Proteolytic processing regulates receptor specificity and activity of VEGF-C, *European Molecular Biology Organization Journal*, **16**, 3898–3911 (1997).

25. Jussila, L.: Ph.D. Thesis: VEGFR-3 in angiogenesis and lymphangiogenesis, University of Helsinki, Finland (2001).

26. Jussila, L., and Alitalo, K.: Vascular growth factors and lymphangiogenesis, *Physiological Reviews*, **82**, 673–700 (2002).

27. Karkkainen, M.J., Mäkinen, T., and Alitalo, K.: Lymphatic endothelium: a new frontier of metastasis research, *Nature Cell Biology*, **4**, E2–E5 (2002).

28. Karpanen, T., and Alitalo, K.: Lymphatic vessels as targets of tumor therapy, *Journal of Experimental Medicine*, **194**, F37–F42 (2001).

29. Korpelainen, E.I., and Alitalo, K.: Signaling angiogenesis and lymphangiogenesis, *Current Opinion in Cell Biology*, **10**, 159–164 (1998).

30. Levine, H.A., Sleeman, B.D., and Nilsen-Hamilton, M.: A mathematical model for the role of pericytes and macrophages in the initiation of angiogenesis: I. The role of protease inhibitors in preventing angiogenesis, *Mathematical Biosciences*, **168**, 77–115 (2000).

31. Levine, H.A., Pamuk, S., Sleeman, B.D., and Nilsen-Hamilton, M.: Mathematical modeling of capillary formation and development in tumor angiogenesis: penetration into the stroma, *Bulletin of Mathematical Biology*, **63**, 801–863 (2001).

32. Levine, H.A., Sleeman, B.D., and Nilsen-Hamilton, M.: Mathematical modeling of the onset of capillary formation initiating angiogenesis, *Journal of Mathematical Biology*, **42**, 195–238 (2001).

33. Liotta, L.A., Steeg P.S., and Stetler-Stevenson W.G.: Cancer metastasis and angiogenesis: An imbalance of positive and negative regulation, *Cell*, **64**, 327–336 (1991).

34. Lolas, G.: Ph.D. Thesis: Mathematical modelling of the urokinase plasminogen activation system and its role in cancer invasion of tissue, *University of Dundee, Scotland* (2003).

35. Lolas, G., and Friedman, A.: Lymphangiogenesis in tumors: A mathematical model, submitted for publication, (2007).

36. Mäkinen, T., Veikkola, T., Mustjoki, S., Karpanen, T., Catimel, B., Nice, E.C., Wise, L., Mercer, A., Kowalski, H., Kerjaschki, D., Stacker, S.A., Achen, M.G., and Alitalo, K.: Isolated lymphatic endothelial cells transduce growth, survival

and migratory signals via the VEGF-C/D receptor VEGFR-3, *European Molecular Biology Organization Journal*, **20**, 4762–4773 (2001).

37. Mandriota, S.J., Jussila, L., Jeltsch M., Compagni, A., Baetens, D., Prevo, R., Banerji, S., Huarte, J., Montesano, R., Jackson, D.G., Orci, L., Alitalo, K., Christofori, G., and Pepper, M.S.: Vascular endothelial growth factor-C-mediated lymphangiogenesis promotes tumour metastasis, *European Molecular Biology Organization Journal*, **20**, 672–682 (2001).

38. McCarthy, J.B., Palm, S.L., and Furcht, L.T.: Migration by haptotaxis of a schwann cell tumor line to the basement membrane glycoprotein lamini, *Journal of Cell Biology*, **97**, 772–777 (1983).

39. McCarthy, J.B., and Furcht, L.T.: Laminin and fibronectin promote the haptotactic migration of B16 mouse melanoma cells in vitro, *Journal of Cell Biology*, **98**, 1474–1480 (1984).

40. McCarthy, J.B., Hagen, S.T., and Furcht, L.T.: Human fibronectin contains distinct adhesion- and motility-promoting domains for metastatic melanoma cells, *Journal of Cell Biology*, **102**, 179–188 (1986).

41. McColl, B.K., Baldwin, M.E., Roufail, S., Freeman, C., Moritz, R.L., Simpson, R.J., Alitalo, K., Stacker, S.A., and Achen, M.G.: Plasmin activates the lymphangiogenic growth factors VEGF-C and VEGF-D, *The Journal of Experimental Medicine*, **198**, 863–868 (2003).

42. Nagy, J.A., Vasile, E., Feng, D., Sundberg, C., Brown, L.F., Detmar, M.J., Lawitts, J.A., Benjamin, L., Tan, X., Manseau, E.J., Dvorak, A.M., and Dvorak, H.F.: Vascular permeability factor/vascular endothelial growth factor induces lymphangiogenesis as well as angiogenesis, *Journal of Experimental Medicine*, **196**, 1497–1506 (2002).

43. Oh, C.W., Hoover-Plow, J., and Plow, E.F.: The role of plasminogen in angiogenesis *in vivo*, *Journal of Thrombosis and Haemostasis*, **1**, 1683–1687 (2003).

44. Oh, S-J., Jeltsch, M.M., Birkenhäger, R., McCarthy, J.E.G., Weich, H.A., Christ, B., Alitalo, K., and Wilting, J.: VEGF and VEGF-C: Specific Induction of angiogenesis and lymphangiogenesis in the differentiated avian chorioallantoic membrane, *Developmental Biology*, **188**, 96–109 (1997).

45. Oliver, G.: Lymphatic vasculature development, *Nature Reviews Immunology*, **4**, 35–45 (2004).

46. Oliver, G., and Detmar, M.: The rediscovery of the lymphatic system: Old and new insights into the development and biological function of the lymphatic vasculature, *Genes & Development*, **16**, 773–783 (2002).

47. Orme, M.E., and Chaplain, M.A.J.: Two-dimensional models of tumour angiogenesis and anti-angiogenesis strategies, *IMA Journal of Mathematics Applied in Medicine & Biology*, **14**, 189–205 (1997).

48. Partanen, T.A., Arola, J., Saaristo, A., Jussila, L., Ora, A., Miettinen, M., Stacker, S.A., Achen, M.G., and Alitalo, K.: VEGF-C and VEGF-D expression in neuroendocrine cells and their receptor, VEGFR-3, in fenestrated blood vessels in human tissues, *The FASEB Journal*, **14**, 2087–2096 (2000).

49. Partanen, T.A., and Paavonen, K.: Lymphatic versus blood vascular endothelial growth factors and receptors in humans, *Microscopy Research and Technique*, **55**, 108–121 (2001).

50. Pepper, M.S.: Lymphangiogenesis and tumor metastasis: Myth or reality?, *Clinical Cancer Research*, **7**, 462–468 (2001).

51. Pepper, M.S., Ferrara, N., Orci, L., and Montesano, R.: Vascular endothelial growth factor (VEGF) induces plasminogen activators and plasminogen activator inhibitors-1 in microvascular endothelial cells, *Biochemical and Biophysical Research Communications*, **189**, 824–831 (1991).
52. Pepper, M.S., Wasi, S., Ferrara, N., Orci, L., and Montesano, R.: *In vitro* angiogenic and proteolytic properties of bovine lymphatic endothelial cells, *Experimental Cell Research*, **210**, 298–305 (1994).
53. Pepper, M.S., Mandriota, S.J., Jeltsch, M., Kumar, V., and Alitalo, K.: Vascular endothelial growth factor (VEGF)-C synergizes with basic fibroblast growth factor and VEGF in the induction of angiogenesis in vitro and alters endothelial cell extracellular proteolytic activity, *Journal of Cellular Physiology*, **177**, 439–452 (1998).
54. Pepper, M.S., and Skobe, M.: Lymphatic endothelium: Morphological, molecular and functional properties, *Journal of Cell Biology*, **163**, 209–213 (2003).
55. Pepper, M.S., Tille, J-C., Nisato, R., and Skobe, M.: Lymphangiogenesis and tumor metastasis, *Cell Tissue Research*, **314**, 167–177 (2003).
56. Plate, K.H.: From angiogenesis to lymphangiogenesis, *Nature Medicine*, **7**, 151–152 (2001).
57. Podgrabinska, S., Braun, P., Velasco, P., Kloos, B., Pepper, M.S., Jackson, D.G., and Skobe, M.: Molecular characterization of lymphatic endothelial cells, *Proceedings of the National Academy of Sciences*, **99**, 16069–16074 (2002).
58. Rakic, J.M., Maillard, C., Jost, M., Bajou, K., Masson, V., Devy, L., Lambert, V., Foidart, J.M., and Nöel, A.: Role of plasminogen activator-plasmin system in tumor angiogenesis, *Cellular and Molecular Life Sciences*, **60**, 463–473 (2003).
59. Reis-Filho, J.S., and Schmitt, F.C.: Lymphangiogenesis in tumors: What do we know?, *Microscopy Research and Technique*, **60**, 171–180 (2003).
60. Ristimäki, A., Narko, K., Enholm, B., Joukov, V., and Alitalo, K.: Proinflammatory cytokines regulate expression of the lymphatic endothelial mitogen vascular endothelial growth factor-C, *The Journal of Biological Chemistry*, 8413–8418 (1998).
61. Ruoslahti, E.: How cancer spreads, *Scientific American*, **275**, 72–77 (1996).
62. Schoppmann, S.F., Birner, P., Stöckl, J., Kalt, R., Ullrich, R., Caucig, C., Kriehuber, E., Nagy, K., Alitalo, K., and Kerjaschki, D.: Tumor-associated macrophages express lymphatic endothelial growth factors and are related to peritumoral lymphangiogenesis, *American Journal of Pathology*, **161**, 947–956 (2002).
63. Shayan, R., Achen, M.G., and Stacker, S.A.: Lymphatic vessels in cancer metastasis: Bridging the gaps, *Carcinogenesis*, **27**, 1729–1738 (2006).
64. Sidenius, N., and Blasi, F.: The urokinase plasminogen activator system in cancer: Recent advances and implication for prognosis and therapy, *Cancer and Metastasis Reviews*, **22**, 205–222 (2003).
65. Skobe, M., Hamberg, L.M., Hawighorst, T., Schirner, M., Wolf, G.L., Alitalo, K., and Detmar, M.: Concurrent induction of lymphangiogenesis, angiogenesis, and macrophage recruitment by vascular endothelial growth factor-C in melanoma, *Americal Journal of Pathology*, **159**, 893–903 (2001a).
66. Skobe, M., Hawighorst, T., Jackson, D.G., Prevo, R., Janes, L., Velasco, P., Riccardi, L., Alitalo, K., Claffey, K., and Detmar, M.: Induction of tumor lymphangiogenesis by VEGF-C promotes breast cancer metastasis, *Nature Medicine*, **7**, 192–198 (2001b).

67. Sleeman, J.P.: The lymph node as a bridgehead in the metastatic dissemination of tumors, in: Schlag P.M., Veronesi U. (Eds.), *Lymphatic Metastasis and Sentinel Lymphonodectomy*, Springer, New York, 55–81 (2000).

68. Stacker, S.A., Stenvers, K., Caesar, C., Vitali, A., Domagala, T., Nice, E., Roufail, S., Simpson, R.J., Moritz, R., Karpanen, T., Alitalo, K., and Achen, M.G.: Biosynthesis of vascular endothelial growth factor-D involves proteolytic processing which generates non-covalent homodimers, *Journal of Biological Chemistry*, **274**, 32127–32136 (1999).

69. Stacker, S.A., Achen, M.G., Jussila, L., Baldwin, M.E., and Alitalo, K.: Lymphangiogenesis and cancer metastasis, *Nature Reviews*, **2**, 573–583 (2002a).

70. Stacker, S.A., Baldwin, M.E., and Achen, M.G.: The role of tumor lymphangiogenesis in metastatic spread, *The FASEB Journal*, **16**, 922–934 (2002b).

71. Swartz, M.A., and Skobe, M.: Lymphatic function, lymphangiogenesis, and cancer metastasis, *Microscopy Research and Technique*, **55**, 92–99 (2001).

72. Taraboletti, G., Roberts, D.D., and Liotta, L.A.: Thrombospondin-induced tumor cell migration: Haptotaxis and chemotaxis are mediated by different molecular domains, *Journal of Cell Biology*, **105**, 2409–2415 (1987).

73. Tille, J-C., Wang, X., Lipson, K.E., McMahon, G., Ferrara, N., Zhu, Z., Hicklin, D.J., Sleeman, J.P., Eriksson, U., Alitalo, K., and Pepper, M.S.: Vascular endothelial growth factor (VEGF) receptor-2 signaling mediates $VEGF-C_{\Delta N \Delta C}$- and VEGF-A-induced angiogenesis in vitro, *Experimental Cell Research*, **285**, 286–298 (2003).

74. Valtola, R., Salven, P., Heikkilä, P., Taipale, J., Joensuu, H., Rehn, M., Pihlajaniemi, T., Weich, H., deWaal, R., and Alitalo, K.: VEGFR-3 and its ligand VEGF-C are associated with angiogenesis in breast cancer, *American Journal of Pathology*, **154**, 1381–1390 (1999).

M for Invasion: Morphology, Mutation and the Microenvironment

Alexander R. A. Anderson

Division of Mathematics, University of Dundee, Dundee DD1 4HN, UK
anderson@maths.dundee.ac.uk

11.1 Introduction

Cancer is a complex, multiscale process, in which genetic mutations occurring at a subcellular level manifest themselves as functional changes at the cellular and tissue scales. The importance of tumour cell/microenvironment interactions is currently of great interest to both the biological and the modelling communities. Both the immediate microenvironment (e.g. cell-cell signalling or cell-matrix interactions) and the extended microenvironment (e.g. nutrient supply or a host tissue structure) are thought to play crucial roles in both tumour progression and suppression. In this chapter we focus on tumour invasion, as defined by the emergence of a fingering morphology. We present a hybrid discrete-continuum (HDC) mathematical model that considers the tumour as a collection of many individual cancer cells that interact with and modify the environment through which they grow and migrate. The HDC model we develop focuses on four key variables implicated in the invasion process: tumour cells, host tissue (extracellular matrix), matrix-degradative enzymes and oxygen. We will use this model to investigate how cell metabolism (the intrinsic rate of nutrient consumption and cell resistance to starvation) influences the growing tumour. We will also discuss the evolutionary influence that the microenvironment, via extreme changes in nutrient supply, has upon the tumour's genetic makeup. Finally we will discuss other applications of the HDC technique, its advantages and limitations.

11.1.1 Biology of Tumour Invasion

The development of a primary solid tumour (e.g. a carcinoma) begins with a single normal cell becoming transformed as a result of mutations in certain key genes. This transformed cell differs from a normal one in several ways, one of the most notable being its escape from the body's homeostatic mechanisms, leading to inappropriate proliferation. An individual tumour cell has

N. Bellomo et al. (eds.), *Selected Topics in Cancer Modeling*,
DOI: 10.1007/978-0-8176-4713-1_11, © Springer Science+Business Media, LLC 2008

the potential, over successive divisions, to develop into a cluster (or nodule) of tumour cells. Further growth and proliferation lead to the development of an avascular tumour consisting of approximately 10^6 cells. Since the tumour is dependent on diffusion as the only means of receiving nutrients and removing waste products its growth is limited. For any further development to occur the tumour must initiate angiogenesis—the recruitment of blood vessels from a pre-existing vascular network. Once angiogenesis is complete, the perfused vascular network can supply the tumour with the nutrients it needs to grow further. There is also now the possibility of tumour cells finding their way into the circulatory system (via the vascular network) and being deposited at distant sites in the body, resulting in metastases (secondary tumours). Angiogenesis is therefore key for metastatic invasion (see Fig. 11.1).

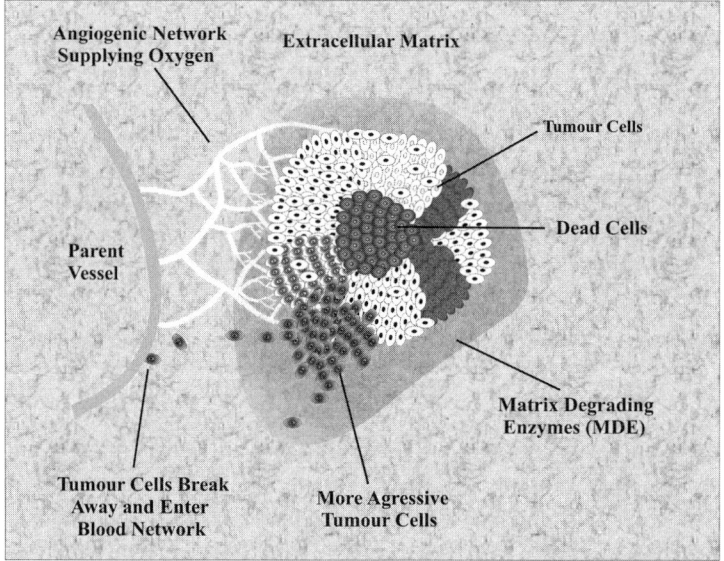

Fig. 11.1. Schematic diagram showing the key variables involved in solid tumour growth: tumour cells, extracellular matrix, matrix-degrading enzyme and oxygen. The tumour contains a heterogeneous population of cells with varying degrees of aggressiveness.

Another crucial part of the invasive process is the ability of the cancer cells to degrade the surrounding tissue or *extracellular matrix* (ECM) [51]. This is a complex mixture of macromolecules (MM). Some, like the collagens, play a structural role and others (such as laminin, fibronectin and vitronectin) are important for cell adhesion, spreading and motility. We note that all of these macromolecules are *bound* within the tissue, i.e. they are non-diffusible. The ECM can also sequester growth factors and itself be degraded to release fragments which can have growth-promoting activity. Thus, while the ECM may have to be physically removed in order to allow a tumour to spread, its degradation may, in addition, have biological effects on tumour cells.

A number of *matrix degradative enzymes* (MDEs) such as the large family of *matrix metalloproteinases* (MMPs) have been described [36] and have been repeatedly implicated in tumour invasion. In addition to opening migratory pathways, MDEs can alter cell adhesion properties regulated through several classes of cell surface receptors. These receptors, including cadherins, CD44, integrins and receptors for fibronectin, laminin and vitronectin, negatively regulate cell motility and growth through cell-cell and cell-matrix interactions [51]. Molecules which facilitate interactions between cells and between cells and the ECM, known as cell adhesion molecules, are now thought to be central to the invasive process [28]. Therefore it is important for any model that considers tumour invasion to include both cell-cell and cell-matrix interactions.

Tumour heterogeneity at the genetic level is well known and the "Guardian of the Genome," the p53 gene, is widely considered as a precursor to much wider genetic variation [32]. Loss of p53 function (e.g. through mutation) allows for the propagation of damaged DNA to daughter cells [32]. Once the p53 mutation occurs many more mutations can easily accrue, and these changes in the tumour cell genotype ultimately express themselves as behavioural changes in cell phenotype. As a step towards the inclusion of true tumour heterogeneity we shall consider a tumour that has phenotypic heterogeneity. The tumour cell phenotype will be defined here in terms of cell traits including cell-cell adhesiveness, proliferation, degradation and migration rates (further details will be discussed below).

The importance of the tumour microenvironment is currently of great interest to both the biological and the modelling communities. In particular, both the immediate microenvironment (cell-cell or cell-matrix interactions) and the extended microenvironment (e.g. vascular bed or nutrient supply) are thought to play crucial roles in both tumour progression and suppression (see the recent series of papers in *Nature Reviews Cancer* for further details [2, 14, 41]). Aggressive tumours are often described as having an invasive phenotype, characterised by fingering margins as opposed to more benign tumours which are characterised by smooth non-invasive margins. Recently it has been shown that not only can the microevironment promote tumour progression but it can also drive the invasive tumour phenotype. The work of Weaver [42] focuses on the impact of tissue tension in driving the invasive phenotype and clearly correlates higher tension in the tissue (a harsher environment) with an invasive phenotype. Similarly Pennacchietti [44] has shown a relationship between a hypoxic tumour microenvironment (again a harsher environment) and the invasive phenotype.

11.1.2 Fingering Morphology

Fingering and branched patterns can be found in a variety of animate [13] and inanimate [31] systems. One large class of non-living systems that exhibit fingering patterns are those obeying diffusion-limited growth. These include viscous fingering [17], electro-chemical deposition [37] and crystal growth [12]. Morphologies similar to those encountered in diffusion-limited growth can be observed in microbial colonies during stressed growth conditions [38] and in fungal growth in low nutrient concentrations [33]. It is notable that in both these examples the finger-like morphology does not seem to arise due to cell cooperation, but rather emerges from the underlying physical properties of the microenvironment.

Branched or fingered morphologies have also been observed in several models of tumour growth, and again appear to be driven by the microenvironment. Ferreira and collaborators [21] presented a hybrid reaction-diffusion model of tumour growth. By varying the consumption rate of an essential nutrient in their model they obtained a variety of morphologies, ranging from compact to fingered and disconnected. The impact of the ECM on tumour morphology was investigated by Anderson using a hybrid discrete-continuous model [8, 9]. He showed that growth in a heterogeneous ECM gives rise to a fingered morphology and, moreover, that such a morphology can also be induced by lowering the oxygen concentration in a homogeneous ECM, highlighting the importance of oxygen availability in determining tumour structure. Anderson also established a key link between the tumour morphology and the more aggressive phenotypes of the tumour cell population. This was subsequently refined by Gerlee and Anderson [25, 26] using an evolutionary hybrid cellular automaton model that considered the genotype to phenotype mapping using a neural network. This work also linked low nutrient availability with a fingered tumour morphology, and showed that tumours with irregular shapes are more likely to contain aggressive phenotypes. Cristini and colleagues [16, 23] have also looked at the role of nutrient gradients in driving morphological instability of tumour spheroids, both from a mathematical and an experimental point of view. Using a reaction-diffusion model for tumour growth and considering a discrete vasculature he showed that a disordered tumour vascular network caused simulated tumours to grow smaller with a fragmented or fingered morphology. A further model that considered individual deformable elastic cells interacting with a surrounding fluid and nutrients has been used by Rjniak in [47, 48]. She showed that the emergence of tumor microregions characterised by different cell subpopulations and distinct nutrient concentrations subsequently leads to the formation of finger-like tumor morphologies where long tissue extensions are created as result of cell competition for resources in the tumor vicinity.

11.2 Hybrid Discrete-Continuum Technique

When deciding which model should be used, the number and scale of the organisms being modelled arc important and the manner in which the organisms interact with their environment and each other is also important. Discrete, stochastic interactions between organisms cannot be captured by the continuum approach and likewise global population interactions cannot be captured by the discrete approach. Therefore the most appropriate modelling technique depends on both the number of organisms and the scale at which they are being studied.

Over the last ten years or so many mathematical models of tumour growth, both temporal and spatio-temporal, have appeared in the research literature (see [11] for a review of many of these). Deterministic reaction-diffusion equations have been used to model the spatial spread of tumours both at early stages of growth [49, 53, 15] and at later invasive stages [39, 24, 45, 5, 52]. Typical solutions observed in all these models [39, 24, 45] appear as invading travelling waves of cancer cells. Other mathematical techniques used to model the cumulative growth of tumours are based on boundary-integral, finite-element and level-set methods [55, 35]. Whilst these models are able to capture the tumour structure at the tissue level, they fail to describe the tumour at the cellular level and subsequently the subcellular level. On the other hand, single-cell-based models provide such a description and allow for a more realistic stochastic approach at both the cellular and subcellular levels. Several different discrete models of tumour growth have been developed recently, including cellular automata models [1, 18, 20, 30, 46, 50, 43], Potts models [29], lattice free cell-centered models [19] and agent-based models [54]. For a review on many different single-cell-based models applied to tumour growth and other biological problems see [10].

The model presented here we classify as "hybrid," since a continuum deterministic model (based on a system of reaction-diffusion-haptotaxis equations) controls the chemical/ECM dynamics and a discrete cellular automata like model (based on a biased random-walk model) controls the cell migration and interaction. Initially we define a system of coupled nonlinear partial differential equations to model tumour invasion of surrounding tissue. We then use a discretised form of the partial differential equation governing cell migration as the basis for the hybrid discrete-continuum model. This then enables specific cell properties to be modelled at the level of the individual cell. We shall consider proliferation, death, cell-cell adhesion, mutation and production/degradation at the individual cell level. The crucial point of this technique is that it allows cells to be treated as discrete individuals and the cell processes to be modelled at the level of the cell whilst allowing the chemicals/ECM to be treated as continuous. A detailed discussion on the types of systems to which this technique is applicable is given in [6]. Applications of the technique can be found in [3]–[9].

In the last few years there has been a rapid development in such hybrid models in application to tumour growth. The work of Deutsch [18], Deisboeck [54] and Alarcon [1] have all coupled individual tumour cells with continuous chemical dynamics. However, none of these works has explicitly modelled the direct impact of the microenvironment upon both the tumour cell population at the phenotype scale and the resulting changes in tumour geometry at the organ scale.

The aim of this chapter is to show how the tumour microenvironment impacts directly upon both tumour morphology and tumour heterogeneity. By using a combination of different nutrient microenvironments with different cell metabolisms we will show how aggressiveness of the tumour population and the formation of finger-like invasive morphologies are intimately linked.

11.3 The Continuum Model

We will base our mathematical model on the growth of a generic three-dimensional solid tumour. We will model a two-dimensional slice through this, one cell diameter thick. We choose to focus on four key variables involved in tumour invasion, thereby producing a minimal model: tumour cell density (denoted by n), MDE concentration (denoted by m), MM concentration (denoted by f) and oxygen concentration (denoted by c), see Fig. 11.1. Initially we define a system of coupled nonlinear partial differential equations to model tumour invasion of surrounding tissue and use these as the basis for the *hybrid discrete-continuum* (HDC) technique.

The complete system of equations describing the interactions of the tumour cells, MM, MDEs and oxygen is

$$\frac{\partial n}{\partial t} = \overbrace{D_n \nabla^2 n}^{random\ motility} - \overbrace{\chi \nabla \cdot (n \nabla f)}^{haptotaxis},$$

$$\frac{\partial f}{\partial t} = - \overbrace{\delta m f}^{degradation},$$

$$\frac{\partial m}{\partial t} = \overbrace{D_m \nabla^2 m}^{diffusion} + \overbrace{\mu n}^{production} - \overbrace{\lambda m}^{decay},$$

$$\frac{\partial c}{\partial t} = \overbrace{D_c \nabla^2 c}^{diffusion} + \overbrace{\beta f}^{production} - \overbrace{\gamma n}^{uptake} - \overbrace{\alpha c}^{decay},$$

(11.1)

where D_n, D_m and D_c are the tumour cell, MDE and oxygen diffusion coefficients respectively, χ is the haptotaxis coefficient and δ, μ, λ, β, γ and α are positive constants. We should also note that cell-matrix adhesion is modelled here by the use of haptotaxis in the cell equation, i.e. directed movement up gradients of MM. Therefore χ may be considered as relating to the strength of the cell-matrix adhesion. Since this model has already been published [8, 9] we will not discuss its derivation here. However, some explanation should be given regarding the manner in which oxygen is modelled. Oxygen is assumed to diffuse into the MM, decay naturally and be consumed by the tumour. For simplicity oxygen production is proportional to the MM density, and this might be considered as modelling the pre-existing blood supply. This is a crude way of modelling an angiogenic oxygen supply, see [4, 34] for a more appropriate way of modelling the angiogenic network. Since oxygen production is directly proportional to MM density, as the MM is degraded the oxygen production will drop.

The above system is considered to hold on a square of tissue Ω of length L, with appropriate initial conditions for each variable. We assume that the MM, oxygen, tumour cells and consequently the MDEs, remain within the domain of tissue under consideration and therefore no-flux boundary conditions are imposed on $\partial\Omega$, the boundary of Ω. We rescale distance with an appropriate length scale L (e.g. the maximum invasion distance of the cancer cells at this early stage of invasion, approximately 1 cm), and time with the average time taken for mitosis to occur, approximately 16 hrs. Full details on the model non-dimensionalisation and subsequent parameterisation can be found in [8].

11.4 The Discrete Model

Now that we have defined the continuum model of tumour invasion we can implement the HDC technique (see [3]–[9]) which will allow us to follow the paths of individual tumour cells. This first involves discretising (using standard finite-difference methods) the system of partial differential equations (11.1). We then use the resulting coefficients of the finite-difference stencil to generate the probabilities of movement of an individual cell in response to its local milieu (see Appendix of [5] for the full discrete system). Once the movement probabilities have been defined we then consider the specific individual-based processes that we will incorporate into the model.

As an illustration of the technique we only consider the tumour cell equation and discretise Eq. (11.1) in two spatial dimensions using central finite-difference approximations to obtain the following:

$$n_{i,j}^{q+1} = n_{i,j}^q P_0 + n_{i+1,j}^q P_1 + n_{i-1,j}^q P_2 + n_{i,j+1}^q P_3 + n_{i,j-1}^q P_4 , \qquad (11.2)$$

where the subscripts specify the location on the grid and the superscripts the time steps. That is, $x = ih$, $y = jh$ and $t = qk$ where i, j, k, q and h are positive parameters. In a numerical simulation of the continuous model Eq. (11.1), the purpose of the discrete equation Eq. (11.2) is to determine the tumour cell density at grid position (i, j), and time $q + 1$, by averaging the density of the four surrounding neighbours at the previous time step q. However, for the HDC technique, we will use the five coefficients P_0 to P_4 from Eq. (11.2) to generate the motion of an individual tumour cell. The central assumption of the HDC technique is that these five coefficients can be thought of as being proportional to the probabilities of a cell being stationary (P_0) or moving west (P_1), east (P_2), south (P_3) or north (P_4) one grid point (h) at each time step (k).

The coefficient P_0, which is proportional to the probability of no movement, has the form

$$P_0 = 1 - \frac{4kD_n}{h^2} - \frac{k\chi}{h^2} \left(f^q_{i+1,j} + f^q_{i-1,j} - 4f^q_{i,j} + f^q_{i,j+1} + f^q_{i,j-1} \right), \qquad (11.3)$$

and the coefficients P_1, P_2, P_3 and P_4, which are proportional to the probabilities of moving west, east, south and north respectively, have the forms

$$\begin{aligned}
P_1 &= \frac{kD}{h^2} - \frac{k\chi}{4h^2} \left[f^q_{i+1,j} - f^q_{i-1,j} \right], \\
P_2 &= \frac{kD}{h^2} + \frac{k\chi}{4h^2} \left[f^q_{i+1,j} - f^q_{i-1,j} \right], \\
P_3 &= \frac{kD}{h^2} - \frac{k\chi}{4h^2} \left[f^q_{i,j+1} - f^q_{i,j-1} \right], \\
P_4 &= \frac{kD}{h^2} + \frac{k\chi}{4h^2} \left[f^q_{i,j+1} - f^q_{i,j-1} \right],
\end{aligned} \qquad (11.4)$$

where the subscripts specify the location on the grid and the superscripts the time steps, all parameters are positive and are as discussed above. From these we see that if there were no MM the values of P_1 to P_4 would be equal, with P_0 smaller (or larger, depending on the precise values chosen for the space and time steps). That is, there is no bias in any one direction and the tumour cell is less (more) likely to be stationary—approximating an unbiased random walk. However, if there are gradients in the MM, haptotaxis contributes to the migration process and the coefficients P_1 to P_4 will become biased towards the direction of increased MM concentration. The equation P_0 represents the probability of a cell being stationary and takes into account the situation when a single cell does not experience a gradient between neighbouring points because they contain equal concentrations of MM; if neighbouring points contain higher (lower) MM concentrations, the probability of being stationary is diminished (increased) by the sign and magnitude of the term $\left(f^q_{i+1,j} + f^q_{i-1,j} - 4f^q_{i,j} + f^q_{i,j+1} + f^q_{i,j-1} \right)$. See Anderson [8] for a full derivation. The motion of an individual cell is therefore governed by its interactions with the matrix MM in its local environment. Of course the motion will also be modified by interactions with other tumour cells.

11.4.1 Individual-Based Processes

Since we model individual tumour cells we have the ability to incorporate individual-based processes. We now discuss in detail the processes each tumour cell will experience as it migrates through the MM field driven by the movement probabilities defined above. As a step towards the inclusion of true tumour heterogeneity we shall consider a tumour that has phenotypic heterogeneity. The tumour cell phenotype will be defined here by a collection of cell-specific traits, i.e. a combination of its cell-cell adhesiveness, proliferation, degradation and migration rates (see mutation paragraph below). We have chosen these specific traits based on the current views of the invasive phenotype [27]. In the following paragraphs we discuss some of the key processes and traits involved in the HDC model of invasion (see [8] for a more detailed discussion).

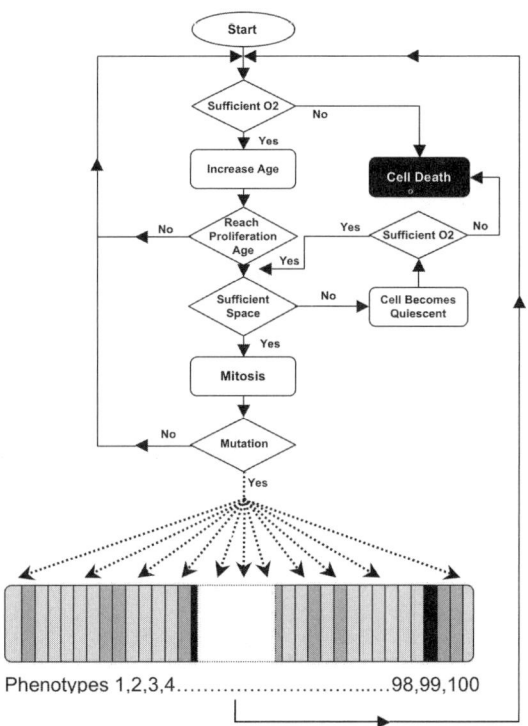

Fig. 11.2. Flowchart of the tumour cell life cycle within the HDC simulation.

Fig. 11.2 shows a flowchart of a tumour cell's "life cycle" within the HDC simulation. At each time step a tumour cell will initially check if it can move with regards to cell-cell adhesion restrictions (see the next paragraph for criteria); if it can, then the movement probabilities (above) are calculated and the cell is moved. A check is then made to see if there is sufficient oxygen for the cell to survive (see the paragraph on necrosis). If not, the cell dies. If there is sufficient oxygen, the cell's age is increased and a check is performed to see if it has reached proliferation age. If it has not reached this age then it starts the whole loop again. If proliferation age has been reached then a check is made to see if the criteria for proliferation are satisfied (see proliferation paragraph for details). If proliferation criteria are not met then the cell becomes quiescent. If they are satisfied then we check to see if this mitosis results in a mutation. All mutations in a particular simulation are assumed to occur in a random (Fig. 11.2) manner (see mutation paragraph for details). This whole process is repeated at each time step of the simulation.

Cell-Cell Adhesion. To model cell-cell adhesion explicitly we assume each cell has its own internal adhesion value (A_i) i.e. the number of neighbours that it will preferentially adhere to. We therefore examine the number of external neighbours each cell has (A_e) and if $A_e \geq A_i$ then the cell is allowed to migrate, otherwise it remains stationary.

Necrosis. For the tumour cell to survive it requires sufficient oxygen. Since some tumour cells have been found to survive in very poorly oxygenated environments, we make the assumption that the concentration has to drop to σ for cell death to occur. This assumption is also applied to quiescent tumour cells.

Proliferation. An individual cell will produce two daughter cells as a result of mitosis provided: (i) the parent cell has reached maturity (see mutation paragraph) and (ii) there is sufficient space surrounding the parent cell for the two new daughter cells to occupy. In order to satisfy condition (ii), we assumed that one daughter cell replaces the parent cell and the other daughter cell will move to any one of the parent cell's four orthogonal neighbours that is empty. If no empty neighbours exist then the cell becomes quiescent and proliferation is delayed until space becomes available. Quiescent cells are assumed to consume half the oxygen of normal cells.

Production/Degradation. Since we are modelling individual tumour cells we must consider production and consumption of MDE and oxygen at the level of a single cell. In the continuum model Eq. (11.1) we have these rates as being proportional to the tumour cell density. Now these terms will only be active at a specific lattice point if a tumour cell is occupying that point (i.e. we take $n = 1$), otherwise they will be zero (i.e. we take $n = 0$).

Mutation. Here we shall consider 100 randomly defined phenotypes, each phenotype has an equal probability of being selected. A cell's phenotype consists of a randomly selected, proliferation age ($Phen_{age} = 8$–16 hrs), O_2 consumption ($Phen_{O_2} = \gamma$-4γ), MDE production ($Phen_{mde} = \mu$-4μ), haptotaxis coefficient ($Phen_{taxis} = \chi$-4χ) and adhesion value ($Phen_A = 0$-3). In most cases the ranges of values each parameter can take to define the phenotype were chosen to represent biologically realistic limits. Each cell is initially assigned the values of one of the hundred randomly selected phenotypes and for each subsequent proliferation there is a small probability (P_{mutat}) of further mutations occurring which will lead to another randomly selected phenotype and so on.

11.4.2 Simulation Process for the Hybrid Discrete-Continuum Model

Each time step of the simulation process involves solving the discrete form of the system (11.1) numerically to generate the five coefficients P_0 to P_4. We then normalise these coefficients to obtain five corresponding final probabilities of motion, where normalisation simply means division by the total of the five coefficients. Probability ranges are then computed by summing the coefficients to produce 5 ranges. We then generate a random number between 0 and 1, and depending on the range in which this number falls, the current individual tumour cell under consideration will remain stationary or move to one of its orthogonal neighbours at each time step. This is provided the conditions imposed by cell-cell adhesion are satisfied. Once movement has occurred then the other individual-based processes are considered and may result in cell death or proliferation and mutation.

11.4.3 Parameters

The time step in the simulation was set to $k = 5 \times 10^{-4}$ and the space step to $h = 2.5 \times 10^{-3}$ giving a grid size of $(i, j) = (400, 400)$. The mutation probability is set to $P_{mutat} = 0.01$. The background oxygen concentration was set to $c_0 = 1.7 \times 10^{-8}$ mol O_2 cm^{-2} [8] and and the base oxygen consumption rate was taken to be $\gamma_0 = 2.3 \times 10^{-16}$ mol cell^{-1} s^{-1} [22]. The necrotic switch level σ_0 is assumed to be 5 % of the initial oxygen concentration. For a complete list of parameters and how they were chosen see [8].

11.5 Morphology and Metabolism

Now that we have discussed the HDC model of tumour invasion in detail we shall use it to examine the key role that nutrients play in driving changes in tumour morphology. In particular, we will investigate how changes in cell metabolic parameters influence the structure of the developing tumour. Specifically we explore the parameter space of oxygen consumption rate γ versus the oxygen threshold level σ at which cells become necrotic. We explore this two-dimensional parameter space (γ, σ) by selecting 4 values for each parameter and then simulating the growth of the tumour at these $4 \times 4 = 16$ points. We chose to vary the parameters as follows: oxygen consumption rate $\gamma = \{\gamma_0, 3\gamma_0, 5\gamma_0, 7\gamma_0\}$ and the threshold value $\sigma = \{\sigma_0, 2\sigma_0, 3\sigma_0, 4\sigma_0\}$.

All simulations have initially uniform oxygen, MM and MDE concentrations of $c_0 = 1, f_0 = 1$ and $m_0 = 0$ and are initiated with 50 tumour cells in the centre of the domain each with a randomly assigned phenotype. After

200 time steps the tumour cell distributions for each parameter combination (γ, σ) produced were collected to generate Fig. 11.3. Since the tumour population has the potential to mutate (via mitosis) to one of a hundred randomly defined phenotypes the constraint on consumption is only a lower bound and can vary from γ–4γ.

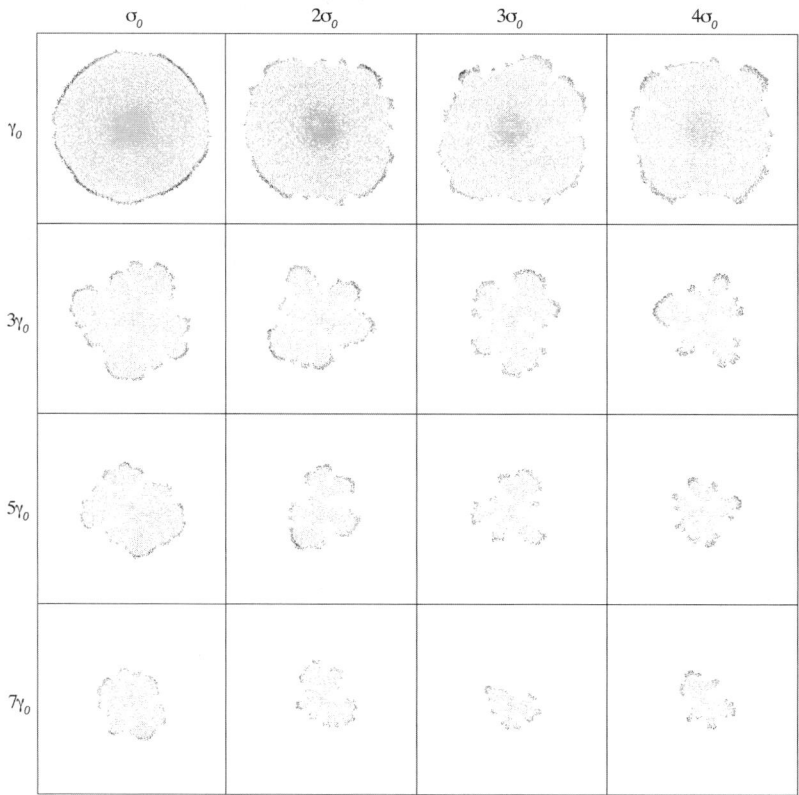

Fig. 11.3. Tumour cell distributions at the end of 200 time steps for different combinations of the parameters (γ, σ). Both parameters influence the morphology of the tumour: increasing γ reduces size and produces fingering, increasing σ has a similar but more subtle effect. Colouration represents cell type: black (living); grey (dead).

From Fig. 11.3 we see a diversity of tumour morphologies that share several common features. They consist of mainly dead (grey) and living (black) cells which are mostly located on the outer rim of each tumour. We can clearly see the emergence of a fingering morphology as both the consumption rate and the threshold level are increased. Increasing the consumption rate also appears to decrease the overall size of the tumour in contrast to a more or less constant size as the threshold level is increased. Increasing the threshold level appears to cause the emerging fingers to take on thinner, more elongated, structures. If we examine the figures that run along the diagonal we see that the tumour becomes smaller and more fingered as we move from (γ_0, σ_0) to $(7\gamma_0, 4\sigma_0)$ which is consistent with the above statements. These results clearly show that there is a direct correlation between the oxygen consumption rate and necrosis threshold value and tumour morphology.

One of the problems with showing the end result of the simulations is that the whole growth process that produced these results is missing. However, for all of the simulations in Fig. 11.3 the same growth process occurs and is of course dependent upon available oxygen levels. During the initial abundance of oxygen the tumour grows as a small round mass with smooth margins, further growth leads to more consumption of the available oxygen. In the HDC model oxygen is produced proportionally to the MM density (under the assumption of a background vascular network) and therefore as the tumour grows and degrades the MM it is also destroying its own oxygen source. This results in necrosis and a dead central core forms within the tumour mass which is now surrounded by a thin rim of proliferating cells that continue to grow at the boundary of the tumour. When there is little consumption or the threshold level is low this rim of cells grows in a more or less symmetric manner, but as these parameters are increased this symmetry is broken.

The time at which the necrotic core forms seems to be important as it is one of the first differences seen between the results collected in Fig. 11.3 (before the more obvious morphological changes occur). What we observe is that the earlier the appearance of the core the more likely fingering will occur—therefore the core in (γ_0, σ_0) forms much later than in $(5\gamma_0, \sigma_0)$. The reason for this apparent relationship is mainly due to competition for available oxygen as a means of avoiding death. As the nutrient consumption is increased and the threshold level increased the competition for the little available oxygen becomes dominant and one cell (or a small cluster of cells) will live at the expense of others by consuming the only oxygen that is left. Looking at the most fingered structures in Fig. 11.3 it is clear that none of them really has any large necrotic circular cores. Other differences relate to the evolutionary dynamics of the fingering versus the non-fingering tumour population, but we will discuss this in more detail in Section 11.6.

When the consumption rate is high compared to the oxygen concentration at the boundary of the tumour the cells have to rely on the flux of oxygen to survive long enough to go into mitosis. This implies that only at the points on the boundary where the flux of oxygen is sufficient do we observe growth of the tumour. This effect can be seen in Fig. 11.4, which shows the magnitude of the oxygen gradient along the tumour boundary as vertical bars. From this plot we can observe that only at the tips of the fingers, where the living cells reside, is the flux non-zero.

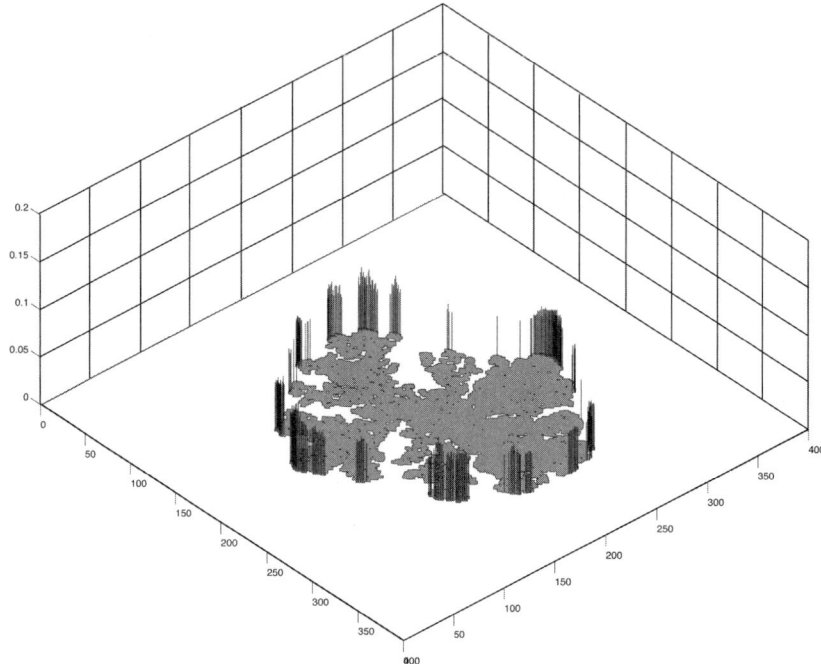

Fig. 11.4. The vertical bars show magnitude of the flux of oxygen at the boundary of the tumour shown in grey (see Fig. 11.3 with $(5\gamma_0, \sigma_0)$ for the original simulation result). Only where living cells reside do we observe a non-zero flux.

11.6 Mutation and the Microenvironment

It is clear from the previous results that nutrient starvation leads to a fingering morphology. Proliferating cells are located on the tumour fingertips, and thus exposed to higher concentrations of oxygen, grow at the expense of their closest neighbours causing starvation and necrosis. This, in turn, amplifies the growth advantage of cells at the leading edge and further enhances the invasion of surrounding tissue. Whether cell starvation is a result of high cell metabolism or of limited oxygen supply (note that reducing the amount of available oxygen gives similar effects to increasing the consumption rate of the cells), it creates a microenvironment dependent pressure for selection of the most aggressive cells capable of survival. Thus, since a harsh microenvironment induces tumour fingering, whereas a mild microenvironment gives rise to tumours with smooth margins, is it possible to reverse the fingering morphology by simply increasing the available oxygen levels and if so how will this effect the growth and evolutionary dynamics of the tumour population?

To test the oxygen switch hypothesis we implemented the following scenario: we grew the tumour using the parameters $(5\gamma_0, \sigma_0)$, see Fig. 11.3, initially in an oxygen rich environment $(c = c_0)$ until $t = 60$. We then dropped the oxygen concentration ($c = 0.25c_0$) until $t = 160 - 220$ where it is set to high ($c = c_0$) again and then finally for $t = 220 - 320$ we impose the low oxygen environment ($c = 0.25c_0$). This imposes two different forms of competition upon the tumour cells—for space and nutrients in the poor oxygen microenvironment, and for space only in the oxygen rich microenvironment. To show that the tumour morphologies are typical for each phase, we use a double switch in concentration of supplied oxygen: high-low-high-low (similair to that used in [9]). During the high oxygen phases, the tumour cells also consume oxygen but it is always replaced.

11.6.1 Morphology

Fig. 11.5 shows the simulation results with the tumour cell distributions at $t = 60$, 160, 220 and 320. After the first period of high oxygen the smooth circular tumour contains a mixed population of proliferating and quiescent cells and obviously does not contain any necrotic cells. However, as soon as the oxygen level drops we immediately see the emergence of the fingering morphology from the circular necrotic core. The population is now dominated by necrosis with only a few proliferating cells, on the tips of the fingers, and no quiescent cells. Increasing the oxygen level again results in the fingers filling out and merging such that the boundary of the tumour becomes smooth again. We also see the remergence of the quiescent population. When the oxygen level is dropped for the final time we again see small fingers protruding from the smooth necrotic mass. The quiescent tumour population again becomes extinct and is dominated by necrotic and proliferating cells. The outcome is clear: under harsh conditions, when oxygen is in short supply, the morphology of the tumour is invasive ($t = 160$; $t = 320$). In mild conditions, the morphology is non-invasive ($t = 60$; $t = 220$).

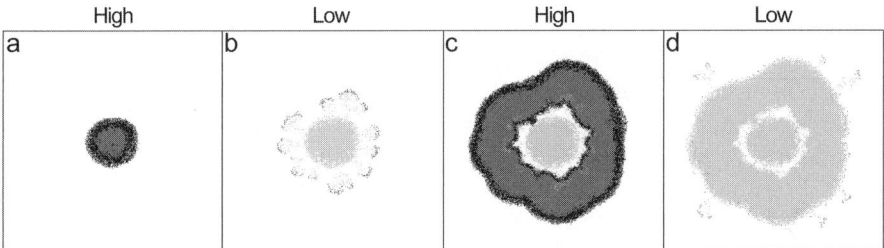

Fig. 11.5. Tumour cell distributions at the end of each switch in oxygen concentration: a. High ($t = 60$); b. Low ($t = 160$); c. High ($t = 220$); d. Low ($t = 320$). Colouration represents cell type: black (proliferating); dark grey (quiescent); light grey (dead).

These results also indicate a relationship between the invasive morphology and the quiescent tumour cell population. To investigate this we tracked the three tumour subpopulations (proliferating, quiescent and necrotic) over time and found that during the oxygen poor regimes there are almost no quiescent cells and in the oxygen rich regimes there are a large proportion of quiescent cells. To some extent this seems logical as within the nutrient rich environment all of the tumour population has the potential to proliferate and therefore space becomes a limiting constraint leading to the growth of the quiescent population. However, in the nutrient poor environment only the select few cells on the boundary of the tumour have the chance to proliferate and this is precisely where no space constraints exist. This may have some important implications for the treatment of real invasive tumours if valid, since a large percentage of chemotherapeutic drugs specifically target proliferating cells. If this were true though, treatment success would be more likely for invasive tumours which is generally not the case and therefore implies that other factors must play a key role. The evolutionary ability of the tumour population could be such a key factor.

11.6.2 Mutation

An important benefit of using an individual-based simulation approach is that at the same time as we simulate tumour growth we also track the numbers of the different phenotypes in the population. Fig. 11.6 shows a plot of the numbers of each cell phenotype over the time of this simulation. During the first high oxygen period all of the phenotypes are more or less equally represented with no single dominant clone. However, as soon as the oxygen level is dropped we see the emergence of a single aggressive phenotype (with phenotype number, PN, 12). This phenotype slowly grows to completely dominate the population in the low oxygen phase and as a result of this it also dominates the following high oxygen phase. It should be noted that other phenotypes are emerging during this second high oxygen phase, but their influence is small in comparison to that of the dominant clone. In the final low oxygen phase the same aggressive phenotype (PN 12) dominates again. An aggressive phenotype here is defined as one with a low proliferation age, high MDE production rate, zero cell-cell adhesion value and high haptotaxis coefficient.

What is interesting from these results is the fact that the same aggressive phenotype (PN 12) dominates in the latter three phases (i.e. the low, high and low oxygen levels) and during the high oxygen phase no fingering is observed. The implication of these results is that an invasive outcome appears to be co-dependent upon the appropriate cell phenotype in combination with the right kind of microenvironment. In this case the phenotype is an aggressive one and the microenvironment is a harsh one. The cooperation, or more accurately the competition, that these two invasive properties confer upon the tumour population create a fingered invasive tumour. Potentially other combinations may lead to the same outcome (e.g. heterogeneous ECM, see [8]); however,

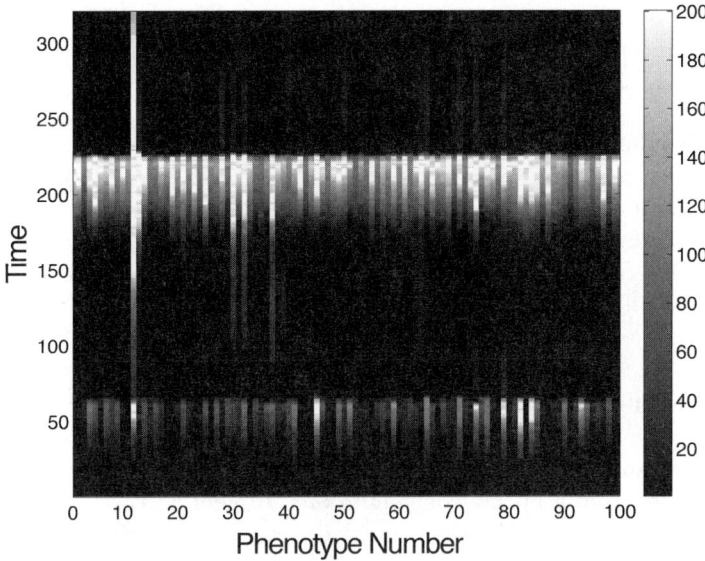

Fig. 11.6. The time evolution of each of the 100 phenotypes for the oxygen switch simulation shown in Fig. 11.5. Greyscale colouration signifies phenotype abundance: high (white), low (grey).

within the nutrient dependent context of these simulations this is the only combination that results in invasion.

11.7 Conclusion

In this chapter we have examined in detail the intimate relationship between the tumour nutrient microenvironment and the emergence of an invasive tumour morphology. In particular we considered the effects of changing metabolism parameters and nutrient availability. In both of these situations we observed tumour fingering, when metabolism was high or when nutrient availability was low.

However, what should be emphasised is the fact that the emergence of tumour fingering also went hand in hand with the selection of more aggressive phenotypes. The evolutionary dynamics produced several intriguing results, and most of these were from the oxygen switch computations of Section 11.6. During the initial phase of these simulations whilst all cells are capable of proliferating only those on the outer boundary actually proliferate, due to the physical constraints of space availability. Even so the tumour population contains many phenotypes with varying degrees of aggressiveness. This all changes when the first low oxygen switch occurs, as this results in a large percentage of the population becoming necrotic. The remaining living cells are mainly dominated by a single aggressive phenotype which rapidly takes over and produces the fingering morphology typical of the low nutrient environment. As expected a smooth non-invasive morphology develops during the second high oxygen switch. However, unexpectedly the non-invasive tumour population continues to be dominated by the same aggressive phenotype that produced the fingering morphology. In the final low oxygen phase, fingering reappears and again the same aggressive phenotype dominates. One important implication from these results is that tumour invasion, as represented by fingering, will only emerge if the right combination of tumour phenotypes and microenvironment occurs, i.e. context matters.

11.8 Discussion

We have presented a simple technique for deriving a hybrid discrete-continuum (HDC) model from a purely continuum one. In general this technique is useful for mathematical models that involve variables on different scales and in particular consider organism migration. It is the migration terms in the continuum model (e.g. diffusion, chemotaxis, convection) that drive the movement probabilities of the HDC technique. In effect, we derive a biased random walk governing the motion of an organism based on a system of partial differential equations (PDEs). This may seem somewhat back-to-front, as random-walk models are often used to derive continuum approximations. Othmer and Stevens [40] do precisely this; in particular, the transition probabilities of their gradient model are very similar to the probabilities of movement that were derived in this chapter. They show that in the continuum limit such transition probabilities result in a diffusion chemotaxis equation, and the same sort of analysis can be carried out on the cell movement probabilities defined here (see [6] for further details). However, it should be noted that such continuum approximations are only valid for individual organisms that do not interact with one another. Deriving continuum limit approximations for populations of interacting organisms is much more difficult and ultimately reflects the fact that these models should be developed at the scale of the individual organism.

One question which might arise from using the HDC technique is: why derive a discrete model from the continuum PDE model instead of starting with a discrete model in the first place? There are two main reasons for this: (i) when modelling the migration of cells that are influenced by stimuli at different scales it is easier to model these initially at the continuum level; (ii) since the movement probabilities, in the HDC technique, have been derived from a numerical discretisation of the PDE (governing cell migration), the space and time steps for the individuals already match those for the numerical solution of the "continuous" variables (the external stimuli) and therefore make interactions between these discrete and continuous variables much more straightforward.

Due to the derivation of the discrete model being based on a finite difference approximation of a PDE there is some restriction in the choice of the space (h) and time (k) steps in order to insure stability. A basic rule for stability of a diffusion driven model requires that the constants h and k should satisfy the condition $\dfrac{4kD}{h^2} < 1$ where D is the diffusion coefficient. Since in general the spatial grid size (h) will be fixed by the scale of the organism (this need not always be the case), the time step (k) must be chosen sufficiently small in order to satisfy the above condition. This could result in slower computations.

In conclusion, whilst the HDC technique will not be applicable to every migration system, the idea of using standard numerical techniques for solving PDEs to derive individual-based models is clearly a very simple way of obtaining a hybrid model of individual organism migration. Indeed, the HDC technique provides a powerful means of linking microscale events to macroscale events, and individual behaviour to population behaviour and is therefore intrinsically multiscale and can easily incorporate a range of scales, i.e. genetic, subcellular, cellular and tissue. The HDC technique has potential application to a wide range of problems in mathematical biology and has already been applied to several. It was initially developed in application to nematode migration in heterogeneous microenvironments [3] and has subsequently been applied to endothelial cell migration in both two- and three-dimensional tumour induced angiogenesis [4, 34] and has also been used to model amoebae migration in *Dictyostelium discoideum* aggregation [7].

References

1. Alarcon, T., Byrne, H. M., and Maini, P. K.: A multiple scale model for tumor growth. *Multiscale Model Simul.* **3**, 440–475 (2005).
2. Albini, A., and Sporn, M. B.: The tumour microenvironment as a target for chemoprevention. *Nature Rev. Cancer*, **7**, (2007), doi:10.1038.
3. Anderson, A. R. A., Sleeman, B. D., Young, I. M., and Griffiths, B. S.: Nematode movement along a chemical gradient in a structurally heterogeneous environment: II. Theory. *Fundam. appl. Nematol.*, **20**, 165–172 (1997).
4. Anderson, A. R. A. and Chaplain, M. A. J.: Continuous and discrete mathematical models of tumour-induced angiogenesis. *Bull. Math. Biol.*, **60**, 857–899 (1998).
5. Anderson, A. R. A., Chaplain, M. A. J., Newman, E. L., Steele, R. J. C., and Thompson, A. M.: Mathematical modelling of tumour invasion and metastasis. *J. Theoret. Med.*, **2**, 129–154 (2000).
6. Anderson, A. R. A.: A hybrid discrete-continuum technique for individual based migration models, in *Polymer and Cell Dynamics*, eds. W. Alt, M. Chaplain, M. Griebel, J. Lenz, Birkhauser, Boston, MA, 2003.
7. Anderson, A. R. A., and Pitcairn, A.: Application of the hybrid discrete-continuum technique, in *Polymer and Cell Dynamics*, eds. W. Alt, M. Chaplain, M. Griebel, J. Lenz, Birkhauser, Boston, MA, 2003.

8. Anderson, A. R. A.: A hybrid mathematical model of solid tumour invasion: The importance of cell adhesion. *IMA J. Math. Med. and Biol.*, **22**, 163–186 (2005).

9. Anderson, A. R. A, Weaver, A. M., Cummings, P. T., and Quaranta, V.: Tumor morphology and phenotypic evolution driven by selective pressure from the microenvironment. *Cell*, **127**, 905–915 (2006).

10. Anderson, A. R. A., Chaplain, M. A. J., and Rejniak, K. A.: *Single-Cell-Based Models in Biology and Medicine*. Birkhauser, Boston, MA, (2007).

11. Araujo, R. P., and McElwain, D. L. S.: A history of the study of solid tumour growth: The contribution of mathematical modeling. *Bull. Math. Biol.* **66**, 1039–1091 (2004).

12. Ben-Jacob, E., and Garik, P.: The formation of patterns in non-equilibrium growth. *Nature*, **343**, 523–530 (1990).

13. Ben-Jacob, E., Cohen, I., and Levine, H.: Cooperative self-organization of microorganisms. *Advances in Physics*, **49**, 395–554 (2000).

14. Bierie, B., and Moses, H. L.: Tumour microenvironment: TGF: the molecular Jekyll and Hyde of cancer. *Nature Rev. Cancer*, **6**, 506–520 (2006).

15. Chaplain, M. A. J., Graziano, L., and Preziosi, L.: Mathematical modelling of the loss of tissue compression responsiveness and its role in solid tumour development, *Mathematical Medicine and Biology*, **23**:197–229 (2006).

16. Cristini, V., Frieboes, H. B., Gatenby, R., Caserta, S., Ferrari, M., and Sinek, J.: Morphologic instability and cancer invasion. *Clin Cancer Res*, **127**, 6772–6779 (2005).

17. Daccord, G., Nittmann, J., and Stanley, H. E.: Radial viscous fingers and diffusion-limited aggregation: Fractal dimension and growth sites. *Phys. Rev. Lett.*, 56(4), 336–339 (1986).

18. Dormann, S., and Deutsch, A.: Modeling of self-organzied avascular tumor growth with a hybrid cellular automaton. *In Silico Biology,* **2**, 0035 (2002).

19. Drasdo, D., and Höhme, S.: Individual-based approaches to birth and death in avascular tumors, *Mathematical and Computer Modelling*, **37**, 1163–1175 (2003).

20. Düchting, W.: Tumor growth simulation. *Comput. & Graphics,* **14**, 505–508 (1990a).

21. Ferreira, S. C., Martins, M. L., and Vilela, M. J.: Reaction-diffusion model for the growth of avascular tumor. *Physical Review E*, **65**, 021907 (2002).

22. Freyer, J. P., and Sutherland, R. M.: A reduction in the in situ rates of oxygen and glucose consumption of cells on EMT6/Ro spheroids during growth. *J. Cell Physiol.* **124**, 516–524 (1985).

23. Frieboes, H. B., Zheng, X., Sun, C., Tromberg, B., Gatenby, R., and Cristini, V.: An integrated computational/experimental model of tumor invasion. *Cancer Res*, **66**, 1597–1604 (2006).

24. Gatenby, R. A., and Gawlinski, E. T.: A reaction-diffusion model of cancer invasion. *Cancer Research,* **56**, 5745–5753 (1996).

25. Gerlee, P., and Anderson, A. R. A.: An evolutionary hybrid cellular automaton model of solid tumour growth. *Journal of Theoretical Biology,* **246**(4), 583–603 (2007)a.

26. Gerlee, P., and Anderson, A. R. A.: Stability analysis of a hybrid cellular automaton model of cell colony growth. *Physical Review E,* **75**, 051911 (2007)b.

27. Hanahan, D., and Weinberg, R. A.: The hallmarks of cancer. *Cell,* **100**, 57–70 (2000).

28. Hynes, R. O.: Integrins: versatility, modulation, and signalling in cell adhesion. *Cell,* **69**, 11–25 (1992).
29. Jiang, Y., Pjesivac-Grbovic, J. A., Cantrell, C., and Freyer, J. P.: A multiscale model for avascular tumour growth. *Biophys. J.,* **89**, 3884–3894 (2005).
30. Kansal, A. R., Torquato, S., Harsh, G. R., Chiocca, E. A., and Deisboeck, T. S.: Simulated brain tumor growth using a three-dimensional cellular automaton, *J. Theor. Biol.* **203**, 367–382 (2000).
31. Kessler, D. A., Koplik, J., and Levine, H.: Pattern selection in fingered growth phenomena. *Advances in Physics,* **37**, 255–339 (1988).
32. Lane, D. P.: The regulation of p53 function. Steiner Award Lecture. *Int. J. Cancer* **57**, 623–627 (1994).
33. Lopez, J. M. and Jensen, H. J.: Generic model of morphological changes in growing colonies of fungi. *Physical Review E,* **65**(2), 021903 (2002).
34. McDougall, S., Anderson, A. R. A., and Chaplain, M. A. J.: Mathematical modelling of dynamic adaptive tumour-induced angiogenesis: Clinical implications and therapeutic targeting strategies. *J. Theo. Biol.,* **241**, 564–589 (2006).
35. Macklin, P., and Lowengrub, J. S.: Evolving interfaces via gradients of geometry-dependent interior Poisson problems: Application to tumor growth, *J. Comput. Phys.,* **203**(1), 191–220 (2005).
36. Matrisian, L. M.: The matrix-degrading metalloproteinases. *Bioessays,* **14**, 455–463 (1992).
37. Matsushita, M., Sano, M., Hayakawa, Y., Honjo, H., and Sawada, Y.: Fractal structures of zinc metal leaves grown by electrodeposition. *Phys. Rev. Lett.,* **53**(3), 286–289 (1984).
38. Matsushita, M., Wakita, J., Itoh, H., Watanabe, K., Arai, T., Matsuyama, T., Sakaguchi, H., and Mimura, M.: Formation of colony patterns by a bacterial cell population. *Physica A,* **274**, 190–199 (1999).
39. Orme, M. E., and Chaplain, M. A. J.: A mathematical model of vascular tumour growth and invasion. *Mathl. Comp. Modelling,* **23**, 43–60 (1996).
40. Othmer, H., and Stevens, A.: Aggregation, blowup and collapse: The ABCs of taxis and reinforced random walks. *SIAM J. Appl. Math.,* **57**, 1044–1081 (1997).
41. Overall, C. M., and Kleifeld, O.: Tumour microenvironment opinion: Validating matrix metalloproteinases as drug targets and anti-targets for cancer therapy. *Nature Rev. Cancer,* **6**, 227–239 (2006).
42. Paszek, M. J., Zahir, N., Johnson, K. R., Lakins, J. N., Rozenberg, G. I., Gefen, A., Reinhart-King, C. A., Margulies, S. S., Dembo, M., Boettiger, D., Hammer, D. A., and Weaver, V. M.: Tensional homeostasis and the malignant phenotype. *Cancer Cell,* **8**, 241–254 (2005).
43. Patel, A. A., Gawlinski, E. E., Lemieux, S. K., and Gatenby, R. A.: A cellular automaton model of early tumor growth and invasion: The effects of native tissue vascularity and increased anaerobic tumor metabolism, *J. Theoret. Biol.,* **213**, 315–331 (2001).
44. Pennacchietti, S., Michieli, P., Galluzzo, M., Mazzone, M., Giordano, S., and Comoglio, P. M.: Hypoxia promotes invasive growth by transcriptional activation of the met protooncogene. *Cancer Cell,* **3**, 347–361 (2003).
45. Perumpanani, A. J., Sherratt, J. A., Norbury, J., and Byrne, H. M.: Biological inferences from a mathematical model of malignant invasion. *Invasion and Metastases,* **16**, 209–221 (1996).
46. Qi, A., Zheng, X., Du, C., and An, B.: A cellular automaton model of cancerous growth. *J. Theor. Biol.,* **161**, 1–12 (1993).

47. Rejniak, K. A.: A single-cell approach in modeling the dynamics of tumor microregions. *Math. Biosci. Eng.*, **2**, 643–655 (2005).
48. Rejniak, K. A.: An immersed boundary framework for modelling the growth of individual cells: An application to the early tumour development. *J. Theor. Biol.*, **247**, 186–204 (2007).
49. Sherratt, J. A., and Nowak, M. A.: Oncogenes, anti-oncogenes and the immune response to cancer: A mathematical model. *Proc. R. Soc. Lond. B*, **248**, 261–271 (1992).
50. Smolle, J., and Stettner, H.: Computer simulation of tumour cell invasion by a stochastic growth model. *J. Theor. Biol.*, **160**, 63–72 (1993).
51. Stetler-Stevenson, W. G., Aznavoorian, S., and Liotta, L. A.: Tumor cell interactions with the extracellular matrix during invasion and metastasis. *Ann. Rev. Cell Biol.*, **9**, 541–573 (1993).
52. Swanson, K. R., Bridge, C., Murray, J. D., and Alvord Jr., E. C.: Virtual and real brain tumors: Using mathematical modeling to quantify glioma growth and invasion. *J. Neuro. Sci.*, **216**, 1–10 (2003).
53. Ward, J. P., and King, J. R.: Mathematical modelling of avascular-tumour growth II: Modelling growth saturation. *IMA J. Math. Appl. Med. Biol.*, **16**, 171–211 (1999).
54. Zhang, L., Athale, C. A., and Deisboeck, T. S.: Development of a three-dimensional multiscale agent-based tumor model: Simulating gene-protein interaction profiles, cell phenotypes and multicellular patterns in brain cancer. *J. Theo. Biol.* **244**, 96–107 (2007).
55. Zheng, X., Wise, S. M, and Cristini, V.: Nonlinear simulation of tumour necrosis, neo-vascularization and tissue invasion via an adaptive finite-element/level-set method. *Bull. Math. Biol.*, **67**, 211–256 (2005).

12

Methods of Stochastic Geometry, and Related Statistical Problems in the Analysis and Therapy of Tumour Growth and Tumour-Driven Angiogenesis

Vincenzo Capasso,[1] Elisabetta Dejana,[2,3] and Alessandra Micheletti[1]

[1] Dipartimento di Matematica, Università degli Studi di Milano, Via C. Saldini 50, 20133 Milano, Italy
Vincenzo.Capasso@unimi.it, Alessandra.Micheletti@unimi.it
[2] Dipartimento di Scienze Biomolecolari e Biotecnologie, Università degli Studi di Milano, via Celoria 26, 20133 Milano, Italy
[3] IFOM - Fondazione Istituto FIRC di Oncologia Molecolare, via Adamello 16, 20139 Milano, Italy
elisabetta.dejana@ifom-ieo-campus.it

12.1 Introduction

Many processes of interest in the study of tumour growth and tumour-driven angiogenesis may be modelled as birth-and-growth processes (germ-grain models), which are composed of two processes, birth (nucleation, branching, etc.) and subsequent growth of spatial structures (cells, vessel networks, etc.), which, in general, are both stochastic in time and space. These structures induce a random division of the relevant spatial region, known as random tessellation. A quantitative description of the spatial structure of a tessellation can be given in terms of the mean densities of interfaces (n-facets; $n = 0$ for vertices, $n = 1$ for lines—edges, fibres, etc.—$n = 2$ for facets, and so on, up to the full dimension d of the relevant space).

In this context, an understanding of the principles and the dominant mechanisms underlying tumour growth is an essential prerequisite for identifying optimal control strategies, in terms of prevention and treatment. Predictive mathematical models which are capable of producing quantitative morphological features of developing tumour and blood vessels can contribute to this.

The study of angiogenesis has such potential for providing new therapies that it has received enthusiastic interest from the pharmaceutical and biotechnology industries. Many of the compounds now under investigation inhibit angiogenesis and thus the growth of the cancer.

In a detailed description, all these processes can be modelled as birth (branching)-and-growth processes strongly coupled with underlying fields.

N. Bellomo et al. (eds.), *Selected Topics in Cancer Modeling*,
DOI: 10.1007/978-0-8176-4713-1_12, © Springer Science+Business Media, LLC 2008

Tumor growth develops due to the nutritional underlying field, driven by blood circulation (and thus enhanced by angiogenesis) [Folk74]. On the other hand angiogenesis is activated by the presence of chemicals released by the tumour mass. Tumour-induced angiogenesis is believed to occur when normal tissue vasculature is no longer able to support growth of an avascular tumour. At this stage the tumour cells, lacking nutrients and oxygen, become hypoxic. This is assumed to trigger cellular release of tumour angiogenic factors (TAFs) which start to diffuse into the surrounding tissue and approach endothelial cells (ECs) of nearby blood vessels [FK87]. ECs subsequently respond to the TAF concentration gradients by forming sprouts, dividing and migrating towards the tumour. A summary of these mechanisms can be found in the recent paper by Carmeliet [JC01] (see also Figs. 12.1–12.4 where examples of real or simulated vascular networks are depicted).

All these kinds of phenomena are subject to random fluctuations, together with underlying fields, because of intrinsic reasons or because of the coupling with the stochasticity of the growth process itself.

In developing mathematical models of angiogenesis, the hope is to be able to provide a deeper insight into the underlying mechanisms which cause the process.

An important goal would then be the integration of mathematical models for angiogenesis and tumour growth, but the existing unsolved complexity of the individual models has prevented such an integration.

A satisfactory mathematical modelling of angiogenesis and of many other fibre processes requires a theory of stochastic fibre processes, evolving in time, and strongly coupled with underlying fields. In this case the theory of birth-and-growth processes, developed for volume growth [BCS02, BCM04], cannot be applied to analyze realistic models, due to intrinsic mathematical difficulties.

A major difficulty derives from the strong coupling of the kinetic parameters of the relevant birth-and-growth (or branching-and-growth) process with the geometric spatial densities of the existing tumour, or the capillary network itself, via various underlying fields [CM06, McDou06].

All these aspects induce stochastic time and space heterogeneities, thus motivating a more general analysis of the stochastic geometry of the process. The formulation of an exhaustive evolution model which relates all the relevant features of a real phenomenon dealing with different scales, and a stochastic domain decomposition at different Hausdorff dimensions, is a problem of high complexity, both analytically and computationally. Methods for reducing complexity include homogenization at larger scales, thus leading to hybrid models (deterministic at the larger scale, and stochastic at smaller scales, possibly at the level of individual cells or vessels). A widely used method for reducing complexity is based on the homogenization at larger scales, e.g. by (locally) averaging the stochastic cell or vessel densities in the evolution equations of the underlying fields, while keeping stochasticity at lower scales. The simple stochasticity of the geometric processes of birth (branching) and growth is

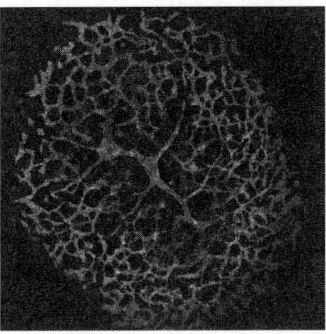

Fig. 12.1. Vascularization of an allantoid (from [CFD99]).

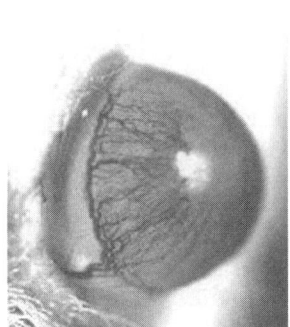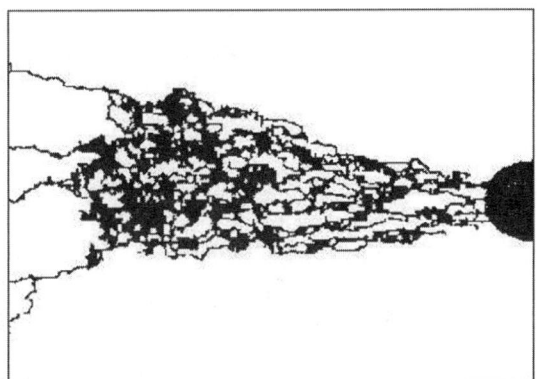

Fig. 12.2. Angiogenesis on a rat cornea [Credit: Dejana et al. [CZD02]] (left). A simulation of an angiogenesis due to a localized tumour mass (black region on the right) (from [CA99])(right).

maintained , by reducing the local dependence of the relevant kinetic parameters upon deterministic mean underlying fields. These kinds of models are known as hybrid models (see e.g. [BCP05, CM06, Harr06]). As an example we present a simplified stochastic geometric model for a spatially distributed angiogenic process, strongly coupled with a set of relevant underlying fields.

Statistical methods for the estimation of geometric densities may offer significant tools for diagnosis and dose/response analysis in medical treatments.

The aim of this paper is to offer a mathematical framework for modelling random geometric structures, so as to define in a rigorous way the geometric densities of such structures. Correspondingly we propose statistical estimators

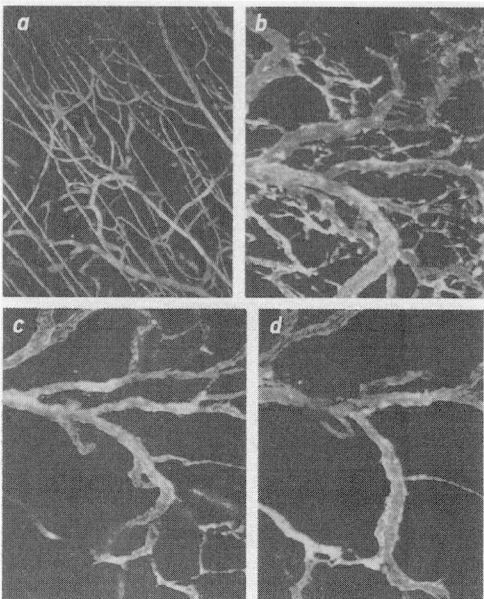

Fig. 12.3. Response of a vascular network to an antiangiogenic treatment (from [JC01]).

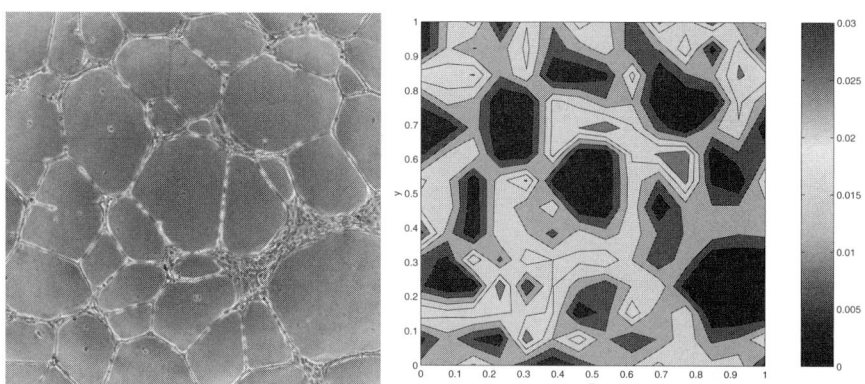

Fig. 12.4. Left figure: A real picture showing a spatial tessellation due to vascularization of a biological tissue: endothelial cells form a vessel network (from [Ser03]). Right figure: an estimate of the spatial density of the length of the fibres forming the network. See also Fig. 12.8 for a simulation of a stochastic tessellation generated by a birth-and-growth process.

of such densities which, in general, are not spatially homogeneous as required by most of the available literature on the subject (see e.g. [BR04]).

In the modelling and statistical analysis of the above-mentioned systems it is of great importance to handle random closed sets of different (although integer) Hausdorff dimensions, usually smaller than the dimension $d \in \mathbb{N}$ of the relevant space.

Here an original approach is reported, recently proposed by the authors, who have suggested coping with these problems by introducing generalized densities (distributions) *à la Dirac–Schwartz*, for both the deterministic case and the stochastic case. In this last one, mean generalized densities are meaningful [CV07, ACV06].

For our applications of interest, the *delta formalism* provides a natural framework for deriving evolution equations for mean densities at all (integer) Hausdorff dimensions, in terms of the local relevant kinetic parameters of birth (branching) and growth.

Section 12.9 is devoted to the presentation of an original statistical approach for estimating geometric densities of stochastic fibre systems, that characterize the morphology of a real vascular system.

In Section 12.10 a series of experimental results are reported, which show the power of this approach for the estimation of such densities for vascular systems, either real or simulated.

12.2 Stochastic Geometry

A relevant aspect of stochastic geometry is the analysis of the spatial structure of objects which are random in location and shape. Given a random object $\Sigma \in \mathbb{R}^d$, a first quantity of interest is for example the probability that a point x belongs to Σ, or more in general the probability that a compact set K intersects Σ.

The theory of Choquet–Matheron [Mat75, SKM95] shows that it is possible to assign a unique probability law P_Σ associated with a *RACS* (*random closed set*) $\Sigma \in \mathbb{R}^d$ on the measurable space $(\mathcal{F}, \sigma_\mathcal{F})$ of the family of closed sets in $\mathbb{R}^d$ endowed with the σ-algebra generated by the hit-or-miss topology, by assigning its *hitting functional* T_Σ. Given a probability space $(\Omega, \mathcal{A}, P)$, a RACS Σ is a measurable function

$$\Sigma : (\Omega, \mathcal{A}) \longrightarrow (\mathcal{F}, \sigma_\mathcal{F}).$$

The hitting functional of Σ is defined as

$$T_\Sigma : K \in \mathcal{K} \longmapsto P(\Sigma \cap K \neq \emptyset),$$

where $\mathcal{K}$ is the family of compact sets in $\mathbb{R}^d$.

Actually we may consider the restriction of T_Σ to the family of closed balls $\{B_\varepsilon(x); x \in \mathbb{R}^d, \varepsilon \in \mathbb{R}_+ - \{0\}\}$.

We shall denote by $\mathbb{E}_\Sigma$, or simply by $\mathbb{E}$, the expected value with respect to the probability law P_Σ.

12.3 The Hazard Function

In the dynamical case, such as a birth-and-growth process, the RACS Θ^t may depend upon time so that a second question arises, i.e. *when* is a point $x \in E$ reached (*captured*) by a growing stochastic region Θ^t; or vice versa, up to when does a point $x \in E$ survive capture?

In this respect the *degree of crystallinity* (now also depending on time) $V_V(x,t) = P(x \in \Theta^t)$ may be seen as the probability of capture of point $x \in E$, by time $t > 0$. In this sense the complement to 1 of the crystallinity, also known as the *porosity*

$$p_x(t) = 1 - V_V(x,t) = P(x \notin \Theta^t) \qquad (12.1)$$

represents the *survival function* of the point x at time t, i.e. the probability that the point x is not yet covered by the random set Θ^t.

With reference to the growing RACS Θ^t we may introduce the (random) time $\tau(x)$ of survival of a point $x \in E$ with respect to its capture by Θ^t, such that

$$p_x(t) = P(\tau(x) > t).$$

See Fig. 12.5.

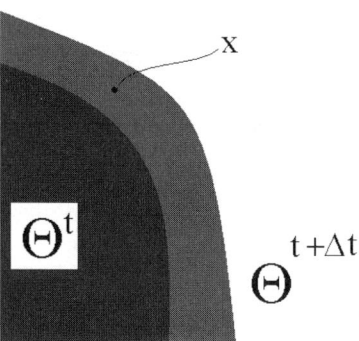

Fig. 12.5. Capture of a point x during time Δt.

More in general, especially for RACS Θ^t of lower dimension with respect to the dimension d of the full relevant space $\mathbb{R}^d$ (as for fibre systems such as capillaries), it is more convenient to analyze *when a compact $K \subset E$ is* reached by the invading stochastic region Θ^t.

In this respect we may introduce the (random) hitting time $\tau(K)$ of a compact $K \subset E$ by Θ^t. It will be such that the corresponding survival function is given by

$$S_K(t) := P(\tau(K) > t) = P(\Theta^t \cap K = \emptyset) = 1 - T_{\Theta^t}(K).$$

The functional

$$T_{\Theta^t}(K) = P(\Theta^t \cap K \neq \emptyset)$$

is called the *hitting functional* of the RACS Θ^t. Correspondingly a *hazard function* $h(K, t)$ can be defined as the hitting rate of the process Θ^t, i.e.

$$h(K, t) = \lim_{\Delta t \to 0} \frac{P(\Theta^{t+\Delta t} \cap K \neq \emptyset | \Theta^t \cap K = \emptyset)}{\Delta t}.$$

Under sufficient regularity,

$$h(K, t) = \frac{1}{1 - T_{\Theta^t}(K)} \lim_{\Delta t \to 0} \frac{T_{\Theta^{t+\Delta t}}(K) - T_{\Theta^t}(K)}{\Delta t}$$

$$= -\frac{d}{dt} \ln(1 - T_{\Theta^t}(K)). \tag{12.2}$$

If at time $t = 0$ the relevant space is empty, then $T_{\Theta^0}(K) = 0$, so that at any other time $t \geq 0$,

$$T_{\Theta^t}(K) = 1 - \exp\left\{ -\int_0^t h(K, s)ds \right\}.$$

This expression provides an important link between the hitting functional and the hazard function.

Finally, we may observe that whenever we may directly estimate the hitting functional $T_{\Theta^t}(K)$, for a sufficiently large family of compact sets K and for different time instants t, we may recover an estimator of the hazard function, via expression (12.2)

$$\hat{h}(K, t) = -\frac{d}{dt} \ln(1 - \hat{T}_{\Theta^t}(K)).$$

Since h is related to the probability that, at a given time, a fixed spatial region is reached by the growing sets, in cases in which the growing sets are vessels, it is an important instrument for estimating the probability that a given part of the human body is reached by angiogenesis by a given time. See Fig. 12.6 for an application to a naive simulated example; the hitting functional has been estimated by dividing the windows of observation into (locally) homogeneous subwindows, and by overlapping to any of them a lattice of points $x_1, \ldots, x_n$ such that $(K \oplus x_i) \cap (K \oplus x_j) = \emptyset$, for any $i \neq j$. For each subwindow we computed the following estimator:

$$\hat{T}_{\Theta^t}(K) = \frac{1}{n} \sum_{i=1}^{n} \mathbf{1}_{[(K \oplus x_i) \cap \Theta^t \neq \emptyset]}.$$

This is a generalization of a classical estimator of $\hat{T}_{\Theta^t}(\{x\})$ proposed in the relevant literature (see e.g. [SKM95]).

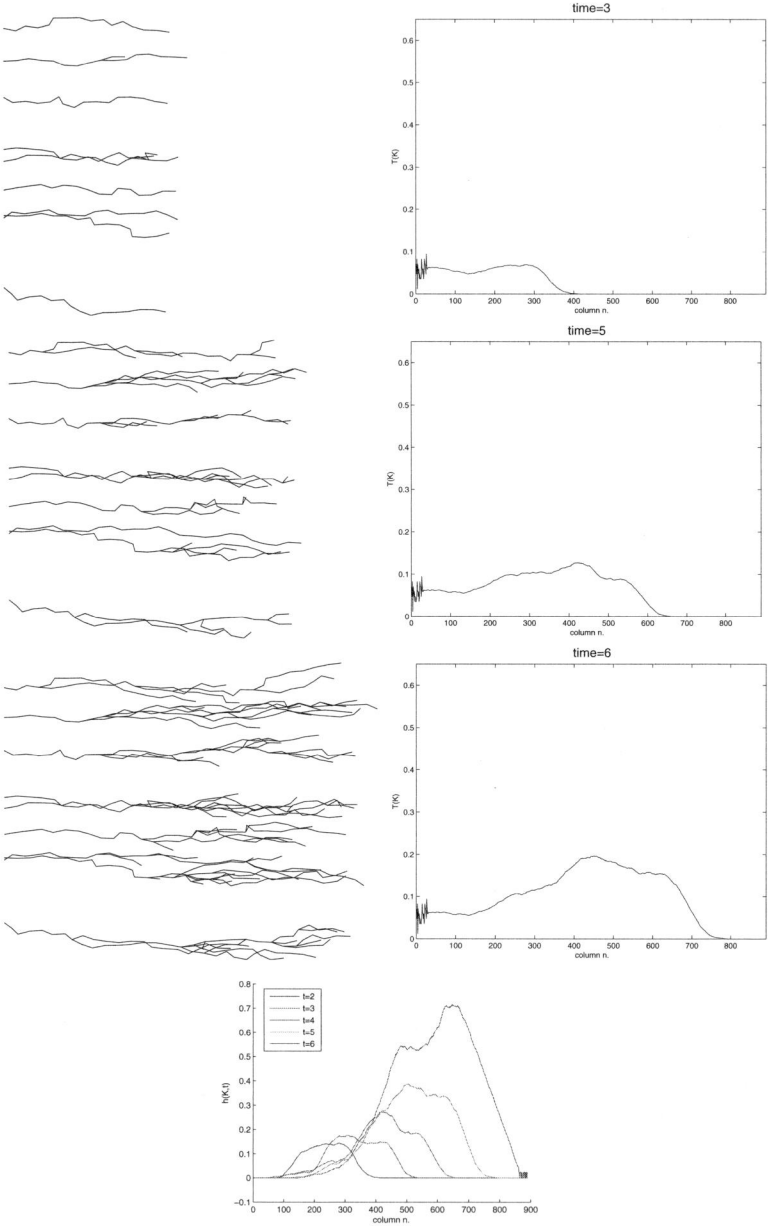

Fig. 12.6. Estimate of the hitting functional $\hat{T}_{\Theta^t}(K)$ for different instants t of a (naive) simulation of an angiogenesis, whose vessels develop from the left to the right. The chosen compact set K is a vertical segment of length 6 pixels, which has been moved into vertical stripes in the pictures, which show a vertical spatial homogeneity. In the bottom picture an estimate of the evolution of the hazard function for different times $t = 2, \ldots, 6$ is shown. The estimate is based on relation (12.2)(discretized by finite differences) applied to $\hat{T}_{\Theta^t}(K)$.

In several real applications it is of interest to study random closed sets of different Hausdorff dimensions (see Section 12.6). For definitions and basic properties of Hausdorff measure and Hausdorff dimension see, e.g., [AFP00, Fal85, Fed96]. Denoting by $\mathcal{H}^n$ the n-dimensional Hausdorff measure, we recall that $\mathcal{H}^0$ is the usual counting measure; for any Borel set $B \subset \mathbb{R}^d$, $\mathcal{H}^d(B)$ coincides with the usual d-dimensional Lebesgue measure of B; for $1 \leq n < d$ integer, $\mathcal{H}^n(B)$ coincides with the classical n-dimensional measure of B if $B \in \mathcal{B}_{\mathbb{R}^d}$ (the Borel σ-algebra of $\mathbb{R}^d$) is contained in a C^1 n-dimensional manifold embedded in $\mathbb{R}^d$. Further, we recall that the Hausdorff dimension of a set $A \subset \mathbb{R}^d$ is defined as

$$\dim_{\mathcal{H}}(A) := \inf\{0 \leq s < \infty \,|\, \mathcal{H}^s(A) = 0\},$$

so that, in particular, a point has Hausdorff dimension 0, a curve (or a fibre) has Hausdorff dimension 1, and a hypersurface in $\mathbb{R}^d$ has Hausdorff dimension $d - 1$. Note that the Hausdorff dimension of a set A need not be an integer (e.g., consider the Cantor set), and $\dim_{\mathcal{H}}(A) = s$ does not imply that $\mathcal{H}^s(A)$ is positive and finite (we may have $\dim_{\mathcal{H}}(A) = s$ and $\mathcal{H}^s(A) = 0$, or $\mathcal{H}^s(A) = \infty$).

We say that a random closed set Θ has Hausdorff dimension n if $\dim_{\mathcal{H}}\Theta(\omega) = n$ for a.e. $\omega \in \Omega$; in such a case we also write Θ_n to remember its Hausdorff dimension.

Depending on its regularity, a random closed set Θ_n with Hausdorff dimension n may induce a random Radon measure

$$\mu_{\Theta_n}(\cdot) := \mathcal{H}^n(\Theta_n \cap \cdot)$$

on $\mathbb{R}^d$, and, as a consequence, an *expected (mean) measure*

$$\mathbb{E}[\mu_{\Theta_n}](\cdot) := \mathbb{E}[\mathcal{H}^n(\Theta_n \cap \cdot)]$$

(for a discussion about the measurability of $\mathcal{H}^n(\Theta_n)$ we refer to [BM97, Zah82]).

12.4 Generalized Densities

In the sequel we will refer to a class of sufficiently regular random closed sets in the Euclidean space $\mathbb{R}^d$, of integer dimension n. We denote by $B_r(x)$ the ball with center x and radius r.

Definition 1 (n-regular set). *Given an integer $n \in [0, d]$, we say that a closed subset A_n of $\mathbb{R}^d$ is n-regular if it satisfies the following conditions:*

(i) $\mathcal{H}^n(A_n \cap B_r(0)) < \infty$ *for any $r > 0$;*

(ii) $\lim\limits_{r \to 0} \dfrac{\mathcal{H}^n(A_n \cap B_r(x))}{b_n r^n} = 1$ *for $\mathcal{H}^n$-a.e. $x \in A_n$.*

Here b_n is the volume of the unit ball in $\mathbb{R}^n$.

Remark 1. Note that condition (ii) is related to a characterization of the $\mathcal{H}^n$-rectifiability of the set S ([Fal85, p. 256,267], [AFP00, p. 83]).

We may observe that if A_n is an n-regular closed set in $\mathbb{R}^d$, we have

$$\lim_{r \to 0} \frac{\mathcal{H}^n(A_n \cap B_r(x))}{b_n r^n} = \begin{cases} 1 & \mathcal{H}^n\text{-a.e. } x \in A_n, \\ 0 & \forall x \notin A_n. \end{cases}$$

As a consequence (by assuming $0 \cdot \infty = 0$), for $0 \leq n < d$ we have

$$\lim_{r \to 0} \frac{\mathcal{H}^n(A_n \cap B_r(x))}{b_d r^d} = \lim_{r \to 0} \frac{\mathcal{H}^n(A_n \cap B_r(x))}{b_n r^n} \frac{b_n r^n}{b_d r^d}$$

$$= \begin{cases} \infty & \mathcal{H}^n\text{-a.e. } x \in A_n, \\ 0 & \forall x \notin A_n. \end{cases}$$

It is known that every positive Radon measure μ on $\mathbb{R}^d$ can be represented in the form

$$\mu = \mu_{\ll} + \mu_{\perp},$$

where $\mu_{\ll}$ and $\mu_{\perp}$ are the absolutely continuous part with respect to ν^d, and the singular part of μ, respectively. We may notice that, if A_n is an n-regular closed set in $\mathbb{R}^d$ with $n < d$, then the measure

$$\mu_{A_n}(\cdot) := \mathcal{H}^n(A_n \cap \cdot)$$

is a singular measure with respect to ν^d, and so the Radon–Nikodym derivative of $\mu_{A_n \ll}$ is zero ν^d-a.e.

Even if, usually, by "density of μ" it is understood the usual Radon–Nikodym derivative of μ with respect to ν^d, and so it is meant that μ is absolutely continuous, in analogy with the usual Dirac delta function $\delta_{x_0}(x)$ associated with a point $x_0 \in \mathbb{R}^d$ (a 0-regular closed set), we may introduce the following definition [KF70].

Definition 2 (generalized density). *We call the* generalized density *(or, briefly,* density*) associated with A_n, the quantity δ_{A_n}, defined by*

$$\delta_{A_n}(x) := \lim_{r \to 0} \frac{\mathcal{H}^n(A_n \cap B_r(x))}{b_d r^d},$$

finite or not.

In this way $\delta_{A_n}(x)$ can be considered as the *generalized density* (or the *generalized Radon–Nikodym derivative*) of the measure μ_{A_n} with respect to the d-dimensional Lebesgue measure ν^d.

Define the function

$$\delta_{A_n}^{(r)}(x) := \frac{\mathcal{H}^n(A_n \cap B_r(x))}{b_d r^d},$$

and correspondingly the associated measure

$$\mu_{A_n}^{(r)}(B) := \int_B \delta_{A_n}^{(r)}(x)\,dx, \qquad B \in \mathcal{B}_{\mathbb{R}^d}.$$

With an abuse of notation, we may introduce the linear functionals $\delta_{A_n}^{(r)}$ and δ_{A_n} associated with the measures $\mu_{A_n}^{(r)}$ and μ_{A_n}, respectively, as follows:

$$(\delta_{A_n}^{(r)}, f) := \int_{\mathbb{R}^d} f(x)\mu_{A_n}^{(r)}(dx),$$

$$(\delta_{A_n}, f) := \int_{\mathbb{R}^d} f(x)\mu_{A_n}(dx),$$

for any $f \in C_c(\mathbb{R}^d, \mathbb{R})$, having denoted by $C_c(\mathbb{R}^d, \mathbb{R})$ the space of all continuous functions from $\mathbb{R}^d$ to $\mathbb{R}$ with compact support.

It can be proven (see [CV06b]) that the sequence of measures $\mu_{A_n}^{(r)}$ weakly* converges to the measure μ_{A_n}; in other words, the sequence of linear functionals $\delta_{A_n}^{(r)}$ weakly* converges to the linear functional δ_{A_n}, i.e. $(\delta_{A_n}^{(r)}, f) \to (\delta_{A_n}, f)$ for any $f \in C_c(\mathbb{R}^d, \mathbb{R})$.

In analogy with the classical Dirac delta, we may regard the continuous linear functional δ_{A_n} as a generalized function on the usual test space $C_c(\mathbb{R}^d, \mathbb{R})$, and, in accordance with the usual representation of distributions in the theory of generalized functions, we formally write

$$(\delta_{A_n}, f) = \int_{\mathbb{R}^d} f(x)\mu_{A_n}(dx) =: \int_{\mathbb{R}^d} f(x)\delta_{A_n}(x)\,dx.$$

Consider now random closed sets.

Definition 3 (n-regular random set). *Given an integer n, with $0 \le n \le d$, we say that a random closed set Θ_n in $\mathbb{R}^d$ is n-regular if it satisfies the following conditions:*

(i) for almost all $\omega \in \Omega$, $\Theta_n(\omega)$ is an n-regular set in $\mathbb{R}^d$;
(ii) $\mathbb{E}[\mathcal{H}^n(\Theta_n \cap B_R(0))] < \infty$ for any $R > 0$.

If Θ_n is a random closed set in $\mathbb{R}^d$, the measure

$$\mu_{\Theta_n}(\cdot) := \mathcal{H}^n(\Theta_n \cap \cdot)$$

is a random measure, and consequently δ_{Θ_n} is a *random linear functional* (i.e. (δ_{Θ_n}, f) is a real random variable for any test function f).

By extending the definition of expected value of a random operator à la Pettis (or Gelfand–Pettis) [AG80, Bosq00], we may define the *expected (mean) linear functional* $\mathbb{E}[\delta_{\Theta_n}]$ associated with δ_{Θ_n} as follows:

$$(\mathbb{E}[\delta_{\Theta_n}], f) := \mathbb{E}[(\delta_{\Theta_n}, f)], \tag{12.3}$$

and the *mean generalized density* $\mathbb{E}[\delta_{\Theta_n}](x)$ of $\mathbb{E}[\mu_{\Theta_n}]$ by the formal integral representation

$$\int_A \mathbb{E}[\delta_{\Theta_n}](x)\, dx := \mathbb{E}[\mathcal{H}^n(\Theta_n \cap A)],$$

with

$$\mathbb{E}[\delta_{\Theta_n}](x) := \lim_{r \to 0} \frac{\mathbb{E}[\mathcal{H}^n(\Theta_n \cap B_r(x))]}{b_d r^d}.$$

It can be shown [CV06b] that an equivalent definition of (12.3) can be given in terms of the expected measure $\mathbb{E}[\mu_{\Theta_n}]$ by

$$(\mathbb{E}[\delta_{\Theta_n}], f) := \int_{\mathbb{R}^d} f(x)\mathbb{E}[\mu_{\Theta_n}](dx),$$

for any f such that the above integral makes sense.

By using the integral representation of (δ_{Θ_n}, f) and $(\mathbb{E}[\delta_{\Theta_n}], f)$, Equation (12.3) becomes

$$\int_{\mathbb{R}^d} f(x)\mathbb{E}[\delta_{\Theta_n}](x)\, dx = \mathbb{E}\left[\int_{\mathbb{R}^d} f(x)\delta_{\Theta_n}(x)\, dx\right];$$

so that, formally, we may exchange integral and expectation.

We wish to stress the fact that it is not always true that the mean measure $\mathbb{E}[\mu_\Theta]$ admits a classical function as density, so that the need of introducing a concept of absolute continuity for random closed sets arises in a natural way. Thus, it is of interest to distinguish between random closed sets which induce an absolutely continuous expected measure, and random closed sets which induce a singular one. To this aim we have introduced the concept of *absolutely continuous* random closed set, coherently with the classical 0-dimensional case, in order to propose an extension of the standard definition of absolutely continuous random variable (for preliminary definitions and results see also [CV06a]).

Thus, for any lower dimensional random closed set Θ_n in $\mathbb{R}^d$, while it is clear that $\mu_{\Theta_n(\omega)}$ is a singular measure, when we consider the expected measure $\mathbb{E}[\mu_{\Theta_n}]$, it may happen that it is absolutely continuous with respect to ν^d, and so it may have a classical Radon–Nikodym derivative, so that $\mathbb{E}[\delta_{\Theta_n}](x)$ is a classical real-valued integrable function on $\mathbb{R}^d$ (see [CV06b] and [CV06a]).

The case of interest in applications [BR04, Mol92, Hahn99] is the one in which the mean measure does admit a density (a classical function) with respect to the usual Lebesgue measure ν^d in $\mathbb{R}^d$.

When $n = d$, integral and expectation can really be exchanged by the Fubini theorem. Since in this case $\delta_{\Theta_d}(x) = \mathbf{1}_{\Theta_d}(x)$, ν^d-a.s., it follows that $\mathbb{E}[\delta_{\Theta_d}](x) = \mathbb{P}(x \in \Theta_d)$. In particular, in material science, the density $V_V(x) := \mathbb{P}(x \in \Theta_d)$ is known as the *(degree of) crystallinity* [Avr39, K37].

If $n = 0$ and $\Theta_0 = X_0$ is an absolutely continuous random point with probability density function (pdf) p_{X_0}, then $\mathbb{E}[\mathcal{H}^0(X_0 \cap \cdot)] = \mathbb{P}(X_0 \in \cdot)$ is absolutely continuous, and its density $\mathbb{E}[\delta_{X_0}](x)$ is just the pdf $p_{X_0}(x)$.

In a tessellation (see Section 12.6), $\mathbb{E}[\delta_{\Theta_n}(x)]$ is known as *n-facet density*, for any other integer $0 \leq n \leq d - 1$; for fibre processes ($n = 1$) we speak of fibre density, etc. (see e.g. Fig. 12.4). Fig. 12.7 shows the estimation of the evolution of the vessel density for the simulation in Fig. 12.2, by means of the estimators proposed in Section 12.10.

To avoid pathologies, as discussed later, we introduce now a class of random sets, which, in particular, include all random sets we will be interested in.

Definition 4 ($\mathcal{R}$ class). *We say that a random closed set Θ in $\mathbb{R}^d$ belongs to the class $\mathcal{R}$ if*

$$\dim_{\mathcal{H}}(\partial\Theta) < d \quad and \quad \mathbb{P}(\mathcal{H}^{\dim_{\mathcal{H}}(\partial\Theta)}(\partial\Theta) > 0) = 1.$$

Definition 5 (strong absolute continuity). *We say that a random closed set Θ is* (strongly) *absolutely continuous if $\Theta \in \mathcal{R}$ and*

$$\mathbb{E}[\mu_{\partial\Theta}] \ll \nu^d \tag{12.4}$$

on $\mathcal{B}_{\mathbb{R}^d}$.

Notation: Without any further specification, in the following we will write "absolutely continuous random set" to mean a "strongly absolutely continuous random set".

Note that, if $\Theta \in \mathcal{R}$ with $\dim_{\mathcal{H}}(\Theta) = d$ is sufficiently regular so that $\dim_{\mathcal{H}}(\partial\Theta) = d-1$, then it is absolutely continuous if $\mathbb{E}[\mathcal{H}^{d-1}(\partial\Theta \cap \cdot)] \ll \nu^d(\cdot)$.

Remark 2. In the particular case that $\Theta = X$ is a random variable, Definition 5 coincides with the usual definition of absolute continuity of a random variable. In fact, $\dim_{\mathcal{H}} X = 0$, $\partial X = X$, and $\mathbb{E}[\mathcal{H}^0(X)] = \mathbb{P}(X \in \mathbb{R}^d) = 1$, so $X \in \mathcal{R}$ and then Condition (12.4) is equivalent to

$$\mathbb{E}[\mathcal{H}^0(X \cap \cdot)] = \mathbb{P}(X \in \cdot) \ll \nu^d.$$

12.5 Approximation of Mean Densities

In many real applications (see e.g. [BR04] and [SKM95]), it is of interest to estimate the local mean density $\mathbb{E}[\delta_{\Theta_n}]$ of a lower dimensional random closed set such as a fibre process of dimension $n = 1$ in a space of dimension $d > 1$.

For facing the problem of the zero ν^2-measure for points or lines in $\mathbb{R}^2$ it is natural to make use of their 2D box approximations. As a matter of fact, a computer graphic representation is usually provided in terms of pixels, which can only offer a 2D box approximation of points or lines in $\mathbb{R}^2$.

Thus, given a random closed set Θ_n with Hausdorff dimension $n < d$, we will consider the enlarged set $\Theta_{n_{\oplus r}}$, which is now of dimension d, and hence of nontrivial measure ν^d.

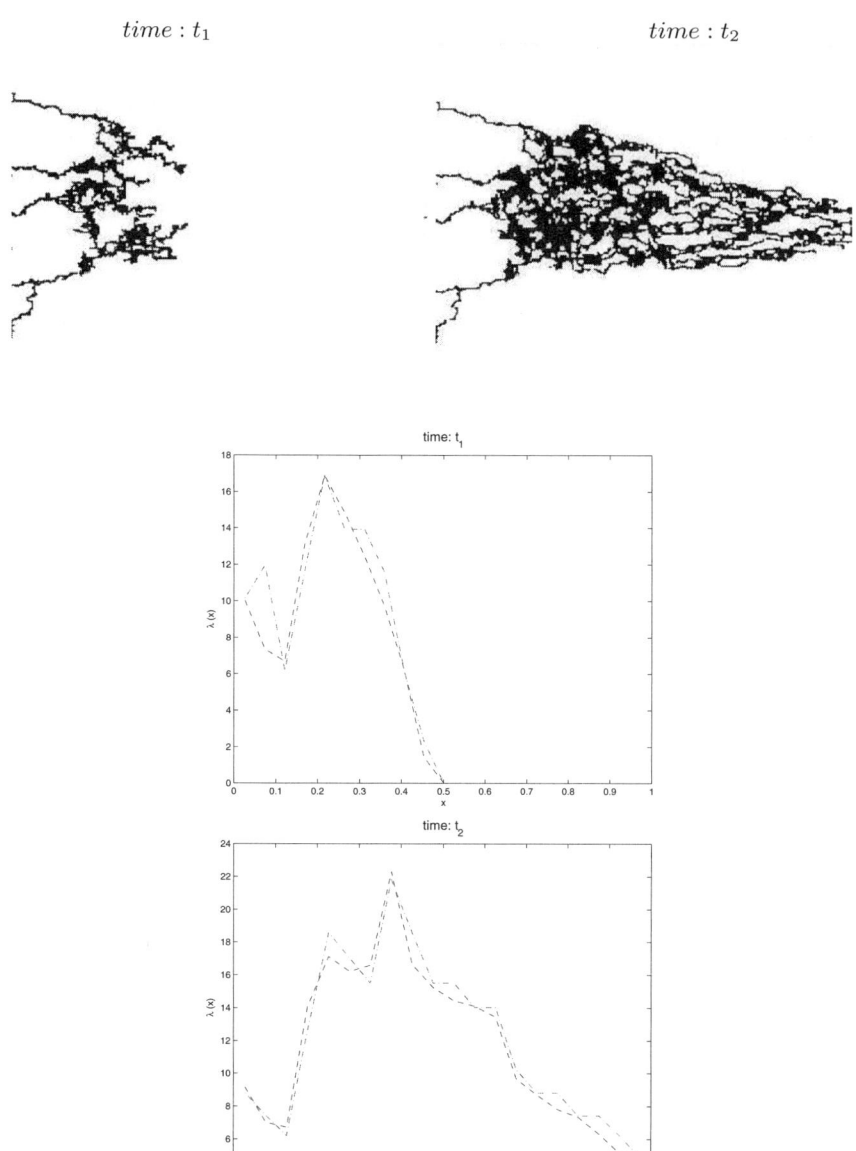

Fig. 12.7. Estimate of the density (mean length per unit area) of fibres, at two different instants of a simulation of a tumour-driven angiogenesis, taken from [CA99]. The estimators are described in Section 12.10. Dashed line $= \hat{\lambda}^1_{k,r,p}$, dotted-dashed line $= \hat{\lambda}^2_{k,r,p}$.

On the other hand, we may observe that $\mathbb{P}(x \in \Theta_{n \oplus r}) = T_{\Theta_n}(B_r(x))$, where T_{Θ_n} is the hitting functional associated to Θ_n, which characterizes the probability structure of the random set Θ_n. Let us now report the following proposition, proven in [ACV06] (see also [CV06a] for the related definitions).

Proposition 1. *Let Θ_n be a regular random closed set with an integer Hausdorff dimension n, and $A \in \mathcal{B}_{\mathbb{R}^d}$ such that $\mathbb{P}(\mathcal{H}^n(\Theta_n \cap \partial A) > 0) = 0$. If*

$$\lim_{r \to 0} \frac{\mathbb{E}[\nu^d(\Theta_{n \oplus r} \cap A)]}{b_{d-n} r^{d-n}} = \mathbb{E}[\mathcal{H}^n(\Theta_n \cap A)], \tag{12.5}$$

then

$$\mathbb{E}[\mathcal{H}^n(\Theta_n \cap A)] = \lim_{r \to 0} \int_A \frac{T_{\Theta_n}(B_r(x))}{b_{d-n} r^{d-n}} \, dx.$$

Sufficient conditions for (12.5) have been given in [ACV06].

According to [CV06a], if Θ_n is an absolutely continuous regular random closed set, then there exists an integrable function λ_{Θ_n} (the Radon–Nikodym derivative) such that, for all $A \in \mathcal{B}_{\mathbb{R}^d}$,

$$\mathbb{E}[\mathcal{H}^n(\Theta_n \cap A)] = \int_A \lambda_{\Theta_n}(x) \, dx.$$

So, in this case, we have that

$$\lim_{r \to 0} \int_A \frac{T_{\Theta_n}(B_r(x))}{b_{d-n} r^{d-n}} \, dx = \int_A \lambda_{\Theta_n}(x) \, dx. \tag{12.6}$$

If Θ_n is a stationary random closed set, then $T_{\Theta_n}(B_r(x))$ is independent of x and the expected measure $\mathbb{E}[\mu_{\Theta_n}]$ is motion invariant, i.e. it is absolutely continuous with density $\lambda_{\Theta_n}(x) = L \in \mathbb{R}_+$ for ν^d-a.e. $x \in \mathbb{R}^d$. It follows that

$$\lim_{r \to 0} \frac{T_{\Theta_n}(B_r(0))}{b_{d-n} r^{d-n}} = L.$$

12.6 Mean Densities of Stochastic Tessellations

Stochastic tessellations are a natural consequence of the random division of space due to the establishment of a vessel network in vasculogenesis (see Fig. 12.4). A random subdivision of space needs further information to be characterized. In this case the spatial region in $\mathbb{R}^d$ where the relevant process occurs is randomly divided into cells (random Johnson–Mehl tessellation [JM39, Mol92]; see also [Mol94]), and interfaces (n-facets, $n = 0, 1, \ldots, d$) at different Hausdorff dimensions (cells, faces, edges, vertices) appear (for a planar process, see Fig. 12.8).

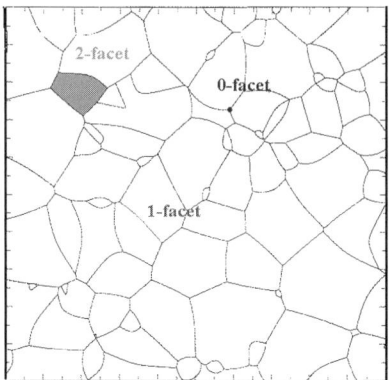

Fig. 12.8. n-facets for a tessellation in $\mathbb{R}^2$.

As above, we may describe quantitatively the tessellation by means of mean densities of the n-facets with respect to the d-dimensional Lebesgue measure [Mol92].

We may call a **cell** of a random tessellation any element of a family of RACSs partitioning the region E in such a way that any two distinct elements of the family have an empty intersection of their interiors. It is clear that this last definition may also be used in the static (time independent) case.

Let us now introduce a rigorous concept of "interface" at different Hausdorff dimensions.

Definition 6. *An* **n-facet** *at time t $(0 \leq n \leq d)$ is the non-empty intersection between $m + 1$ cells, with $m = d - n$.*

Note that in the previous definition

- $d =$ dimension of the space in which the tessellation takes place
- $n =$ Hausdorff dimension of the interface under consideration
- $m + 1 =$ number of cells that form such an interface
- for $n = d$ a d-facet is simply a cell

(see also Fig. 12.8).

Consider now the union of all n-facets at time t, $\Xi_n(t)$. For any Borel set B in $\mathbb{R}^d$ one can define the *mean n-facet content* of B at time t as the measure

$$\mathcal{M}_{d,n}(t, B) = \mathbb{E}\left[\mathcal{H}^n(B \cap \Xi_n(t))\right] \tag{12.7}$$

where $\mathcal{H}^n$ is the n-dimensional Hausdorff measure.

Suppose that the process is such that $\mathcal{M}_{d,n}$ admits a density $\mu_{d,n}(t, x)$ with respect to ν^d, the standard d-dimensional Lebesgue measure on $\mathbb{R}^d$, i.e. for any Borel set B

$$\mathcal{M}_{d,n}(t, B) = \int_B \mu_{d,n}(t, x)dx, \tag{12.8}$$

then the following definition is meaningful.

Definition 7. *The function $\mu_{d,n}(t,x)$ defined by (12.8) is called the local mean n-facet density of the tessellation at time t.*

In particular $\mu_{d,d-1}(t,x)$ is the surface density of the cells.

It is still an open problem, in general, to obtain evolution equations for these densities.

12.7 Birth-and-Growth Processes

Figs. 12.1–12.4 show a family of real processes from biology and medicine. In a detailed description, all these processes can be modelled as birth-and-growth processes. In tumour growth abnormal cells are randomly activated and develop due to a nutritional underlying field driven by blood circulation (angiogenesis); in crystallization processes such as sea shells [Ubu03] and polymer solidification [Cap03], etc., nucleation and growth may be due to a biochemical underlying field, or temperature cooling, etc.

All these kinds of phenomena are subject to random fluctuations, together with the underlying field, because of intrinsic reasons or because of the coupling with the growth process.

12.7.1   The Birth Process: Nucleation or Branching

A birth process can be modelled as a stochastic marked point process (MPP) N, defined as a random measure on $\mathcal{B}_{\mathbb{R}_+} \times \mathcal{E}$ by

$$N = \sum_{j=1}^{\infty} \epsilon_{(T_j, X_j)} \,,$$

where

- $\mathcal{E}$ denotes the sigma-algebra of the Borel subsets of E, a bounded subset of $\mathbb{R}^d$, the physical space;
- T_j is an $\mathbb{R}_+$-valued random variable representing the time of birth of the nth nucleus,
- X_j is an E-valued random variable representing the spatial location of the nucleus born at time T_j,
- $\epsilon_{t,x}$ is the Dirac measure on $\mathcal{B}_{\mathbb{R}_+} \times \mathcal{E}$ such that for any $t_1 < t_2$ and $B \in \mathcal{E}$,

$$\epsilon_{t,x}([t_1, t_2] \times B) = \begin{cases} 1 & \text{if } t \in [t_1, t_2], x \in B, \\ 0 & \text{otherwise .} \end{cases}$$

The (random) number of nuclei born during A, in the region B is given by

$$N(A \times B) = \sharp\{T_j \in A, X_j \in B\}, A \in \mathcal{B}_{\mathbb{R}_+}, B \in \mathcal{E}.$$

12.7.2 Stochastic Intensity

The *stochastic intensity* of the nucleation process provides the probability that a new nucleation event occurs in the infinitesimal region $[x, x + dx]$, during the infinitesimal time interval $[t, t + dt]$, given its past history $\mathcal{F}_{t-}$, i.e. the σ-algebra generated by all random variables of the process, up to time t,

$$\nu(dx \times dt) := P[N(dx \times dt) = 1 \mid \mathcal{F}_{t-}]$$
$$= E[N(dx \times dt) \mid \mathcal{F}_{t-}].$$

In many cases, such as in a crystallization process, or in tumour growth, we have *volume growth models*. If the nucleation events occur at

$$\{(T_j, X_j) \mid 0 \leq T_1 \leq T_2 \leq \ldots\}$$

the relevant phase (crystals or total tumour mass) at time $t > 0$ is described by a random set

$$\Theta^t = \bigcup_{T_j \leq t} \Theta_j^t, \tag{12.9}$$

given by the union of all grains born at times T_j and locations X_j and freely grown up to time t. In this case Θ^t has the same dimension d as the physical space.

If we wish to impose that no further nucleation event may occur in the occupied space, we have to assume that the stochastic intensity is of the form

$$\nu(dx \times dt) = \alpha(x, t)(1 - \delta_{\Theta^{t-}}(x))dt \ dx,$$

where δ_{Θ^t} denotes the indicator function of the set Θ^t, according to a formalism that will be discussed later; so that the term $(1 - \delta_{\Theta^{t-}}(x))$ is responsible for the fact that no new nuclei can be born at time t in the region already occupied by existing grains (see [CM06], and references therein).

The parameter α, also known as the *free space nucleation rate*, is a suitable real-valued measurable function on $\mathbb{R}_+ \times E$, such that $\alpha(\cdot, t) \in \mathcal{L}^1(E)$, for all $t > 0$ and such that

$$0 < \int_0^T dt \int_E \alpha(x, t)dx < \infty$$

for any $0 < T < \infty$, and

$$0 < \int_0^\infty dt \int_E \alpha(x, t)dx = \infty.$$

We will denote by

$$\nu_0(dx \times dt) = \alpha(x, t)dtdx$$

the *free space intensity*. If $\alpha(x, t)$ is deterministic, this corresponds to a space-time (inhomogeneous) Poisson process, in the free space.

12.7.3 Angiogenic Processes

An angiogenic process can be modelled as a branching-and-growth process at dimension 1. Such processes are usually called *fibre systems* [BR04] or *network systems*.

Now the marked counting process modelling the branching processes, called again N, refers to the offspring of a new capillary from already existing vessels, i.e. from a point of the stochastic fibre system Θ^t, now with Hausdorff dimension 1, so that the branching rate is given by

$$\mu(dx \times dt) = P(N(dx \times dt) = 1|\mathcal{F}_{t-}) = \alpha(x,t)\delta_{\Theta^{t-}}(x)dxdt. \qquad (12.10)$$

This case, which may provide a model for the stochastic branching of vessels, illustrated in Fig. 12.2, requires a much more complicated growth model, as do many other so-called fibre processes, or fibre systems; we refer to [CA99, TY01, Sun05a, PA06] for the modelling aspects, and to [BR04] for the (also non-trivial) statistical aspects. This case will be discussed in more detail below.

The growth model

In a model of birth (branching) and growth we need to define a suitable growth mechanism. Volume growth models have been studied more extensively since the pioneering work of [K37]. For our own applications to biomedicine we refer to [CM06].

As far as fibre growth is concerned, as in angiogenesis, we need to model the movement of tips until they meet another vessel (anastomosis), in which case growth stops and a loop is created [PK89].

12.8 Interaction with Underlying Fields

In tumour-induced angiogenesis the organization of endothelial cells and vessels is described by detailed stochastic processes, while various underlying fields (such as TAFs, inhibitors, and extracellular matrix constituents, such as fibronectin or the matrix degrading enzyme (MDE)) are usually described by continuum concentrations governed by partial differential equations (PDEs) [CA99, TY01, Sun05a, PS03].

Indeed, in real processes there is a strong coupling between the geometric structures of the birth (branching)-and-growth processes and such underlying fields. It is a matter of fact that random space-time heterogeneities are induced on the kinetic parameters of the relevant birth (branching)-and-growth processes because of their dependence upon such underlying fields, or their spatial gradients; in turn, the evolution equations of the underlying fields depend upon the evolving geometry of the vessel network produced by the birth (branching)-and-growth process.

Such strong coupling between the underlying fields and the stochastic geometry of the vessel network makes the processes of birth (branching) and growth doubly stochastic, which leads to a non-trivial analytical and computational problem. A way to reduce complexity is based on a possible multiple scale approach, which may lead to a hybrid system including deterministic PDEs for concentrations at the larger scale, and simply stochastic birth (branching)-and-growth processes at the cellular (vascular) scale, by means of averaging techniques.

As an example we propose here a model for tumour-induced angiogenesis proposed in [CMo07] and based on various papers in the literature (see e.g. [CA99, Harr06, Sun05a, PA06, PS03]).

A blood vessel network is generated in response to TAFs, which are released from hypoxic cells within a solid tumour.

The main features of the process of the movement of cells in the formation of the network are

i)   vessel branching;
ii) vessel extension;
iii) chemotaxis in response to a generic TAF, released by tumour cells;
iv) haptotaxis in response to fibronectin gradient, emerging from the extracellular matrix and through degradation and production by endothelial cells themselves;
v)   anastomosis, when a capillary tip meets an existing vessel.

12.8.1 The Vessel Network

Let $N(t) \in \mathbb{N}$ denote the random number of tips at time t, $X^i(t) \in \mathbb{R}^d$ denote the random location of the ith tip at time t, and $T_i \in \mathbb{R}_+$ denote the random birth time of the ith tip.

Sprout extension is modelled by tracking the random trajectory of individual capillary tips, so that

$$X(t) = \bigcup_{i=1}^{N(t)} \{X^i(s), T_i \leq s \leq t\}$$

is the random network of endothelial cells, i.e. the union of the random trajectories described by all existing tips.

From the theory of stochastic distributions presented in the previous sections, $\delta_{X^i(t)}(x)$ is the random distribution (Dirac density) localized at the tip $X^i(t)$, for $i = 1, \ldots, N(t)$, while $\delta_{X(t)}(x)$ is the random distribution localized at the whole network $X(t)$; $X^i(t)$ is a random closed set of Hausdorff dimension zero, and $X(t)$ is a random closed set of Hausdorff dimension one. Whenever the above random sets are absolutely continuous with respect to the usual Lebesgue measure on $\mathbb{R}^d$ [CV06a], the expected value of the Dirac deltas $\delta_{X^i(t)}$ is the usual probability density distribution of tips, while the expected value of the Dirac delta $\delta_{X(t)}$, describing the vessels, is the mean vessel density.

12.8.2 The Underlying Fields

The kinetic parameters of the branching and growth of capillaries are coupled with some underlying fields. Indeed from the literature [PS03, GK06] we know the following. TAFs and fibronectin activate the migration of cells. When activated, cells produce an MDE, which makes cells able to attach to fibronectin contained in the extracellular matrix. Let us denote by $C(x, t)$, $f(x, t)$, and $m(x, t)$ the spatial concentrations of TAFs, fibronectin, and MDE respectively. The chemotactic field TAF diffuses, and it decreases where endothelial cells are present. Two models of interaction may be adopted.

In a first model, the consumption, i.e. the receptor mediated binding, is due to all the cells of the network, in which case the model can be

$$\frac{\partial}{\partial t}C(t, x) = C_1 \delta_A(x) + C_2 \triangle C(t, x) - \eta C(t, x) \frac{1}{N}(\delta_{X(t)} * V_\epsilon)(x). \quad (12.11)$$

In an alternative model, consumption is due to the additional endothelial cells producing vessel extensions. It is proportional to the velocity $v_i, i = 1, \ldots,$ of the tips

$$\frac{\partial}{\partial t}C(t, x) = C_1 \delta_A(x) + C_2 \triangle C(t, x) - \eta C(t, x) \frac{1}{N} \sum_{i=1}^{N(t)} (v_i(t)\delta_{X^i(t)} * V_\epsilon)(x). \quad (12.12)$$

The parameters $C_1, C_2, \eta \in \mathbb{R}^+$ represent the rate of production of a source located in a region $A \subset \mathbb{R}^d$, modelling e.g. a tumour mass, the diffusivity, and the rate of consumption, respectively.

As far as the consumption terms are concerned, i.e. $\frac{1}{N}(\delta_{X(t)} * V_\epsilon)(x)$, and

$\frac{1}{N} \sum_{i=1}^{N(t)} (v_i(t)\delta_{X^i(t)} * V_\epsilon)(x)$, a rescaling by N has been included in order to

consider the dependence upon the (mollified) empirical distribution of either the existing vessels in the first case, or the variation in length of the existing vessels, per unit time. Convolution with a kernel $V_\epsilon(x)$ provides a mollified version of the relevant random distributions; from a modelling point of view this may correspond to a nonlocal reaction with the interacting fields (see e.g. [Sun05b]). The mollifier kernel V_ϵ is chosen such that $\lim_{\epsilon \to 0} V_\epsilon(x) = \delta_0(x)$. Furthermore $\epsilon << 1/N$, so that

$$\lim_{N \to \infty} V_\epsilon(x) = \delta_0(x).$$

Specific choices about the dependence of the kernel V_ϵ upon N will allow the convergence to the corresponding densities, for N tending to infinity, by means of suitable laws of large numbers [Oel89].

Fibronectin is attached to the extracellular matrix and does not diffuse [BBT80]. Degradation of fibronectin, characterized by a coefficient γ, depends on the concentration of MDE, produced by the cells [McDou06]:

$$\frac{\partial}{\partial t} f(t,x) = \beta \frac{1}{N} \sum_{i=1}^{N(t)} (\delta_{X^i(t)} * V_\epsilon)(x) - \gamma m(x,t) f(t,x).$$

The MDE, once produced, diffuses locally with a diffusion coefficient ϵ_1, and is spontaneously degraded at a rate ν:

$$\frac{\partial}{\partial t} m(t,x) = \epsilon_1 \triangle m(t,x) + \nu \frac{1}{N} \sum_{i=1}^{N(t)} (\delta_{X^i(t)} * V_\epsilon)(x) - \nu m(t,x).$$

These equations are subject to suitable boundary and initial conditions. They are random PDEs since the source terms depend upon the stochastic geometric process $X(t)$ of the vessel network. The underlying fields are thus stochastic; a direct consequence is the stochasticity of the kinetic parameters of branching and growth, as we will soon discuss.

12.8.3 The Branching Process

We shall assume for simplicity that only tips may branch, so that the relevant stochastic intensity of the branching process, depending upon the TAFs concentration $C(x,t)$ [CA99, PS03, Harr06], is given by

$$\mu(dt \times dx) = P(N(dt \times dx) = 1 | \mathcal{F}_{t-}) = \alpha(t,x) dx\, dt$$
$$= \alpha_1(C(t,x)) \sum_{i=1}^{N(t)} \delta_{X^i(t-)}(x) dx\, dt.$$

We assume that, when a tip located in x branches, the initial value of the state of the new tip is $\left(X^{N(t)+1}, v^{N(t)+1} \right) = (x, v_0)$, where v_0 is a non-random velocity.

12.8.4 Vessel Extension

As far as movement (elongation) is concerned, we take the Langevin model

$$dX^i(t) = (1 - p_a \mathbb{I}_{X(t)})(X^i(t)) dt,\ t > T^i,$$
$$dv^i(t) = a(X^i(t), v^i(t), t) dt + \sigma dW^i(t),\ t > T^i, \tag{12.13}$$

where the drift $a^i(x,t)$ is a function of the concentrations $C(x,t)$ and $f(x,t)$ and/or their gradients. In particular

$$a(X^i(t), v^i(t), t) = -kv^i(t) + F\left(C(X^i(t), t), f(X^i(t), t)\right), \quad (12.14)$$

i.e. we consider an inertial component and a bias due to the underlying fields,

$$F\left(C(X^i(t), t), f(X^i(t), t)\right) = d_C(C(X^i(t), t)) \, \nabla C(X^i(t), t)$$
$$+ d_f(f(X^i(t), t)) \, \nabla f(X^i(t), t). \quad (12.15)$$

d_C, d_f, are turning coefficients, measuring the ability of a cell of reorienting itself. We consider the following models:

$$d_C(C(X^i(t), t)) = d_1 \frac{\left|\nabla C(X^i(t), t)\right|}{(1 + \gamma C(X^i(t), t))^q}$$
$$d_f(f(X^i(t), t)) = d_2 \left|\nabla f(X^i(t), t)\right| \quad (12.16)$$

where $\gamma, q \geq 0$, so that the reorientation of the cells increases depending on the magnitude of the chemotactic, haptotatic gradient. Furthermore cells become desensitized to chemotactic gradients at high attractant concentrations, as pointed out in [AC98] and [Lev01].

The term $(1 - p_a \mathbb{I}_{X(t)})(X^i(t))$ models the phenomenon of impingement; $\mathbb{I}_{X(t)}$ denotes the indicator function associated with the existing vessel network $X(t)$.

From these facts we can derive the double stochasticity of the branching-and-growth process.

A complete mathematical analysis becomes very difficult and the detailed computational costs of numerical simulations tend to be very high.

Multiple scales and hybrid models

For many practical tasks, the stochastic models presented above, which are able to describe the full process, are too sophisticated. In many real situations multiple scales can be identified (see e.g. [BDEP04]). As a consequence it suffices to use averaged quantities at the larger scale, while still using stochastic quantities at the lower scales. The advantage of using averaged quantities at the larger scale is convenience, from both a theoretical and a computational point of view [PS03, Sun05b].

Under typical conditions, we may assume that the typical scale for diffusion of the underlying field (*macroscale*) is much larger than the typical scale of the growing material (vessels, cells, etc.) (*microscale*). This allows us to approximate the full stochastic model by a hybrid system, as follows. Under these conditions a *mesoscale* may be introduced, which is sufficiently small with respect to the macroscale of the underlying field and sufficiently large with respect to the typical grain size. First this means that the substrate may be considered approximately homogeneous at this mesoscale. A typical size x_{meso} on this mesoscale satisfies

$$x_{micro} << x_{meso} << x_{macro},$$

where x_{micro} and x_{macro} are typical sizes for single grains and for the field diffusion. This typical feature of the process is illustrated in Fig. 12.9.

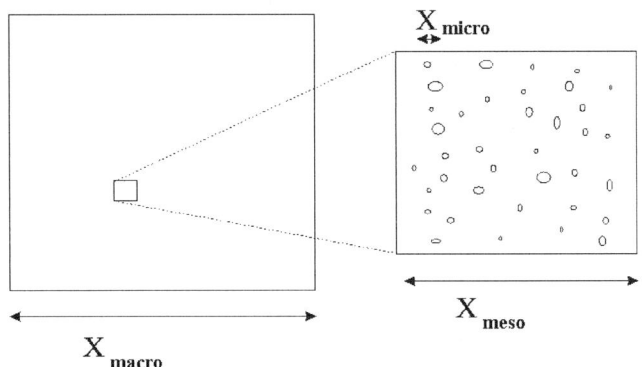

Fig. 12.9. Typical scales in the birth-and-growth process.

It makes sense to consider a discretization of the whole space in subregions $B_i, i = 1, \ldots, L$ at the level of the mesoscale, i.e. small enough that the spatial variation of the underlying fields inside B_i may be denied, but large enough to include a large number of endothelial cells participating in the vessel network; at this scale we may approximate (*law of large numbers*) the contribution due to the vascularization process by local mean values, in the equations for $C(x,t)$, $f(x,t)$, and $m(x,t)$.

If we now substitute all stochastic quantities in the equations for the underlying fields by their corresponding mean values, we may derive the following deterministic equations for the relevant underlying fields:

$$\frac{\partial}{\partial t}\widetilde{C}(t,x) = C_1\delta_A(x) + C_2\triangle\widetilde{C}(t,x) - \eta\widetilde{C}(t,x)w(x,t);$$

$$\frac{\partial}{\partial t}\widetilde{f}(t,x) = \beta\widetilde{p}(x,t) - \gamma m(x,t)\widetilde{f}(t,x);$$

$$\frac{\partial}{\partial t}\widetilde{m}(t,x) = \epsilon_1\triangle\widetilde{m}(t,x) + \nu\widetilde{p}(x,t) - \nu\widetilde{m}(t,x)$$

subject to suitable boundary and initial conditions.

Here $w(x,t) = \mathbb{E}[\delta_{X(t)}(x)]$ in model (12.11), while $w(x,t) = \mathbb{E}[v_i(t)\delta_{X_i(t)}(x)]$ in model (12.12); $\widetilde{p}(x,t) = \mathbb{E}[\delta_{X_i(t)}(x)]$. In the sequel we shall refer only to model (12.12); model (12.11) is subject to further investigation. In order to close the above system, evolution equations for such mean densities are now needed.

We may notice that the above system now provides deterministic fields $\widetilde{C}(x,t)$, $\widetilde{f}(x,t)$ and $\widetilde{m}(x,t)$. Consequently, we are given deterministic fields for the branching parameter $\alpha(x,t)$ and the extension parameter $a(x,v,t)$.

With these parameters, the branching-and-growth process is now again stochastically simple.

This approach is called "hybrid", since we have substituted all stochastic underlying fields by their "averaged" counterparts; most of the current literature could now be reinterpreted along these lines.

Indeed, one has to check that the hybrid system is fully compatible with a rigorous derivation of the evolution equations for the vessel densities. Nonlinearities in the full model are a big difficulty in this direction; a heuristic derivation will be offered below, while a rigorous mathematical analysis requires further investigation. We stress that substituting mean geometric densities of tips or of full vessels for the corresponding stochastic quantities leads to an acceptable coefficient of variation (percentage error) only when a law of large numbers can be applied, i.e. whenever the relevant numbers per unit volume are sufficiently large. Otherwise, stochasticity cannot be avoided, and in addition to mean values, the mathematical analysis and/or simulations should provide confidence bands for all quantities of interest [BCP05].

Empirical distributions and densities

A simplified case is the one in which the equations for concentrations do not depend on the random distribution of the full vessel network $\delta_{X(t)}(x)$, but on the random empirical distribution of tips (see e.g. [PS03]); here we refer to the evolution equations for the relevant densities of the model presented above [CMo07].

The global random empirical measure of the process $\{(X^k(t),v^k(t)),k=1,\ldots,N(t)\}_t$ is

$$Q_N(t) = \frac{1}{N} \sum_{i=1}^{N(t)} \epsilon_{(X^i(t),v^i(t))} \, .$$

The random empirical distribution of active tips is

$$T_N(t) = \frac{1}{N} \sum_{i=1}^{N(t)} \epsilon_{X^i(t)};$$

so that

$$T_N(t) = Q_N(t)(\cdot \times \mathbb{R}^d).$$

The empirical velocity distribution is given by

$$V_N(t) = \frac{1}{N} \sum_{i=1}^{N(t)} v_i(t)\epsilon_{X^i(t)};$$

consequently

$$V_N(t)(B_1) = \int_{B_1 \times \mathbb{R}^d} v \, Q_N(t)(d(x,v)).$$

In order to proceed with the asymptotics of the empirical measures, we also rescale the counting process $N(t)$ with respect to the scaling parameter N, i.e.

$$Z_N(t) := \frac{N(t)}{N};$$

which is now a jump process with jumps of size $1/N$, occurring at a rate $\alpha(t, x)$.

Heuristically, if we suppose that, for $N \to \infty$

$$Q_N(t) \longrightarrow Q_\infty(t)(d(x,v)) = p(t, x, v)d(x, v),$$

then also the empirical processes T_N and V_N will converge to

$$T_\infty(t)(dx) = \tilde{p}(t, x)dx,$$

and

$$V_\infty(t)(dx) = w(t, x)dx,$$

respectively.

Due to the known relations between all these densities, we have

$$\tilde{p}(t, x) = \int p(t, x, v)dv$$

$$w(t, x) = \int v \, p(t, x, v)dv.$$

Hence it is sufficient to provide an evolution equation for $p(t, x, v)$ in order to close the approximate evolution equations for the whole system.

Such an equation has been derived in [CMo07] by a suitable convergence of empirical processes (see e.g. [Oel89] and [MCO05]); the desired PDE for the joint density $p(t, x, v)$ is

$$\frac{\partial}{\partial t}p(t, x, v) = -v \cdot \nabla_x p(t, x, v) + k\nabla_v \cdot (vp(t, x, v)) + \alpha(t, x)p(t, x, v_0)$$

$$-\nabla_v \cdot [F\left(C(t, x), f(t, x)\right) p(t, x, v)] + \frac{\sigma^2}{2}\Delta_v p(t, x, v).$$

Inverse and optimal control problems

In presence of relevant data on the spatial density of the vessel network during a time interval, inverse roblems regarding the functional dependence of the kinetic parameters of the angiogenesis upon the underlying fields might be faced, as the authors did for problems of polymer crystallization (see [BCE99]).

Moreover, treatment of angiogenesis by means of anti-angiogenic chemicals, such as angiostatin, as discussed in [PS03], can be faced as an optimal control problem (see e.g. [BCM04]), once a suitable cost functional can be given.

12.9 Statistical Methods for Fibre Systems

In this and in the following sections we will describe some statistical methods which furnish a quantitative description of the mean geometric characteristics of random fibre systems, which, at a suitable scale where the width of the fibres can be neglected (i.e. fibres have Hausdorff dimension 1), may represent networks of vessels generated by angiogenesis or vasculogenesis, or also other networks, for example of neurons, lymph vessels, etc. Since in most cases such networks have a spatially non homogeneous structure, statistical methods which may put into evidence and compare quantitatively spatial inhomogeneities are a valid tool both for medical doctors, for diagnosis and dose/response analysis and thus therapy, and for mathematicians, to validate mathematical models by comparison of simulated and real data. One of the first descriptors of the mean geometry of a random fibre system is its mean length density, also called *intensity*, of which here we will describe some estimators.

Let Γ be a stochastic $1-$regular closed set in $\mathbb{R}^d$ that we will call *random fibre system*.

Note that

$$T_\Gamma(B_r(x)) = \mathbb{P}(x \in \Gamma_{\oplus r}) = \mathbb{P}(\Gamma \cap B_r(x) \neq \emptyset)$$

thus we may rewrite Equality (12.6), for $\Theta_n = \Gamma$ and $n = 1$, in the following way

$$\int_A \lambda_1(x)dx = \lim_{r \to 0} \int_A \frac{T_\Gamma(B_r(x))}{b_{d-1}r^{d-1}} dx \tag{12.17}$$

$$= \lim_{r \to 0} \int_A \frac{\mathbb{P}(x \in \Gamma_{\oplus r})}{b_{d-1}r^{d-1}} dx \tag{12.18}$$

$$= \lim_{r \to 0} \int_A \frac{\mathbb{P}(\Gamma \cap B_r(x) \neq \emptyset)}{b_{d-1}r^{d-1}} dx \tag{12.19}$$

Equalities (12.17)-(12.19) provide a way to introduce estimators of $\lambda_1(x)$ for a random fibre, or fibre system Γ, provided that the limit and the integrals in the right-hand terms of (12.17)-(12.19) can be exchanged, by estimating the quantities

$$\frac{T_\Gamma(B_r(x))}{b_{d-1}r^{d-1}} = \frac{\mathbb{P}(x \in \Gamma_{\oplus r})}{b_{d-1}r^{d-1}} = \frac{\mathbb{P}(\Gamma \cap B_r(x) \neq \emptyset)}{b_{d-1}r^{d-1}}.$$

We will call them *histogram-like* estimators, since the "enlargement" $\Gamma_{\oplus r}$ of the set Γ via the Minkowski addition of a d-dimensional ball, which approximates the fibre with a d-dimensional set, imitates the procedure used when we estimate the p.d.f. of a real random variable from an i.i.d. sample using moving histograms or kernels (see [Hard91, Pest98, Silv86] for details), where we "enlarge" the Dirac-delta's measures concentrated on the sample points, approximating them with classical and sufficiently regular functions.

According to the definitions introduced in the previous sections, the density of Γ is defined by

$$\lambda(x) := \lambda_1(x) = \mathbb{E}[\delta_\Gamma](x) = \lim_{r \to 0} \frac{\mathbb{E}(\mathcal{H}^1(\Gamma \cap B_r(x)))}{r^d b_d}.$$

In the following we will provide two estimators for the density of a random fibre system Γ, based on the estimate of $T_\Gamma(B_r(x))$ or of $\mathbb{P}(\Gamma \cap B_r(x) \neq \emptyset)$.

Basic assumptions for the estimation procedure

Suppose to have one or more images of the random fibre system Γ under study and that the window $W \subseteq \mathbb{R}^d$ where Γ is observed can be divided in a partition of subwindows $\{A_k\}_{k=1,\dots,K}$ such that

A1 $A_j \cap A_k = \emptyset, \ \forall j \neq k$
A2 $\bigcup_{k=1}^{K} A_k = W$
A3 in each window A_k limit and integral in (12.6) can be exchanged when
    $\Theta_n = \Gamma$
A4 the density $\lambda(x)$ can be locally well approximated by piecewise constant
    functions, assuming different constant values in each window A_k.

Note that Assumption A3 is satisfied if in A_k the fibre system is (*locally*) stationary at a suitable mesoscale (see [ACV06] for a discussion of this problem).

12.9.1 Estimators of the density

Let us assume A1-A4; then for all $x \in A_k$, let us denote by

$$\lambda_k := \lim_{r \to 0} \frac{\mathbb{E}(\nu^1(\Gamma \cap B_r(x)))}{b_d r^d}$$
$$= \lim_{r \to 0} \frac{\mathbb{P}(x \in \Gamma_{\oplus r} \cap A_k)}{2r}$$
$$= \lim_{r \to 0} \frac{T_\Gamma(B_r(x))}{2r}$$

the (constant) density of the random fibre system in the subwindow A_k. We have explicited all the previous equalities since we will obtain different estimators, based on the estimate of the quantities

1. $\mathbb{P}(x \in \Gamma_{\oplus r} \cap A_k)$
2. $T_\Gamma(B_r(x))$,

respectively.

Fattening fibres

Let us build first an estimator based on the estimate of $\mathbb{P}(x \in \Gamma_{\oplus r} \cap A_k)$. Let us overlap to A_k a grid of points $z_1, \ldots, z_p \in A_k$ and build the set $\Gamma_{\oplus r} \cap A_k$. Then a first estimator of λ_k is

$$\hat{\lambda}^1_{k,r,p} : = \frac{1}{2rp} \sum_{i=1}^{p} \mathbf{1}_{z_i \in \Gamma_{\oplus r} \cap A_k} \tag{12.20}$$

where $\mathbf{1}_{z_i \in \Gamma_{\oplus r} \cap A_k}$ are Bernoulli random variables assuming value one with probability $\mathbb{P}(x \in \Gamma_{\oplus r} \cap A_k)$ which is independent of $x \in A_k$ in our assumptions.

The asymptotic unbiasedness and other relevant statistical properties of this estimator can be proven (see [CM07] for the proofs, and a discussion on edge effects).

Fattening points

Let us now introduce an estimator based on the estimate of $T_\Gamma(B_r(x)), x \in A_k$.

Let us again consider a grid of points $z_1, \ldots, z_p$ overlapped on the window A_k, such that $B_r(z_i) \subseteq A_k$ for all $i = 1, \ldots, p$ (this assumption has the aim of reducing the edge effects). We then define

$$\hat{\lambda}^2_{k,r,p} : = \frac{1}{2rp} \sum_{i=1}^{p} \mathbf{1}_{\Gamma \cap B_r(z_i) \neq \emptyset} \tag{12.21}$$

where again $\mathbf{1}_{\Gamma \cap B_r(z_i) \neq \emptyset}$ is a Bernoulli random variable assuming value 1 with probability $\mathbb{P}(\Gamma \cap B_r(z_i) \neq \emptyset) = T_\Gamma(B_r(z_i)) = T_\Gamma(B_r(x)), \forall x \in A_k$.

Again this is an asymptotically unbiased estimator (see [CM07]).

Both estimators can be computed by overlapping either a grid of deterministic and equally spaced points $z_1, \ldots, z_p$, or a random grid of points uniformly distributed on a window of observation. For a discussion of the advantages of either methods see [CM07].

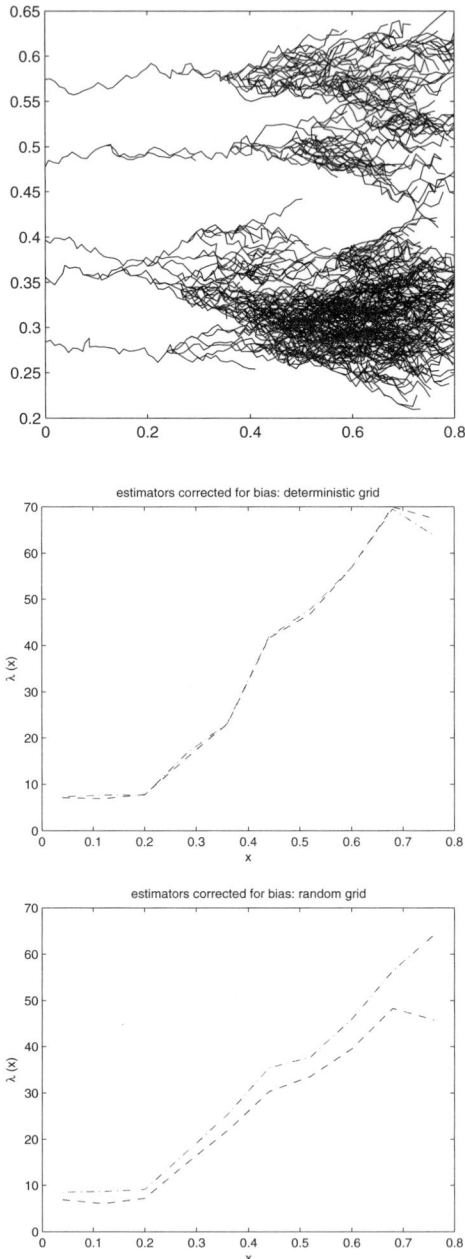

Fig. 12.10. Estimate of the fibre density of an angiogenic process with a chemotactic field having a gradient in the x direction. Middle figure: estimate with a deterministic grid; bottom figure: estimate with a random grid of 2000 points. Dashed line= $\hat{\lambda}^1_{k,r,p}$, dotted-dashed line= $\hat{\lambda}^2_{k,r,p}$

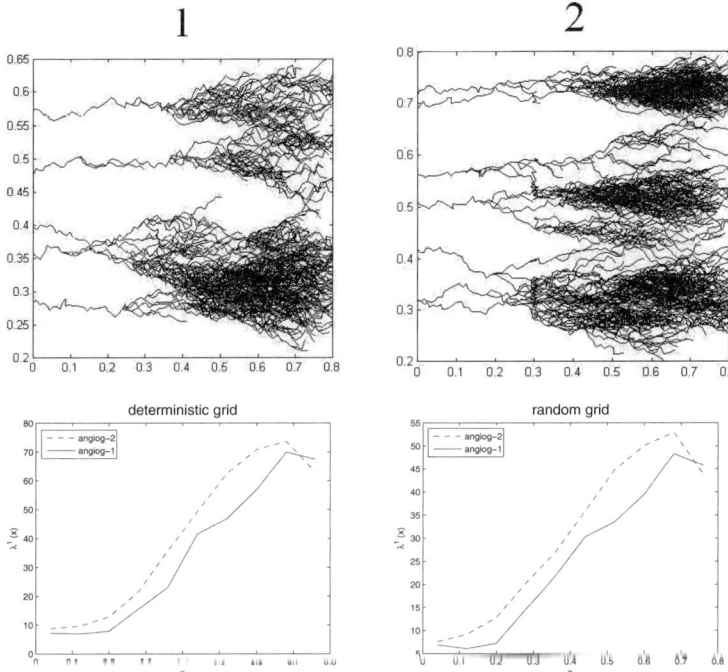

Fig. 12.11. Comparison between the two simulated angiogenic processes depicted in the top line. Bottom left: comparisons of $\hat{\lambda}^1_{k,r,p}$ for the two processes estimated with a deterministic grid; bottom right: comparisons of $\hat{\lambda}^1_{k,r,p}$ for the two processes estimated with a random grid. In both cases the first process reveals a density lower than the second, and this was really the case in the performed simulation.

12.10 Application of the Estimators to Simulated Angiogenic Processes

The estimators have then been applied to some (naive) simulations of real fibre processes , where the true density simulation of the generation and branching of vessels driven by a chemotactic field generated by a tumor is reported. The tumor is located on the right hand side of the window and the vessels start growing and branching from the left hand side of the window in the right direction. The chemotactic field has a gradient in the x direction and influences both the speed of growth and the branching of the vessels. The density has been estimated both with a deterministic and a random grid, by dividing the observation window into 10 vertical stripes of the same width. The results are reported in Figure 12.10. In Figure 12.11 two simulations are reported where the intensities of branching where different. The difference is not much evident by simply looking at the patterns, but the estimate of the density reveals that the pattern on the left has a lower density than the

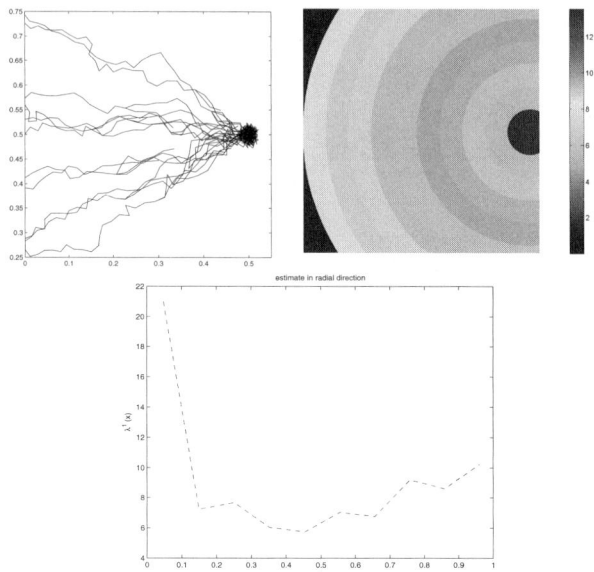

Fig. 12.12. Estimate of the fibre density of an angiogenic process driven by a chemotactic field with a spherical symmetry. Top line: the fibre process and an estimate of $\hat{\lambda}^1_{k,r,p}$ using a random grid and dividing the window into 10 spherical shells centered at the tumor; bottom: plot of $\hat{\lambda}^1_{k,r,p}$ with respect to the radial coordinate, centered at the tumor

pattern on the right for any value of x, and this was really the case, since the frequency of branching and speed of growth was settled higher in the right hand pattern. This is thus an example where quantitative analysis is essential for the characterization and differentiation of the geometry.

In Figure 12.12 an analogous process but driven by a chemotactic field with a spherical symmetry around a point-shaped tumor is reported. Because of the observed symmetry, in this case the window of observation has been divided into 10 spherical shells centered at the tumor location. Both the estimated values in each subregion in a 2D visualization and the plot of the estimated density with respect to the radial coordinate are reported. In this case, since the subwindows are spherical shells, only estimator $\hat{\lambda}^1_{k,r,p}$ has been computed, since it is more easily computable for non-rectangular regions (see [CM07]).

In Figure 12.13 estimator $\hat{\lambda}^1_{k,r,p}$ has been computed on three images of vascular networks generated in allantoids (see [CM06] for a discussion of the relevance of these studies in tumor treatment). Two of the three allantoids have been treated with two different doses of an antiangiogenic substance, which should inhibit the formation of vessels. The figure on the left refers to an untreated control allantoid. Because of the spherical symmetry of the images, also in this case the observation window has been divided into spherical shells

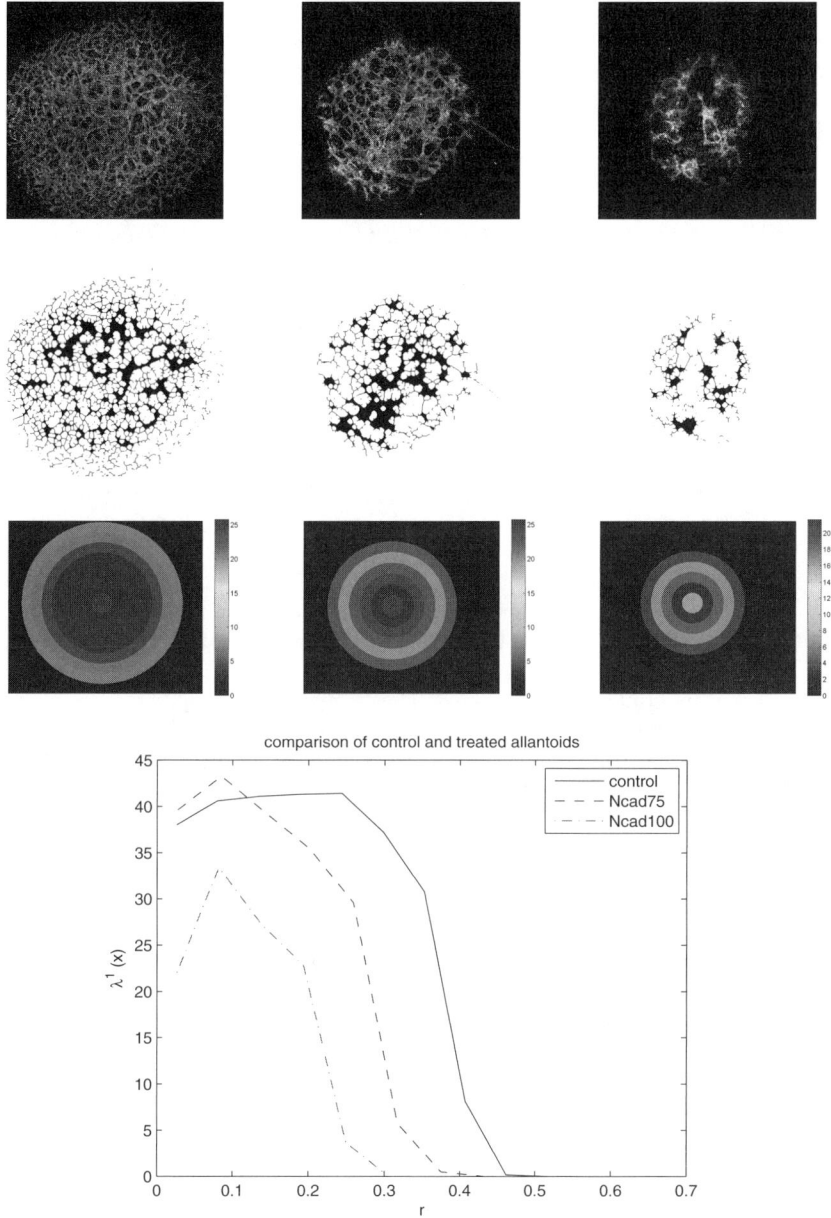

Fig. 12.13. Vascularization in allantoids. First line, from left to right: control experiment (untreated), treated with 0.75 mg of antiangiogenic substance, treated with 1 mg of antiangiogenic substance [Credit: [CFD99]]. Second line: scheletonization of the upper images. Third line: 2D representation of the density estimate of the fibres in the skeletons; the space has been divided into 10 spherical concentric shells. Bottom line: comparison of the radial estimates of the intensities of the 3 allantoids

centered at the centroid of the allantoid. The results of the estimate reveal, in a quantitative way, that the increase of the dose of the substance results in a less widespread network and in a lower density of length of the vessels.

Acknowledgments

It is a pleasure to acknowledge useful discussions with many colleagues at different universities and research centres. Particular thanks are due to Professor Martin Burger (Münster), Dr. Daniela Morale (Milan), and Dr. Elena Villa (Milan).

References

[ACV06]   Ambrosio, L., Capasso, V., Villa, E.: On the approximation of geometric densities of random closed sets. RICAM Report N. 2006–14, Linz, Austria (2006).

[AFP00]   Ambrosio, L., Fusco, N., Pallara, D.: Functions of Bounded Variation and Free Discontinuity Problems. Clarendon Press, Oxford (2000).

[AC98]   Anderson, A.R.A., Chaplain, M.: Continuous and discrete mathematical models of tumour-induced angiogenesis. Bull. Math. Biol., **60**, 857–899 (1998).

[AG80]   Araujo, A., Giné, E.: The Central Limit Theorem for Real and Banach Valued Random Variables. John Wiley & Sons, New York (1980).

[Avr39]   Avrami, M.: Kinetics of phase change. Part I, J. Chem. Phys., **7**, 1103–112 (1939).

[BM97]   Baddeley, A.J., Molchanov, I.S.: On the expected measure of a random set. In: Proceedings of the International Symposium on Advances in Theory and Applications of Random Sets (Fontainebleau, 1996). World Sci. Publishing, River Edge, NJ, 3–20 (1997).

[BDEP04]   Bellomo, N., De Angelis, E., Preziosi L.: Multiscale modelling and mathematical problems related to tumour evolution and medical therapy. J. Theor. Med., **5**, 111–136 (2004).

[BR04]   Beneš, V., Rataj, J.: Stochastic Geometry. Kluwer, Dordrecht (2004).

[BBT80]   Birdwell, C., Brasier, A., Taylor, L.: Two-dimensional peptide mapping of fibronectin from bovine aortic endothelial cells and bovine plasma. Biochem. Biophys. Res. Commun., **97**, 574–581 (1980).

[Bosq00]   Bosq, D.: Linear Processes in Function Spaces. Theory and Applications, Lecture Notes in Statistics, **149**, Springer-Verlag, New York (2000).

[BCE99]   Burger, M., Capasso, V., Engl, H.: Inverse problems related to crystallization of polymers. Inverse Problems, **15**, 155–173 (1999).

[BCM04]   Burger, M., Capasso, V., Micheletti, A.: Optimal control of polymer morphologies. Journal of Engineering Mathematics, **49**, 339–358 (2004).

[BCP05] Burger, M., Capasso, V., Pizzocchero, L.: Mesoscale averaging of nucleation and growth models. Multiscale Modeling and Simulation: a SIAM Interdisciplinary Journal. **5**, 564–592 (2006).

[BCS02] Burger, M., Capasso, V., Salani, C.: Modelling multi-dimensional crystallization of polymers in interaction with heat transfer. Nonlinear Analysis: Real World Application, **3**, 139–160 (2002).

[Cap03] Capasso, V. (ed): Mathematical Modelling for Polymer Processing. Polymerization, Crystallization, Manufacturing. Mathematics in Industry, Vol. 2, Springer-Verlag, Heidelberg (2003).

[CM06] Capasso, V., Micheletti, A.: Stochastic geometry and related statistical problems in Biomedicine. In: A. Quarteroni et al. (eds.) Complex Systems in Biomedicine. Springer, Milano, 36–69 (2006).

[CM07] Capasso, V., Micheletti, A.: Kernel-like estimators of the mean density of inhomogeneous fibre processes. In preparation (2007).

[CMo07] Capasso, V., Morale, D.: Stochastic modelling of tumour-induced angiogenesis. Preprint (2007).

[CV06a] Capasso, V., Villa, E.: Continuous and absolutely continuous random sets. Stoch. Anal. Appl., **24**, 381–397 (2006a).

[CV06b] Capasso, V., Villa, E.: On the geometric densities of random closed sets. Stoch. Anal. Appl. 2007. In press.

[CV07] Capasso, V., Villa, E.: On mean densities of inhomogeneous geometric processes arising in material science and medicine. Image Analysis and Stereology, **26**, 23–36 (2007).

[CA99] Chaplain, M.A.J., Anderson, A.R.A.: Modelling the growth and form of capillary networks. In: Chaplain, M.A.J. et al. (eds.) On Growth and Form. Spatio-temporal Pattern Formation in Biology. John Wiley & Sons, Chichester (1999).

[CZD02] Corada, M., Zanetta, L., Orsenigo, F., Breviario, F., Lampugnani, M.G., Bernasconi, S., Liao, F., Hicklin, D.J., Bohlen, P., Dejana, E.: A monoclonal antibody to vascular endothelial-cadherin inhibits tumor angiogenesis without side effects on endothelial permeability. Blood. **100**, 905–911 (2002).

[CFD99] Crosby, C.V., Fleming, P., Zanetta, L., Corada, M., Giles, B., Dejana, E., Drake, C.: VE-cadherin is essential in the de novo genesis of blood vessels (vasculogenesis) in the allantoids. Blood, **105**, 2771–2776 (2005).

[Fal85] Falconer, K.J.: The Geometry of Fractal Sets. Cambridge University press, Cambridge (1985).

[Fed96] Federer, H.: Geometric Measure Theory. Springer, Berlin (1996).

[Folk74] Folkman, J.: Tumour angiogenesis. Adv. Canc. Res., **19**, 331–358 (1974).

[FK87] Folkman, J., Klagsbrun, M.: Angiogenic factors. Sci., **235**, 442–447 (1987).

[GK06] Gabrial, A.S., Krasnow, M.A.: Social interactions among epithelial cells during tracheal branching morphogenesis. Nature, **441**, 746–749 (2006).

[Hahn99] Hahn, U., Micheletti, A., Pohlink, R., Stoyan, D., Wendrock, H.: Stereological analysis and modeling of gradient structures. J. of Microscopy, **195**, 113–124 (1999).

[Hard91]   Hardle, W.: Smoothing Techniques. With Implementation in S, Springer-Verlag, New York (1991).

[Harr06]   Harrington, H.A., et al.: A hybrid model for tumor-induced angiogenesis in the cornea in the presence of inhibitors (2006). Preprint.

[JC01]   Jain, R.K., Carmeliet, P.F.: Vessels of Death or Life. Scientific American **285**, 38–45 (2001).

[JM39]   Johnson, W.A., Mehl, R.F.: Reaction kinetics in processes of nucleation and growth. Trans. A.I.M.M.E., **135**, 416–458 (1939).

[K37]   Kolmogorov, A.N.: On the statistical theory of the crystallization of metals. Bull. Acad. Sci. USSR, Math. Ser. **1**, 355–359 (1937).

[KF70]   Kolmogorov, A.N., Fomin, S.V.: Introductory Real Analysis, Prentice-Hall, Englewood Cliffs, NJ, (1970).

[Lev01]   Levine, H.A., Pamuk, S., Sleeman, B.D., Nilsen-Hamilton, M.: A mathematical model of capillary formation and development in tumour angiogenesis: penetration into the stroma. Bull. Math. Biol., **63**, 801–863 (2001).

[Mat75]   Matheron, G.: Random Sets and Integral Geometry. John Wiley & Sons, New York (1975).

[McDou06]   McDougall, S.R., Anderson, A.R.A., Chaplain, M.A.J.: Mathematical modelling of dynamic tumour-induced angiogenesis: clinical implications and therapeutic targeting strategies. J. Theor. Biology, **241**, 564–589 (2006).

[Mol92]   Møller, J.: Random Johnson-Mehl tessellations. Adv. Appl. Prob., **24**, 814–844 (1992).

[Mol94]   Møller, J.: Lectures on Random Voronoi Tessellations. Lecture Notes in Statistics, Springer-Verlag, New York (1994).

[MCO05]   Morale, D., Capasso, V., Ölschlaeger, K.: An interacting particle system modelling aggregation behavior: from individuals to populations, J. Math. Bio. **50**, 49–66 (2005).

[Oel89]   Oelschläger, K.: On the derivation of reaction-diffusion equations as limit dynamics of systems of moderately interacting stochastic processes. Prob. Th. Rel. Fields. **82**, 565–586 (1989).

[PK89]   Paweletz, N., Kneirim, M.: Tumour related angiogenesis. Crit. Rev. Oncol. Haematol., **9**, 197–242 (1989).

[Pest98]   Pestman, W.R.: Mathematical Statistics. An Introduction, Walter de Gruyter, Berlin, (1998).

[PS03]   Planck, M.J., and Sleeman, B.D.: A reinforced random walk model of tumour angiogenesis and anti-angiogenic strategies. Math Med Biology, **20**, 135–181 (2003).

[PA06]   Preziosi, L., Astanin, S.: Modelling the formation of capillaries. In: A. Quarteroni et al.(eds.) Complex Systems in Biomedicine. Springer, Milano, 109–145 (2006).

[Ser03]   Serini, G., et al.: Modeling the early stages of vascular network assembly. EMBO J., **22**, 1771–1779 (2003).

[Silv86]   Silverman, B.W.: Density Estimation for Statistics and Data Analysis, Chapman & Hall, London (1986).

[SKM95]   Stoyan, D., Kendall, W.S., Mecke, J.: Stochastic Geometry and Its Application. John Wiley & Sons, New York (1995).

[Sun05a]   Sun, S., et al.: Nonlinear behaviors of capillary formation in a deterministic angiogenesis model. Nonlinear Analysis, **63**, e2237–e2246 (2005).

[Sun05b]   Sun, S., et al.: A multiscale angiogenesis modeling using mixed finite element methods. SIAM J. on Multiscale Model Simul., **4**, 1137–1167 (2005).

[TY01]   Tong, S., and Yuan, F.: Numerical simulations of angiogenesis in the cornea. Microvascular Research, **61**, 14–27 (2001).

[Ubu03]   Ubukata, T.: Computer modelling of microscopic features of molluscan shells. In: Sekimura, T. et al. (eds.) Morphogenesis and Pattern Formation in Biological Systems. Springer-Verlag, Tokyo, 355–368 (2003).

[Zah82]   Zähle, M.: Random processes of Hausdorff rectifiable closed sets. Math. Nachr., **108**, 49–72 (1982).

13

Mathematical Modelling of Breast Carcinogenesis, Treatment with Surgery and Radiotherapy, and Local Recurrence

Heiko Enderling[1] and Jayant S. Vaidya[2]

[1] Center of Cancer Systems Biology, Caritas St. Elizabeth's Medical Center, Tufts
University School of Medicine, 736 Cambridge Street, Boston, MA 02135, USA
heiko.enderling@tufts.edu
[2] Division of Surgery and Molecular Oncology, Ninewells Hospital and Medical
School, University of Dundee, Dundee DD1 9SY, UK
j.s.vaidya@dundee.ac.uk

13.1 Introduction

Breast cancer is the single commonest cause of death of women in forties and
fifties [V07]. In the last decade, we have seen a considerable decline in breast
cancer mortality [B00]. This mainly reflects wider and improved implementation of therapies that were already known and proven to be useful in reducing
mortality from the disease, rather than novel paradigms of disease. There have
been many attempts at discovering and inventing new approaches to therapy
with only a few successes. One was herceptin—an antagonist of the growth
receptor HER-2/neu [PG05, RP05]. The other major success was the proof of
benefit of the aromatase inhibitor Arimidex resulting from one of the largest
randomised controlled trials (the ATAC trial). One cannot let this decline in
mortality lead to complacence as it is may not continue much longer. For further improvements in breast cancer outcomes one needs to synthesise newer
models of disease that incorporate new molecular biology information. This is
not only important in understanding its natural history, but also in simulating
new therapies, which are increasingly difficult and time consuming to test in
a clinical setting.

In this chapter, we shall be looking at the development of new models of
breast cancer initiation and progression and its local treatment with surgery
and radiotherapy. It is generally accepted that breast cancer arises in the pre-
menopausal period and is stimulated to grow at some point in the woman's
life time. By the age of 55, about a third of women harbour occult cancer
in their breasts—only a third of which become clinically manifest. We shall
not be considering other dormant cancers in this chapter, but it is important

N. Bellomo et al. (eds.), *Selected Topics in Cancer Modeling*,
DOI: 10.1007/978-0-8176-4713-1_13, © Springer Science+Business Media, LLC 2008

to acknowledge their existence and put in perspective the clinically manifest cancer.

As regards the local treatment, there are some important facts to be rehearsed.

(a) Adequate local treatment of breast cancer does not necessarily need to be very radical. The difference between the local control rates achieved by mastectomy and breast conserving surgery plus whole breast radiotherapy are essentially equivalent.

(b) However, local control of the disease is important both for patient symptomatic and psychological welfare and for its effects on overall survival. It is clear from the overview analysis that for every 4% absolute reduction in local control at 5 years, there is about 1% reduction in mortality at 15 years.

(c) The main determinant of patient survival is distant disease which is mainly affected by systemic therapy (and early local control).

Systemic therapies have been the subject of considerable research, and far more clinical trials have been conducted on systemic therapies (which also attract big pharmaceutical interests) than on local therapies, which are mainly academically driven.

Local treatment of breast cancer involves either wide local excision (lumpectomy) or mastectomy and some type of axillary surgery which today takes the form of a limited axillary sampling usually guided by a radioactive dye injection (sentinel node) in the first instance [KJ04, VD05]. An essential component of the package of local treatment is radiotherapy using ionizing radiation. This is essential in almost all cases of surgery that conserve the breast and is frequently given to patients who have had a mastectomy and have a high risk of local recurrence due to advanced or aggressive disease.

Radiotherapy has been used for treatment of cancer almost since it was discovered. For breast cancer its value was firmly established in 1985, with the publication of the Oxford overview for breast conserving surgery, and in 2005 for post-mastectomy use [C05]. However, the principles that guide radiotherapy treatment planning, though based on sound foundations, have remained the same for the last three decades. There is a lack of complex models that describe irradiation and tissue/tumour interaction, and most clinic treatment plans are based on empirical knowledge and wisdom. Briefly, and with a risk of oversimplification, they are the following: irradiation causes damage to cellular DNA machinery; this damage is usually repairable by normal cells, but not cancer cells with a faulty repair mechanism; smaller doses allow easier repair and have a greater therapeutic ratio, leading to the common practice of fractionated doses of radiotherapy—typically about 2 Gy per fraction for 25 to 30 fractions. It is also known that different tissues react at different times after radiotherapy and late reacting tissues are more sensitive to larger single fractions of radiotherapy. The problem with the latter is that normal tissues also react poorly and can undergo severe fibrosis and scarring if they are not in some way protected by a more targeted therapy. Recent literature suggests that breast cancer may react in a way similar to late reacting tissues so single fractions may have a greater therapeutic effect. Their side effects could in turn be reduced if the target volume is low and accurately includes the tissues at highest risk of local recurrence.

The exact mechanism of radiotherapy effects as an adjuvant to surgery is not clear. The main assumption is that radiotherapy would eradicate microtumours or single stray cancer cells that remain after surgery. One other concern about radiotherapy is that in breast cancer it is effective in reducing local recurrence by about two-thirds [C05]. This proportional reduction in local recurrence does not vary with the extent of primary surgery or whether there were tumour cells at the histological margin of surgical excision or not, and this is puzzling [VT04]. Although tumour cells present at the margin of the primary excision increase the risk, it is reduced by radiotherapy by the same proportional extent as that when there are no tumour cells present at the margin, suggesting that radiotherapy may be working in ways other than by killing actual tumour cells [VT04]. The effect of radiotherapy is likely to be a combination of effects on peri-tumoural breast tissues and on residual tumour cells. One effect could be altering the internal milieu of the tumour bed, making it less conducive to tumour growth and tumour cell migration [VT04, MB06]. There is translational research evidence that radiotherapy could reduce the stimulatory effect of surgical wound fluid on cancer cells [MB06]. Another possibility could be an effect on cells that are not morphologically abnormal, but harbour genetic abnormalities.

Finally, novel technology has allowed radiotherapy to be delivered with smaller and less expensive machines that can be easily transported to the operation theatre and easily manipulated to enable good targeting of the tumour bed at the time of operation. However, the schedules for the new techniques that take into consideration the newer biological understanding of disease are difficult to test in randomised trials. This is where mathematical modeling could be of considerable value.

If we develop a mathematical model that simulates growth and recurrence of breast cancer and therapeutic radiotherapy schedules and validate the model with clinical trial results, then it could be used to simulate new therapeutic strategies and guide the development of intelligent randomised clinical trials, avoiding those trials that are unlikely to give a useful result. Furthermore, inclusion of newer biological parameters in the model may allow us to develop more individualised treatment for a particular patient.

13.1.1 Mathematical Models of Cancer

Over the last few decades or so the number of mathematical models of cancer initiation, promotion, and progression has dramatically increased [AC00, TS02, AM04, SB04]. With more biological information on cancer development becoming available, more detailed models can be designed that can be used to ask specific questions. In recent years mathematical models have become more accepted by biologists and clinicians, resulting in improved communication with mathematicians. Building on this interface, interdisciplinary multi-scale models could be developed with the potential to steer the direction of future research.

Mathematical models have the power to simulate different possible setups and investigate various clinically plausible parameter sets simultaneously to identify key mechanisms involved in the process under consideration. This will become increasingly important for predicting the outcome of possible treatment strategies or designing new treatment protocols. Based on simple mathematical and biological information on how different therapeutic agents, such as those administered in chemotherapy or radiotherapy, affect healthy and tumour cells, different doses and treatment protocols can be simulated without harming a single patient. The number of interesting interdisciplinary studies to improve cancer therapy (using chemotherapy and/or radiotherapy) has increased noticeably in recent years [PA95, SH01, BW02, SA02, DS04, AM06, DH06, K06, MN06, MO06, RC06, PK07]. The information resulting from mathematical models becomes available within minutes or hours compared to the long time periods of trial design, patient recruitment, and followup times to investigate late effects. The persisting rate of local and distant recurrence after apparently adequate treatment shows the need to investigate the disease further and identify how and when the treatment fails, and most importantly to design new treatment strategies that may provide better tumour control, reduce patient inconvenience, and maybe reduce logistic and financial burdens in current cancer treatment facilities.

Mathematical models were used to address the basis of sequential chemotherapy given in cycles—the hamster lymphoma model is more than 40 years old but is still the model used for most chemotherapy regimens. In many ways, it falls short of simulating the natural history of solid tumours and this corroborates well with the failure of non-specific chemotherapy to make a significantly large impact on solid tumour mortality. New models that take into account the different biology of a solid tumour are necessary for progress in this field. With a knowledge of how different agents interact with the cells and induce death and the reasons for possible survival of healthy cells, mathematical models could be used to investigate the benefits of combining different agents and determine which administration sequence has the highest promise of providing tumour control. In this chapter we shall not be discussing models for chemotherapy further, but will concentrate on models for local growth, radiotherapy, and recurrence.

13.1.2 Interaction of Ionizing Radiation with DNA

Ionizing radiation interacts with the DNA of the cell and causes different kinds of damage (Fig. 13.1). Single base damages and single-strand breaks are repairable with time as the complementary base information is available.

DNA double-strand breaks as induced by ionizing radiation, however, are repaired either by homologous recombination or non-homologous end-joining mechanisms [SLB04], which can result in crucial DNA alterations and cell death.

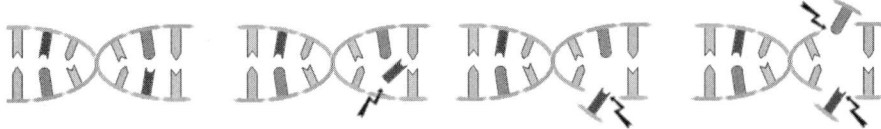

DNA double helix   *single base damage*   *single-strand break*   *double-strand break*

Fig. 13.1. Cartoon of DNA and possible radiation-induced damage. Single base damage and single-strand breaks are repairable as the complement information on the other strand is still available. Double-strand breaks can be misrepaired if the wrong DNA endings are joined.

Normal DNA-repair mechanisms at different check points during the cell cycle are able to detect and to repair most low-dose radiation-induced damage [O01] in a relatively short time (approximately 70.2 min, [BA98]). The therapeutic index of radiotherapy relies on the fact that cancer cells lack such efficient DNA-repair mechanisms and therefore genetic damage is carried on. If the resulting unrepaired mutations in cancer cells limit the cell's ability to survive, which is the case in about 12% of all radiaton-induced double-strand breaks [TC03], a proportion dies with every small dose of radiation. The traditional aim of radiotherapy has been to achieve a therapeutic index by inducing tumour cell death while limiting the damage to nearby healthy cells. Most radiobiological reaction-rate models lead to linear-quadratic (LQ) relations [SH97]. The biologically effective dose (BED) can be obtained from this relation, i.e.

$$BED: \quad \frac{E}{\alpha} = nd(1 + \frac{d}{\alpha/\beta}), \tag{13.1}$$

where E denotes the effectiveness of irradiation, d is the physical dose delivered per fraction, n is the total number of fractions, and α and β are positive constants describing single-hit DNA damage and the combination of two independent single hits, respectively [O01].

With the known BEDs for healthy cells and cancer cells one can calculate the surviving probability S [GAL03] as

$$S = \exp(-\alpha BED), \tag{13.2}$$

which can then be used to predict the outcome of a treatment.

In this chapter we will present a complex model of breast cancer initiation and its progression, treatment with breast conserving surgery and adjuvant radiotherapy, and local recurrence. The development of cancer cells occurs on a scale of months, years, or even decades. Once a cancer cell is established, the formation of a tumour can be seen in a relatively short time compared to the development of a cancer cell. Tumour and tissue interactions, however, such as production and diffusion of matrix degrading enzymes, occur on a much smaller time scale, i.e. hours or minutes. When the tumour has reached a clinically detectable size it is treated within days or weeks.

Spatially we scale our model to represent the macroscopic tumour level that is present at time of detection and treatment. Therefore we choose a continuous approach and describe the system dynamics using differential equations. At the end we will discuss the limitations of a continuous model and motivate the development of a discrete or hybrid discrete-continuous model.

13.2 A Continuous Mathematical Model of Breast Cancer Initiation and Progression

Tumours are highly heterogeneous and feature millions of different mutations, not only from patient to patient, but also organ specific. Cells are subject to mutations whenever they divide, as the reading of DNA and encoding of proteins does not occur without any mistakes. The probability that one gene suffers such a mutation during mitosis is generally assumed to be 10^{-7} [T01, MIN04]. Other mutations can occur when the cell receives environmental insults, such as radiation exposure. [HW00] have reviewed that there are six crucial mutations that each cell has to accumulate before the transformation into a cancer cell is complete. These mutations are (i) limitless replicative potential, (ii) evasion of apoptosis, (iii) self-sufficiency in growth signals, (iv) insensitivity to anti-growth signals, (v) sustained angiogenesis, and (vi) tissue invasion and metastasis. However, it is generally assumed that differentiated somatic cells do not live long enough to acquire all these mutations. In recent years the role of stem cells as initiators for carcinogenesis became more of interest, as stem cells have two of the crucial probabilities of cancer cells already established: evading apoptosis and limitless replicative potential [AHW03, SA03, WC05]. Stem cells therefore live long enough to accumulate several mutations.

Different kinds of genes are involved in cancer development: oncogenes and tumour suppressor genes. Each gene is composed of two alleles inherited from the paternal and maternal gene (Fig. 13.2). Oncogenes contribute to carcinogenesis if one of their two alleles is mutated, whereas both alleles in tumour suppressor genes have to be inactivated for the gene to lose its functionality. If only one of the two alleles is mutated the bi-fold information is lost, a feature known as loss of heterozygosity (LOH) on a tumour suppressor gene.

Stem cells play a crucial role especially in the female breast, which develops relatively late in life through clonal expansion of a small number of stem cells. These stem cells are subject to mutations pre-puberty, and if a crucial

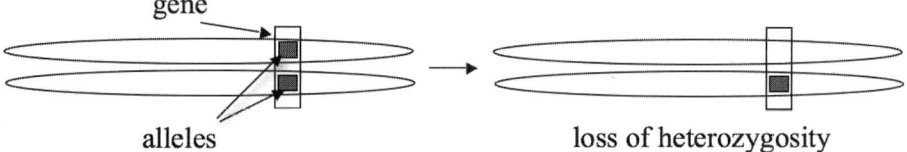

Fig. 13.2. Schematic of a chromosome (left) with a gene encoded by two alleles. After having received a mutative hit the chromosome on the right features a phenomena known as loss of heterozygosity.

mutation such as LOH on a tumour supressor gene (TSG) occurs, then during puberty this mutation will be present in all daughter cells and thus spread throughout the breast (Fig. 13.3). These fields of mutated cells result in a large number of cells susceptible to further mutative hits.

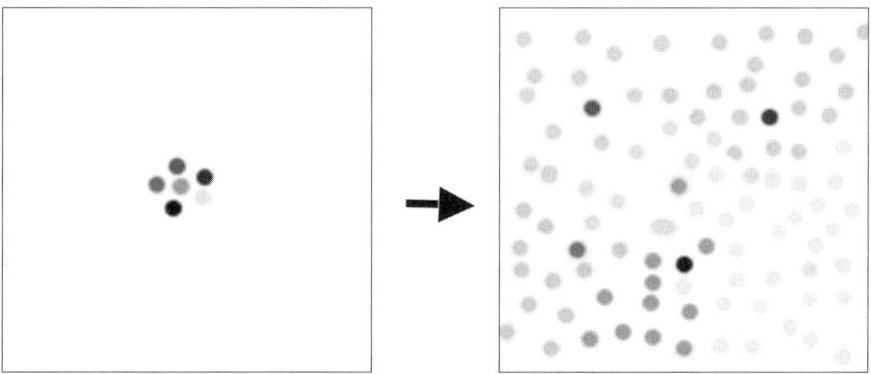

Fig. 13.3. Schematic of the clonal formation of the breast from only a few stem cells (left). The panel on the right shows fields of cells with identical genetic material formed from the initial stem cells.

In our model of tumour initiation and development we assume that the inactivation of two TSGs is sufficient to give rise to a fully developed cancer cell. For simplicity we ignore oncogenes in our study as the activation of oncogenes is much more likely than the inactivation of a TSG, for which two independent hits are necessary. We denote a healthy TSG with $TSG_i^{+/+}$, a TSG with LOH $TSG_i^{+/-}$, and an inactivated TSG with $TSG_i^{-/-}$. The mutation pathway from a cell with two healthy TSGs, i.e. $TSG_1^{+/+}TSG_2^{+/+}$, to a cancer cell with both TSGs inactivated is

$$TSG_1^{+/+}TSG_2^{+/+} \xrightarrow{p_1} TSG_1^{+/-}TSG_2^{+/+} \xrightarrow{p_2} TSG_1^{-/-}TSG_2^{+/+}$$
$$\xrightarrow{p_3} TSG_1^{-/-}TSG_2^{+/-} \xrightarrow{p_4} TSG_1^{-/-}TSG_2^{-/-} .$$

We have estimated the probabilities of the primary and subsequent mutations (p_1–p_4) in line with the studies by [TNB96, MIN04, NMK04]. The probability p_1 of mutating one allele of a normal cell is widely assumed to be 2×10^{-7} per gene per cell division ([TNB96, NMK04]), and the subsequent mutation rates follow from this value. This value for p_1 is widely used in the literature, and variation of it would result in a faster or delayed mutation acquisition. After the first LOH on a TSG, the mutation probability increases by a factor of magnitude 10^1–10^2 and hence we assume $p_2 = 10^{-6} - 10^{-5}$. Once two mutations accumulate within a cell, the possibility of further mutations increases to about $p_3 = 10^{-3}$, and the final mutation probability rate p_4 in the model increases as above and hence is assumed to be about $p_4 = 10^{-2}$ [EC07].

In an ordinary differential equation form the mutation pathway is as follows:

$$\text{tissue} \qquad \frac{df}{dt} = \overbrace{-\theta f}^{f \to TSG_1^{+/-}}$$

$$TSG_1^{+/-} \qquad \frac{dq}{dt} = \overbrace{\theta f}^{f \to TSG_1^{+/-}} - \overbrace{p_2 q}^{TSG_1^{+/-} \to TSG_1^{-/-}}$$

$$TSG_1^{-/-} \qquad \frac{dr}{dt} = \overbrace{p_2 q}^{TSG_1^{+/-} \to TSG_1^{-/-}} - \overbrace{p_3 r}^{TSG_1^{-/-} \to TSG_2^{+/-}}$$

$$TSG_2^{+/-} \qquad \frac{ds}{dt} = \overbrace{p_3 r}^{TSG_1^{-/-} \to TSG_2^{+/-}} - \overbrace{p_4 s}^{TSG_2^{+/-} \to n} \qquad (13.3)$$

$$\text{tumour} \qquad \frac{\partial n}{\partial t} = \overbrace{p_4 s}^{TSG_2^{+/-} \to n}$$

with f denoting healthy cells (i.e. $TSG_1^{+/+}TSG_2^{+/+}$), and q, r, s, and n denoting pre-malignant subpopulations and tumour cells (i.e. $TSG_1^{-/-}TSG_2^{-/-}$), respectively. For the purpose of this model we assume that breast cancer is a spatial phenomenon within a highly heterogeneous breast tissue. The female breast is composed of different structures with different physical properties, and therefore the spatial interaction of tumour cells with their environment plays a crucial role. We therefore introduce spatial tumour migration, i.e. random diffusion and migration up hatotactic gradients within the heterogeneous breast tissue. Furthermore, all pre-malignant subpopulations as well as tumour cells have a selective advantage over non-mutated cells, which we implement in the mutation rates p_i. With many cells competing for space, tumour cells have the ability to release matrix degrading enzymes such as matrix metalloproteinases and urokinase [M92, CL05] that diffuse throughout the tissue and degrade the environment upon contact. This results in steep haptotactic gradients that guide tumour cell migration as well as space for these cells to migrate and proliferate into. Tumour cells are known to create an acidic environment that makes it difficult for non-tumour cells to survive. For simplicity we have not included oxygen and glucose in our model, but have modelled pre-malignant cell death dependent on adjacent tumour cell density. Factors such as oxygen and glucose, however, can be incorporated in a model such as ours as done for example in [A05] and [SG05]. The described dynamics and spatial components lead to the following set of ordinary and partial differential equations ([E06, EC07]):

$$
\text{tissue} \quad \frac{df}{dt} = \overbrace{\mu_f\, f(f_0 - A)}^{\text{repopulation}} - \overbrace{\kappa_f\, mf}^{\text{degradation}} - \overbrace{\theta f}^{f \to \text{TSG}_1^{+/-}}
$$

$$
\text{TSG}_1^{+/-} \quad \frac{dq}{dt} = \overbrace{\mu_q q(1 - A)}^{\text{proliferation}} - \overbrace{\kappa_q\, nq}^{\text{death}} + \overbrace{\theta f}^{f \to \text{TSG}_1^{+/-}} - \overbrace{p_2 q}^{\text{TSG}_1^{+/-} \to \text{TSG}_1^{-/-}}
$$

$$
\text{TSG}_1^{-/-} \quad \frac{dr}{dt} = \overbrace{\mu_r r(1 - A)}^{\text{proliferation}} - \overbrace{\kappa_r\, nr}^{\text{death}} + \overbrace{p_2 q}^{\text{TSG}_1^{+/-} \to \text{TSG}_1^{-/-}} - \overbrace{p_3 r}^{\text{TSG}_1^{-/-} \to \text{TSG}_2^{+/-}}
$$

$$
\text{TSG}_2^{+/-} \quad \frac{ds}{dt} = \overbrace{\mu_s s(1 - A)}^{\text{proliferation}} - \overbrace{\kappa_s\, ns}^{\text{death}} + \overbrace{p_3 r}^{\text{TSG}_1^{-/-} \to \text{TSG}_2^{+/-}} - \overbrace{p_4 s}^{\text{TSG}_2^{+/-} \to n} \quad (13.4)
$$

$$
\text{tumour} \quad \frac{\partial n}{\partial t} = \overbrace{\mu_n n(1 - A)}^{\text{proliferation}} + \overbrace{D_n \nabla^2 n}^{\text{random motility}} - \overbrace{\nabla \cdot (\chi n \nabla f)}^{\text{haptotaxis}}
$$

$$
+ \overbrace{p_4 s}^{\text{TSG}_2^{+/-} \to n}
$$

$$
\text{MDE} \quad \frac{\partial m}{\partial t} = \overbrace{D_m \nabla^2 m}^{\text{diffusion}} + \overbrace{\xi n(1 - m)}^{\text{production}} - \overbrace{\omega m}^{\text{decay}},
$$

where $A = n + f + q + r + s$ represents the total tissue and cell population including cancer cells and θ is the product of the normal mutation probability p_1, the proportion of stem cells within the tissue, and the number of TSGs. We note that healthy tissue (f) is degraded by the enzymes (m) released by the tumour, whereas nearby cells (q, r, s) only suffer from the presence of tumour cells (n) which create an unfavourable environment. We scaled the carrying capacity of the breast tissue, and $A = n + f + q + r + s \leq 1$ represents the total tissue and cell population including cancer cells. If the tissue density decreases compared to its initial density f_0 we assume the tissue to repopulate with factor μ_f. We assume that the tumour grows inside the breast without reaching the outer boundary—the skin. Hence we neglect the anatomically correct breast geometry and introduce a "heterogeneous tissue" represented by a 2-dimensional (2D) domain initialized with a combination of *sine* and *cosine* functions with frequency variations in the x and y directions (Fig. 13.4).

We assume that the tumour grows inside that domain of breast tissue, and therefore our system is considered to hold in a 2D spatial domain Ω (a region of tissue) with appropriate initial conditions for each variable. We assume that all pre-malignant and tumour cells, and consequently the matrix degrading enzymes (MDEs), remain within the domain of tissue under consideration and therefore no-flux boundary conditions are imposed on $\partial\Omega$, the boundary of Ω.

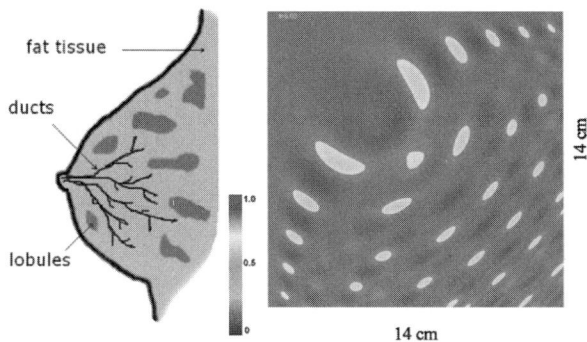

Fig. 13.4. a) Schematic of the female breast, showing different internal structures such as ducts, lobules, and fat tissue. b) Heterogeneous breast tissue used as initial condition for all subsequent simulations. Tissue heterogeneity is colour-coded, with dark gray representing a very dense tissue, and lighter gray tissue with a compactness of 0.5. We have used a combination of *sine* and *cosine* functions with frequency variations in x and y directions to account for heterogeneity. The average density is 0.75 as estimated in [N05].

In order to solve the system numerically, we first of all non-dimensionalise the equations in the standard way. We rescale distance with an appropriate length scale L (i.e. the size of the breast $= 14$ cm [BS04]), time with $t = 1$ year, tumour cell density with n_0, healthy tissue density with f_0, $TSG_1^{+/-}$ density with q_0, $TSG_1^{-/-}$ density with r_0, $TSG_2^{+/-}$ density with s_0, and MDE concentration with m_0 (where n_0, f_0, q_0, r_0, s_0, m_0 are appropriate reference density and concentration variables). Therefore setting

$$\tilde{f} = \frac{f}{f_0}, \; \tilde{q} = \frac{q}{q_0}, \; \tilde{r} = \frac{r}{r_0}, \; \tilde{s} = \frac{s}{s_0}, \; \tilde{n} = \frac{n}{n_0}, \; \tilde{m} = \frac{m}{m_0}, \; \tilde{\tau} = \frac{t}{\tau_0}$$

in (13.4) and dropping the tildes for notational convenience, we obtain the scaled system of equations:

$$\frac{df}{dt} = \overbrace{\lambda_f f(f_0 - A)}^{\text{repopulation}} - \overbrace{\eta_f\, mf}^{\text{degradation}} - \overbrace{l_1 f}^{f \to \text{TSG}_1^{+/-}}$$

$$\frac{dq}{dt} = \overbrace{\lambda_q q(1 - A)}^{\text{proliferation}} - \overbrace{\eta_q\, nq}^{\text{death}} + \overbrace{l_1 f}^{f \to \text{TSG}_1^{+/-}} - \overbrace{\rho_2 q}^{\text{TSG}_1^{+/-} \,\to\, \text{TSG}_1^{-/-}}$$

$$\frac{dr}{dt} = \overbrace{\lambda_r r(1 - A)}^{\text{proliferation}} - \overbrace{\eta_r\, nr}^{\text{death}} + \overbrace{\rho_2 q}^{\text{TSG}_1^{+/-} \to \text{TSG}_1^{-/-}} - \overbrace{\rho_3 r}^{\text{TSG}_1^{-/-} \to \text{TSG}_2^{+/-}}$$

$$\frac{ds}{dt} = \overbrace{\lambda_s s(1 - A)}^{\text{proliferation}} - \overbrace{\eta_s\, ns}^{\text{death}} + \overbrace{\rho_3 r}^{\text{TSG}_1^{-/-} \to \text{TSG}_2^{+/-}} - \overbrace{\rho_4 s}^{\text{TSG}_2^{+/-} \to n} \qquad (13.5)$$

$$\frac{\partial n}{\partial t} = \overbrace{\lambda_n n(1 - A)}^{\text{proliferation}} + \overbrace{d_n \nabla^2 n}^{\text{random motility}} - \overbrace{\nabla \cdot (\gamma n \nabla f)}^{\text{haptotaxis}} + \overbrace{\rho_4 s}^{\text{TSG}_2^{+/-} \to n}$$

$$\frac{\partial m}{\partial t} = \overbrace{d_m \nabla^2 m}^{\text{diffusion}} + \overbrace{\alpha n(1 - m)}^{\text{production}} - \overbrace{\beta m}^{\text{decay}}.$$

We have solved the above model numerically using a finite difference scheme implemented in Java, and all simulation results shown in this chapter are also generated in Java.

In our first simulation, we have initialized our model with a healthy cell density as shown in Fig. 13.4. All pre-malignant and tumour populations are initially zero, i.e. $q_0 = r_0 = s_0 = n_0 = 0$. We have solved the model and simulated more than 100 years until the development of a tumour up to clinically realistic size, i.e. 1.5 cm in diameter [VVH05], could be observed. These results lead to two different assumptions: (i) the normal mutation rate during mitosis is not sufficient to give rise to a tumour within a patient's life span, and therefore external factors that may act as mutagens play a major role in cancer initiation, or (ii) there are fields of pre-malignant subclones in the female breast after puberty. We will focus on the latter case. As discussed above, the female breast develops relatively late in life during puberty (Fig. 13.3). We assume that there is a pool of stem cells responsible for the formation of the female breast during puberty that were subject to mutations pre-puberty. If one of these stem cells received a mutative hit, such as LOH in a TSG, then all clonal daughter cells harbour this mutation, too. This leaves a field with a large number of pre-malignant cells susceptible to further mutative hits, which may ultimately lead to the development of a tumour (Fig. 13.5).

We now introduce such a field of mutated cells into our initial conditions. We again believe that only stem cells live long enough to accumulate all necessary mutations and hence only a small fraction of these pre-malignant cells are considered. Fig. 13.6 (left panel) shows the initialized breast tissue as well as a small area with a very low density of cells with LOH in a TSG. The numerical solution of these conditions then leads to the development of a tumour within 58 years (Fig. 13.6, center and right panels). 58 years after puberty will translate into patients of a very high age. However, as mentioned

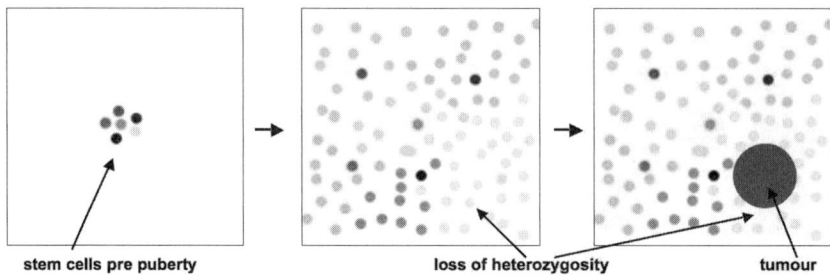

stem cells pre puberty   **loss of heterozygosity**   **tumour**

Fig. 13.5. Development of a tumour (solid circle, right panel) from a field of pre-malignant cells, i.e. cells with LOH in a tumour suppressor gene (TSG1+/-TSG2+/+) formed after clonal expansion of a mutated stem cell (light gray, cells in bottom right corner) pre-puberty.

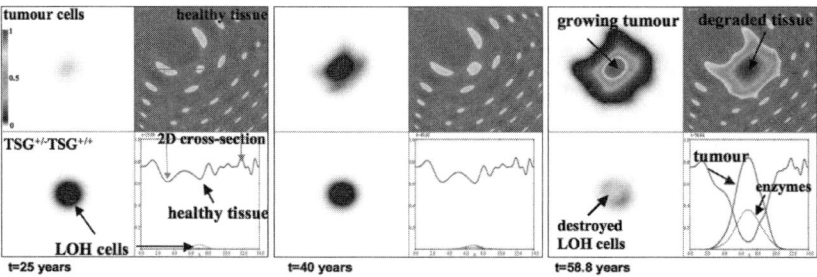

Fig. 13.6. Development of a tumour (top left panels) from a field of cells with LOH in a TSG, i.e. $TSG_1^{+/-}$ (bottom left panels) within the healthy tissue (top right panels). As time evolves (left to right, 25 years, 40 years, 58.8 years) the tumour grows and invades the domain. As the tumour grows it releases MDEs that destroy the cells with LOH in a TSG as well as healthy tissue to make space for the tumour to grow into. A cross section through the domain and all data sets is shown in the bottom right panels.

before, we have not considered any external mutagens in our model, which are likely to increase the transformation of normal cells towards cancer cells. We can estimate that such external factors to scale the cancer onset time to be in line with clinical findings.

We have transferred the tumour progression model into three special dimensions to solve it in a biologically more realistic environment [EA06b]. Similar to the 2D results discussed in Fig. 13.6, we use a combination of *sine* and *cosine* functions with frequency variations in the x, y, and z directions to model tissue heterogeneity. Fig. 13.7 shows the growth of a tumour in a heterogeneous 3D domain. Initially a small tumour is located in the center of the domain. As time evolves it invades the tissue, and due to haptotaxis it grows towards areas of high tissue density (elliptic areas throughout the domain, lighter gray represents higher density than lower gray, Fig. 13.7a

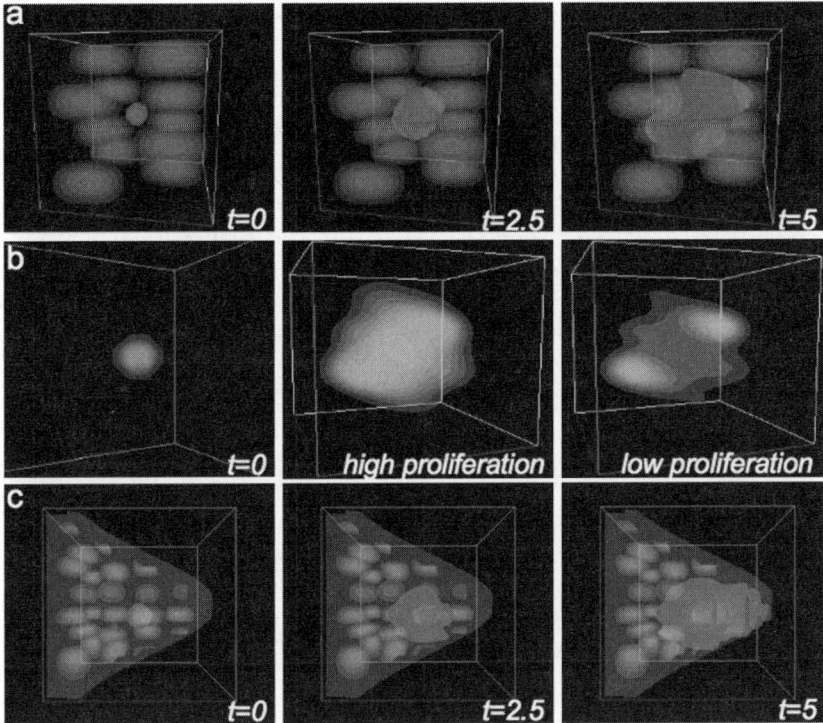

Fig. 13.7. Growth of a tumour in a heterogeneous 3D domain. a) A small tumour cell density is initially placed at the center of the domain. Areas of high tissue densities throughout the domain are shown where an intense gray represents a higher tissue density than a less intense gray (shown only $f(x, y, z) > 0.7; 0.8; 0.9$). As time evolves the tumour grows and invades the domain. Due to haptotaxis it grows towards areas of higher tissue density. b) Study of the impact of proliferation on internal tumour density. With a high proliferation rate the tumour core is very dense (center). With a low proliferation rate diffusion and haptotaxis define the tumour with the highest density being located at the edge of the tumour near areas of high tissue density (right). c) A tumour that grows and invades a breast-like shaped domain.

and 13.7c). Fig. 13.7b shows the impact of tumour cell proliferation on the internal tumour density distribution. With a high proliferation rate the core of the tumour is very dense (center panel). With a low proliferation rate diffusion and haptotaxis are dominant and hence the tumour has denser regions near its boundary where the tissue density is highest (right panel).

13.3 Modelling Surgery and Radiotherapy

The conventional treatment of patients with early stage breast cancer is breast conserving surgery (i.e. lumpectomy) and adjuvant fractionated external beam radiotherapy. About 30% of patients treated with lumpectomy alone develop a local recurrence within 10 years of primary treatment. Radiotherapy reduces the local recurrence rates by about two-thirds, yet leaves behind a persisting rate of local recurrence of about 10% [C05]. In this section we will apply our model of breast cancer development and extend it with a model of surgery and radiotherapy. With this approach we aim to identify why conventional treatment fails and how future treatments can be designed to prevent local recurrence.

In Figs. 13.6 and 13.7 we have shown the simulation of tumour initiation and progression. Breast tumours are dense lumps within less dense breast tissue. Norton has estimated a tumour compactness of 0.98 compared to a 0.75 breast tissue density [N05]. The average breast cancer detection size is about 1.5 cm in diameter [VVH05]. In the simulation shown in Fig. 13.6 the tumour core has reached a density of 0.75 and more. We stopped the simulation once the tumour diameter above the 0.75 density threshold reached 1.5 cm in diameter (Fig. 13.6, right panel). Additionally to the core lump there are low tumour densities at the outer surface of the tumour within the adjacent tissue.

We assume the surgeon to remove the detected dense tumour as well as a 1 cm margin around it. Fig. 13.8 then shows that in our simulation of this procedure some small tumour cell densities may reside in the tumour bed. During surgery biopsies from the tissue in the tumour bed are taken, and if single tumour cells are found, then another margin will be excised. However, there is a possibility that microscopic tumours or single stray cells remain undetected. If we re-initialize our model with this setup then a new tumour will form from these residual tumour cells within 10 years of surgery (Fig. 13.8). This is in line with the local recurrences observed in the clinic after treatment with surgery alone. Simulations of our model support the understanding that residual tumour cells or microscopic tumours in the tumour bed could be the cause for a local recurrence post breast conserving surgery.

With the possibility of single tumour cells or microscopic tumours straying beyond the surgical margin, radiotherapy is now standard as adjuvant treatment post-surgery for early stage breast cancer patients. Adjuvant radiotherapy has been shown to reduce local recurrence in about two-thirds of patients [C05]. Conventional external beam radiotherapy (EBRT) is given in 25 fractions of 2 Gy (1 Gy = 1 Joule/kg). After surgery, the patient returns to the hospital each day for 5 weeks to receive the treatment. The time between the fractions gives the healthy tissue enough time to repair the radiation-induced damage and recover from irradiation. Tumour cells, however, lack efficient repair mechanisms and hence accumulate damage, which may ultimately lead to the death of cancer cells. The tumour bed is exposed to significant stress

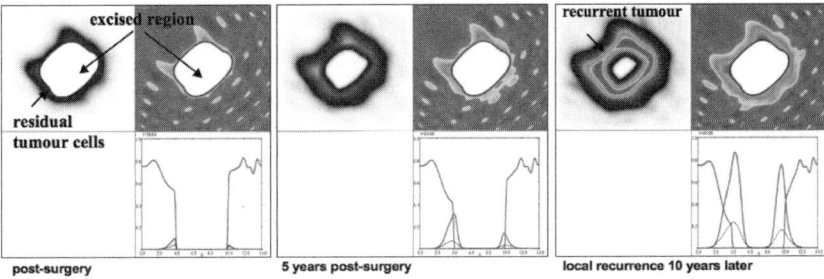

Fig. 13.8. Simulation of surgery of the tumour (development shown in Fig. 13.5) and local recurrence after treatment if a small tumour density resides in the tissue post surgery. The recurrence becomes clinically apparent in our simulations within 5 to 10 years after primary treatment.

post-surgery. During the process of wound healing, a burst of growth factors, angiogenesis, and increased proliferation can be observed [MB06]. We therefore believe that all tumour cells in the tumour bed are likely to be radiosensitive at the time of irradiation delivery. In Fig. 13.9 we show the simulation of 25×2 Gy EBRT to the post-surgical tissue shown in Fig. 13.8a. The dose is delivered uniformly to the whole breast. At simulated days of treatment (excluding the weekends) we apply the introduced LQ model (13.2) to estimate the survival fractions of each subpopulation in the tissue at each grid point in the computational domain. In between fractions we solve the continuous cancer development and progression model (13.5) to account for inter-fraction repopulation and migration dynamics. For the continuous model we assume the same tumour doubling time as before. Due to re-oxygenation and space availability in the tumour bed the tumour cell doubling time may reduce. We will discuss this later and motivate the development of a discrete or hybrid model. However, assuming no increase in doubling time, then as shown in Fig. 13.9 all tumour cells are likely to be eradicated. In our simulations, the largest tumour cell density is the tumour bed post-surgery of 0.001 reduces to 10^{-9}. Given the discussed assumptions, our model suggests that radiotherapy is likely to achieve tumour control.

13.3.1 Genetically Mutated Cells in the Tumour Bed and Targeted Intra-Operative Radiotherapy

In the previous section we have shown a biological setup where breast conserving surgery and adjuvant radiotherapy provided sufficient tumour control. However, clinical data shows that about 10% of patients will face a local recurrence within 10 years of primary treatment [C05]. About 92% of local recurrences occur at the side of the primary tumour. The current standard adjuvant EBRT protocols hence include additionally a boost to the tumour bed.

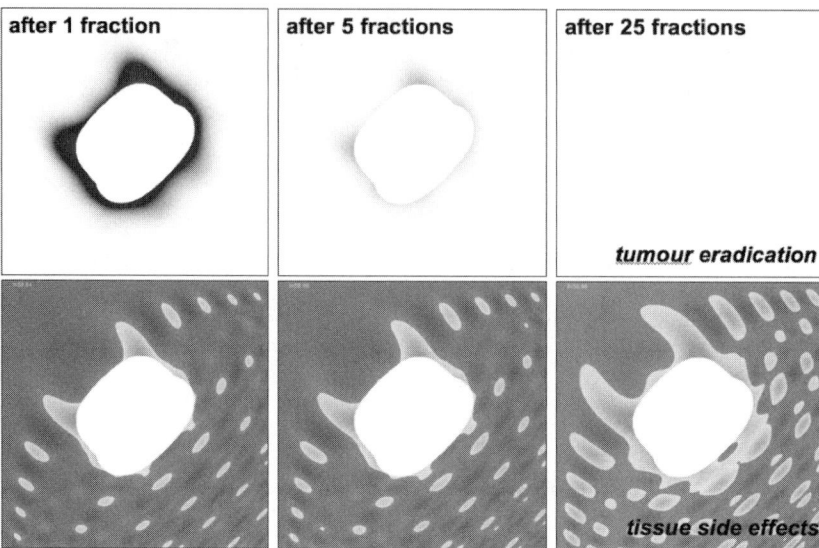

Fig. 13.9. Simulation of external beam radiotherapy (EBRT) as adjuvant treatment after breast conserving surgery for early breast cancer. The three columns show the effect of the delivery of the first, fifth, and the final 25th fraction of irradiation, respectively on the tumour (top row) and healthy tissue (bottom row). With every dose many tumour cells are eradicated while the majority of the healthy tissue survives. At later fractions (right column) a proportion of healthy tissue has suffered from irradiation as well.

A different approach of delivering radiotherapy to the tumour bed is called targeted intra-operative radiotherapy (TARGIT). If the tumour bed is the most likely source of local recurrence it might be sufficient to target irradiation to this area. During TARGIT, a single high dose of irradiation is delivered intra-operatively in the operating theatre while the patient is still anaesthetized. The applicator head is placed into the tumour bed formed after wide local excision of the primary tumour. Since the applicator is placed directly into the tumour bed, a "geographical miss" is avoided (Fig. 13.10a). The tumour bed wraps around the radiation source, so that the breast tissue that was previously close to the tumour is now close to the spherical applicator and therefore receives the highest dose of radiotherapy [VB01]. An electron-beam driven X-ray source is used for TARGIT. This point source emits low energy (50 kV) X-rays isotropically and gives a uniform dose rate at the applicator surface. There is rapid attenuation of the dose within the tissues that absorb the radiation energy and thus there is only a small high-dose region and distant normal tissues are spared [VB01]. Fig. 13.10b shows the experimentally measured loss of energy of soft X-rays over short distances as well as an approximated function $f(x)$ of this exponential decay. The data is normalised to 5 Gy at 1 cm distance from the applicator surface. The highest radiation dose of about 20 Gy is located close to the source, whereas at a distance of 2.7 cm from the source only a dose of 1 Gy remains. The approximated dose can be used to compute the BED and survival fractions for any area in the tissue.

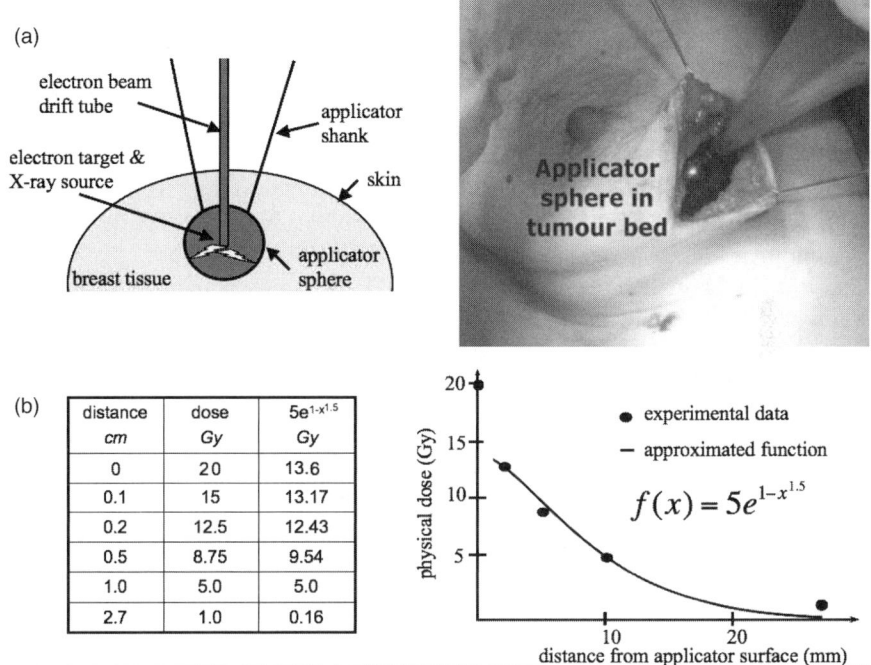

Fig. 13.10. a) Diagrams showing the TARGIT system. Left: schematic diagram of the intra-beam system. X-rays are generated when electrons that are accelerated along the drift tube hit the tip. These X-rays are modulated by the spherical applicator delivering a uniform dose of radiation at the surface of the applicator sphere. Right: The applicator being placed in the tumour bed, immediately after the excision of the tumour. b) TARGIT observed radiation dose over distance [VB01] and its approximation with a function $f(x)$ with exponential decay. The rapid attenuation reduces the treatment area to tissue close to the tumour bed.

We now focus again on the breast tissue setup to investigate the impact of fields of pre-malignant cells in the tumour bed on local recurrence. In Fig. 13.5 we sketched the development of a tumour from a field of pre-malignant cells, i.e. cells with LOH in a tumour suppressor gene (i.e. $TSG_1^{+/-}TSG_2^{+/+}$) that formed after clonal expansion of a mutated stem cell pre-puberty. In our simulations (Fig. 13.6) presented above we have seen a tumour developing from such a field. As the tumour progressed and invaded the tissue it grew beyond the margin of this field of pre-malignant cells, and hence after surgery none of these cells were left in the tissue. In our continuous model the tumour always develops from the center of the field of pre-malignant cells where the cell density is highest. By the time the tumour has reached a clinically detectable size it has grown beyond the margin of this field harbouring pre-malignant cells. Various studies, however, have reported fields adjacent to the tumour with cells with similar mutations as inside the tumour [DL96, D98, FL01]. To ensure in our simulations that a small fraction of such mutated cells reside in the tumour bed after surgery, we initialize a small tumour cell density at the border of the initial field of mutated cells (Fig. 13.11a, left panel). The tumour grows in a similar manner as before, but by the time the tumour reaches a clinically detectable size there remains a small fraction of cells with LOH in a TSG outside the tumour (Fig. 13.11a, center panel). Even after surgical excision of the tumour with a 1 cm margin some of these cells reside in the tumour bed. Fig. 13.11b shows that conventional EBRT will eradicate the tumour population again, yet fails to eradicate the residual pre-malignant cells with LOH in a TSG. Cells with LOH have not shown a reduced repair capacity and hence survive low-dose fractionated irradiation treatment as well as healthy cells. The high dose directed at the tumour delivered with TARGIT, however, eradicates all tumour cells as before, but also eradicates pre-malignant cells in the tumour bed (Fig. 13.11c).

In the Introduction we have presented the puzzling phenomenon that radiotherapy reduces local recurrence to the same extent whether or not cancer cells are found in the tumour bed. Given the discussed set of assumptions, our model attempts to explain why conventional radiotherapy may fail in a certain percentage of patients. An additional boost to the tumour bed—for example given with TARGIT—delivers a high dose of irradiation to the tissue of high risk harbouring morphologically normal pre-malignant cells. Such a boost eradicates healthy cells as well as those genetically mutated cells, which can result in a better tumour control [V07b].

13.4 Discussion

In this chapter we have presented a continuous model of breast carcinogenesis, progression, and treatment. For the initiation of the cancer cells we assumed a multi-step linear mutation pathway implemented in a system of ordinary differential equations. We assumed the normal mutation rate that occurs during cell division to be the sole source of genetic aberrations. With our model we were able to show that breast tumours are likely to develop from a field of pre-malignant cells. Such fields can arise during puberty, when the breast is formed by clonal expansion of a small number of stem cells. A large number of stem cells results in a higher possibility that one cell has received a mutation. A smaller number of stem cells, however, may result in larger fields of daughter cells with identical genetic code. Our model of cancer growth and invasion includes production of matrix degrading enzymes and consequently matrix degradation, which enables tumour progression. We have modelled surgical

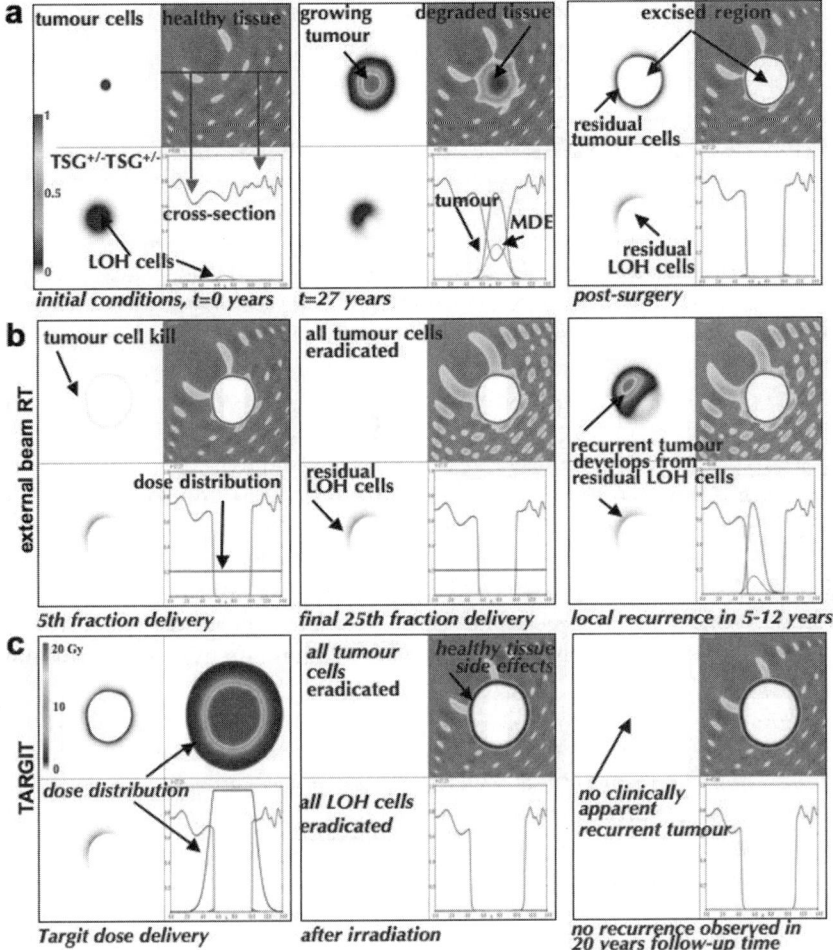

Fig. 13.11. Simulation of tumour growth at the margin of a field of cells with LOH in a TSG (top row). When the tumour has reached a clinically detectable size, the core is surgically excised leaving some stray tumour cells as well as LOH cells behind in the tumour bed (top right panel. EBRT eradicates the tumour cells but fails to kill residual LOH cells from which a tumour can develop a local recurrence within 5–12 years of primary treatment (center row). The high dose delivered with TARGIT eradicates all tumour cells and all LOH cells in the vicinity of the primary tumour providing a relapse-free survival for the simulated 20 years follow-up time (bottom row).

excision of the tumour, and our model suggests that residual cancer cells can cause local recurrence within a clinically realistic time. If we assume wound healing in the tumour bed post-surgery and subsequently a burst of growth factors, it is likely that all cells in the tumour bed are active after primary surgery. With this assumption in mind our model suggests that adjuvant radiotherapy may be sufficient to provide total control over stray single cancer cells or microscopic tumours in the vicinity of the primary disease.

However, if the tumour bed harbours genetically mutated, i.e. premalignant cell that have not lost their DNA damage repair ability, then fractionated irradiation protocols that use low-dose fractions are likely to spare those cells. However, a single or a few high and targeted doses could eradicate pre-malignant cells. If, as set up in our simulations, residual tumour cells and pre-malignant cells are located in the vicinity of the primary tumour, then novel treatment strategies such as targeted intra-operative radiotherapy (TARGIT) can provide similar tumour control than conventional treatment. With TARGIT a single high dose of irradiation is delivered directly to the tumour bed. The rapid dose fall-off over distance spares distant tissues which could provide a better cosmetic outcome for the patients. Additionally the patient's inconvenience is reduced significantly, as the five-week course of daily irradiation is replaced by a single 20-minute boost during primary surgery.

The results presented in this chapter are based on a specific set of assumptions. Most of our model is based on biologically plausible setups of which only little is known to date. The fraction of breast stem cells as well as the impact of single stem cells on the breast architecture are unknown. Our model and simulations suggest that fields of pre-malignant cells in the tumour bed are candidates for treatment failure. However, the size of such fields is unknown as is the number of possible mutations resulting in crucial loss of heterozygosity in tumour suppressor genes. In our simulations the size of the residual field of pre-malignant cells was sufficiently small and located close to the applicator surface applied in TARGIT. In this scenario the high dose delivered with TARGIT to the tumour bed eradicated those cells and hence could provide a longer relapse-free survival. However, if such fields are found to be larger, the short range of high-dose irradiation may not be sufficient to eradicate pre-malignant cells, and more radical treatment protocols may have to be implemented.

The model presented here is designed to explain the macroscopic behaviour of breast tumours and tumour-tissue interactions. Tumour initiation and early progression, however, occur on a much smaller scale and in individual cells. Mutative hits are stochastic events, and cells that receive a mutation have to compete with their environment to successfully pass on the aberration. Such random and single cell events are difficult to capture in a continuous model. Similarly, the response to radiotherapy is dependent on different factors in individual cells. Such factors are amongst others availability of nutrients and oxygen or hypoxia, or position in the cell-cycle [DS04, RC06]. To capture cell specific individual behaviour, future models of tumour initiation and response to treatment such as chemotherapy or irradiation must aim for individual cell or agent-based descriptions.

For simulating radiotherapy schedules other than the standard or single dose schedules, we would also need to incorporate the duration of the inter-fraction time as well as the tumour cell repopulation. To model radiotherapy successfully and use mathematical models to design new treatment strategies healthy tissue response has to be taken into consideration. A model such as the one presented in this chapter can serve as a basis for this simulation. Despite increasing the dose delivered to the tumour the side effects of treatment need to remain minimal. With more and more biological data on tumour and tissue response to irradiation becoming available, mathematical models of treatment protocols have the potential to predict the success or hazards of novel treatment protocols without harming any patient.

Despite many biological uncertainties and a long list of simplifying assumptions, our model has successfully simulated early stage breast cancer growth, treatment, and potential treatment failure. Furthermore we have shown that novel techniques could provide a better treatment outcome if certain biological setups are found to be true. Mathematical models such as those presented in this chapter are still far from providing a tool for treatment planning. Yet we have shown that by reducing the complexities and new biological insights of breast cancer development, treatment, and recurrence to a small set of equations and probabilities, we can guide biologists and clinicians into areas of further research to understand and improve breast cancer treatment.

Acknowledgments

The authors would like to thank Dr Alexander Anderson and Prof Mark Chaplain for their contribution and fruitful discussions, and Cancer Research UK for financial support in form of a Pilot Project Research Grant.

References

[AM06]   Abbot, L.H., Michor, F.: Mathematical models of targeted cancer therapy. Br. J. Cancer, 95(9), 1136–1141 (2006).

[AHW03]   Al-Hajj, M., Wicha, M.S., Benito-Hernandez, A., Morrison, S.J., Clarke, M.F.: Prospective identification of tumorigenic breast cancer cells. PNAS, 100(7), 3983–3988 (2003).

[AC00]   Anderson, A.R.A., Chaplain, M.A.J., Newman, E.L., Steele, R.J.C., Thompson, A.M.: Mathematical modelling of tumour invasion and metastasis. J. Theoret. Med, 2, 129–154 (2000).

[A05]   Anderson, A.R.A.: A hybrid mathematical model of solid tumour invasion: The importance of cell adhesion. Math. Med. Biol., 22, 163–186 (2005).

[AM04]   Araujo, R.P., McElwain, D.L.S.: A history of the study of solid tumour growth: The contribution of mathematical modelling. Bull. Math. Biol., 66, 1039–1091 (2004).

[BW02]   Beil, D.R., Wein, L.M.: Sequencing surgery, radiotherapy and chemotherapy: Insights from a mathematical analysis. Breast Cancer Res. Treat., 74(3), 279–286 (2002).

[BS04]   Boone, J.M., Shah, N., Nelson, T.R.: A comprehensive analysis of DgNCT coefficients for pendant-geometry cone-beam breast computed tomography. Med. Phys., 31(1), 226–235 (2004).

[BA98]   Brenner, D., Armour, E., Corry, P., Hall, E.: Sublethal damage repair times for a late-responding tissue relevant to brachytherapy (and external-beam radiotherapy): Implications for new brachytherapy protocols. Int. J. Radiat. Oncol. Biol. Phys., 41(1), 135–138 (1998).

[B00]   Brwon, P.: UK death rates from breast cancer fall by a third. BMJ, 321(7265), 849 (2000).

[CL05]   Chaplain, M.A.J., Lolas, G.: Mathematical modelling of cancer cell invasion of tissue: The role of the urokinase plasminogen activation system. Math. Modell. Methods Appl. Sci., 15, 1685–1734 (2005).

[C05]   Clarke, M., Collins, R., Darby, S., Davies, C., Elphinstone, P., Evans, E., Godwin, J., Gray, R., Hicks, C., James, S., MacKinnon, E., McGale, P., McHugh, T., Peto, R., Taylor, C., Wang, Y.: Effects of radiotherapy, of differences in the extent of surgery for early breast cancer on local recurrence, 15-year survival: An overview of the randomised trials. Lancet, 366(9503), 2087–2106 (2005).

[D98]   Dairkee, S.H.: Allelic loss in normal lobules adjacent to breast cancer. Cancer Detection and Prevention, 22(1), 135A (1998).

[DH06]   Dawson, A., Hillen, T.: Derivation of the tumour control probability (TCP) from a cell cycle model. Comput. Math. Meth. in Medicine, 7, 121–142 (2006).

[DL96]   Deng, G., Lu, Y., Zlotnikov, G., Thor, A.D., Smith, H.S.: Loss of heterozygosity in normal tissue adjacent to breast carcinomas. Science, 274, 2057–2059 (1996).

[DS04]   Dionysiou, D.D., Stamatakos, G.S., Uzunogly, N.K., Nikita, K.S., Marioli, A.: A four-dimensional simulation model of tumour response to radiotherapy in vivo: Parametric validation considering radiosensitivity, genetic profile, fractionation. J. Theor. Biol., 230, 1–20 (2004).

[E06]   Enderling, H.: Mathematical modelling of breast cancer development, local treatment, recurrence. PhD Thesis, Dundee University, Dundee (2006).

[EA06]   Enderling, H., Anderson, A.R.A., Chaplain, M.A.J., Munro, A.J., Vaidya, J.S.: Mathematical modelling of radiotherapy strategies for early breast cancer. J. Theor. Biol., 241(1), 158–171 (2006).

[EA06b]   Enderling, H., Anderson, A.R.A., Chaplain, M.A.J., Rowe, G.W.: Visualisation of the numerical solution of partial differential equation systems in three space dimensions and its importance for mathematical models in biology. Math. Biosci. Eng., 3(4), 571–582 (2006).

[EC07]   Enderling, H., Chaplain, M.A.J., Anderson, A.R.A., Vaidya, J.S.: A mathematical model of breast cancer development, local treatment, recurrence. J. Theor. Biol., 264(2), 245–259 (2007).

[FL01]   Försti, A., Louhelainen, J., Söderberg, M., Wijkström, H., Hemminki, K.: Loss of heterozygosity in tumour-adjacent normal tissue of breast and bladder cancer. Eur. J. Cancer, 37, 1372–1380 (2001).

[GAL03]   Guerrero, M., Allen Li, X.: Analysis of a large number of clinical studies for breast cancer radiotherapy: Estimation of radiobiological parameters for treatment planning. Phys. Med. Biol., 48(20), 3307–3326 (2003).

[HW00]   Hanahan, D., Weinberg, R.A: The hallmarks of cancer. Cell, 100, 57–70 (2000).

[K06]   Komarova, N.: Stochastic modeling of drug resistance in cancer. J Theor. Biol., 239(3), 351–366 (2006).

[KJ04]   Krag, D.N., Julian, T.B., Harlow, S.P., Weaver, D.L., Ashikaga, T., Bryant, J., Single, R.M., Wolmark, N.: NSABP-32: Phase III, randomized trial comparing axillary resection with sentinal lymph node dissection: A description of the trial. Ann. Surg. Oncol., 11(3 Suppl), 208S–210S (2004).

[MB06]   Massarut, S., Baldassare, G., Belleti, B., Reccanello, S., D'Andrea, S., Ezio, C., Perin, T., Reccanello, S., Roncadin, M., Vaidya, J.S.: Intraoperative radiotherapy impairs breast cancer cell motility induced by surgical wound fluid. J. Clin. Oncol., 24(18S), 10611 (2006).

[M92]   Matrisian, L.N.: The matrix-degrading metalloproteinases. Bioessays, 14, 455–463 (1992).

[MO06]   McAneney, H., O'Rourke, SFC.: Investigation of various growth mechanisms within the linear-quadratic model for radiotherapy. Phys. Med. Biol., 52, 1039–1054.

[MIN04]   Michor, F., Iwasa, Y., Nowak, M.A.: Dynamics of cancer progression. Nat. Rev. Can., 4, 197–205 (2004).

[MN06]   Michor, F., Nowak, M.A., Iwasa, Y.: Evolution of resistance to cancer therapy. Curr. Pharm. Des., 12(3), 161–271 (2006).

[N05]   Norton, L.: Conceptual, practical implications of breast tissue geometry: Toward a more effective, less toxic therapy. Oncologist, 10(6), 370–381 (2005).

[NMK04]   Nowak, M.A., Michor, F., Komarova, N.L., Iwasa, Y.: Evolutionary dynamics of tumor suppressor gene inactivation. PNAS, 101(29), 10635–10638 (2004).

[O01]   Oldham, M.: Radiation physics, applications in therapeutic medicine. Phys. Educ., 36, 460–467 (2001).

[PA95]   Panetta, J.C., Adam, J.: A mathematical model of cycle-specific chemotherapy. Math. Comp. Modell., 22(2), 67–82 (1995).

[PG05]   Piccart-Gebhart, M.J., Procter, M., Leyland-Jones, B., Goldhirsch, A., Untch, M., Smith, I., Gianni, L., Baselga, J., Bell, R., Jackisch, C., Cameron, D., Dowsett, M., Barrios, C.H., Steger, G., Huang, C.S., Andersson, M., Inbar, M., Lichinitser, M., Lang, I., Nitz, U., Iwata, H., Thomssen, C., Lohrisch, C., Suter, T.M., Ruschoff, J., Suto, T., Greatorex, V., Ward, C., Straehle, C., McFadden, E., Dolci, M.S., Gelber, R.D.: Herceptin adjuvant (HERA) trial study team. Trastuzumab after adjuvant chemotherapy in HER2-positive breast cancer. N. Engl. J. Med., 353(16), 1659–1672 (2005).

[PK07]   Powathil, G., Kohandel, M., Sivaloganathan, S., Oza, A., Milosevic, M.: Mathematical modeling of brain tumors: Effects of radiotherapy, chemotherapy. Phys. Med. Biol., 52, 3291–3306 (2007).

[RC06]   Ribba, B., Colin, T., Schnell, S.: A multiscale mathematical model of cancer, its use in analyzing irradiation therapies. Theor. Biol. Med. Model, 3(7), (2006).

[RP05]   Romond, E.H., Perez, E.A., Bryant, J., Suman, V.J., Geyer, C.E. Jr, Davidson, N.E., Tan-Chiu, E., Martino, S., Paik, S., Kaufman, P.A.,

Swain, S.M., Pisansky, T.M., Fehrenbacher, L., Kutteh, L.A., Vogel, V.G., Visscher, D.W., Yothers, G., Jenkins, R.B., Brown, A.M., Dakhil, S.R., Mamounas, E.P., Lingle, W.L., Klein, P.M., Ingle, J.N., Wolmark, N.: Trastuzumab plus adjuvant chemotherapy for operable HER2-positive breast cancer. N. Engl. J. Med., 353(16), 1673–1684 (2005).

[SH97]   Sachs, R.K., Hahnfeld, P., Brenner, D.J.: The link between low-LET dose-response relations, the underlying kinetics of damage production/repair/misrepair. Int. J. Biol., 72(4), 351–374 (1997).

[SH01]   Sachs, R.K., Hlatky, L.R., Hahnfeldt, P.: Simple ODE models of tumour growth, anti-angiogenic or radiation treatment. Math. Comput. Modelling, 33, 1297–1305 (2001).

[SLB04]   Sancar, A., Lindsey-Boltz, L.A., Ünsal-Kaçmaz, K., Linn, S.: Molecular mechanisms of mammalian DNA repair, the DNA damage checkpoints. Annu. Rev. Biochem., 73, 39–85 (2004).

[SG05]   Smallbone, K., Gavaghan, D.J., Gatenby, R.A., Maini, P.K.: The role of acidity in solid tumour growth, invasion. J. Theor. Biol., 235, 476–484 (2005).

[SA03]   Smalley, M. and Ashworth, A.: Stem cells and breast cancer: A field in transit. Nat. Rev. Can., 3, 832–844 (2003).

[SB04]   Spencer, S.L., Berryman, M.J., Garcia, J.A. , Abbott, D.: An ordinary differential equation model for the multistep transformation to cancer. J. Theor. Biol, 231, 515–524 (2004).

[SA02]   Swanson, K.R., Alvord, E.C. Jr, Murray, J.D.: Quantifying efficacy of chemotherapy of brain tumors with homogeneous, heterogeneous drug delivery. Acta Biotheor., 50(4), 223–237 (2002).

[TNB96]   Tomlinson, I.P.M., Novelli, M.R., Bodmer, W.F.: The mutation rate, cancer. PNAS, 93(25), 14800–14803 (1996).

[T01]   Tomlinson, I.P.M.: Mutations in normal breast tissue, breast tumours. Breast Cancer Res., 3(5), 299–303 (2001).

[TC03]   Turesson, I., Carlsson, J., Brahme, A., Glimelius, B., Zackrisson, B., Stenerlöw, B.: Biological response to radiation therapy. Acta Oncologica, 42(2), 92–106 (2003).

[TS02]   Turner S., Sherrat, J.A.: Intercellular adhesion and cancer invasion: A discrete simulation using the extended Potts model. J. Theor. Biol., 216, 85–100 (2002).

[VB01]   Vaidya, J.S., Baum, M., Tobias, J.S., D'Souza, D.P., Naidy, S.V., Morgan, S., Metaxas, M., Harte, K.J., Sliski, A.P., Thomson, E.: Targeted intra-operative radiotherapy (Targit): An innnovative method of treatment for early breast cancer. Annals of Oncology, 12, 1075–1080 (2001).

[VD05]   Vaidya, J.S., Dewar, J.A., Brown, D.C., Thompson, A.M.: A mathematical model for the effect of a false-negative sentinel node biopsy on breast cancer mortality: A tool for everyday use. Breast Cancer Res., 7(5), 225–227 (2005).

[VT04]   Vaidya, J.S., Tobias, J.S., Baum, M., Keshtgar, M., Joseph, D., Wenz, F. et al.: Intraoperative radiotherapy for breast cancer. Lancet Oncol., 5(3), 165–173 (2004).

[V07]   Vaidya, J.S.: Breast cancer: An artistic view. Lancet Oncol., 8(7), 583–558 (2007).

[V07b]   Vaidya, J.S.: Partial breast irradiation using targeted intraoperative radiotherapy (Targit). Nat. Clin. Pract. Oncol., 4(7), 384–385 (2007).

[VVH05]   Verschraegen, C., Vinh-Hung, V., Cserni, G., Gordon, R., Royce, M.E., Vlastos, G., Tai, P., Storme, G.: Modeling the effect of tumor size in early breast cancer. Annals of Surgery, 241, 309–318 (2005).

[WC05]   Woodward, W.A., Chen, M.S., Behbod, F., Rosen, J.M: On mammary stem cells. J. Cell Science, 118, 3585–3594 (2005).

14

Predictive Models in Tumor Immunology

Pier-Luigi Lollini,[1] Arianna Palladini,[1] Francesco Pappalardo,[2] and
Santo Motta[2]

[1] Sezione di Cancerologia, Dipartimento di Patologia Sperimentale
Università di Bologna, Italy
{pierluigi.lollini,arianna.palladini}@unibo.it
[2] Dipartimento di Matematica e Informatica
Università di Catania, Italy
{francesco,motta}@dmi.unict.it

14.1 Introduction

The role of the immune system in tumor surveillance is clearly established, and tumor immunologists are actively working to devise preventive and therapeutical vaccines against cancer; however, the growth of biological knowledge is still too slow to win the war against cancer as soon as possible. Mathematical models are quantitative representations of phenomena developed in the framework of a theory using the language of mathematics. Living organisms are natural complex systems and their modeling may play a crucial role since models can also be built with approximate and imperfect knowledge of a phenomenon, and model parameters (initial data, entities, relations between entities) can be adjusted to fit modeling results to experimental measurements. Such models can then be used to understand the general behavior of the phenomenon in different situations, to perform model experiments or simulations to study the role of single constituents and relations, to plan new experiments, and to test theoretical assumptions and suggest theory modifications. In this chapter we present a success story of scientific cooperation between tumor immunologists and applied mathematicians. We developed a model of the effects of a vaccine designed to prevent mammary carcinoma in transgenic mice. This model faithfully summarizes not only the outcome of the vaccination experiments, but also the dynamics of the immune responses elicited by the vaccine. We then used a genetic algorithm to search for an optimal vaccination schedule. The predicted schedules are currently being tested *in vivo*. The model plays the role of a virtual laboratory, performing in a few minutes *in silico* experiments that would take years *in vivo*.

N. Bellomo et al. (eds.), *Selected Topics in Cancer Modeling*,
DOI: 10.1007/978-0-8176-4713-1_14, © Springer Science+Business Media, LLC 2008

14.2 Tumor Immunology

The immune system protects the host from cancer. This apparently straightforward and simple statement has been the subject of considerable scientific debate and conflicting experiments over several decades. A clear demonstration was obtained only recently, thanks to the availability of appropriate genetically modified mouse models. Therefore, a brief outline of the controversies seems appropriate in the context of a book devoted to (mathematical) modeling, as it clearly illustrates key critical issues of biological, in particular *in vivo,* models in cancer research.

The earliest evidence of antitumor immune reactivity was obtained in the 1940s and 1950s by showing that inbred mice vaccinated against syngeneic tumors rejected a subsequent challenge with the same tumor (immune memory), but succumbed to the growth of an antigenically unrelated tumor (immune specificity). This kind of evidence led to the formulation of the "immune surveillance" theory, postulating that protection of the host from carcinogenesis and tumor development was a fundamental function of the immune system [27]. Two testable consequences of this theory are that a) tumor incidence should be significantly higher in immunodeficient hosts, and b) the immunogenicity of tumors that eventually grow in immunocompetent hosts must be very low to escape immune defenses. The latter was easily demonstrated for a variety of murine model systems, and in general applies to most human tumors as well, thus explaining the intrinsic difficulties in devising effective approaches to cancer immunotherapy and the unescapable need for powerful new approaches to stimulate immune responses *in vivo* against poorly immunogenic tumor cells [27].

The main problem haunting the immune surveillance theory for many years was the lack of a clear demonstration of an increased tumor incidence in immunodeficient hosts. On the contrary, experiments in athymic "nude" mice showed that long-term, spontaneous tumors arose with the same frequency as in immunocompetent (euthymic) control mice [27]. It must be recalled that the mutation harbored by nude mice does not directly affect lymphocytes, rather it blocks the development of the epithelial component of the thymus, hence the generation of T cell precursors in the bone marrow is normal, but their maturation and selection are severely hampered by the absence of a functional thymus. A fact poorly appreciated at the time was that T cells can also mature (with low efficiency and without proper selection) in extrathymic sites, hence over time nude mice accumulate a sizeable T cell response, and aged nude mice, when spontaneous tumors begin to appear, are no longer fully immunodeficient, as attested also by the high incidence of autoimmune diseases. In practice young nude mice are a reliable model of immunodeficiency, but this is no longer true for old nude mice.

The advent of genetically modified mice with knocked-out specific genes directly controlling immune development definitively vindicated immune surveillance, allowing a clear-cut demonstration that truly immunodeficient models indeed have an enormously higher occurrence of tumors than the corresponding immunocompetent mice [27]. In conclusion the current unanimous view is that the immune surveillance theory was indeed correct in postulating defense from tumor onset as a fundamental function of the immune system.

Genetically modified mouse models also shed additional light on the issue of tumor immunogenicity. It was shown that tumors arising in immunodeficient knockout mice are mostly immunogenic, hence the poor immunogenicity of tumors arising in immunocompetent mice is a consequence of the competition between the growing tumor and the immune system of the host, leading to the elimination of immunogenic tumor cell populations and to the selection of less immunogenic cell variants, a phenomenon now defined as "immunoediting" [27].

14.2.1 Tumor Antigens

The search for tumor antigens was conducted for several decades with strategies similar to that of the man who lost his keys in a dark alley and kept looking for them under a lamppost because at least there was some light. One typical example was the discovery of tumor antigens using antibodies induced by vaccination of rodents with human neoplastic tissues. This approach has two fundamental drawbacks: it misses most antigens recognized by T cell receptors and unveils many molecules recognized by rodent immune systems because of human-rodent species differences. Such molecules may be essentially nonantigenic in the species of origin, i.e. useless as immunotherapy targets, even though they might be useful as tumor markers for diagnostic purposes and for monitoring patients at risk of tumor relapse.

The 1980s saw the advent of molecular technologies allowing the direct cloning of tumor antigens recognized by the human immune system, in particular by T cells, eventually leading to the discovery of hundreds of true tumor antigens that could be targeted by specific immunotherapeutic endeavors [20]. Tumor antigens can be divided into four major classes: *cancer-testis antigens* (also called *melanoma-testis antigens*), a previously unknown class of testicular molecules of uncertain physiological function, expressed by melanomas and various other tumor types, a typical example is the MAGE family of antigens; *differentiation antigens*, expressed by a given cell type and by tumor cells derived from the same differentiation line, for example melanoma cells express antigens derived from components of the melanin synthesis pathway; *shared tumor antigens*, expressed by diverse tumor types, like the HER-2/neu oncoprotein and telomerase (TERT); *unique tumor antigens*, so called because antigenic specificities of individual patients are frequently non-crossreacting. Unique antigens can result from random mutational events (*e.g.* point mutations and chromosome translocations) affecting oncogenes like RAS or tumor suppressor genes like p53; this class includes also the idiotype of neoplastic B and T cell clones.

A prominent feature is that, with the exception of unique antigens, tumor antigens lack true tumor specificity because they are also expressed by normal, non-neoplastic cells. Hence most antitumor immune responses are actually autoimmune responses, triggered by inappropriate or excessive expression of the antigen by tumor cells and by the massive apoptotic and necrotic cell death that frequently accompanies tumor growth. Two important consequences are that a successful antitumor immune response against such self-antigens requires a break of immune tolerance, and that a certain degree of immune damage to normal cells expressing the antigen is unavoidable. Some autoimmune responses cause only a limited damage to normal tissues and are surrogate markers of an efficacious antitumor reaction, as in the case of autoimmune vitiligo (patches of non-pigmented skin) caused by destruction of normal melanocytes in melanoma patients undergoing antitumor vaccinations.

14.2.2 The Mechanisms of Tumor Immunity

The mechanisms that mediate tumor rejection have been investigated in depth over several decades through the dissection of individual immune responses occurring during vaccination and rejection of tumors, and through the selective abrogation of specific cells and molecules by means of monoclonal antibodies and drugs, or in immunodeficient hosts. The whole picture is now coherent and quite complete.

- Phagocytic cells, like granulocytes and particularly macrophages, have a dual role, as they attack and destroy tumor cells and simultaneously generate cell degradation products that can be picked up by antigen-presenting cells (APCs). Current research is also focused on myeloid suppressor cells that can be induced by cytokines secreted by tumor cells and inhibit antitumor immune responses.
- Dendritic cells (DCs) are professional APCs that pick up tumor antigens in the periphery, then migrate to lymph nodes to present antigens to T cells. Antigen presentation and release of cytokines (interleukin 12, IL-12) by DCs are a *conditio sine qua non* for the initiation of all primary immune responses.
- All types of T cells play fundamental roles in tumor immunity. After antigen presentation helper T (Th) cells proliferate and secrete cytokines to activate cytotoxic T (Tc) cells that in turn can directly kill tumor cells. Cytokines, besides their role as internal mediators of the immune system, can also directly affect tumor cells; for example, interferons inhibit cell proliferation. Regulatory T (Treg) cells, physiologically involved in the control of autoimmunity, can inhibit antitumor responses, and many endeavors now aim at inhibiting Treg to enhance the activity of immunotherapy.
- B cells, antibodies and complement play only a marginal role in the immune responses against solid tumors. Most solid tumors are in fact pro-

tected from lysis by antibodies and complement by the expression of inhibitory molecules such as CD55 and CD59. B cells can even downregulate T cell responses and facilitate tumor growth, a phenomenon known as enhancement.

14.2.3 T Cells *vs.* Antibodies: The Great Contradiction of Tumor Immunology

The analysis described above leads to the conclusion that T cells are the major antitumor mechanism deployed by the immune system, and this fact has not only shaped basic research, but also the translation of experimental results to clinical approaches. The ingenuity of tumor immunologists had no limits in devising new therapeutic strategies, and literally hundreds of different approaches were clinically tested over the years. Currently the most popular ones are based on therapeutic vaccines (i.e. vaccines administered to cure a condition rather than to prevent its onset), possibly coupled with drugs to inhibit Treg cells, and on various maneuvers to enhance tumor antigen presentation by DCs.

Unfortunately the clinical results of decades of massive T cell-centric clinical efforts are on the whole disappointing [24]. One clear benchmark of clinical success is the acceptance of a new therapeutic approach as a standard therapy for a given oncological condition. At present none of the attempts described above can be considered as a standard therapy. Hence mainstream tumor immunology remains an unfulfilled promise in the clinical arena.

An independent clinical development came from the technology of monoclonal antibodies (MAbs), which allows the large-scale production *in vitro* of immunoglobulin molecules of predefined specificity. The clinical use of antitumor antibodies was led by MAbs developed against cell surface molecules expressed by lymphomas which, unlike solid tumors, are sensitive to lysis by antibodies and complement. Now anti-CD20 MAbs are standard therapy against B cell lymphomas [25, 28].

An unanticipated clinical success came from the trial of a MAb directed against HER-2, a cell surface oncoprotein expressed by about one fourth of all breast cancer cases. Molecular studies showed that this type of therapy is based on multiple mechanisms. In addition to direct cytotoxicity mediated by complement and other immune mechanisms, which could play a minor role against resistant tumor cells, antibodies inhibit the function of the target antigen HER-2, which is causally involved in the maintenance of the tumorigenic ability of breast carcinoma cells. The anti-HER-2 MAb rapidly became a therapeutic standard and promoted the development of many other therapeutic MAbs directed against conceptually similar target antigens which are rapidly being developed and approved for clinical use [25, 28].

In conclusion the clinical development of cancer immunotherapy was, and still is, contradictory, with basic research and most translational groups on the one side working on therapeutic vaccines, DCs, and other ingenious but disappointing approaches that still have an unfulfilled potential, whereas "Big Pharma" industry on the other side is now massively focused on monoclonal antibodies thanks to a series of striking clinical successes.

14.3 Cancer Immunoprevention

Cancer immunoprevention is a fresh approach based on the idea that stimulation of the immune response could be used to prevent tumor onset in healthy individuals at risk of cancer. The theory of immune surveillance (see above) clearly shows that spontaneous immune responses are effective in preventing a sizeable proportion of incipient tumors, however the very existence of progressive malignant tumors demonstrates that the efficiency of spontaneous immune surveillance is below 100%. Hence the question is whether vaccines or other immune stimuli can significantly raise the bar.

We already have mass vaccinations that effectively prevent cancer in humans. The first example was the vaccine against hepatitis B virus (HBV) which, in a minority of patients, gives rise to a chronic form of hepatitis that can eventually foster the onset of liver cancer. Human populations vaccinated against HBV are protected not only from hepatitis, but also from post-hepatitis liver carcinoma [4]. Papilloma viruses (HPVs) are the most prevalent carcinogenic viruses in humans, and the ensuing tumors (carcinoma of the uterine cervix and others) account for one tenth of all human cancers. Recently approved vaccines against HPV prevented near 100% of cervical carcinomas in early clinical trials [26] and hold the promise to completely eliminate this tumor, much as the smallpox vaccine did for a deadly infective disease.

Altogether the proportion of human tumors directly or indirectly caused by infectious agents is about 15%. The challenge now for tumor immunologists is to develop strategies that could prevent the remaining 85% of tumors, unrelated to infectious agents.

14.3.1 Cancer Immunoprevention in Preclinical Mouse Models

Clear demonstrations of the principles of cancer immunoprevention for non-viral tumors were mostly obtained in cancer-prone mouse models either as a consequence of a genetic modification of a cancer gene, or in mice treated with chemical carcinogens. Three different types of immunological approaches were used: a) passive administration of monoclonal antibodies directed against surface oncoproteins like HER-2, b) non-specific immunomodulators such as cytokines or bacterial products and c) antigen-specific vaccines made of whole cells, proteins, peptides or DNA encoding the target antigen [10, 11].

These pioneering studies provided the proof of principle that stimulation of the immune system in healthy hosts at risk of cancer can effectively affect cancer incidence later in life. One limit was that in most early studies tumor onset was merely delayed, and most mice eventually succumbed to cancer.

14.3.2 The Triplex Vaccine Completely Prevents Mammary Carcinoma

To improve the efficacy of cancer immunoprevention we designed a vaccine named Triplex because it combined three immune stimuli: the target antigen and two powerful non-specific adjuvants. The target antigen in our case was the HER-2/neu rat oncoprotein expressed by transgenic mice prone to mammary carcinoma, the biologic adjuvants were interleukin 12 (IL-12) and class I allogeneic histocompatibility antigens, which stimulate a broad polyclonal T cell response. The first formulation of the vaccine consisted of allogeneic transgenic mammary carcinoma cells expressing HER-2/neu coupled with systemic administration of IL-12 [17], then we transduced IL-12 genes into mammary carcinoma cells to obtain a single cell type expressing all three components at once [8]. As both formulations proved equally effective, we will not further distinguish the two in the following description of the results.

Chronic, lifelong administration of the Triplex vaccine resulted in the complete prevention of mammary carcinoma in HER-2/neu transgenic mice [8, 17]. All control mice developed multiple progressive mammary carcinomas by six months of age, but almost all vaccinated mice were alive and tumor-free at one year of age, when experiments were usually terminated. Microscopic analysis revealed that the mammary glands of one-year-old mice were free from microscopic carcinomas and resembled the glands of young HER-2/neu transgenic mice, with small preneoplastic foci. Tumors of control mice showed a high expression of HER-2/neu, whereas the mammary epithelial cells of vaccinated mice were mostly negative. In practice the Triplex vaccine "froze" neoplastic development at the preneoplastic level of six-week-old mice, when vaccinations started [17].

14.3.3 The Immune Mechanisms of Cancer Immunoprevention

The Triplex is a powerful vaccine that induces a large array of diverse cellular and humoral immune responses when administered chronically to immunocompetent mice. The notable absence of cytotoxic T cell (CTL) responses was unexpected [17], given their importance in many antitumor immune responses. However it must be kept in mind that such responses are mostly short lived, because a chronic CTL activity is highly toxic for the host, thus it is logical that long-term protection from tumor onset in our system could not be supported by a chronic activation of CTL.

To dissect protective immune mechanisms from less relevant immune responses we crossed HER-2/neu transgenic mice with immunodepressed knockout mice selectively lacking the ability to produce γ-interferon, the main cytokine released by Th cells in response to IL-12, and with antibody-deficient mice. In both cases we found a complete loss of protection from tumor onset [16], thus demonstrating that both γ-interferon and antibodies were essential for cancer immunoprevention. Some antibody subclasses (e.g. IgG2a) strongly elicited by the Triplex vaccine in immunocompetent mice were missing in γ-interferon deficient mice, because the relevant isotypic switch is induced by γ-interferon, whereas antibody-deficient mice retained the ability to produce γ-interferon in response to the vaccine. This indicates that the main function of γ-interferon after vaccination was the induction of specific anti-HER-2/neu antibodies.

In summary the Triplex vaccine induces strong Th responses polarized toward γ-interferon production, but no CTL response. In turn γ-interferon induces IgG2a antibodies directed against p185, the protein product of HER-2/neu. Such antibodies have multiple antitumor activities, including direct inhibition of p185 oncoprotein expression and function, complement-dependent cytotoxicity and antibody-dependent cell-mediated cytotoxicity (ADCC), altogether resulting in the long-term block of HER-2/neu oncogenicity. In conclusion the protective immune responses of cancer immunoprevention were quite different from the CTL responses usually investigated in short-term immunotherapy of tumors. It is interesting to note that a similar dichotomy occurs in infectious immunity: the clearance of acute viral infections is operated by CTL responses, whereas long-term protection from subsequent infections and the prophylactic activity of vaccines are mediated by neutralizing antibodies [1].

14.3.4 Lessons from Cancer Immunoprevention: The Oncoantigens

It is important to note that the results obtained with the Triplex vaccine were replicated by several other laboratories using different vaccines and different oncological mouse models (reviewed in [10]). The major variable controlling the level of protection from tumor onset attained using different combinations appeared to be the target antigen, rather than the type of vaccine. For example Guido Forni and Federica Cavallo (University of Turin) using DNA vaccines against HER-2/neu obtained results closely matching those reported above for the Triplex vaccine [23], whereas we obtained a much lower level of protection in prostate cancer-prone TRAMP mice with a cell vaccine against the large T SV40 antigen formulated according to the Triplex concept [7]. This led us to critically appraise the reasons for the success of the Triplex vaccine in cancer prevention, and eventually to reconsider the notion of tumor antigen in the light of the current lack of clinical impact [12].

T cells recognize tumor antigens in the form of peptidic fragments processed by tumor cells and exposed on their surface by class I MHC molecules, whereas antibodies bind to three dimensional conformational epitopes of intact molecules. Two major reasons for a loss of T cell recognition are the selection of "escape" tumor cell variants lacking expression of either the antigen or class I MHC. In the HER-2/neu transgenic system the loss of HER-2/neu expression was accompanied by a loss of tumorigenicity *in vivo* [18], because HER-2/neu is at the same time the target antigen and the oncogene driving tumor development. Therefore, this route of escape was blocked for HER-2/neu mammary carcinoma development, whereas most other tumor antigens, like MAGE or CEA, do not control tumor cell growth and a loss of expression does not impinge on tumorigenicity. In HER-2/neu mice class I MHC loss variants appeared frequently *in vivo* [14], and this further explains why CTLs do not play a significant role in the system, however this did not alter recognition of tumor cells by antibodies which bind whole HER-2/neu molecules on the cell surface. Many other tumor antigens are not expressed on the cell surface, hence a loss of MHC expression abrogates any possibility of immune recognition.

We proposed to define "oncoantigens" as those tumor antigens that share with HER-2/neu the two properties of being indispensable for tumor growth and expressed on the cell surface [10]. Most known tumor antigens [20] do not fulfill the definition of oncoantigen, hence they are easily prone to lack of immune recognition because of antigen and/or class I MHC loss. We advocate a major effort toward the molecular and immunological definition of new oncoantigens, starting with tyrosine kinase receptors similar to HER-2/neu, and of powerful vaccines like the Triplex to elicit immune responses against oncoantigens, not only for cancer immunoprevention, but also for cancer immunotherapy.

14.3.5 Clinical Translation of Cancer Immunoprevention and the Need for Mathematical Models

The application to humans of the principles of cancer immunoprevention defined in mice will face many hurdles that were discussed elsewhere in greater detail [10, 11] and include the precise definition of individuals at risk of cancer, the evaluation of potentially harmful side effects, such as the induction of autoimmune responses, and the implementation of early clinical trials in advanced cancer patients to evaluate feasibility and toxicity.

One specific issue of relevance for the present discussion is the scheduling of vaccine administrations for maximal prevention of tumor onset. A complete prevention of mammary carcinoma in HER-2/neu transgenic mice was obtained when the Triplex vaccine was administered chronically for the entire lifetime of the mouse, however shorter (three months) vaccination protocols significantly delayed tumor onset, but all mice eventually succumbed to cancer [8, 11].

It is obvious that the compliance of humans undergoing this type of vaccination would be enhanced by a sizeable reduction in the number of vaccine administrations, however the sheer number of possible schedules to be tested, combined with the extremely long duration of each experiment, forbids a brute force biological approach. The solution of this issue was instrumental first in the implementation of the simulator and then in the design of the genetic algorithm described here.

14.4 The Model

As shown in the previous sections cancer-immune system competition is a very complex process to describe and consequently modeling it is a very hard task. All the crucial entities (cells, molecules, adjuvants, cytokines and so on) that biologists recognize as relevant have to be included in the model. In our case, the choice of entities was driven by the experimental data on the Triplex vaccine, where the relevant entities (the cells and molecules) have mechanical and biological states—*viz.* position, lifetime, internal states and specificity. Position and lifetime apply to all, but internal states only to cellular entities, and specificity to both cellular and molecular entities.

The Catania Mouse Model (CMM), previously described in detail in [15, 21] was implemented in a simulator called SimTriplex using a lattice Boltzmann-like approach, including the entities (cells and molecules) of the adaptive and natural immune system, the cancer cells and the vaccine. This approach is the computational counterpart of the generalized Boltzmann approach [3, 2, 6].

In designing so complex a model, and in particular to eliminate semantic misunderstandings between biologists, mathematicians and computer scientists, it is necessary to list the most important and frequently used concepts coherently defined, to provide an exact, semantic specification of the concepts used in an existing schema and to manage and annotate existing database entries consistently.

The use of an ontology is the best way to describe the biological entities and concepts. An ontology formally describes basic concepts in a domain and defines relations among them. Basic building blocks of ontology design include:

- classes or concepts;
- properties of each concept describing various features and attributes of the concept (slots, sometimes called roles or properties);
- restrictions on slots (facets, sometimes called role restrictions).

The immune system entities included in the model are B lymphocytes (B), Plasma cells (P), Helper T lymphocytes (TH), Cytotoxic T lymphocytes (TC), Macrophages (M), Dendritic cells (DC), Interleukin 2 (IL-2), Immunoglobulins (IG), Danger signal (D), Major histocompatibility complex class I (MHCI), Major histocompatibility complex class II (MHCII), Immunocomplexes (IC), Natural killer cells (NK). Cancer cells and vaccine components are Cancer cells (CC), Tumor associated antigens (TAA), Vaccine cells (VC), and Interleukin 12 (IL-12). All of the various classes of immune functional activity, such as phagocytosis, immune activation, opsonization, infection and cytotoxicity are described using probability functions and translated into computational rules. Fig. 14.1 shows a subset of the ontology for the Identification concept used in CMM.

The ontology "Identification" concept has been developed as a "class diagram". A concept identifies a class. A class defines the attributes and the

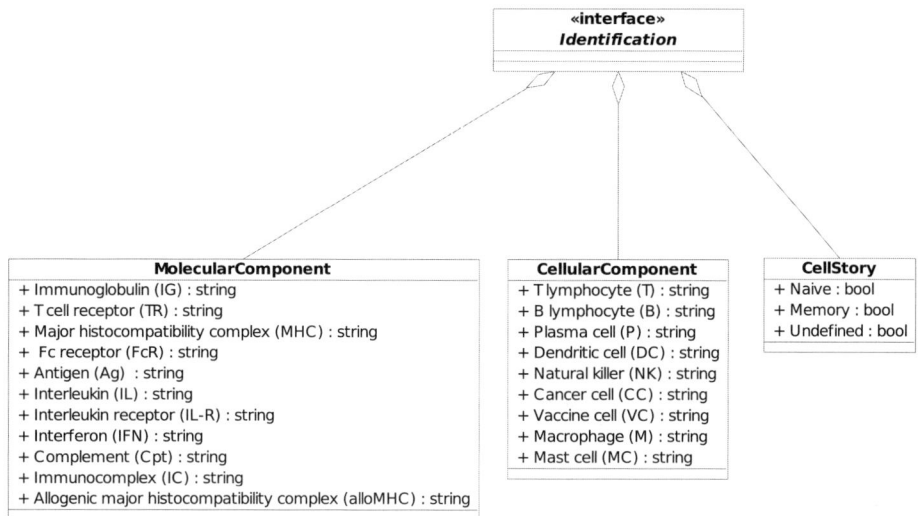

Fig. 14.1. Identification concept of entities in the ontology of the model.

methods of a set of objects. All objects of this class (instances of this class) share the same behavior, and have the same set of attributes (each object has its own set). Classes are represented by rectangles, with the name of the class, and can also show the attributes and operations of the class in two other "compartments" inside the rectangle. Interfaces are abstract classes which means instances cannot be directly created from them. They can contain operations but no attributes.

An interaction between two entities is a complex stochastic event, which eventually may bring about a change in the state of one or both entities. Interactions can be *specific* or *aspecific*. Specific interactions need a *recognition phase* between the two entities (*e.g.* B ↔ TAA). Recognition is based on the Hamming distance and affinity function, and is eventually enhanced by adjuvants. Aspecific interactions do not have a recognition phase.

Biological interactions occur by contact between entities. In a lattice gas scheme this implies that only entities present in the same lattice site are candidates for interactions. Moreover biological interactions are state-dependent events, i.e. an interaction may occur only if one or both entities are in the appropriate state. When those conditions are satisfied the interaction will occur according to a probabilistic law. Both specific and aspecific interactions are stochastically determined using a probability function, which depends on different parameters, computed via random number generators. Changing the seed of the random number generator yields a different sequence of probabilistic events. This mimics biological differences between individuals who share the same event probabilities.

An overall scheme of the interactions included in the CMM is shown in Fig. 14.2. The "Interactions" concept has been modelled in CMM-Ontology using component diagrams. They show the components (either component technologies or sections of the system which are clearly distinguishable) and the artifacts they are made of such as source code files, or relational database tables. Components can have interfaces (i.e. abstract classes with operations) that allow associations between components.

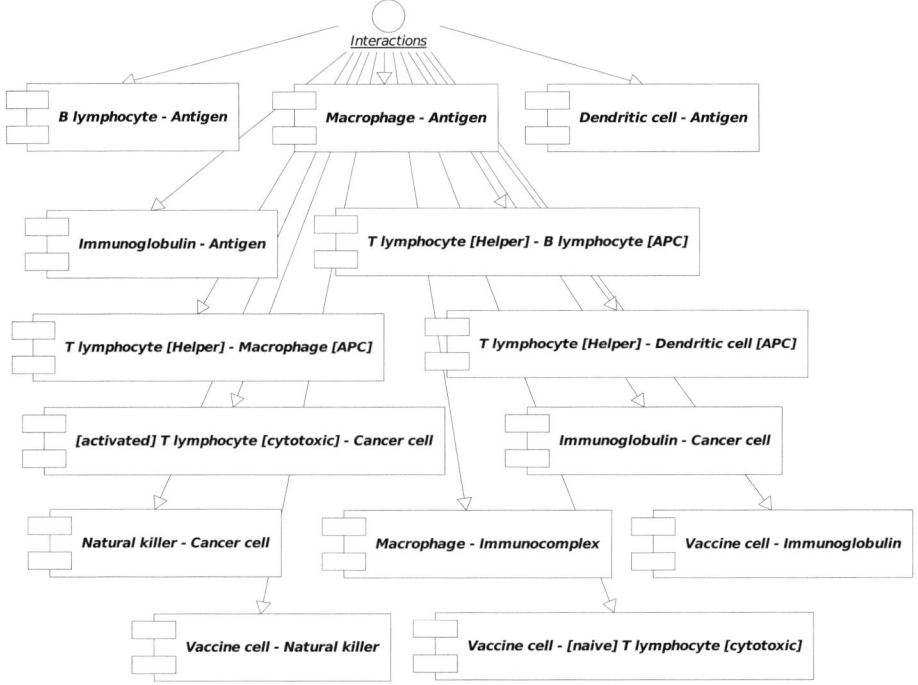

Fig. 14.2. The full set of interactions in the model.

Fig. 14.3 shows the ontology of a specific interaction (specific antibody directed against a cancer cell) modeled in CMM.

SimTriplex simulator computes the main biological entities of the cancer-immune system-vaccine competition. If the number of cancer cells is greater than 10^5, then the simulator recognizes carcinoma in situ (CIS) formation and simulation ends at the time that has been reached. We will refer to this time as the mouse survival time. The 10^5 limit was a value agreed with biologists to approximate the threshold of emipirical tumor detectability *in vivo* under realistic conditions.

The CMM and its simulator have been compared using data from *in vivo* experiments, showing good agreement [21].

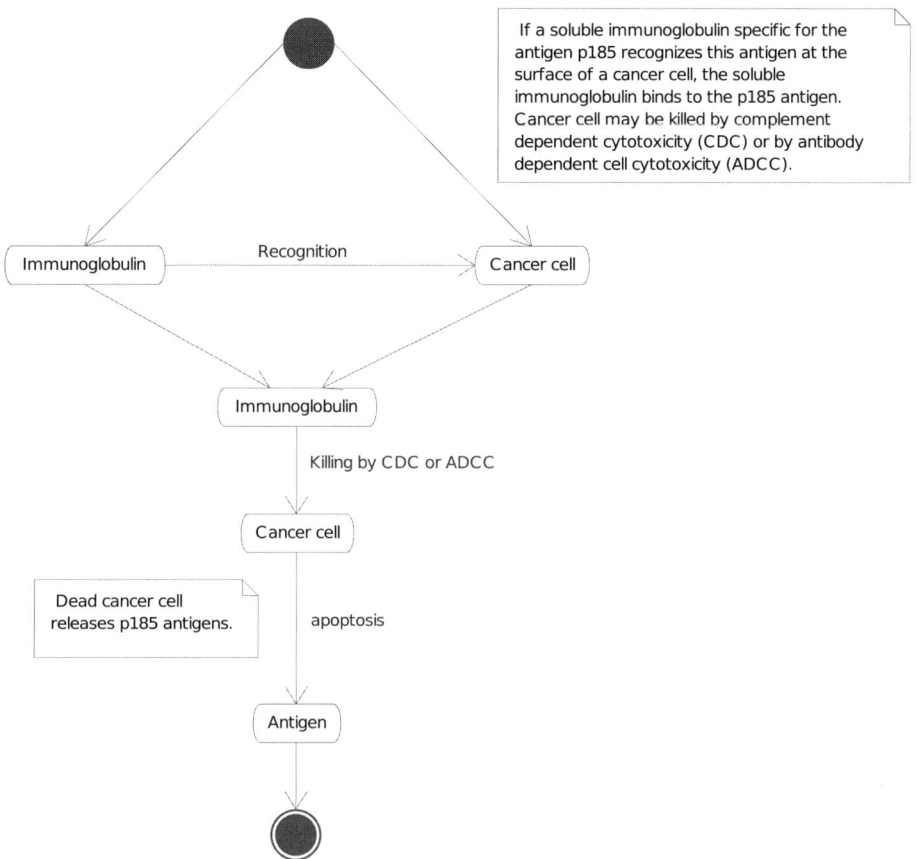

Fig. 14.3. Ontology of a specific soluble immunoglobulin directed against a cancer cell.

14.5 The Optimal Scheduling Problem

From the immunological point of view, an optimal schedule is a schedule which maintains its efficacy with a minimum number of vaccine administrations. However, due to the biological diversity of individuals, a schedule which works well for one individual may not be effective for a different individual. In designing therapies medical doctors face the problem of finding a *standard treatment* which will be effective for a high percentage of patients.

This is usually achieved by a *consensus* technique, a public statement on a particular aspect of medical knowledge available at the time it was written, and that is generally agreed upon as the evidence-based, state-of-the-art (or state-of-science) knowledge by a representative group of experts in that area. Progress in scientific knowledge requires periodic updating of consensus on standard treatments.

In what follows we describe a mathematical-based quantitative approach to the former problem. This attempt is based on the previously described model/simulator of the immune response induced by the vaccine. In mathematical terms the simulator defines a vector function from the set of initial data and parameters to the set of the results.

The function f is built using the biological rules underlying the action of the vaccine.

To translate the biological concept of *effectiveness of a vaccination schedule* let us consider a time interval $[0, T]$ in which we study the action of the schedule on a set of mice S. The time T is the duration of the *in vivo* experiment. We discretize the given time interval in $N - 1$ equally spaced subintervals of width Δt, i.e. $\{t_1 = 0, \ t_2, \ \ldots, t_i, \ \ldots, \ t_N = T\}$. The time interval $\Delta t = 8$ hrs corresponds to the time step of the simulator. Vaccine can only be administrated at time t_i.

Let $\mathbf{x} = \{x_1, x_2, \ldots, x_i, \ldots x_N\}$ be a binary vector representing the sequence of vaccine schedule where $x_i = 0/1$ means respectively administration/no-administration of the vaccine. The label i represents the time t_i of the vaccine administration and t_N the end of the vaccination period. The number of vaccine administrations is given by $n = \sum_{i=1}^{N} x_i$.

Let $\tau(\mathbf{x}, \lambda_j)$ be mouse survival time, i.e. the time of CIS formation. This is a function of the vaccination schedule $\mathbf{x}$ administered to the mouse $j \in S$ and a parameter λ_j which describes the biological diversity. If $\tau < t_N$ the simulator will return a time τ, otherwise, as the simulation stops at $t = T_N$, the simulator sets $\tau = T_N$. A vaccine schedule is effective if $\tau = T_N$. This definition can be applied either to a single mouse or to a set of mice.

14.5.1 Optimal Schedule for a Single Mouse

The simplest case is the unconstrained optimization problem for a single mouse. Using the quantities defined above we can formulate this optimization problem as follows.

Problem 1. Find a binary vector $\overline{\mathbf{x}}$ such that

$$\tau(\overline{\mathbf{x}}, \lambda_j) = \ max\{\tau(\mathbf{x}, \lambda_j)\} \tag{14.1}$$

$$(\overline{\mathbf{x}}) = \ min\{n(\mathbf{x})\}. \tag{14.2}$$

This is a multi-objective discrete optimization problem. The search space D has cardinality 2^N. For $T = 360$ days, and reducing the problem to only one vaccine administration per day, the cardinality is $2^{360} \sim 10^{108}$ which prevents any chance of an exhaustive search. The function τ depends on the response of the stimulated immune system. Such a function cannot be expressed in an analytical form and $\tau(\mathbf{x}, \lambda_j)$ can only be computed through the simulator described in Sect. 14.4.

Assuming that there is no conflict between the two objective functions, the standard technique to find a solution of a multi-objective optimization problem, $min(g_1)$ and $min(g_2)$, is to transform the problem into a single-objective problem for a new function $f(g_1, g_2)$. The simplest case is to consider a linear combination $f = g_1 + \alpha g_2$, where α is a *weight* parameter. However a linear combination is not appropriate for our problem. As a general guideline for identifying a new objective function f to minimize we note that: i) any objective function which just takes into consideration (14.1) will increase if the number of vaccine administrations increases (increasing number of vaccine administrations implies later formation of CIS), i.e. $n(\mathbf{x})$ increases; ii) conversely if one considers just (14.2), then f increases for schedules with a lower number of vaccine administrations. To consider both (14.1) and (14.2) the objective function must be at least a two-variable function of type $f(n(\mathbf{x}), \tau(\mathbf{x}, \lambda_j), \ldots)$ which satisfies the following two properties:

$$f(n, \tau, \ldots) < f(n, \tau', \ldots) \text{ if } \tau > \tau' \qquad (14.3)$$
$$f(n, \tau, \ldots) > f(n', \tau, \ldots) \text{ if } n > n'. \qquad (14.4)$$

A simple function which satisfies these requirements is

$$f_j(n(\mathbf{x}), \tau(\mathbf{x}, \lambda_j)) = \frac{[n(\mathbf{x})]^2}{\tau(\mathbf{x}, \lambda_j)} \qquad (14.5)$$

and problems (14.1) and (14.2) reduce to the following.

Problem 1.a   Find $\overline{\mathbf{x}}$ such that

$$f_j(n(\overline{\mathbf{x}}), \tau(\overline{\mathbf{x}}, \lambda_j)) = min\ \{f_j(n(\mathbf{x}), \tau(\mathbf{x}, \lambda_j))\}. \qquad (14.6)$$

Integer optimization is, in general, a difficult problem. A variety of methods and algorithms are available, i.e. branch and bound, general cutting edge, dynamic Programming, heuristic algorithms, decomposition algorithms [19] and evolutionary algorithms [9]. To modify the problem according to biological requirements we choose to adopt a genetic algorithm (GA) approach which appears to be the most flexible with respect to our requirements.

To solve (14.6) with a GA, we have to provide a fitness function that ranks the chromosomes with respect to (14.1) and (14.2). In most cases of the single-objective optimization problem the fitness function coincides with the objective function. We used (14.5) as the fitness function for the GA search.

This problem was solved in [22]. However the solution was biologically unsatisfactory because the optimal schedule $\overline{x}$ yielded very high peaks in cancer cells. Even if a CIS is not yet formed, a high number of cancer cells may induce, by overstimulation, an anergic state of T lymphocytes, depleting in this way the immune system response and enhancing the risk of carcinogenesis. Moreover due to biological variability the optimal schedule found for mouse j was able, as expected, to prevent CIS formation only in a small fraction ($\sim 20\%$) of mice of the set S. So the problem formulated for a single mouse is not appropriate for finding an optimal schedule for a population of mice as tested in *in vivo* experiments.

To overcome the first point we add to the problem (14.6) two constraints on the maximum allowed number of cancer cells. This, as suggested by biologists, should prevent an anergic state of T lymphocytes. Let $M_1(\mathbf{x}, \lambda_j)$ and $M_2(\mathbf{x}, \lambda_j)$ respectively be the maximum number of cancer cells in $[0, T_{in}]$ (cell-mediated controlled phase) and in $[T_{in}, T]$ (humoral-mediated controlled phase) where $T_{in} \sim T/3$. Let γ_1 and γ_2 be, respectively, the cancer cells threshold in $[0, T_{in}]$ and in $[T_{in}, T]$. Our optimization problem (14.6) now becomes

Problem 1.b   Find $\overline{\mathbf{x}}$ such that

$$
\begin{cases}
f_j(n(\overline{\mathbf{x}}), \tau(\overline{\mathbf{x}}, \lambda_j)) = min \left\{ f_j(n(\mathbf{x}), \tau(\mathbf{x}, \lambda_j)) \right\} \\
\text{subject to:} \\
M_1(\overline{\mathbf{x}}, \lambda_j) \leq \gamma_1, \ t \in [0, T_{in}] \\
M_2(\overline{\mathbf{x}}, \lambda_j) \leq \gamma_2, \ t \in [T_{in}, T]
\end{cases}
\tag{14.7}
$$

At variance with usual methods in continuous optimization, the optimal search performed using GA translates the constraints into *penalties* in the fitness function. Solutions which do not satisfy the constraints are still accepted but with lower ranking; hence the optimal solution found by a GA may not satisfy all the constraints.

14.5.2 Optimal Schedule for a Set of Mice

We now extend the previous formulation to solve the problem of finding the optimal schedule for a set S of mice. For this we need to reformulate the optimization problem. Let $\{j_1, j_2, \ldots, j_m\} \subset S$, with $m = 8$, a random chosen subset of *in silico* mice. The optimization problem is

Problem 2   Find $\overline{\mathbf{x}}$ such that

$$
\begin{cases}
f_{j_1}(n(\overline{\mathbf{x}}), \tau(\overline{\mathbf{x}}, \lambda_{j_1})) = min \left\{ f_{j_1}(n(\mathbf{x}), \tau(\mathbf{x}, \lambda_{j_1})) \right\} \\
f_{j_2}(n(\overline{\mathbf{x}}), \tau(\overline{\mathbf{x}}, \lambda_{j_2})) = min \left\{ f_{j_2}(n(\mathbf{x}), \tau(\mathbf{x}, \lambda_{j_2})) \right\} \\
\vdots \\
f_{j_8}(n(\overline{\mathbf{x}}), \tau(\overline{\mathbf{x}}, \lambda_{j_8})) = min \left\{ f_{j_8}(n(\mathbf{x}), \tau(\mathbf{x}, \lambda_{j_8})) \right\} \\
\text{subject to:} \\
M_1(\overline{\mathbf{x}}, \lambda_j) \leq \gamma_1, \ t \in [0, T_{in}] \quad j = \{j_1, j_2, \ldots, j_8\} \\
M_2(\overline{\mathbf{x}}, \lambda_j) \leq \gamma_2, \ t \in [T_{in}, T] \quad j = \{j_1, j_2, \ldots, j_8\}
\end{cases}
\tag{14.8}
$$

This is again a multi-objective optimization problem. We can reduce it to a standard problem by defining the new objective function as a linear combination of $f_{j_1}, \ldots, f_{j_8}$, i.e.

$$
f(n, \tau_{j_1}, \tau_{j_2}, \ldots, \tau_{j_8}) = \sum_{k=1}^{8} \alpha_k \, f_{j_k}(n, \tau_{j_k}),
\tag{14.9}
$$

where we set all $\alpha_k = 1$ as the mice are equiweighted.

Problem 2.a   Find $\bar{\mathbf{x}}$ such that

$$
\begin{cases}
f(n(\bar{\mathbf{x}}), \tau(\bar{\mathbf{x}}, \lambda_{j_1}, \ldots, \lambda_{j_8})) = min\, \{f(n(\mathbf{x}), \tau(\mathbf{x}, \lambda_{j_1}, \ldots, \lambda_{j_8}))\} \\
\text{subject to:} \\
M_1(\bar{\mathbf{x}}, \lambda_j) \leq \gamma_1,\ t \in [0, T_{in}] \quad j = \{j_1, j_2, \ldots, j_8\} \\
M_2(\bar{\mathbf{x}}, \lambda_j) \leq \gamma_2,\ t \in [T_{in}, T] \quad j = \{j_1, j_2, \ldots, j_8\}
\end{cases}
\tag{14.10}
$$

The solution of this problem [13] is an optimal schedule which prevents CIS formation for 85% of the *virtual mice* $\in S$. This is a *predictive solution* that can be validated with *in vivo* experiments.

14.5.3 Wet Biology Constrained Genetic Algorithm Search

There still is a big gap between mathematical solutions and *in vivo* experiments that applied mathematicians should carefully take into consideration in the analysis of the problem. We faced this aspect when we proposed our schedule to the wet biologists group for testing *in vivo*. We discovered that our optimal schedule was not suitable for experiments as it did not take into account the procedures that were used in the actual laboratory experiments. The most important of these requirements was the fact that vaccine administrations were performed only twice a week (Monday and Thursday). This is considered a very intensive vaccination schedule from an immunological point of view and it is also labor intensive, because it requires the preparation of fresh cells to make the vaccine twice weekly.

In our GA a chromosome in the population of chromosomes represents a vaccine schedule (see the discussion ealier in the section). *In silico* experiments last usually for 400 days. Taking into account that the time step of the simulator is 8 hrs and assuming that one could administer the vaccine up to three times a day, this leads to a chromosome with 1200 alleles. Without any constrain on vaccine administration each allele can take the two instances 0/1.

The wet biologist requirements drastically reduce the number of alleles which can take two instances. These constraints cannot be translated into penalties in the fitness function because they must be completely satisfied. Therefore we used a different strategy to constrain the optimal search.

As pointed out these constraints drastically reduce the search space as a large number of alleles are forced to have the value 0. The number of such alleles can be easily computed as 1200 time steps which corresponds to 400 days; 400 days are 57 weeks plus 1 day. Assuming that weeks run from Monday to Sunday this leads to 115 days in which the vaccine can be administered. Thus the cardinality of the new search space $\overline{\mathbf{D}}$ reduces to 2^{115} (while the complete search space $\mathbf{D}$ was 2^{1200}).

As the simulator, which computes the function τ, runs with a time step of 8 hrs we need to map the new search space into the old one. A function $i(k)$ which maps a 115 day schedule into 1200 time steps is

$$i(k) = 9 \cdot k + 3 \cdot \left\lfloor \frac{k}{2} \right\rfloor + 1 \,,$$

where $k \in [1, 115]$ represents the available days (genes) for the vaccination administration in the GA. $i(k) \in [1, 1200]$ returns the corresponding time step. With this function the GA will only search two days within a week. Using this set of constraints our GA search found that a 37 vaccination schedule gave a survival of 88% of mice *in silico*.

To check how much this solution depends on the number of days allowed for the vaccine administration we searched for a different optimal schedule using a three day (Mondays, Wednesdays, Fridays) constrained GA. In this experiment we found a schedule with 37 vaccine administrations and a survival rate of 90%. These two results are almost equivalent as produced in the day-unconstrained GA model both in terms of the number of injections required and the survival rate reached. The schedule constrained with two days per week of vaccine administrations is currently under *in vivo* testing.

In Fig. 14.4 we show the schedules that are currently under *in vivo* testing.

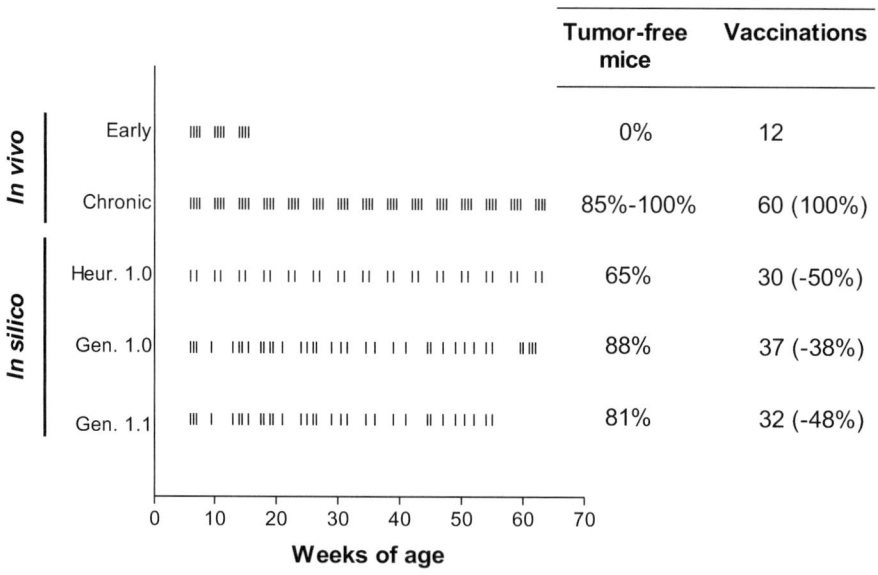

Fig. 14.4. Full story of optimal vaccination schedule search.

The "Heur 1.0" one refers to an immunologist suggestion to keep the number of administrations equal to the *in silico* proposed one. The "Gen. 1.0" represents the GA's protocol output constrained to 2 days; the Gen. 1.1 represents the GA's protocol without the last five vaccine administrations, which have been cut out by our expert biologist as the last period of mouse life is not important for the evaluation of the protocol efficacy.

Finally we show in Figs. 14.5 and 14.6 the behavior *in silico* of the main immune entities during the Gen. 1.0 optimal vaccination schedule.

Fig. 14.5 shows that the cancer cells are kept under a safe threshold (indicated by the line above the curves) by the GA proposed vaccination protocol. The safe threshold is the same one envisaged by the *in vivo* "Chronic" schedule.

Fig. 14.6 shows the behavior of B lymphocytes during the vaccine administrations (showed as vertical small lines). The vaccine administrations elicit a humoral response showed by specific B lymphocytes that differentiate into plasma cells secreting specific immunoglobulins against cancer cells and tumor associated antigens. The high humoral response elicited *in silico* suggests that the proposed vaccination schedule should work for cancer immunoprevention *in vivo*. Fig. 14.6 also shows that the GA proposed vaccination schedule elicits a cytotoxic response as one can appreciate from the two bottom panels of the figure.

14.6 Conclusion

We presented here the results of an ongoing close collaboration between mathematicians and biologists that is leading to sequential improvements both to mathematical and computational *in silico* models of the immune system, and to *in vivo* models of immune system-tumor competition and of vaccines to prevent tumor onset.

Our successful experience with this collaborative interdisciplinary approach suggests that vaccine research and development can be accelerated by using appropriate models of vaccine-induced immune responses. Further applications of this approach are in progress and results will be published in due course.

Mathematical and computational models have proven to be the right instruments to overcome the inherent difficulties of biological models. They have been applied in the last century in many different areas of engineering and applied science. To further extend this experience to biosciences we need a close collaboration between mathematicians and biologists. In particular we need to share a common basic language to describe the biological processes into a mathematical and computational model.

Acknowledgments

This work was supported under the EC contract FP6-2004-IST-4, No. 028069 (ImmunoGrid). PLL acknowledges financial support from the Italian Association for Cancer Research (AIRC), the University of Bologna, the Department

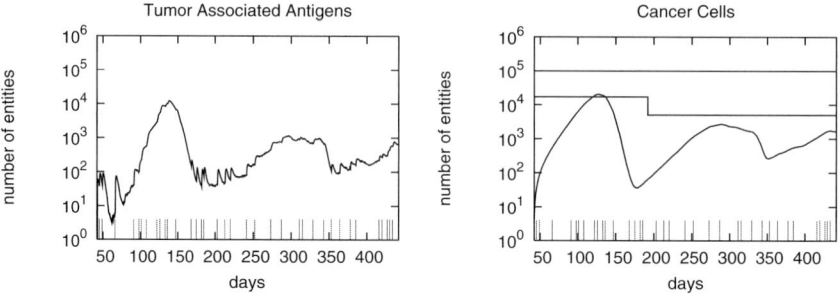

Fig. 14.5. Cancer cells' behavior (right panel) and tumor associated antigens (left panel). Small vertical lines indicate the time of vaccine administrations.

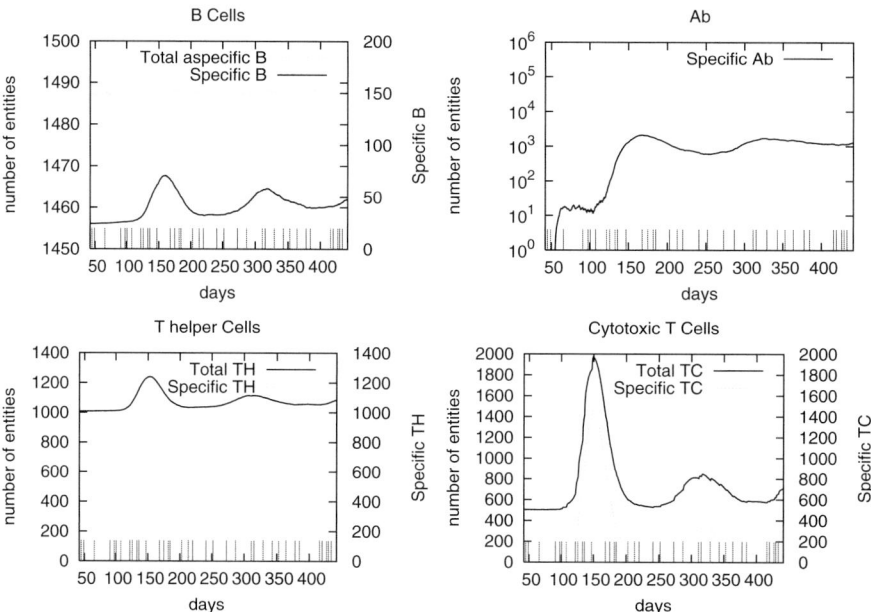

Fig. 14.6. Total aspecific B lymphocytes and specific B lymphocytes against tumor associated antigen (top, left panel); total specific immunoglobulins against cancer cells and tumor associated antigens (top, right panel). Specific cytotoxic T lymphocytes (against peptide/major histocompatibility class I complex) and specific helper T lymphocytes (against peptide/major histocompatibility class II complex) respectively showed in right and left, lower panel. Small vertical lines indicate the time of vaccine administrations.

of Experimental Pathology ("Pallotti" fund), and MIUR. AP is in receipt of a fellowship from the Italian Foundation for Cancer Research (FIRC). FP and SM acknowledge partial support from the University of Catania research grant and MIUR PRIN 2006.

References

1. Ada, G.L.: The immunological principles of vaccination. Lancet, **335:8688**, 523–526 (1990).
2. Arlotti, L., Bellomo, N., De Angelis, E.: Generalized kinetic (Boltzmann) models: mathematical structures and applications. Mathematical Models and Methods in Applied Science, **12:4**, 567–591 (2002).
3. Bellomo, N., Preziosi, L.: Modelling and mathematical problems related to tumor evolution and its interaction with the immune system. Math. Comp. Model., **32**, 413–452 (2000).
4. Chang, M.H., Shau, W.Y., Chen, C.J., Wu, T.C., Kong, M.S., Liang, D.C., Hsu, H.M., Chen, H.L., Hsu, H.Y., Chen, D.S.: Hepatitis B vaccination and hepatocellular carcinoma rates in boys and girls. JAMA, **284:23**, 3040–3042 (2000).
5. Croci, S., Nicoletti, G., Landuzzi, L., De Giovanni, C., Astolfi, A., Marini, C., Di Carlo, E., Musiani, P., Forni, G., Nanni, P., Lollini, P.-L.: Immunological prevention of a multigene cancer syndrome. Cancer Research, **64**, 8428–8434 (2004).
6. De Angelis, E., Jabin, P.-E.: Mathematical models of therapeutical actions related to tumour and immune system competition. Math. Meth. Appl. Sci., **28:17**, 2061–2083 (2005).
7. De Giovanni, C., Croci, S., Nicoletti, G., Landuzzi, L., Palladini, A., Pannellini, T., Borgia, L., Iezzi, M., Di Carlo, E., Orengo, A.M., Kennedy, R.C., Lollini, P.-L., Nanni, P., Musiani, P.: Inhibition of prostate carcinogenesis by combined active immunoprophylaxis. Int. J. Cancer, **121:88**, (2007).
8. De Giovanni, C., Nicoletti, G., Landuzzi, L., Astolfi, A., Croci, S., Comes, A., Ferrini, S., Meazza, R., Iezzi, M., Di Carlo, E., Musiani, P., Cavallo, F., Nanni, P., Lollini, P.-L.: Immunoprevention of HER-2/neu transgenic mammary carcinoma through an interleukin 12-engineered allogeneic cell vaccine. Cancer Research, **64:11**, 4001–4009 (2004).
9. Dorne, C., Dorigo, M., Glover, F.: New ideas in optimization. Advanced Topics in Computer Science, McGraw-Hill, New York (1999).
10. Lollini, P.-L., Cavallo, F., Nanni, P., Forni, G.: Vaccines for tumour prevention. Nat. Rev. Cancer, **6:3**, 204–216 (2006).
11. Lollini, P.-L., De Giovanni, C., Pannellini, T., Cavallo, F., Forni, G., Nanni, P.: Cancer immunoprevention. Future Oncol., **1:1**, 57–66 (2005).
12. Lollini, P.-L., Forni, G.: Cancer immunoprevention: tracking down persistent tumor antigens. Trends Immunol., **24:2**, 62–66 (2003).
13. Lollini, P.-L., Motta, S., Pappalardo, F.: Discovery of cancer vaccination protocols with a genetic algorithm driving an agent based simulator. BMC Bioinformatics, **7:352**, doi:10.1186/1471-2105-7-352 (2006).
14. Lollini, P.-L., Nicoletti, G., Landuzzi, L., De Giovanni, C., Rossi, I., Di Carlo, E., Musiani, P., Muller, W.J., Nanni, P.: Down regulation of major histocompatibility complex class I expression in mammary carcinoma of HER-2/neu transgenic mice. Int. J. Cancer, **77:6**, 937–941 (1998).
15. Motta, S., Lollini, P.-L., Castiglione, F., Pappalardo, F.: Modelling vaccination schedules for a cancer immunoprevention vaccine. Immunome Research, **1:5**, doi:10.1186/1745-7580-1-5 (2005).

16. Nanni, P., Landuzzi, L., Nicoletti, G., De Giovanni, C., Rossi, I., Croci, S., Astolfi, A., Iezzi, M., Di Carlo, E., Musiani, P., Forni, G., Lollini, P.-L.: Immunoprevention of mammary carcinoma in HER-2/neu transgenic mice is IFN-gamma and B cell dependent. J. Immunol., **173:4**, 2288–2296 (2004).

17. Nanni, P., Nicoletti, G., De Giovanni, C., Landuzzi, L., Di Carlo, E., Cavallo, F., Pupa, S.M., Rossi, I., Colombo, M.P., Ricci, C., Astolfi, A., Musiani, P., Forni, G., Lollini, P.-L.: Combined allogeneic tumor cell vaccination and systemic interleukin 12 prevents mammary carcinogenesis in HER-2/neu transgenic mice. J. Exp. Med., **194:9**, 1195–1205 (2001).

18. Nanni, P., Pupa, S.M., Nicoletti, G., De Giovanni, C., Landuzzi, L., Rossi, I., Astolfi, A., Ricci, C., De Vecchi, R., Invernizzi, A.M., Di Carlo, E., Musiani, P., Forni, G., Menard, S., Lollini, P.-L.: p185(neu) protein is required for tumor and anchorage-independent growth, not for cell proliferation of transgenic mammary carcinoma. Int. J. Cancer, **87:2**, 186–194 (2000).

19. Nemhauser, G.L., Wolsey, L.A.: Integer and combinatorial optimization. Wiley, New York (1988).

20. Novellino, L., Castelli, C., Parmiani, G.: A listing of human tumor antigens recognized by T cells: March 2004 update. Cancer Immunol. Immunother., (2004).

21. Pappalardo, F., Lollini, P.-L., Castiglione, F., Motta, S.: Modelling and simulation of cancer immunoprevention vaccine. Bioinformatics, **21:12**, 2891–2897 (2005).

22. Pappalardo, F., Mastriani, E., Lollini, P.-L., Motta, S.: Genetic algorithm against cancer. Lecture Notes in Computer Science, **3849**, 223–228 (2006).

23. Quaglino, E., Iezzi, M., Mastini, C., Amici, A., Pericle, F., Di Carlo, E., Pupa, S.M., De Giovanni, C., Spadaro, M., Curcio, C., Lollini, P.-L., Musiani, P., Forni, G., Cavallo, F.: Electroporated DNA vaccine clears away multifocal mammary carcinomas in Her-2/neu transgenic mice. Cancer Res., **64:8**, 2858–2864 (2004).

24. Rosenberg, S.A., Yang, J.C., Restifo, N.P.: Cancer immunotherapy: moving beyond current vaccines. Nat. Med., **10:9**, 909–915 (2004).

25. Ross, J.S., Gray, K., Gray, G.S., Worland, P.J., Rolfe, M.: Anticancer antibodies. Am. J. Clin. Pathol., **119:4**, 472–485 (2003).

26. Sawaya, G.F., Smith-McCune, K.: HPV vaccination–more answers, more questions. N. Engl. J. Med., **356:19**, 1991–1993 (2007).

27. Smyth, M.J., Dunn, G.P., Schreiber, R.D.: Cancer immunosurveillance and immunoediting: the roles of immunity in suppressing tumor development and shaping tumor immunogenicity. Adv. Immunol., **90**, 1–50 (2006).

28. Waldmann, T.A., Morris, J.C.: Development of antibodies and chimeric molecules for cancer immunotherapy. Adv. Immunol., **90**, 83–131 (2006).

15

Dynamically Adaptive Tumour-Induced Angiogenesis: The Impact of Flow on the Developing Capillary Plexus

Steven R. McDougall

Institute of Petroleum Engineering, Heriot-Watt University, Edinburgh, EH14
4AS, Scotland
Steve.Mcdougall@pet.hw.ac.uk

15.1 Introduction

Uncontrolled or excessive blood-vessel formation is an essential accompaniment to solid tumour growth, beginning with the rearrangement and migration of endothelial cells from a pre-existing vasculature and culminating in the formation of an extensive network, or bed, of new capillaries [40]. Although the precise molecular cascades associated with a given instance of angiogenesis may differ from case to case, a common sequence of events associated with tumour-induced angiogenesis has been broadly identified and well documented.

The process begins when the oxygen demands of cancerous cells within a solid tumour are unable to be adequately met via diffusion from nearby capillaries. These cells consequently become hypoxic and this is assumed to trigger cellular release of tumour angiogenic factors (TAFs) [16], which start to diffuse into the surrounding tissue and approach the endothelial cells of nearby blood vessels. These endothelial cells subsequently respond to the TAF concentration gradient by releasing a number of matrix degrading enzymes (including matrix metalloproteinases), which degrade the surrounding tissue leading to the formation of new capillary sprouts. These then migrate towards the tumour [67] [5] [70] and the resulting vascular connection subsequently provides all the nutrients and oxygen required for continued tumour growth. Initially, the sprouts arising from the parent vessel grow in an essentially parallel manner. However, once the finger-like capillary sprouts have reached a certain distance from the parent vessel, they are seen to incline toward each other [48], leading to numerous tip-to-tip and tip-to-sprout fusions known as anastomoses. Such anastomoses result in the fusing of the finger-like sprouts into a network of poorly perfused loops or arcades. Following this process of anastomosis, the first signs of circulation can be recognised and, from the primary loops,

N. Bellomo et al. (eds.), *Selected Topics in Cancer Modeling*,
DOI: 10.1007/978-0-8176-4713-1_15, © Springer Science+Business Media, LLC 2008

new buds and sprouts emerge repeating the angiogenic sequence of events and providing for the further extension of the new capillary bed.

Most modelling studies dealing with the process of angiogenesis have tended to concentrate upon the way in which the new capillary bed is initiated and migrates in response to various chemical stimuli and mechanical forces affiliated with the tumour and host tissue. However, relatively few theoretical studies have examined the important role played by blood perfusion during angiogenesis and fewer still have explored the ways in which a dynamic bed architecture can affect the distribution of flow within it. This is clearly an important feature of angiogenesis, as capillary size and bed architecture are key determinants of not only oxygen delivery to the tumour during growth, but also chemotherapy delivery during treatment. It is reasonable to assume that an aberrant tumour vasculature will hinder uniform delivery of therapeutic compounds to the tumour tissue.

Although there have been a number of theoretical models developed to try to better understand vascular architecture in general ([68] [22] [31] [61] [26] *inter alia*) and to examine clinical implications in a broader sense ([15] [29] [63] [32] *inter alia*), there have only been a small number of theoretical studies examining blood flow issues in tumour-induced (micro) capillary networks ([46] [6] [7] [37] [2] [71] [64] [72] [38]). Moreover, most of these studies have tended to focus upon tumour blood flow (i.e. flow within the tumour itself) and have largely neglected the importance of flow in the vicinity of the tumour periphery. The fact that new treatments are being tailored to specifically target vascular endothelium associated with tumour-induced plexuses suggests that it would be of some benefit to understand the coupling between vascular structure and perfusion more fully in a range of different situations.

This chapter begins with a review of previous models associated with the key phenomena of solid tumour growth, capillary migration and microcirculatory vessel adaptation, together with a discussion of recent *coupled* angiogenesis models that have attempted to address these issues simultaneously. The strengths and weaknesses of different approaches are discussed. Section 15.3 then focuses upon one particular coupled migration-flow model (the DATIA model of [38]). The sensitivity of the model to changes in a number of physical and biochemical parameters is examined in detail and results clearly demonstrate the impact of dynamic remodelling and shear-induced vessel branching upon global network architecture. A new extension of this adaptive model to three dimensions is also presented. The effects of dynamic vessel adaptation and system dimensionality upon the delivery of chemotherapeutic agents to the tumour surface are presented in Section 15.4. Results from the full DATIA model not only highlight the need for incorporating vessel adaptations into any angiogenesis model involving transport issues, such as chemotherapeutic or anti-vascular intervention, but also show that three-dimensional modelling is required if quantitative predictions are to be made. The chapter concludes with a discussion section summarising all the main results and offering directions for future model development and study.

15.2 Angiogenesis and Perfusion: A Brief Review

Although very few hybrid mathematical models currently exist that deal with capillary plexus formation coupled to blood flow in the context of solid tumour growth, it should be noted that a great deal of research *has* been undertaken on related topics over the past decade. Continuous models mimicking aspects of avascular and vascular tumour growth have existed for over 50 years: from the early paper of [76] Thomlinson and Gray (1955) dealing with simple diffusive transport of oxygen in tumour cords, through the surface tension approxima- tion of [24] [25] and the inhibitor switches of [21] and [1], to the inclusion of chemotactic responses of tumour cells [39] and multi-species models exam- ining the nutrient dependency of tumour heterogeneity [78] [79] [52]. Indeed, further refined models of tumour growth continue to be produced, highlighting a wide range of new mechanisms and possible targets for therapeutic inter- vention (see, for example, [69] [54] [10] [19] [17]). However, whilst continuous formulations of vascular tumour growth are illuminating in their own right, they are by definition unable to resolve the fine detail associated with the ar- chitecture of vascular beds: detail that can prove extremely important when considering quantitative comparisons with available experimental data. In or- der to consider such detail, discrete formulations of the differential equations must be considered and some degree of rule-based simulation employed.

One of the first attempts at constructing discrete vascular structures was presented by Stokes and Lauffenburger [74], who considered the migration of endothelial tip cells due to random motility, viscous damping, and a chemo- tactic response. This model produced vascular branching patterns similar to those observed experimentally but no cell biology was included locally at the sprout tip (only average features were considered along a sprout length). At around the same time, a deterministic formulation of vessel migration was published by Gottlieb [23] and was further extended by Nekka et al. [45]. The latter (rule-based) approach involved the extension, branching, and anasto- mosis of pre-seeded vessels within a mitotically active cellular milieu; vessel subbranches and new sprouts were assumed to migrate towards ischaemic cen- tres within the tissue in an attempt to mimic endothelial cell chemotaxis via angiogenic factor release. Once again, realistic branching structures emerged from the model but the fundamental framework was essentially phenomeno- logical in nature and offered little insight into the underlying biological pro- cesses involved. A more realistic cell tracking methodology was developed by Anderson and Chaplain [4] using a model that built upon concepts derived from earlier work by Othmer and Stevens [47] (reinforced random walks) and Anderson et al. (1997) [3] (nematode movement). This novel hybrid model used a combination of the continuum and probabilistic approaches, combin- ing the strengths of each. The mathematical model focussed on three key variables involved in tumour-induced angiogenesis; namely, endothelial cells, tumour angiogenic factors (TAFs) and fibronectin, each of which has a cru- cial role to play. The model was motivated by the experimental system of

Muthukkaruppan et al. [44], whereby a small solid tumour or fragment of tumour is implanted in the cornea of a test animal close to the limbal vessels of the eye, which are lined with endothelial cells. For the endothelial cells it was assumed that there was a small amount of random motion, and that they responded chemotactically to gradients of TAF and haptotactically to gradients of fibronectin in the matrix. Proliferation of the cells was incorporated at the individual (discrete) level. For the TAF, it was assumed that a (quasi) steady state distribution already existed in the matrix, the TAF having initially been secreted by the tumour cells. As the endothelial cells migrated through the tissue, there was some binding of the TAF to the cells, modelled with a simple uptake function. Endothelial cells are known to produce fibronectin as they migrate and also to degrade the matrix as they progress, and so simple production and loss terms were included in the fibronectin equation to reflect these facts. An extended form of this model will be discussed in greater detail later and the relevant equations are summarised in Appendix A. Later papers in the area of discrete modelling have examined the impact of lattice-free migration [51], TAF diffusion and decay [77], and tissue heterogeneity [75] upon sprout migration. Vascular structures similar to those reported by Anderson and Chaplain were observed.

In all of the models of endothelial migration and capillary formation discussed thus far, one important ingredient has been missing—namely flow. Fortunately, whilst perfusion-free tumour-induced angiogenesis modelling was continuing to develop apace, microvascular researchers were independently developing network models of blood perfusion from the joint perspectives of embryonic development and haemorheology. Two excellent reviews on this subject can be found in [66] and [53]. Although spatially heterogeneous network flows had been studied by researchers in the context of flow through porous media for over 50 years (see [36] for a review), microvascular research had tended to focus upon measurement rather than predictive modelling. One of the first examples of modelling blood flow in microvascular networks was undertaken in [55], which examined the implications of haematocrit partitioning at vessel junctions and haematocrit-radius parameterisation of effective viscosity upon the erythrocyte distribution within a vascular bed. This early model was later extended to incorporate a modified equation for apparent blood viscosity [56] and structural adaptations within the flowing network itself due to a number of physiological and rheological stimuli [57]. All of these studies utilised data from the rat mesentery, but a more recent study [26] has found that an additional stimulus is required in the vessel adaptation equation when considering remodelling of the mouse gracilis artery. This stimulus reflects time-delayed remodelling due to hypoxia and inflammation and may prove to be important in other applications. Further extensions to the Pries model can be found in [60] (which looks at the role played by wall thickness during adaptation) and [62] (which revisits the *in vitro* viscosity model and derives an *in vivo* equivalent in light of new measurements related to the endothelial surface layer). In addition to the Pries models outlined above, there are also a small number of modelling papers in the literature that deal with vascular adaptation in the context of developmental angiogenesis. One of the earliest of these papers is by Honda and Yoshizato [28], who described a simple computational model for simulating the branching pattern of capillaries in the wall of the avian yolk sac. An initial network of identical resistors (representing capillary elements) was established by means of a Voronoi grid and points were chosen at opposite ends of the domain to represent the avian heart (high potential/pressure) and sinus terminalis (low potential/pressure). The network was then switched on (i.e. flowed) and resistors were allowed to adapt according to a simple positive feedback relationship. The network was seen to remodel, with paths of low resistance becoming positively reinforced and high resistance vessels effectively disappearing. The result was a branched capillary plexus that broadly reproduced experimental observations. A more refined model of vascular remodelling, including both arterial and venous structures, was presented by Gödde and Kurz [22]. This successfully reproduced interdigitation between the terminal branches of arterial and venous trees during developmental angiogenesis and explicitly incorporated deterministic vessel degeneration due to wall shear stress and an alternative radius-dependent blood viscosity. In addition, Peclet number-dependent transmural oxygen transport was included: this played no further role in the model, however. Although more refined than the Honda and Yoshizato model, the Gödde and Kurz approach is still rather idealised, in that a fixed branching angle is assumed throughout the simulation and vessel growth is simply approximated by means of adding arterial or venous "tripods" in a probabilistic manner. Furthermore, no continuous process of vessel dilation or constriction is considered and radial variations are accounted for by either applying a modified form of Murray's law to new capillary tips or by removing elements completely if shear stress falls below a certain threshold.

So far, this review has described modelling advances related to vascular and avascular tumour growth at the continuum level, perfusion-free angiogenesis at the discrete level, and concomitant research in interconnected microvascular structures. Attention next turns to a brief summary of recent attempts at coupling some of these approaches in order to better understand the impact of convective vascular transport upon the growth and subsequent treatment of solid tumours. Most of the research in this area has been concentrated upon tumour blood flow (i.e. blood flow within the tumour itself) and very few studies have examined the impact of flow during angiogenesis (see later). One of the earliest papers aimed at coupling blood flow to tumour tissue was published by Netti et al. [46], who described the link between tumour haemodynamics and transvascular fluid exchange. The tumour vasculature was modelled by means of a single permeable and deformable vessel embedded within a fluid medium of uniform pressure. Sensitivities to vessel leakiness, vessel compliance, and tumour pressure were carried out and results compared with *ex vivo* tumours. It was shown that the coupling between vascular and extravascular flow could lead to heterogeneities in tumour blood flow and that this could, in turn, have implications for the treatment of solid tumours. Of course, the main limitation of this model was the fact that blood flow had been approximated by a single conduit, but this assumption was relaxed in two later papers by Baish et al. [6] [7]. In the first of these, a percolation-based network model of tumour blood flow was considered. A variety of capillary networks of differing fractal dimension was examined and the distribution of oxygen tension within the tumour resulting from each was calculated using a steady state diffusion equation. Results showed how the tortuous structure of the percolating network could affect the spatial heterogeneity of oxygen delivery and help explain increases in vascular resistance observed experimentally within solid tumours. The second paper amalgamated this percolation-based formulation with the permeable and compliant vessel used by Netti et al. This model was able to reproduce a high interstitial pressure within the tumour mass and this was subsequently seen to affect the distribution of vascular pressure. It was consequently shown how extravasated fluid became diverted from the tumour centre, preferring a more peripheral path by which to leave the system. A more recent paper by Mollica et al. [42] has extended the approach still further in order to examine temporal heterogeneity in tumour blood flow and has been used to reproduce the oscillatory behaviour of tumour blood flow *in vivo*. A similar, though more dynamic, model of tumour blood flow was described by Alarcon et al. [2]. The aim of this work was also to model the oxygen distribution within a tumour (see [6]) but then go on to determine its influence on the dynamics of a colony of normal and cancerous cells. The novelty of the approach lay in the fact that vessel radii could adapt in response to perfusion, thereby producing variable oxygen sources. Results from computational simulations of the model produced heterogeneous distributions of haematocrit, oxygen tension, and cancer cell density and highlighted the important role played by hypoxic cells during tumour invasion. A similar framework has recently been used to model treatment efficacy for non-Hodgkin's lymphoma [64].

All of the models discussed so far have dealt with vascular flow and transmural transport *within* a tumour mass and no details have been presented relating to models that have incorporated flow via vasculatures feeding the tumour periphery. In the work of McDougall et al. [37], flow simulations through such mature tumour-induced vascular networks were performed to investigate the efficiency of chemotherapy delivery as treatments passed from a nearby parent vessel to the tumour surface via a network of capillary vessels. These vessels had been stimulated to grow by chemical factors secreted by the tumour cells themselves (i.e. tumour-induced angiogenesis). The capillary vessels were generated from an angiogenesis model of Anderson and Chaplain [4] (described earlier). Flow modelling techniques used previously in the context of petroleum engineering to model the flow of water, oil, and gas through the interstices of a porous rock [36] were adapted to model blood and drug flow through these microvascular networks. Although blood was rather crudely considered to be a Newtonian fluid in this early work, results highlighted two important effects that could be responsible for the failure of some therapy regimes. First, it was found that a considerable amount of the drug injected into the parent vessel simply bypassed the tumour by way of the highly interconnected capillary network. The second effect related to the dilution of the drug as it became dispersed throughout the tumour-induced vasculature: the concentration of any drug reaching the tumour became so dilute as to have little effect on the tumour cells. Simulations were then performed to investigate ways to reduce these two detrimental phenomena and thereby optimise the drug uptake by the tumour. Increasing the mean capillary radius of the capillary bed and/or decreasing the blood viscosity both led to a significant increase in the drug uptake. Although these results were interesting from a qualitative perspective, this early model was somewhat naïve, with blood perfusion modelled as the flow of a Newtonian fluid through rigid cylindrical capillaries. The paper of Stéphanou et al. [71] extended the work of McDougall et al. (2002) [37] by examining how the removal of certain capillaries affected the distribution of blood flow in the system. Capillary pruning algorithms were designed to reflect how different anti-vascular and anti-angiogenic drugs were thought to operate *in vivo*. Simulations demonstrated that drug uptake could be increased by up to 130% via the random removal of vessels and this suggested the possibility of developing a new cancer treatment strategy, *viz.*, coupling the administration of an anti-angiogenic drug (to preliminarily optimise the vasculature) prior to chemotherapy treatment (thereby ensuring maximum delivery). This model has been further extended recently to incorporate vascular adaptation processes and non-Newtonian blood rheology [72]. This work considered how adaptive remodelling affected the supply of oxygen and drugs to the tumour periphery. Results clearly demonstrated that the combined effects of blood rheology, network architecture, and vessel compliance should be included in future models of angiogenesis if therapy protocols are to be quantitatively assessed. However, it should be noted that, as in all previous papers on vessel adaptation described in this review, the flow remodelling was carried out *a posteriori*, i.e. after an initial cell migration model had produced a hollow vessel network. The paper of McDougall et al. [38] implemented a number of significant improvements to this approach by considering a network that evolved both spatially and temporally in response to its associated flow distribution, with vessel adaptation occurring as a consequence of primary anastomosis. This model will now be described in greater detail in the following section.

15.3 Dynamic Adaptive Tumour-Induced Angiogenesis (DATIA)

This section begins by briefly describing the salient features of an extended angiogenesis model based upon the earlier formulation of Anderson and Chaplain discussed in the previous section. This is followed by a short summary describing the way in which blood perfusion and vessel dilation/constriction mechanisms have been incorporated into the model. These extensions result in a more realistic model of the angiogenesis process that is both adaptive and dynamic, with the resulting vascular network evolving both temporally and spatially in response to a number of migratory and transport-related cues. Results are presented that demonstrate the importance of these processes in determining global network architecture.

15.3.1 Capillary Migration in the Absence of Flow

The dynamic capillary migration model presented in this section explicitly takes into account the important function of matrix degrading enzymes (such as matrix metalloproteinases, MMPs; urokinase plasminogen activators, uPAs) during angiogenesis in the absence of flow [34] [35] [11]. Mediation in vessel growth via extracellular matrix proteolysis by specific enzymes produced by endothelial cells is also included. A number of recent publications have demonstrated the importance of enzymes from the MMP family and their involvement in the regulation of the various stages of the angiogenic process ([14] [80] [27] [73]). These MMPs are involved in the migration of endothelial cells within the extracellular matrix, endothelial cell proliferation, and the remodelling of the basement membrane of newly formed vessels. Their importance is such that these proteinases and their regulation form new targets for cancer treatment. As the ultimate goal of this work is to propose a global modelling framework within which to further investigate new treatments, it is important to incorporate the MMP effect into the modelling.

All of the vasculatures presented in the remainder of this chapter were generated using a hybrid discrete-continuum model inspired by the tumour-induced angiogenesis model proposed by Anderson and Chaplain [4]. The model assumes that individual endothelial cells at the tips of the new capillary sprouts (vessels) migrate through (i) random motility, (ii) chemotaxis in response to TAFs released by the tumour, and (iii) haptotaxis in response to fibronectin (FN) gradients in the extracellular matrix. A (non-dimensional) equation describing endothelial cell (n) conservation is used to produce movement weightings for discrete tip cells as they leave the parent vessel (see Appendix A and Fig. A.1). The equation is given by

$$\frac{\partial n}{\partial t} = \overbrace{D\nabla^2 n}^{random} - \overbrace{\nabla \cdot (\chi(c)n\nabla c)}^{chemotaxis} - \overbrace{\rho \nabla \cdot (n\nabla f)}^{haptotaxis}. \tag{15.1}$$

In addition to an equation for endothelial cell density, the model also requires equations governing the evolution of angiogenic factor (c), matrix degrading enzyme (m), and the matrix-bound protein associated with the haptotactic response (fibronectin in this case, denoted by f). For the TAF, it is assumed that a (quasi) steady state distribution already exists in the matrix, the TAF having initially been secreted by the tumour cells. As the individual endothelial cells migrate through the tissue, there is some binding of the TAF to the cells and this is modelled with a simple uptake term that is only switched on locally in the presence of a migrating tip cell. Fibronectin exists in the matrix in bound form and therefore there is no diffusion term for fibronectin. Endothelial cells are known to produce fibronectin as they migrate and also to degrade the matrix as they progress. Consequently, simple production and loss terms in the fibronectin equation are switched on wherever an endothelial tip cell exists to reflect these facts. Tumour angiogenesis factors and fibronectin are known to bind to specific membrane receptors on endothelial cells and subsequently trigger molecular cascades inside the endothelial cells, activating cell migratory machinery. One consequence of this activation process is the production by the cells of a matrix degrading enzyme (MDE), which enhances the attachment of the cells to fibronectin contained in the extracellular matrix. The endothelial cells are consequently able to exert the traction forces required to propel themselves during migration. This mechanism is included in the modelling by allowing individual tip cells to produce MDE locally, which then diffuses and degrades within the host tissue. With these modelling assumptions the full (non-dimensional) system of equations can be defined as

$$\frac{\partial c}{\partial t} = -\eta\, n_k\, c,$$

$$\frac{\partial f}{\partial t} = \beta\, n_k - \gamma\, m\, f, \tag{15.2}$$

$$\frac{\partial m}{\partial t} = \alpha\, n_k + \varepsilon \nabla^2 m - \nu\, m,$$

where c represents the TAF concentration, f the fibronectin concentration, m the MDE density, and n_k a Boolean value (1 or 0) that indicates the presence or absence of an endothelial cell at a given position. Details of other parameters together with a brief explanation of the hybrid modelling approach and algorithms for sprout branching and anastomosis are given in Appendix A.

The model for tumour-induced capillary growth described by the system of equations (15.1) and (15.2) was solved numerically on a 100×100 (x, y) square grid. The system of equations (15.2) was solved for each grid point at each time step and the resulting variables c and f were then used to calculate the coefficients P_0–P_4 (2D) appearing in the discretised form of equation (15.1). These coefficients were then used to calculate the migratory direction of each endothelial cell at the vessel tip at each time step of the simulation, i.e. the direction of growth of each sprout.

Fig. 15.1 presents some simulation results associated with an initial linear gradient of TAF. The top panels show the network growth and vascular architecture, whilst the bottom panels show the corresponding MDE concentrations in the extracellular matrix. Observe the stochastic nature of each of the five sprout trajectories as they progress towards the tumour (the surface of which occupies the lower boundary of the domain). Initially, the MDE concentrations are highly localised around the individual sprout tips and the migratory

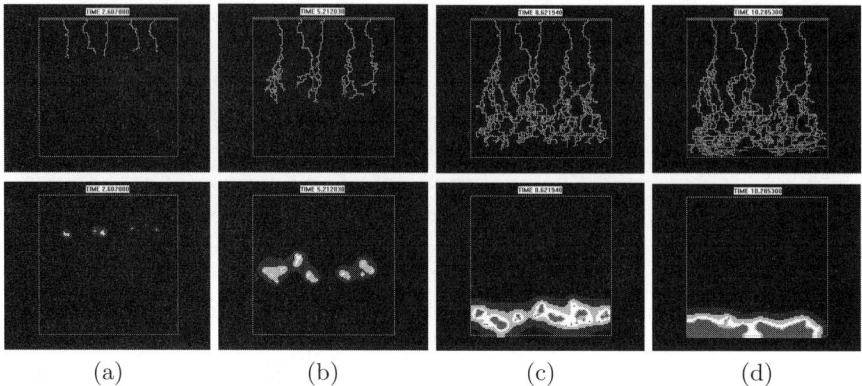

(a)   (b)   (c)   (d)

Fig. 15.1. Spatio-temporal evolution of a developing hollow capillary network and the corresponding MDE concentration in the extracellular matrix. The figure shows the migration of the endothelial cells at the vessel tips and the paths they follow as they migrate through the extracellular matrix in response to TAF gradients (chemotaxis) and FN gradients (haptotaxis). The paths of the tip cells define the subsequent vessel structure. Tip branching and vessel fusion (loop formation or anastomosis) are also included in the model. Pairs of results correspond to dimensionless times $\tilde{\tau} = 2.6, \tilde{\tau} = 5.2, \tilde{\tau} = 8.6$, and $\tilde{\tau} = 10.2$. In the MDE figures, grey corresponds to high MDE concentration and white corresponds to low MDE concentration. Black indicates absence of MDE.

path taken by each vessel is essentially independent of its neighbours. At time $\tilde{\tau} = 2.6$ (corresponding to $t = 3.9$ days), vessels 2 and 3 (numbered from left to right) begin to converge and by $\tilde{\tau} = 5.2$ (7.8 days) some degree of sprout branching and local anastomosis has already taken place for all five sprouts. Vessels 2 and 3 have now formed an anastomosis (loop)—hence perfusion could be expected to occur within the developing capillary bed at this time (as will be described later when discussing the full DATIA model). It takes approximately 10 days for the growth process to be completed, i.e. for the vasculature to connect the tumour to the parent vessel and hence to the blood supply.

The vascular architectures produced by the model at this stage are in good agreement with experimental data [20] [44], but the resulting vascular networks lack any variation in capillary radius (a vital factor when considering treatment efficacy). Moreover, vessel branching at this stage only depends upon the local TAF concentration and is unaffected by perfusion. The following sections present results that address these issues, together with an examination of the roles played by a number of important physical and biochemical parameters.

15.3.2 Capillary Migration Incorporating Flow

Having extended the migration model to account for the key biochemical interactions characterising the angiogenesis process, attention next turns to the incorporation of perfusion-related mechanisms. Previous approaches examining flow through tumour-induced networks [37] [71] had made the rather limiting assumptions of constant capillary radius and invariant blood viscosity, whereas, in reality, biological structures tend to exhibit some degree of compliance and blood is non-Newtonian. This earlier formulation must therefore be extended to account for variable blood viscosity and evolving capillary vessels that may either dilate or constrict both spatially and temporally. The details of how this has been achieved, including a discussion related to the different time scales associated with endothelial cell migration and capillary flow processes, are available in [38] and will only be briefly summarised here.

Blood Rheology
Because of its biphasic nature, blood does not behave as a continuum and the viscosity measured while flowing at different rates in microvessels is not constant. Moreover, direct measurement of blood viscosity in living microvessels is very difficult to achieve with any degree of accuracy. In [56] Pries et al. (1996) proposed an alternative approach, which involves "history matching" the flow distribution in a numerical network (generated by a mathematical model) with similar experimental systems. The relationship which was found to offer the best fit with experimental data from the rat mesentery at the microvascular scale is given by

$$\mu_{rel}(R, H_D) = \left[1 + (\mu_{0.45} - 1) f(H_D) \left(\frac{2R}{2R - 1.1} \right)^2 \right] \left(\frac{2R}{2R - 1.1} \right)^2 , \quad (15.3)$$

where $\mu_{0.45}$ is the viscosity corresponding to the normal average value of the discharge haematocrit ($H_D = 0.45$), R the vessel radius, and $f(H_D)$ a function of the haematocrit. The various terms appearing in (15.3) are defined as follows:

$$\mu_{0.45} = 6e^{-0.17R} + 3.2 - 2.44e^{-0.06(2R)^{0.645}},$$

$$f(H_D) = \frac{(1 - H_D)^C - 1}{(1 - 0.45)^C - 1} , \quad (15.4)$$

$$C = (0.8 + e^{-0.15R}) \left(-1 + \frac{1}{1 + 10^{-11}(2R)^{12}} \right) + \left(\frac{1}{1 + 10^{-11}(2R)^{12}} \right) .$$

The relative viscosity defined by equations (15.3) and (15.4) has been used in an extended form of Poiseuille's law at the scale of a single capillary. Of course, this is only one particular formulation of relative viscosity and any well-founded local flow/pressure-drop relationship could easily be incorporated into the model if alternatives emerge from future experimental studies. The methodology used to model perfusion within a developing network is described more fully in [37] and summarised in Appendix B.

Vessel Adaptation

Blood rheological properties and microvascular network remodelling are interrelated issues, as blood flow creates stresses on the vascular wall (shear stress, pressure, tensile stress) which lead to adaptation of the vascular diameters via either vasodilatation or constriction. In turn, blood rheology (viscosity, haematocrit, etc.) is affected by the new network architecture—consequently, adaptive angiogenesis should be expected to be a highly dynamic process. In this paper, vessel adaptation follows the treatment of [56] [57] [58] and considers a number of stimuli affecting vessel diameter that account for the influence of the wall shear stress (S_{wss}), the intravascular pressure (S_p), and a metabolic mechanism depending on the blood haematocrit (S_m). These stimuli form a basic set of requirements in order to obtain stable network structures with realistic distributions of vessels diameters and flow velocities. The equation used for radial variation as a function of these stimuli is as follows:

$$\Delta R = \left[\underbrace{\log\left(\tau_w + \tau_{ref}\right)}_{S_{wss}} - \underbrace{k_p \log \tau_e(P)}_{S_p} + \underbrace{k_m \log\left(\frac{Q_{ref}}{QH_D} + 1\right)}_{S_m} - k_s \right] R\Delta t.$$

(15.5)

The various terms used in (15.5) are described more fully in [38] and a brief summary is supplied in Appendix B, along with details of a modified branching algorithm that accounts for vessel branching in areas of heightened wall shear stress.

15.3.3 Extension of the Model to 3D

All of the models described thus far have been restricted to two dimensions and this is wholly acceptable when studying qualitative aspects of angiogenesis—moreover, results are far easier to visualise and interpret. However, as will be shown later, quantitative analysis requires the third dimension and so the fully adaptive model should be extended to address this shortcoming.

In theoretical terms this does not pose too much of a problem: the governing equations are simply expanded to include the third spatial variable and two additional endothelial cell movement weightings are retrieved from the 3D equivalent of (15.1) (see Equation (A2) in Appendix A). The main challenges lie in formulating the network flow equations efficiently in three dimensions, designing optimised 3D pressure solution algorithms, and dealing with increased computational demands. However, these challenges are ameliorated somewhat by choosing a regular structure for the underlying flow template (here, a regular cubic geometry), where many of the associated computational issues have already been addressed by a number of authors in the context of multiphase flow through porous media ([12] [41] *inter alia*). Interestingly, it has recently become feasible to simulate flow through irregular 3D network structures reconstructed from physical porous media (see, for example [49] [50]) and this may prove to be a useful starting point for the development of more advanced vascular flow models in the future.

For the 3D model described in this section, legacy code from a petrophysics-based multiphase flow simulator was incorporated into the existing angiogenesis model to deal with non-Newtonian flow and varying capillary radii in three dimensions. This model used an optimised 3D Cholesky conjugate gradient pressure solver and an adapted Haring–Greenkorn clustering algorithm to track changes in vascular topology.

15.3.4 Vascular Bed Comparisons

A comparison of the final vasculatures resulting from the different stages of the model development described above is shown in Fig. 15.2 (2D) and Fig. 15.3 (3D). Fig. 15.2(a) shows a 2D network resulting from the simple migration model, without any flow-related remodelling, whilst Fig. 15.2(b) demonstrates the effect of dynamic remodelling *after growth*. Although the overall architectures from the static and *a posteriori* remodelled approaches are similar, the dilated backbone apparent in the remodelled network will clearly play a dominant role in determining drug delivery to the tumour surface (as will be shown later). Hence, it seems reasonable to infer that the effect of capillary remodelling should be incorporated into angiogenesis models at this scale, if transport issues are to be addressed.

Of course, restricting the remodelling of a capillary bed until after migration is complete is rather artificial, as blood perfusion begins soon after the first capillary arcade has formed. In reality, bed remodelling and capillary dilation/constriction occur as immediate consequences of primary anastomosis and the network resulting from this approach is shown in Fig. 15.2(c). The effect of increased vessel branching in areas of high wall shear stress modifies the bed topology, leading to the formation of dilated arcades closer to the parent vessel accompanied by an overall increase in capillary density. The implications for therapeutic delivery of coupling capillary growth and radial adaptation will be discussed in Section 15.4.

In addition to radial adaptation, the dimensionality of the capillary network itself will also be shown to have a large impact upon treatment delivery. The architecture comparison shown in Fig. 15.3 suggests that drug bypassing could be even more of an issue in three dimensions, with the dilated backbone (Fig. 15.3(c)) branching into many alternative directions and forming a dense brush border as the tumour periphery is approached. It would be reasonable to anticipate that delivery using 2D models would overestimate delivery consid-

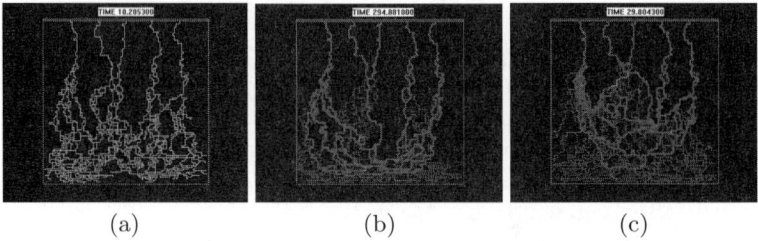

(a)   (b)   (c)

Fig. 15.2. 2D capillary networks formed as endothelial sprouts migrate from a parent vessel at the upper boundary of the domain through the extracellular matrix in response to gradients in TAF (chemotaxis) and FN (haptotaxis). Growth complete after approximately 16 days. (a) Simple migration model without flow-induced remodelling of the capillaries; (b) *a posteriori* remodelling after growth; (c) full DATIA model, including shear-stress-induced branching. Radii vary from 12 μm to 6 μm to 2 μm.

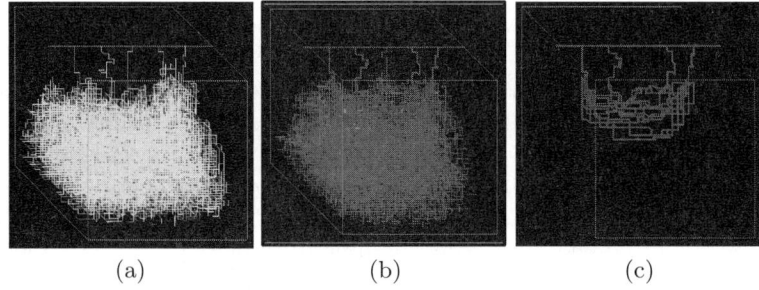

(a)   (b)   (c)

Fig. 15.3. 3D capillary networks formed as endothelial sprouts migrate from a parent vessel at the upper face of the domain through the extracellular matrix. (a) Simple migration model without flow-induced remodelling of the capillaries; (b) full DATIA model, including shear-stress-induced branching; (c) the dilated backbone isolated from (b). Radii vary from 12 μm to 6 μm to 2 μm.

erably and that 3D models should be used for quantitative comparisons with experiment. This issue will be addressed more thoroughly in Section 15.4.

15.3.5 Sensitivity of the DATIA Model to Biological Parameters

Examples of the changes seen in bed topology due to dynamic radial adaptation have been given in Figs. 15.2 and 15.3. The most important aspect of these examples was that they demonstrated how shear-induced branching could lead to earlier formation of dilated anastomoses close to the parent vessel. However, these examples form only a small subset of the possible architectures that can emerge from the angiogenesis model—by varying a number of physical and biochemical parameters, a wide range of network heterogeneity is predicted (Fig. 15.4). See the paper [38] by McDougall et al. (2006) for

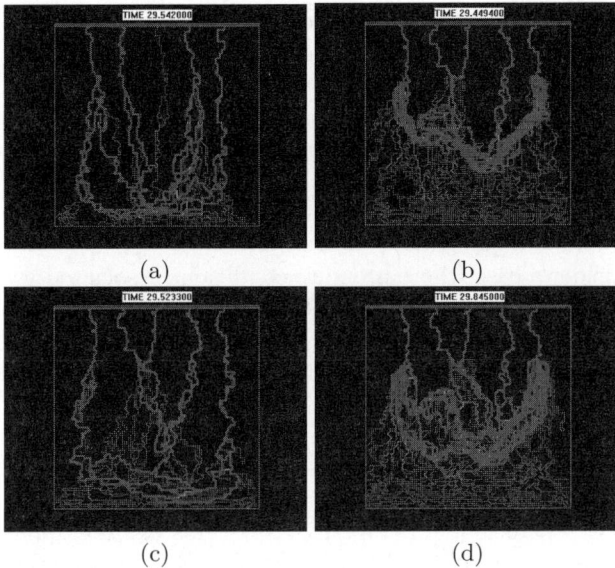

Fig. 15.4. Plots showing the different steady state capillary network structures which have evolved after 48 days due to changes in model parameters. (a) reduced haptotactic coefficient $\rho = 0.16$; (b) reduced input haematocrit $H_D = 0.225$; (c) reduced inlet blood pressure ($P_{in} = 2960$ Pa, $P_{out} = 2060$ Pa); (d) reduced outlet blood pressure ($P_{in} = 3260$ Pa, $P_{out} = 1760$ Pa). Compare with the base case in Fig. 15.1(c).

a fuller discussion and additional results. In order to highlight the importance of including perfusion-related phenomena into angiogenesis models, it may be instructive to analyse two of these sensitivities in a little more detail.

First, as has already been discussed, the migratory direction of any given endothelial cell from the parent vessel to the tumour surface is affected by a number of parameters that incorporate the effects of random, chemotactic, and haptotactic movement (cf. equation (15.1)). Fig. 15.4(a) shows the vasculature that develops when $\rho = 0.16$, i.e. when the strength of the haptotactic response has been reduced. In contrast to the base-case simulation shown in Fig. 15.2(c), where $\rho = 0.28$, the capillary vessels are seen to grow towards the tumour surface in a more directed fashion and lateral migration is reduced. This is not unexpected given the endothelial cell chemotactic response to TAF and is also in line with the results of [4] Anderson and Chaplain (1998). One major consequence of this more directed vessel growth, however, is the delay in the formation of anastomoses and subsequent perfusion from the parent vessel. This result not only highlights the important role played by cell-matrix interactions during angiogenesis, but also emphasises the way in which several apparently unconnected phenomena can interact throughout the process. Although the only direct coupling between perfusion and cell migration in the model is that related to shear-induced branching, the distribution of intravascular pressure and flow is actually affected by the local network architecture, which is, in turn, effectively controlled by the underlying cell biology (through chemotaxis and haptotaxis). Hence, not only does perfusion modify the network topology (through vessel branching), but the evolving topology itself affects the subsequent distribution of shear stresses and new branches—another link is established between perfusion, capillary remodelling, and the biological processes.

Next, consider a case where pressure conditions associated with the parent vessel are varied. Fig. 15.4(c) shows the resulting plexus structure when the inlet blood pressure was decreased by 300 Pa (2.25 mmHg) from the base case to 2960 Pa (22.25 mmHg), whilst the outlet pressure remained fixed at 2060 Pa (15.5 mmHg). In this case, all capillary flows are reduced due to the decrease in the global pressure drop, vessel branching diminishes, and the resulting dilated backbone is less dense than before. In fact, it is interesting to note that the final network architecture is close to that obtained by reducing the haptotactic coefficient (cf. Fig. 15.4(a)). This again emphasises the way in which perfusion can affect the interpretation of the underlying biological processes in an unexpected manner.

So far, this chapter has mainly focused on the variations observed in plexus architecture under different modelling assumptions. However, the resulting topology of a developing plexus is not simply interesting from an anatomical standpoint—the underlying spatial distributions of vessel connectivity and conductivity also play vital roles in determining the evolution of perfused treatments. By quantifying the efficiency of different networks in carrying blood-borne material to the tumour, it is hoped that some insights can be offered into the precise fate of chemotherapeutic agents in the vasculature during treatment and, moreover, that this could lead to the identification of a number of new therapeutic targets and strategies for tumour management (for example, drug-induced normalisation of tumour blood vessels).

15.4 Chemotherapy Delivery via Dynamically Adaptive Capillary Beds

Results presented in this section will show the impact of dynamic remodelling and shear-induced vessel branching upon chemotherapeutic treatment delivery—these highlight a number of new therapeutic targets for tumour management. The initial focus will be on 2D capillary beds, as results are far easier to visualise and interpret. However, quantitative analysis requires the third dimension and so some drug delivery comparisons from 3D simulations will be presented at the end of the section.

In order to assess transport efficacy within a given adapted vessel network, a drug at concentration C_{max} was continuously infused into the inlet of the parent vessel for 500 seconds. The base-case simulation for transport utilised the vasculature shown in Fig. 15.2(c). Fig. 15.5 shows the tracer-drug evolution through the capillary network at a number of different times (in sec-

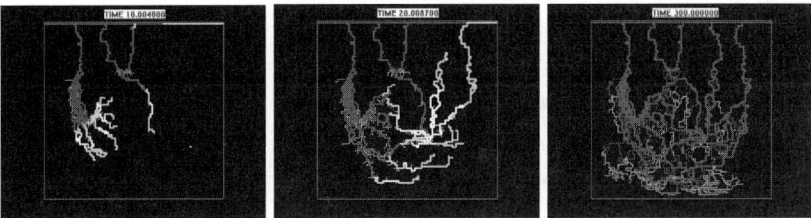

Fig. 15.5. Plots of the tracer-drug concentration distribution in the network shown in Fig. 15.2(c) at different times. Grey corresponds to high concentration and white to low concentration. Black indicates absence of tracer-drug.

onds). It is immediately clear that the bulk (in fact, almost all) of the injected tracer-drug flows through the highly conductive dilated backbone, largely by-passing the tumour and recirculating to the parent vessel. In excess of 250 s of continuous infusion is required before any tracer-drug reaches the tumour surface, and only then in very small concentrations. Fig. 15.6 shows plots of the total drug mass in the system (parent vessel and capillary network) and

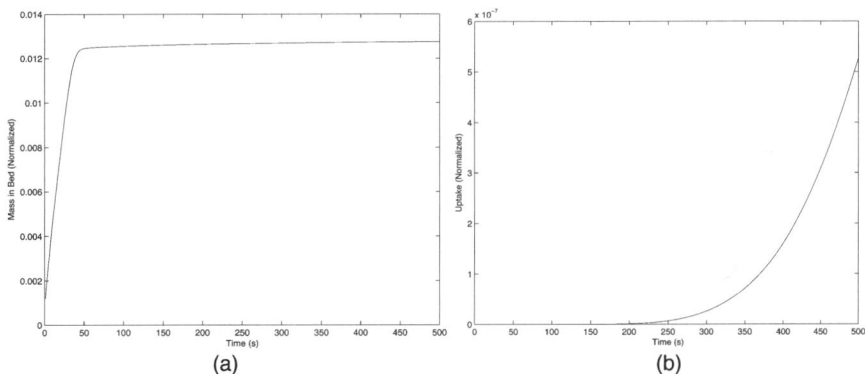

Fig. 15.6. Plots of (a) normalised total drug mass in parent vessel and network over time and (b) normalised delivery reaching the tumour.

delivery to the tumour surface as functions of time. It should be noted that all masses have been normalised to the total mass injected into the parent vessel over the course of the simulation. Only around 1.5% of the infused tracer-drug even enters the capillary network and, although the total mass in the network reaches a plateau after approximately 50 s (transport being essentially governed by steady state flow through the dilated backbone), it takes another 200–250 s before uptake commences. This is because capillaries form-ing part of the brush border close to the tumour surface are narrow and poorly perfused—consequently, only a very small fraction of the injected treatment actually reaches the target. As an aside, it should be noted that, although convective transport through the vessels of the network would be a rather poor delivery mechanism for large molecules (i.e. cytotoxic treatments), the dilated network is sufficiently well developed within a few hundred microme-ters of the tumour surface that diffusion of nutrients (oxygen, glucose) would be relatively efficient over the time scale of tumour growth.

Fig. 15.7(a) shows the uptake using an identical network architecture but with all capillary radii set permanently to 6 μm (the default value given at vessel birth in the model)—uptake values are approximately three orders of magnitude larger than those obtained from the remodelled vasculature. These results clearly demonstrate the impact of network heterogeneity upon treatment efficacy and highlight the need for incorporating vessel adaptations (dilation/constriction) into any angiogenesis model involving transport issues, such as chemotherapeutic intervention. In the absence of vessel size variation, delivery is greatly overestimated.

A possible therapeutic target identified from simulation is the manipu-lation of the haptotactic response of the migrating endothelial cells during angiogenesis, characterised by reduced lateral migration of the vessels and reduced shear-induced branching (Fig. 15.4(a)). The tracer-drug evolution through this vessel network suggests that tumours supplied by this type of vasculature would be well supplied with nutrients and could be expected to grow rapidly. Paradoxically, however, such tumours would also be highly sus-ceptible to infused treatments, with far more cytotoxic agent reaching the tumour than observed in previous cases. This conjecture is supported by the uptake results from the infusion simulation shown in Fig. 15.7(b). Whilst the total mass of tracer-drug entering the supplying vasculature is almost iden-tical to that observed in the base case simulation $\rho = 0.28$, not shown), the drug uptake by the tumour *is fifty times greater* when lateral migration and vessel branching are reduced.

The network shown in Fig. 15.4(b) suggests that a depressed haematocrit can be expected to lead to the formation of highly dilated arcades close to the parent vessel and Fig. 15.7(c) shows the therapeutic implications of this phenomenon—more drug enters the capillary network than entered in the base-case simulation but drug delivery to the tumour *is reduced by more than three orders of magnitude*. In the context of nutrient supply to the tumour, it is proposed here that decreasing local haematocrit could be a possible mech-anism for generating vasculatures that are detrimental to tumour growth.

Fig. 15.7(d) shows the impact upon drug delivery of lowering the pressure at the inlet of the parent vessel by 300 Pa (2.25 mm Hg) prior to angiogen-esis, whilst keeping the outlet pressure unchanged. Delivery is dramatically increased *by more than three orders of magnitude* and tumours characterised by similar vascular architectures are consequently highly likely to be vulner-

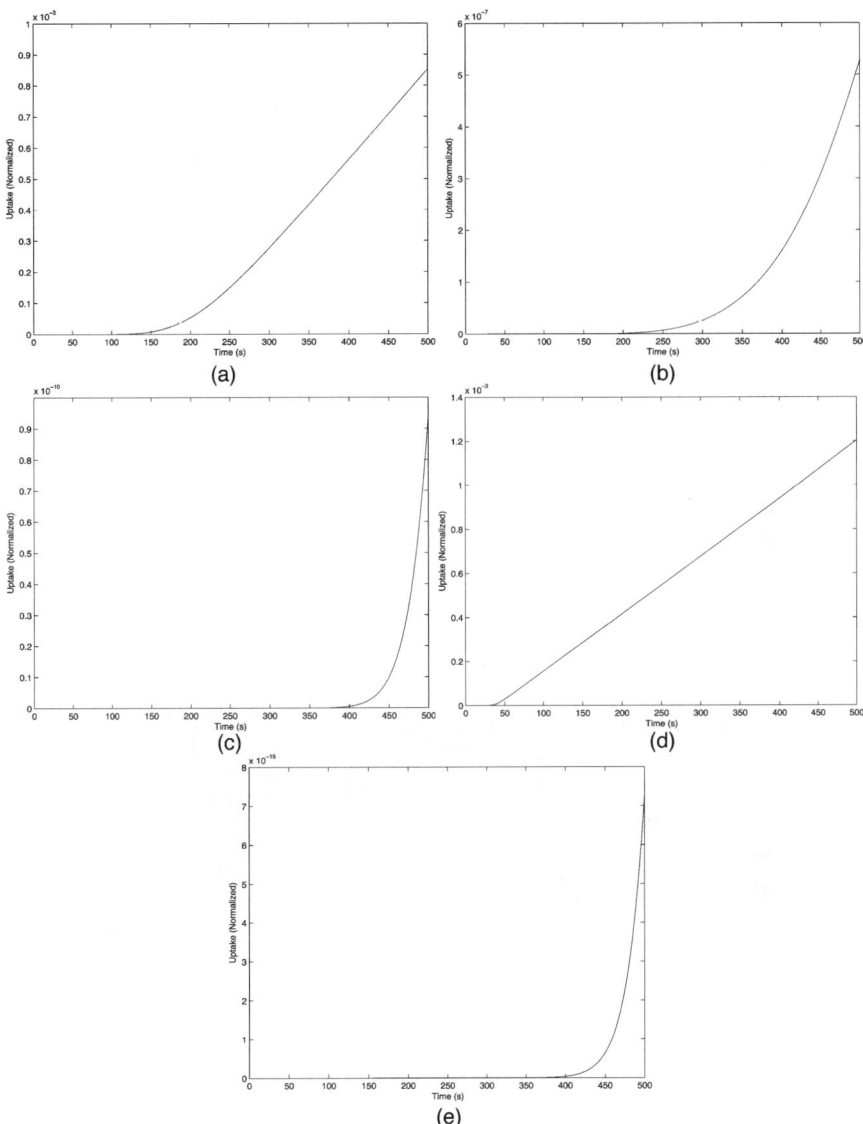

Fig. 15.7. Plot showing the amount of drug reaching the tumour over time under various model assumptions. (a) a network where all vessels have a fixed radius of 6 μm. Note the difference in scale compared to that of Fig. 15.6b, (b) the effect of varying haptotactic sensitivity (magenta line (top) corresponds to $\rho = 0.16$, red line (bottom) corresponds to $\rho = 0.28$), (c) the effect of reduced input haematocrit $H_D = 0.225$, (d) lower pressure at inlet of parent vessel, (e) lower pressure at outlet of parent vessel.

able to chemotherapeutic infusions. Finally, Fig. 15.7(e) shows the uptake
by the tumour supplied by the network in Fig. 15.8(d), where the pressure
gradient across the parent vessel was increased by 300 Pa (2.25 mm Hg)
prior to angiogenesis. Uptake is extremely poor, which is not too surprising
given the presence of highly dilated loops close to the parent vessel. Hence,
intravenous/intra-arterial treatments would be expected to prove ineffective
in this case.

Having examined the role played by vessel adaptation on drug delivery
qualitatively in two dimensions, attention next turns towards quantitative
simulations in three dimensions. Snapshots of the drug evolution through the
3D adaptive bed are shown in Fig. 15.8 and once again demonstrate the dominant role played by the dilated backbone in determining drug bypassing. As
expected, bypassing begins earlier in the adaptive network, with the backbone
effectively at maximum concentration after approximately 100 seconds. Drug
deliveries between 3D-adaptive and 3D-non-adaptive networks and between
2D- and 3D-adaptive networks are correspondingly reduced i.e. the increased
dimensionality and vessel adaptation each reduce delivery by over an order of
magnitude. The importance of the third dimension and the inclusion of adaptive architecture in providing quantitative predictions for comparison with *in
vivo* results is clear.

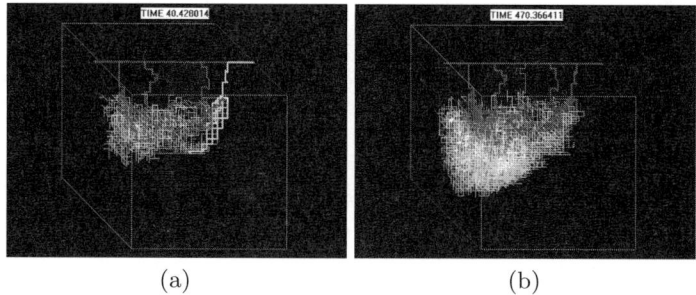

(a)   (b)

Fig. 15.8. Concentration contours for continuous infusion into an adaptive 3D vasculature formed from a linear TAF source. $30 \times 30 \times 30$ domain size. (a) $t = 50$ s,
(b) $t = 500$ s. Grey corresponds to high concentration and white to low concentration. Black indicates abscence of tracer-drug.

15.5 Discussion and Conclusions

This chapter has summarised recent progress towards the development of angiogenesis models that are capable of coupling capillary migration with concomitant blood flow. Although very few hybrid mathematical models currently
exist that deal with such a coupling in the context of solid tumour growth,

a great deal of research *has* been undertaken on related topics over the past decade. In light of this, a number of earlier studies that have addressed issues such as vascular tumour growth at the continuum scale, perfusion-free capillary migration at the discrete level, and adaptation in interconnected microvascular structures have been briefly reviewed. Whilst there have been many modelling studies reported in the literature dealing with the process of angiogenesis itself—i.e. the way in which the new capillary bed is initiated and migrates—there have been relatively few studies examining the important role played by blood perfusion during migration and fewer still examining the delivery of chemotherapeutic compounds through aberrant tumour vasculature. In response to the paucity of transport models in this area, a new 3D framework has been described within which a wide range of therapeutic interventions can be studied. In contrast to previous capillary network flow models reported in the literature ([56] [37] [2] [71] [26] [72]), where the effects of perfusion were evaluated *a posteriori* post-angiogenesis through hollow networks, blood flow in the model described here has been coupled directly to migration. Consequently, the major role played by perfusion during capillary growth has been evaluated, with radial adaptations and vessel remodelling occurring as immediate consequences of primary loop formations (anastomoses). This was achieved by flowing the developing network at regular intervals during the growth process until a steady state vessel structure had been realised. This explicit coupling led to network architectures that differed radically from those found in all previous models.

Simulations using the adaptive model under different parameter regimes highlighted a number of new therapeutic targets for tumour management. For example, reduction of the haptotactic response of the migrating endothelial cells during angiogenesis was shown to reduce lateral migration of the vessels and reduce shear-induced branching. Subsequent evolution of blood perfusion through this network suggested that tumours supplied by this type of vasculature would be well supplied with nutrients and could be expected to grow rapidly. However, such tumours would also be highly susceptible to infused treatments, with cytotoxic agents reaching the tumour surface in higher concentrations than in the base-case simulation. A second set of simulations suggested that a depressed haematocrit could be expected to lead to the formation of highly dilated arcades close to the parent vessel. Although this had the positive effect of causing more drug to enter the capillary network than entered in the base-case simulation, delivery to the tumour was reduced by more than three orders of magnitude. This is a rather negative result in the context of infused treatment, but it also suggests that decreasing local haematocrit could be a possible mechanism for generating vasculatures that are detrimental to further tumour growth.

More generally, it is apparent from the transport simulations presented here that highly dilated loops proximal to the parent vessel remove any possibility of effective treatment via intravenous or intra-arterial infusion. However, if a tumour-induced capillary network could be forced to develop in just such a way, by means of some clinical intervention perhaps, then nutrient supply to the tumour could be effectively curtailed. The DATIA model provides a solid biomechanical framework within which to examine, in some detail, the possibility of normalising tumour blood vessels as a means of effectively treating solid tumours (cf. [65] [33]). Both 2D and 3D simulation results have been presented in this chapter and it has been shown that extending the model to three dimensions reduces chemotherapy delivery to a tumour periphery by an order of magnitude. These results clearly demonstrated that, although 2D studies are valuable in a qualitative sense, 3D angiogenesis modelling appears to be a necessary prerequisite for quantitative prediction for comparison with *in vivo* results. Of course, many more sensitivities could be examined using the framework described here, but one of the main aims has been to demonstrate the need for additional experimental observations to clarify a number of outstanding issues. For example, the key mechanisms governing drug uptake require additional research, as do the metabolic stimuli affecting blood vessel dynamics. It should also be noted that the model described here only addresses transport to the tumour periphery. The fate of nutrients and cytotoxic compounds if they enter the tumour mass can only be properly examined by coupling the present model to one that describes the growth of the tumour itself.

Armed with adjuvant experimental data, it should be possible to refine the model still further; perhaps by including discrete pericyte migration to address the issue of network stability, or by adding a low pressure venous system to examine the implications of arterio-venous coupling. By making regular comparisons between results emerging from an improved mathematical framework and corresponding laboratory experiments, it is hoped that the potential of a range of different chemotherapeutic, anti-angiogenic, and anti-vascular agents can be optimised in the future.

Appendix A: Capillary Growth Details

In the earlier model of Anderson and Chaplain [4], endothelial cell densities and their global influence on TAF and FN concentrations were considered in a continuous formulation. Here, the focus is on local effects and so the influence of each individual cell on its local environment is considered. In order to achieve this, the displacement of each individual endothelial cell, located at the tips of growing sprouts, is given by the discretised form of the endothelial cell mass conservation equation (15.1).

The chemotactic migration is characterised by the function $\chi(c) = \chi/(1+\delta c)$, which reflects the decrease in chemotactic sensitivity with increased TAF concentration. The coefficients D, χ, and ρ characterise the random, chemotactic, and haptotactic cell migration respectively (full details of the nondimensionalisation can be found in [4]). The migration of each cell in 2D is consequently determined by a set of normalized coefficients emerging from this equation (Fig. A.1), which relate to the likelihood of the cell remaining stationary (P_0), or moving left (P_1), right (P_2), up (P_3) or down (P_4) :

$$n_{l,m}^{q+1} = n_{l,m}^{q} P_0 + n_{l+1,m}^{q} P_1 + n_{l-1,m}^{q} P_2 + n_{l,m+1}^{q} P_3 + n_{l,m-1}^{q} P_4 \qquad (A.1)$$

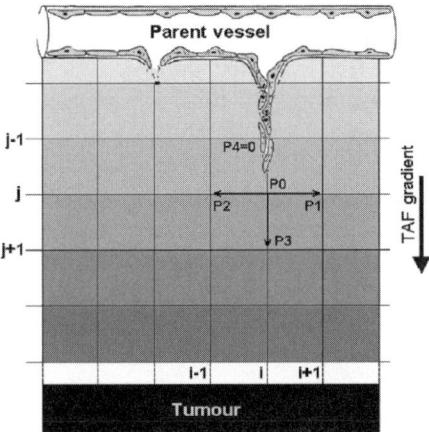

Fig. A.1. Schematic diagram of a section of the 2D grid used in the numerical computation procedure illustrating how the process of the migration of tip endothelial cells, and hence capillary sprout growth, is taken into account in the simulations. At each node, the sprout tip can grow in 3 possible directions in 2D (and 5 possible directions in 3D).

where l and m are positive parameters which specify the position of the endothelial cell on the 2D spatial grid i.e. $x = l\Delta x$ and $y = l\Delta y$ and time discretisation is represented by $t = q\Delta t$. These coefficients P_0–P_4 incorporate the effects of random, chemotactic, and haptotactic movement and depend upon the local chemical environment (FN and TAF concentrations). In 3D, the discretised endothelial equation has the form

$$\begin{aligned} n_{l,m,w}^{q+1} &= n_{l,m,w}^{q} P_0 + n_{l+1,m,w}^{q} P_1 + n_{l-1,m,w}^{q} P_2 + n_{l,m+1,w}^{q} P_3 \\ &+ n_{l,m-1,w}^{q} P_4 + n_{l,m,w+1}^{q} P_5 + n_{l,m,w-1}^{q} P_6 \end{aligned} \qquad (A.2)$$

with additional movement coefficients: in (P_5) or out (P_6). The model is then given by the following set of equations:

$$\frac{\partial n}{\partial t} = \overbrace{D\nabla^2 n}^{random} - \overbrace{\nabla \cdot (\chi(c)n\nabla c)}^{chemotaxis} - \overbrace{\rho \nabla \cdot (n\nabla f)}^{haptotaxis}, \qquad (A.3)$$

$$\frac{\partial c}{\partial t} = -\eta\, n_k\, c,$$

$$\frac{\partial f}{\partial t} = \beta\, n_k - \gamma\, m\, f, \tag{A.4}$$

$$\frac{\partial m}{\partial t} = \alpha\, n_k + \varepsilon \nabla^2 m - \nu\, m,$$

where c represents the TAF concentration, f the FN concentration, m the matrix degrading enzyme (MDE) density, and n_k a Boolean value (1 or 0) that indicates the presence or absence of an endothelial cell at a given position. The parameters β and α characterise the production rate by an individual endothelial cell of FN and MDE respectively and η its TAF consumption rate. The major difference with the earlier model is that degradation of fibronectin f, characterised by the coefficient γ, no longer depends directly on the endothelial cell density n. This now depends upon the MDE density m produced by each individual endothelial cell n_k at rate α. The MDF once produced, diffuses locally with diffusion coefficient ε, and is spontaneously degraded at a rate ν.

Tip and Vessel Branching Probabilities

In earlier work ([4] [37] [71] [72]), branching at the capillary *tips* was assumed to depend only upon the local TAF concentration. This formulation has been used again here and the corresponding tip branching probabilities are shown in Table A.1. In addition to tip branching, however, the physiologically significant process of *vessel* branching is also modelled as part of the current study. In order to implement this effect in the model, we assume that branching along a vessel (i.e. the generation of a new vessel which branches out at some point along an existing vessel wall as distinct from the vessel tip) depends both on the TAF concentration and on the wall shear stress (WSS). Table A.2 shows the dependence of *vessel* branching probability as a function of the combined effects of local wall shear stress and local TAF concentration.

Table A.1. Sprout tip branching probabilities as a function of the local TAF concentration.

TAF Concentration	Sprout Tip Branching Probability
$\leq\ 0.3$	0.0
$]\,0.3 - 0.5\,]$	0.2
$]\,0.5 - 0.7\,]$	0.3
$]\,0.7 - 0.8\,]$	0.4
$>\ 0.8$	1.0

Table A.2. *Vessel* branching probabilities as functions of the local TAF concentration and the magnitude of the local wall shear stress. TAF_{max} is the maximum TAF concentration at $t = 0$ and $\tau_{max} = 2Pa$ (20 dynes/cm^2), the maximum shear stress derived from preliminary flow simulations.

WSS/τ_{max}

	[0, 0.2)	[0.2, 0.4)	[0.4, 0.6)	[0.6, 0.8)	[0.8, 1.0)
[0.0, 0.3)	0.00	0.00	0.00	0.00	0.00
[0.3, 0.5)	0.00	0.02	0.04	0.06	0.08
[TAF]/TAF$_{max}$ [0.5, 0.7)	0.00	0.03	0.06	0.09	0.12
[0.7, 0.8)	0.00	0.04	0.08	0.12	0.16
[0.8, 1.0)	0.00	0.10	0.20	0.30	0.40

One additional constraint on vessel branching is the age of the vessel itself. The time interval within which a vessel can branch has been fixed at [4–8] days in the simulations (i.e. from $\tilde{\tau} = 2.66$ to $\tilde{\tau} = 5.33$). In this interval, the vessel is sufficiently mature for branching to occur yet young enough to ensure that no basal lamina has had time to form (which would contribute considerably to the stabilization of the network [9] [43]).

Initial Conditions

The domain considered for the computational simulation studies is a square of length $L = 2$ mm (2D) or a cube of edge length 0.6 mm (3D) and the parent vessel from which the vascular network grows is located at the upper edge/face of the domain. The tumour surface is located along the lower domain boundary. We assume that the capillary sprouts, TAF, and MDE remain confined within the domain and so no-flux boundary conditions are imposed on the boundaries. Initial TAF and fibronectin profiles are the same as those used in [37], there is initially no MDE present and vascular growth is initialised by distributing five sprouts at regular intervals along the parent vessel.

Cell Migration Parameters

Unless otherwise indicated, the dimensionless parameter values used for the simulations presented in this paper were as follows ([4] [37] [71] [72]):

$$D = 0.00035, \delta = 0.6, \chi = 0.38, \rho = 0.16,$$

$$\eta = 0.1, \beta = 0.05, \gamma = 0.1, \alpha = 10e - 6, \varepsilon = 0.01, \nu = 3.$$

Capillary migration time was scaled as $\tilde{t} = \frac{t}{\tau}$: with $\tau = L^2/D_c$, where $L = 2$ mm (2D) or 0.6 mm (3D) was the length of the domain and $D_c =$

2.9×10^{-7} cm^{2}s^{-1} was taken as the diffusion coefficient for TAF [8]. We note that the time scale associated with the capillary growth process is of the order several days, whereas flow through the parent vessel and capillary network occurs over a time scale of a few seconds to a few minutes. A discussion of how the two time scales are coupled in the full adaptive model is given in [38].

Appendix B: Adaptive Flow Modelling Details

General Model

In its most general form, the flow model developed here consists of a 3D cubic network of *bond elements*. These bonds can be thought of as straight cylindrical capillary elements, although the constraint of cylindrical geometry can easily be relaxed. Now, for a single capillary element i of radius R_i and length L_i, the elemental fluid flow rate in the capillary is given by Poiseuille's law:

$$Q_i = \frac{\pi R_i^4 \Delta P_i}{8\mu L_i},$$

$$(B.1)$$

where μ is the fluid viscosity and ΔP_i the pressure drop across the element. At each node (junction), six elements meet (in 3D) and (assuming incompressible flow) mass conservation means that the sum of all six flows must add up to zero, i.e.

$$\sum_{i=1}^{i=6} Q_i = 0.$$

$$(B.2)$$

Consideration of the whole network then leads to a set of linear pressure equations, the solutions to which (using e.g. successive over-relaxation (SOR), Cholesky conjugate gradient method, Lanczos method) can then be used to calculate elemental flows.

Blood Rheology

When dealing with a non-Newtonian fluid, such as blood, the flow-pressure drop relationship can be approximated by the following Poiseuille-like expression:

$$Q = \frac{\pi R^4 \Delta P}{8\mu_{app}(R, H_D)L},$$

$$(B.3)$$

where $\mu_{app}(R, H_D) = \mu_{rel} \times \mu_{plasma}$ is the apparent blood viscosity, which depends upon the local blood haematocrit, the radius of the vessel through which the blood is flowing, and the underlying plasma viscosity, μ_{plasma}. (See Equations (15.3) and (15.4) in the main text.)

Vessel Adaptation

In this chapter, vessel adaptation follows the treatment of Pries et al. [56] [57] [58]. The model considers a number of stimuli affecting vessel diameter that account for the influence of the wall shear stress (S_{wss}), the intravascular pressure (S_p), and a metabolic mechanism depending on the blood haematocrit (S_m). These stimuli form a basic set of requirements in order to obtain stable network structures with realistic distributions of vessel diameters and flow velocities. A brief description of each now follows.

(i) Wall shear stress. Many studies show that vessels adapt their radius in order to maintain a constant level of wall shear stress ([57] [58] [59] [18]). Hence vessel radius tends to increase with increasing wall shear stress, whilst wall shear stress decreases with increasing radius. The wall shear stress stimulus can be described by a logarithmic law as

$$S_{wss} = \log\left(\tau_w + \tau_{ref}\right),$$

(B.4)

where τ_w is the actual wall shear stress in a vessel segment calculated from

$$\tau_w = \frac{4\mu(R, H_D)}{\pi R^3} |Q|$$

(B.5)

and τ_{ref} is a constant included to avoid singular behaviour at low shear rates [58] (Pries 2001a). Stresses in (B.4) and (B.5) are in dynes/cm². The wall shear stress calculated in the parent vessel of our computational model is of the order 4 Pa (40 dynes/cm²) and capillary values are less than 2 Pa (20 dynes/cm²), in agreement with those measured experimentally in the dog by [30]. Adaptation in response to the wall shear stress stimulus alone tends to reinforce a single path in the network composed of a few well-established fully dilated vessels—corresponding to the main flowing "backbone" of the vasculature—whilst simultaneously eliminating the low-flow paths. However, the resulting network is "unstable" in the sense that there is no consistent balance for the radius and flow distribution achieved when S_{wss} is considered in isolation.

(ii) Intravascular pressure. Intravascular pressure is another key stimulus for vascular adaptation. Pries et al. [56] have experimentally observed on the rat mesentery the dependence of the magnitude of the wall shear stress with the local intravascular pressure (P). They proposed a parametric description of their experimental data, which exhibits a sigmoidal increase of the wall shear stress with increasing pressure through the following:

$$\tau_e(P) = 100 - 86 \cdot \exp\left\{-5000 \cdot [\log\left(\log P\right)]^{5.4}\right\}.$$

(B.6)

Pressure is measured in millimeters of mercury (1 mm Hg = 133 Pa) and stresses are again given in dynes/cm^2. The sensitivity of the corresponding stimulus to intravascular pressure is then described by

$$S_p = -k_P \log \tau_e(P),$$

(B.7)

where k_P is a constant that dictates the relative intensity of the stimulus.

(iii) Metabolic haematocrit-related stimulus. the adapting network by stimulating vessel growth in areas of the vascular bed exhibiting low flow. The stimulus is once again described by a logarithmic law and takes the form

$$S_m = k_m \log \left(\frac{Q_{ref}}{QH_D} + 1 \right),$$

(B.8)

where Q_{ref} is a reference flow. In our simulations, Q_{ref} corresponds to the flow in the parent vessel. H_D represents the discharge haematocrit in the vessels, Q the flow in the vessel under consideration, and k_m is a constant characterising the relative intensity of the metabolic stimulus.

Our theoretical model for vessel adaptation assumes that the change in a flowing vessel radius (ΔR) over a time step Δt is proportional to both the global stimulus acting on the vessel and to the initial vessel radius R, i.e.

$$\Delta R = S_{tot} R \Delta t = (S_{wss} + S_p + S_m) R \Delta t,$$

(B.9)

which leads to Equation (15.5) in the main text. Note that the additional term k_s represents the shrinking tendency of a vessel. This term is interpreted by Pries et al. [57] as reflecting a natural reaction of the basal lamina, which acts to counter any increase in vessel diameter.

Flow Model Parameters

(i) Vessel properties. For the *a posteriori* remodelling simulations presented, the initial radius of each capillary segment was taken to be 6 μm and remodelling of the vessels was permitted within a range, from a minimum radius of 2 μm (essentially eliminating flow) to a maximum radius of 12 μm. During the DATIA simulations, nascent, non-flowing capillaries (i.e. those not yet part of the connected flowing network) were assigned 6μm radii and remodelling was again considered in the range (2, 12) μm. In all simulations, the radius of the parent vessel was kept fixed at 14 μm. These values correspond to vessel radii at the capillary level, where the size of the vessels is very close to the size of the red blood cells [13].

(ii) Adaptation parameters. The parameters used for the base case adaptation model presented in Equation (15.5) were taken to be

$k_s = 0.35$, $k_p = 0.1$, $k_m = 0.07$, $\tau_{ref} = 0.103$, $Q_{ref} = 1.909\mathrm{e}\text{-}11$

(after [71] [72]), where Q_{ref} corresponds to the flow in the parent vessel, calculated from Equation (B.3) with $R = 14$ μm, $L = 2$ mm and $\Delta P = 1200$ Pa (9 mm Hg) (the pressure drop across the parent vessel). The plasma viscosity μ_{plasma} is 1.2×10^{-3}Pa s and this parameterisation gives perfusion velocities in the parent vessel of approximately 3 mm s^{-1}. One of the main determinants of the extent of vascular remodelling is the intravascular pressure (P). In the simulations carried out here, we have chosen inlet and outlet pressures to ensure average intravascular pressures of approximately 20 mm Hg, in accordance with physiological values at the capillary scale.

References

1. Adam, J.A. (1986) A simplified mathematical model of tumour growth. *Math. Biosc.* **81**, 229–244.
2. Alarcon, T., H. Byrne, and P. Maini (2003) A cellular automaton model for tumour growth in inhomogeneous environment. *J. Theor. Biol.* **225**(15.2), 257–274.
3. Anderson, A.R.A., B.D.S. Sleeman, I.M. Young, and B.S. Griffiths (1997) Nematode movement along a chemical gradient in a structurally heterogeneous environment: II Theory. *Fundam. Appl. Nematol.* **20**, 165–172.
4. Anderson, A.R.A., and M.A.J. Chaplain (1998) Continuous and discrete mathematical models of tumor-induced angiogenesis. *Bull. Math. Biol.* **60**, 857–899.
5. Ausprunk, D.H., and J. Folkman (1977) Migration and proliferation of endothelial cells in preformed and newly formed blood vessels during tumour angiogenesis. *Microvasc. Res.* **14**, 53–65.
6. Baish, J.W., Y. Gazit, D.A. Berk, M. Nozue, L.T. Baxter, and R.K. Jain (1996) Role of tumor vascular architecture in nutrient and drug delivery: an invasion percolation-based network model. *Microvasc. Res.* **51**, 327–346.
7. Baish, J.W., P.A. Netti, and R.K. Jain (1997) Transmural coupling of fluid flow in microcirculatory network and interstitium in tumours. *Microvasc. Res.* **53**, 128–141.
8. Bray, D. (1992) *Cell Movements*, Garland Publishing, New York.
9. Benjamin, L.E., I. Hemo, and E. Keshet (1998) A plasticity window for blood vessel remodelling is defined by pericyte coverage of the preformed endothelial network and is regulated by PDGF-B and VEGF. *Development* **125**, 1591–1598.
10. Breward, C.J.W., H.M. Byrne, and C.E. Lewis (2003) A multiphase model describing vascular tumour growth. *Bull. Math. Biol.* **65**, 609–640.
11. Chaplain, M.A.J., and G. Lolas (2005) Mathematical modelling of cancer cell invasion of tissue: the role of the urokinase plasminogen activation system. *Math. Modell. Methods. Appl. Sci.* **15**, 1685–1734.
12. Chatzis, I., and F.A.L. Dullien (1977) Modelling pore structure by 2D and 3D networks with application to sandstone. *J. Can. Pet. Technol.* **16**, 97.
13. Ciofalo, M., M.W. Collins, and T.R. Hennessy (1999) Microhydrodynamics phenomena in the circulation, in Nanoscale Fluid Dynamics in Physiological Processes, A Review Study. WIT Press, Southampton, UK, 219–236.

14. Davis, G.E., K.A. Pintar Allen, R. Salazar, and S.A. Maxwell (2000) Matrix metalloproteinase-1 and –9 activation by plasmin regulates a novel endothelial cell-mediated mechanism of collagen gel contraction and capillary tube regression in three-dimensional collagen matrices. *J. Cell Sci.* **114**, 917–930.

15. El-Kareh, A.W., and T.W. Secomb (1997) Theoretical models for drug delivery to solid tumours. *Crit. Rev. Biomed. Eng.* **25**(6), 503–571.

16. Folkman, J., and M. Klagsbrun (1987) Angiogenic factors. *Science* **235**, 442–447.

17. Franks, S.J., H.M. Byrne, J.R. King, J.C.E. Underwood, and C.E. Lewis (2005) Biological inferences from a mathematical model of comedo ductal carcinoma in situ of the breast. *J. Theor. Biol.* **232**(15.4), 523–543.

18. Fung, Y.C. (1993) *Biomechanics.* Springer-Verlag, New York.

19. Gatenby, R.A., and E.T. Gawlinski (2003) The glycolytic phenotype in carcinogenesis and tumour invasion. Insights through mathematical modelling. *Cancer Res.* **63**, 3847–3854.

20. Gimbrone, M.A., R.S. Cotran, S.B. Leapman, and J. Folkman (1974) Tumor growth and neovascularization: an experimental model using the rabbit cornea. *J. Natl. Cancer Inst.* **52**, 413–427.

21. Glass, L. (1973) Instability and mitotic patterns in tissue growth. *J. Dyn. Syst. Meas. Control.* **95**, 324–327.

22. Gödde, R., and H. Kurz (2001) Structural and biophysical simulation of angiogenesis and vascular remodeling, *Developmental Dynamics* **220**, 387–401.

23. Gottlieb, M.E. (1990) Modelling blood vessels: a deterministic method with fractal structure based on physiological rules. *Proc 12th Int Conf of IEEE EMBS*, 1386–1387, IEEE Press, New York.

24. Greenspan, H.P. (1972) Models for the growth of a solid tumour by diffusion. *Stud. Appl. Math.* **52**, 317–340.

25. Greenspan, H.P. (1976). On the growth and stability of cell cultures and solid tumours. *J. Theor. Biol.* **56**, 229–242.

26. Gruionu, G., J.B. Hoyling, A.R. Pries, and T.W. Secomb (2005) Structural remodelling of mouse gracilis artery after chronic alteration in blood supply. *Am. J. Physiol. Heart. Circ. Physiol.* **288**, 2047–2054.

27. Hidalgo, M., and S.G. Eckkhardt (2001) Development of matrix metalloproteinase inhibitors in cancer therapy. *J. Natl. Cancer Inst.* **93**, 178–193.

28. Honda, H., and K. Yoshizato (1997) Formation of the branching pattern of blood vessels in the wall of the avian yolk sac studied by a computer simulation. *Develop. Growth Differ.* **39**, 581–589.

29. Jackson, T.L. (2002) Vascular tumour growth and treatment: consequences of polyclonality, competition and dynamic vascular support. *J. Math. Biol.* **44**, 201–226.

30. Kamiya, A., R. Bukhari, and T. Togawa (1984) Adaptive regulation of wall shear stress optimizing vascular tree function. *Bull. Math. Biol.* **46**, 127–137.

31. Krenz, G.S., and C.A. Dawson (2002) Vessel distensibility and flow distribution in vascular trees. *J. Math. Biol.* **44**, 360–374.

32. Lankelma, J., R.F. Luque, H. Dekker, W. Shinkel, and H.M. Pinedao (2000) A mathematical model of drug transport in human breast cancer. *Microvasc. Res.* **59**, 149–161.

33. Le Serve, A.W., and K. Hellmann (1972) Metastases and normalization of tumor blood-vessels by icrf 159—new type of drug action. *Br. Med. J.* **1**, 597–601.

34. Levine, H.A., S. Pamuk, B.D. Sleeman, and M. Nielsen-Hamilton (2001) Mathematical modeling of the capillary formation and development in tumor angiogenesis: penetration into the stroma, *Bull. Math. Biol.* **63**(15.5), 801–863.

35. Lolas, G. (2003) Mathematical modelling of the urokinase plasminogen activator system and its role in cancer invasion of tissue. PhD Thesis, University of Dundee.

36. McDougall, S.R., and K. Sorbie (1997) The application of network modelling techniques to multiphase flow in porous media. *Petroleum Geosci.* **3**, 161–169.

37. McDougall, S.R., A.R.A. Anderson, M.A.J. Chaplain, and J.A. Sherratt (2002) Mathematical modelling of flow through vascular networks: implications for tumour-induced angiogenesis and chemotherapy strategies. *Bull. Math. Biol.* **64**(15.4), 673–702.

38. McDougall, S.R., A.R.A. Anderson, and M.A.J. Chaplain (2006) Mathematical modelling of dynamic adaptive tumour-induced angiogenesis: clinical implications and therapeutic targeting strategies. *J. Theor. Biol.* **241**, 564–589.

39. McElwain, D.L.S., and G.J. Pettet (1993) Cell migration in multicell spheroids: swimming against the tide. *Bull. Math. Biol.* **55**, 655–674.

40. Madri, J.A., and B.M. Pratt (1986) Endothelial cell-matrix interactions: in vitro models of angiogenesis. *J. Histochem. Cytochem.* **34**, 85–91.

41. Mohanty, K.K., and S.J. Salter (1982) Multiphase flow in porous media: II Pore-level modelling. SPE 11018 presented at the 57th Annual Conference of the SPE, New Orleans, Louisiana.

42. Mollica, F., R.K. Jain, and P.A. Netti (2003) A model for temporal heterogeneities of tumour blood flow. *Microvasc. Res.* **65**, 56–60.

43. Morikawa, S., P. Baluk, T. Kaidoh, et al. (2002) Abnormalities in pericytes on blood vessels and endothelial sprouts in tumors. *Am. J. Pathol.* **160**, 985–1000.

44. Muthukkaruppan, V.R., L. Kubai, and R. Auerbach (1982) Tumor-induced neovascularization in the mouse eye. *J. Natl. Cancer Inst.* **69,** 699–705.

45. Nekka, F., S. Kyriacos, C. Kerrigan, and L. Cartilier (1996) A model for growing vascular structures. *Bull. Math. Biol.* **58**(15.3), 409–424.

46. Netti, P.A., S. Roberge, Y. Boucher, L.T. Baxter, and R.K. Jain (1996) Effect of transvascular fluid exchange on pressure-flow relationship in tumours: a proposed mechanism for tumour blood flow heterogeneity. *Microvasc. Res.* **52**, 27–46.

47. Othmer, H., and A. Stevens (1997) Aggregation, blowup and collapse. The ABCs of taxis and reinforced random walks. *SIAM. J. Appl. Math.* **57**, 1044–1081.

48. Paweletz, N., and M. Knierim (1989) Tumor-related angiogenesis. *Crit. Rev. Oncol. Hematol.* **9**, 197–242.

49. Piri, M., and M.J. Blunt (2005a) Three-dimensional mixed-wet random pore-scale network modeling of two- and three-phase flow in porous media. I. Model description. *Phys. Rev. E.* **71**, 026301.

50. Piri, M., and M.J. Blunt (2005b) Three-dimensional mixed-wet random pore-scale network modeling of two- and three-phase flow in porous media. II. Results. *Phys. Rev. E.* **71**, 026302.

51. Plank, M.J., and B.D.S. Sleeman (2004) Lattice and non-lattice models of tumour angiogenesis. *Bull. Math. Biol.* **66**(6), 1785–1819.

52. Please, C.P., G.J. Pettet, and D.L.S. McElwain (1998) A new approach to modelling the formation of necrotic regions in tumours. *Appl. Math. Lett.* **11**, 89–94.

53. Popel, A.S., and P.C. Johnson (2005) Microcirculation and haemorheology. *Ann. Rev. Fluid Mech.* **37**, 43–69.

54. Preziosi, L., and A. Farina (2002) On Darcy's law for growing porous media. *Int. J. Non-linear Mechanics.* **37**, 485–491.

55. Pries, A.R., T.W. Secomb, P. Gaehtgens, and J.F. Gross (1990) Blood flow in microvascular networks. Experiments and simulation. *Circulation Res.*, **67**, 826–834.

56. Pries, A.R., T.W. Secomb, and P. Gaehtgens (1996) Biophysical aspects of blood flow in the microvasculature. *Cardiovasc. Res.*, **32**, 654–667.

57. Pries, A.R., T.W. Secomb, and P. Gaehtgens (1998) Structural adaptation and stability of microvascular networks: theory and simulation. *Am. J. Physiol. 275 (Heart Circ. Physiol.* **44**),H349–H360.

58. Pries, A.R., B. Reglin, and T.W. Secomb (2001a) Structural adaptation of microvascular networks: functional roles of adaptive responses. *Am. J. Physiol. Heart Circ. Physiol.* **281**, H1015–H1025.

59. Pries, A.R., B. Reglin, and T.W. Secomb (2001b) Structural adaptation of vascular networks: role of the pressure response. *Hypertension* **38,** 1476–1479.

60. Pries, A.R., B. Reglin, and T.W. Secomb (2005) Remodelling of blood vessels: response of diameter and wall thickness to haemodynamic and metabolic stimuli. *Hypertension* **46,** 725–731.

61. Pries, A.R., and T.W. Secomb (2005) Control of blood vessel structure: insights from theoretical models. *Am. J. Physiol. Heart Circ. Physiol.* **288**, 1010–1015.

62. Pries, A.R., and T.W. Secomb (2005) Microvascular blood viscosity in vivo and the endothelial surface layer. *Am. J. Physiol. Heart Circ. Physiol.* **289**, 2657–2664.

63. Quarteroni, A., M. Tuveri, and A. Veneziani (2000) Computational vascular fluid dynamics: problems, models and methods. *Comput. Visual. Sci.* **2**, 163–197.

64. Ribba, B., K. Marron, Z. Agur, T. Alarcon, and P.K. Maini (2005) A mathematical model of Doxorubicin treatment efficacy for non-Hodgkin's lymphoma. *Bull. Math. Biol.* **67**, 79–99.

65. Salsbury, A.J., K. Burrage, and K. Hellmann (1970) Inhibition of metastatic spread by icrf159—selective deletion of a malignant characteristic. *Br. Med. J.* **4**, 344–346.

66. Schmid-Schönbein, G.W. (1999) Biomechanics of microcirculatory blood perfusion. *Ann. Rev. Biomed. Eng.* **1**, 73–102.

67. Schoefl, G.I. (1963) Studies of inflammation III. Growing capillaries: their structure and permeability. *Virchows Arch. Path. Anat.* **337**, 97–141.

68. Secomb, T.W. (1995) Mechanics of blood flow in the microcirculation. *The Society for Experimental Biology*, 305–321.

69. Sherratt, J.A. and M.A.J. Chaplain (2001) A new mathematical model for avascular tumour growth. *J. Math. Biol.* **43**, 291–312.

70. Sholley, M.M., G.P. Ferguson, H.R. Seibel, J.L. Montour, and J.D. Wilson (1984) Mechanisms of neovascularization. Vascular sprouting can occur without proliferation of endothelial cells. *Lab. Invest.* **51**, 624–634.

71. Stéphanou, A., S.R. McDougall, A.R.A. Anderson, and M.A.J. Chaplain (2005) Mathematical modelling of flow in 2D and 3D vascular networks: applications to anti-angiogenic and chemotherapeutic drug strategies. *Math. Comp. Model.* **41**, 1137–1156.

72. Stéphanou, A., S.R. McDougall, A.R.A. Anderson, and M.A.J. Chaplain (2006) Mathematical modelling of the influence of blood rheological properties upon adaptive tumour-induced angiogenesis. *Math. Comp. Model.* **44**, 96–123.

73. Sternlicht, M.D., and Z. Werb (2001) How matrix metalloproteinases regulate cell behavior. *Annu. Rev. Cell. Dev. Biol.* **17**, 463–516.

74. Stokes, C.L., and D.A. Lauffenburger (1991) Analysis of the roles of microvessel endothelial cell random motility and chemotaxis in angiogenesis. *J. Theor. Biol.* **152**, 377–403.

75. Sun, S., M.F. Wheeler, M. Obeyesekere, and P.W. Charles (2005) A deterministic model of growth factor induced angiogenesis. *Bull. Math. Biol.* **67** (15.2), 313–337.

76. Thomlinson, R.H., and L.H. Gray (1955) The histological structure of some human lung cancers and the possible implications for radiotherapy. *Br. J. Cancer* **9**, 539–549.

77. Tong, S., and F. Yuan (2001) Numerical simulations of angiogenesis in the cornea. *Microvasc. Res.* **61**, 14–27.

78. Ward, J.P., and J.R. King (1997) Mathematical modelling of avascular tumour growth. *IMA J. Math. Appl. Med. Biol.* **14**, 36–69.

79. Ward, J.P., and J.R. King (1999) Mathematical modelling of avascular tumour growth. (ii) Modelling growth saturation. *IMA J. Math. Appl. Med. Biol.* **16**, 171–211.

80. Yan L., M.A. Moses, S. Huang, and D. Ingber (2000) Adhesion-dependent control of matrix metalloproteinase-2 activation in human capillary endothelial cells. *J. Cell Sci.* **113**, 3979–3987.

16

Dynamic Irregular Patterns and Invasive Wavefronts: The Control of Tumour Growth by Cytotoxic T-Lymphocytes

Anastasios Matzavinos

Department of Mathematics, Ohio State University, Columbus, OH 43210, USA
tasos@math.ohio-state.edu

16.1 Introduction

"Cancer dormancy" is an operational term used to describe the phenomenon of a prolonged quiescent state in which tumour cells are present, but tumour progression is not clinically apparent [42, 49, 53]. As a condition, cancer dormancy is often observed in breast cancers, neuroblastomas, melanomas, osteogenic sarcomas, and in several types of lymphomas, and is often found "accidentally" in tissue samples of healthy individuals who have died suddenly [1, 10]. In some cases, cancer dormancy has been found in cancer patients after several years of front-line therapy and clinical remission. The presence of these cancer cells in the body determines, finally, the outcome of the disease. In particular, age, stress factors, infections, the act of treatment itself or other alterations in the host can provoke the initiation of uncontrolled growth of initially dormant cancer cells and subsequent waves of metastases [25, 49]. Recently, some molecular targets for the induction of cancer dormancy and the re-growth of a dormant tumour have been identified [23, 48]. However, the precise nature of the phenomenon remains poorly understood.

One of the main factors (but not the only one) contributing to the induction and maintenance of cancer dormancy is the reaction of the host immune system to the tumour cells [42, 49]. Indeed, tumour-associated antigens can be expressed on tumour cells at very early stages of tumour progression [12] and, as a consequence, during the avascular stage, tumour development can be effectively controlled by *tumour-infiltrating cytotoxic lymphocytes* (TICLs) [33]. The TICLs may be cytotoxic lymphocytes (CD8$^+$ CTLs), natural killer-like (NK-like) cells and/or lymphokine-activated killer (LAK) cells [14, 21, 34, 52].

In recent years several papers have begun to investigate the mathematical modelling of the various aspects of the immune system response to cancer. The development of models which reflect several spatial and temporal aspects of tumour immunology can be regarded as the first step towards an effective computational approach in investigating the conditions under which tumour

N. Bellomo et al. (eds.), *Selected Topics in Cancer Modeling*,
DOI: 10.1007/978-0-8176-4713-1_16, © Springer Science+Business Media, LLC 2008

recurrence takes place and in the optimizing of both spatial and temporal aspects of the application of various immunotherapies. Key papers in this area include [2, 4, 3, 6, 7, 8], which focus on the modelling of tumour progression and immune competition by generalized kinetic (Boltzmann) models, and [39, 40, 41, 45], which focus on the development of tumour heterogeneities as a result of tumour cell and macrophage interactions. Moreover, [51] is concerned with receptor-ligand (Fas-FasL) dynamics, [29] investigates the process of macrophage infiltration into avascular tumours, [11, 31, 32, 36, 35] focus on the dynamics of tumour cell-TICL interactions, and finally [22] and [47] analyze various immune system and immunotherapy models in the context of cancer dynamics.

In this chapter, attention is focused upon a mathematical model of the attack of tumour cells by TICLs, in a small multicellular tumour, without necrosis and at some stage prior to (tumour-induced) angiogenesis. For a particular choice of parameters, the underlying reaction-diffusion-chemotaxis system of partial differential equations is able to simulate the phenomenon of cancer dormancy by depicting a dynamic, irregular pattern of tumour cell arrangement that is characterized by a relatively small total number of tumour cells; a behaviour that is consistent with several immunomorphological investigations. As we will see, the alteration of certain parameters of the model is enough to induce bifurcations into the system, which in turn result in tumour invasion in the form of a standard travelling wave. The latter dynamics and the conditions under which they appear are of great biological importance, since under these conditions the tumour invades the healthy tissue at its full potential, escaping the host's immune surveillance.

In the following section we introduce the mathematical model, the dynamic behaviour of which is the main focus of this chapter. The work presented here is essentially a synthesis of that of [11], [35] and [36].

16.2 The Mathematical Model

16.2.1 Derivation of the Model Equations

We consider a simplified process of a small, growing, avascular tumour which elicits a response from the host immune system and attracts a population of lymphocytes. The growing tumour is directly attacked by TICLs [26, 27, 28] which, in turn, secrete soluble diffusible factors (chemokines). These factors enable the TICLs to respond in a chemotactic manner (in addition to random motility) and migrate towards the tumour cells. Our model will therefore consist of six dependent variables denoted E, T, C, E^*, T^* and α, which are the local densities/concentrations of TICLs, tumour cells, TICL-tumour cell complexes, inactivated TICLs, "lethally hit" (or "programmed-for-lysis") tumour cells and a single (generic) chemokine respectively.

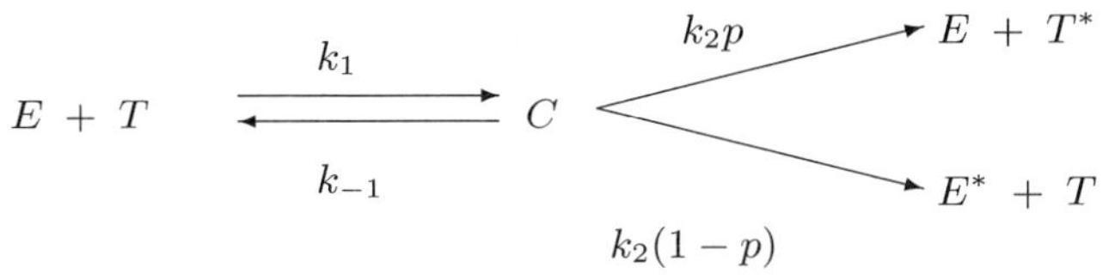

Fig. 16.1. Schematic diagram of local lymphocyte-cancer cell interactions.

The local interactions between the TICLs and tumour cells may be described by the simplified kinetic scheme given in Fig. 16.1 (see [11] and [36] for full details). The parameters k_1, k_{-1} and k_2 are non-negative kinetic constants: k_1 and k_{-1} describe the rate of binding of TICLs to tumour cells and detachment of TICLs from tumour cells *without* damaging cells; k_2 is the rate of detachment of TICLs from tumour cells, resulting in an irreversible programming of the tumour cells for lysis (i.e. death) with probability p or inactivating/killing TICLs with probability $(1-p)$. Using the law of mass action the above kinetic scheme can be "translated" into a system of ordinary differential equations. Furthermore, we consider other kinetic interaction terms between the variables and examine migration mechanisms for the TICLs and tumour cells and also consider diffusion of the chemokines. We assume that there is no "non-linear" migration of cells and no non-linear diffusion of chemokine i.e. all random motility, chemotaxis and diffusion coefficients are assumed constant.

We assume that the TICLs have an element of random motility and also respond chemotactically to the chemokines. There is a source term modelling the underlying TICL production by the host immune system, a linear decay (death) term and an additional TICL proliferation term in response to the presence of the tumour cells. Combining these assumptions with the local kinetics (derived from Fig. 16.1) we have the following partial differential equation for TICLs:

$$\frac{\partial E}{\partial t} = \overbrace{D_1 \nabla^2 E}^{\text{random motility}} \overbrace{- \chi \nabla \cdot (E \nabla \alpha)}^{\text{chemotaxis}} + \overbrace{s \cdot h(\mathbf{x})}^{\text{supply}} + \overbrace{\frac{fC}{g+T}}^{\text{proliferation}}$$

$$\overbrace{- d_1 E}^{\text{decay}} \overbrace{- k_1 ET + (k_{-1} + k_2 p)C}^{\text{local kinetics}}, \tag{16.1}$$

where D_1, χ, s, f, g, d_1, k_1, k_{-1}, k_2 and p are all positive constants. D_1 is the random motility coefficient of the TICLs and χ is the chemotaxis coefficient.

The parameter s represents the "normal" rate of flow of mature lymphocytes into the tissue (non-enhanced by the presence of tumour cells). The function $h(\mathbf{x})$ is a Heaviside function, which aims to model the existence of a subregion of the domain of interest where initially there are only tumour cells and where lymphocytes do not reside. This region of the domain is penetrated by effector cells subsequently through the processes of diffusion and chemotaxis only (see [36] for a full discussion regarding this assumption). The proliferation term $fC/(g+T)$ represents the experimentally observed enhanced proliferation of TICLs in response to the tumour and has been derived through data fitting [32, 36]. This functional form is consistent with a model in which one assumes that the enhanced proliferation of TICLs is due to signals, such as released interleukins, generated by effector cells in tumour cell-TICL complexes. We note that the growth factors that are secreted by lymphocytes in complexes (e.g IL-2) act mainly in an autocrine fashion. That is they act on the cell from which they have been secreted and thus, in our spatial setting, their action can be adequately described by a "local" kinetic term only, without the need to incorporate any additional information concerning diffusivity.

We assume that the chemokines are produced when lymphocytes are activated by tumour cell-TICL interactions. Thus we define chemokine production to be proportional to tumour cell-TICL complex density C. Once produced the chemokines are assumed to diffuse throughout the tissue and to decay in a simple manner with linear decay kinetics. Therefore the partial differential equation (PDE) for the chemokine concentration is

$$\frac{\partial \alpha}{\partial t} = \overbrace{D_2 \nabla^2 \alpha}^{\text{diffusion}} + \overbrace{k_3 C}^{\text{production}} - \overbrace{d_4 \alpha}^{\text{decay}}, \tag{16.2}$$

where D_2, k_3, d_4 are positive parameters.

We assume that migration of the tumour cells may be described by simple random motility and that on the kinetic level the growth dynamics of a solid tumour may be described adequately by a logistic term (see [36] for a full discussion concerning the validity of these assumptions). Hence the PDE governing the evolution of tumour cell density is

$$\frac{\partial T}{\partial t} = \overbrace{D_3 \nabla^2 T}^{\text{random motility}} + \overbrace{b_1(1 - b_2 T)T}^{\text{logistic growth}} \overbrace{- k_1 ET + (k_{-1} + k_2(1-p))C}^{\text{local kinetics}}, \tag{16.3}$$

where D_3 is the random motility coefficient of the tumour cells, and b_1, b_2, k_1, k_{-1}, k_2 and p are positive parameters.

We assume that there is no diffusion of the complexes, only interactions governed by the local kinetics derived from Fig. 16.1. The absence of a diffusion term is justified by the fact that formation and dissociation of complexes occurs on a time scale of tens of minutes, whereas the random motility of the tumour cells, for example, occurs on a time scale of tens of hours. Thus, the cell-cell complexes do not have time to move. Therefore the equation for the complexes is given by

$$\frac{\partial C}{\partial t} = \overbrace{k_1 ET - (k_{-1} + k_2)C}^{\text{local kinetics}}. \tag{16.4}$$

We assume that inactivated and "lethally hit" cells (i.e. cells which will die) are quickly eliminated from the tissue (for example, by macrophages) and do not substantially influence the immune processes being analyzed. Inactivated cells also do not migrate and therefore we have

$$\frac{\partial E^*}{\partial t} = \overbrace{k_2(1-p)C}^{\text{local kinetics}} - \overbrace{d_2 E^*}^{\text{decay}}, \tag{16.5}$$

$$\frac{\partial T^*}{\partial t} = \overbrace{k_2 p C}^{\text{local kinetics}} - \overbrace{d_3 T^*}^{\text{decay}}. \tag{16.6}$$

It is easy to see that equations (16.5) and (16.6) are only coupled to the full system through the complexes C and that neither E^* nor T^* have any effect on the variable C. Thus, equations (16.1), (16.2), (16.3) and (16.4) essentially dictate the behaviour of the complete system.

16.2.2 Initial and Boundary Conditions

The system of equations (16.1), (16.2), (16.3) and (16.4) is closed by applying appropriate boundary and initial conditions. In the one-dimensional case, we define the spatial domain to be the interval $[0, x_0]$ and we assume that there are two distinct regions in this interval—one region entirely occupied by tumour cells, the other entirely occupied by the immune cells. We propose that an initial interval of tumour localization is $[0, l]$, where $l = 0.2x_0$. In this framework the function $h(x)$ (cf. equation (16.1)) is defined by

$$h(x) = \begin{cases} 0, & \text{if } x - l \leq 0, \\ 1, & \text{if } x - l > 0, \end{cases}$$

and the initial conditions are given by

$$E(x,0) = \begin{cases} 0 & \text{if } 0 \leq x \leq l, \\ E_0(1 - \exp(-1000(x-l)^2)) & \text{if } l < x \leq x_0, \end{cases}$$

$$T(x,0) = \begin{cases} T_0(1 - \exp(-1000(x-l)^2)) & \text{if } 0 \leq x \leq l, \\ 0 & \text{if } l < x \leq x_0, \end{cases} \tag{16.7}$$

$$C(x,0) = \begin{cases} 0 & \text{if } x \notin [l - \epsilon, l + \epsilon], \\ C_0 \exp(-1000(x - l)^2) & \text{if } x \in [l - \epsilon, l + \epsilon], \end{cases}$$

$$\alpha(x,0) = 0, \ \forall x \in [0, x_0],$$

where

$$E_0 = \frac{s}{d_1}, \quad T_0 = \frac{1}{b_2}, \quad C_0 = \min(E_0, T_0), \quad 0 < \epsilon \ll 1. \tag{16.8}$$

In addition, zero-flux boundary conditions are imposed on the variables E, α and T.

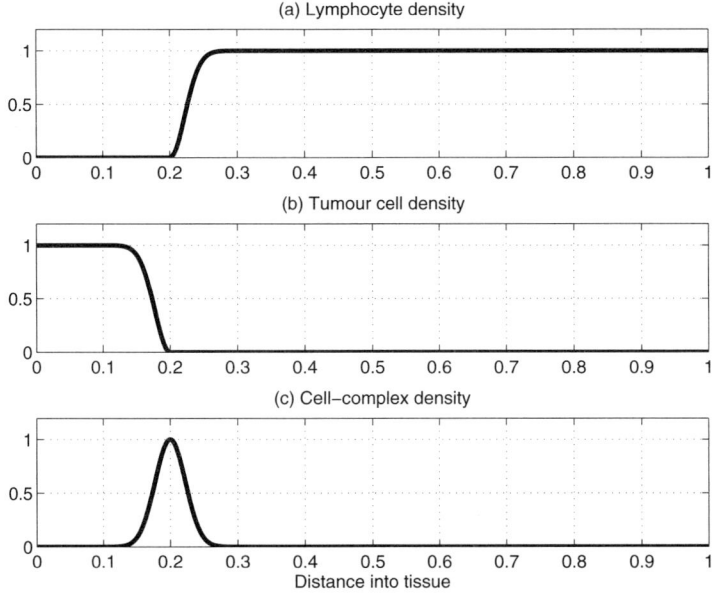

Fig. 16.2. Initial conditions used for the (a) TICLs, (b) tumour cells and (c) cell complexes.

Fig. 16.2 depicts qualitatively the initial conditions described in (16.7) (after the non-dimensionalization of the next section), which shows a front of tumour cells encountering a front of TICLs, resulting in the formation of TICL-tumour cell complexes. A full discussion of the biological interpretation of the particular initial and boundary conditions can be found in [11, 36].

16.2.3 The Non-Dimensionalized System

The closed system is non-dimensionalized by choosing an order-of-magnitude scale for the E, T and C cell densities, of E_0, T_0 and C_0 respectively, as suggested by the initial conditions. The chemokine concentration α is normalized through some reference concentration α_0 discussed in [36]. Time is scaled relative to the diffusion rate of the TICLs, i.e. $t_0 = x_0^2 D_1^{-1}$ and the space variable x is scaled relative to the length of the region under consideration, i.e. $x_0 = 1$ cm. Then, the system of equations (16.1), (16.2), (16.3) and (16.4) may be rewritten in a non-dimensionalized form as

$$\frac{\partial E}{\partial t} = \nabla^2 E - \gamma \nabla(E \nabla \alpha) + \sigma h(x) + \frac{\rho C}{\eta + T} - \sigma E - \mu ET + \epsilon C, \quad (16.9)$$

$$\frac{\partial \alpha}{\partial t} = \delta \nabla^2 \alpha + \kappa C - \xi \alpha, \quad (16.10)$$

$$\frac{\partial T}{\partial t} = \omega \nabla^2 T + \beta_1 (1 - \beta_2 T)T - \phi ET + \lambda C, \quad (16.11)$$

$$\frac{\partial C}{\partial t} = \mu ET - \psi C, \quad (16.12)$$

where

$$\sigma = \frac{st_0}{E_0} = d_1 t_0, \qquad \rho = \frac{ft_0 C_0}{E_0 T_0}, \qquad \mu = \frac{k_1 t_0 T_0 E_0}{C_0} = k_1 t_0 T_0,$$

$$\eta = \frac{g}{T_0}, \qquad \epsilon = \frac{t_0 C_0(k_{-1} + k_2 p)}{E_0}, \quad \omega = \frac{D_3 t_0}{x_0^2} = D_3 D_1^{-1},$$

$$\beta_1 = b_1 t_0, \qquad \beta_2 = b_2 T_0, \qquad \phi = k_1 t_0 E_0,$$

$$\lambda = \frac{t_0 C_0(k_{-1} + k_2(1 - p))}{T_0}, \; \psi = t_0(k_{-1} + k_2), \qquad \gamma = \frac{\chi \alpha_0 t_0}{x_0^2} = \chi \alpha_0 D_1^{-1},$$

$$\delta = \frac{D_2 t_0}{x_0^2} = D_2 D_1^{-1}, \qquad \kappa = \frac{k_3 t_0 C_0}{\alpha_0}, \qquad \xi = d_4 t_0.$$

The boundary and initial conditions are non-dimensionalized accordingly, and in the sections that follow we focus on simulating and analyzing the dynamic behaviour of the system of equations (16.9)–(16.12) and of specific variants of it.

16.3 Numerical Simulation Results

An estimation of the parameters of the system based on experimental data has been obtained in [36]. The experimental data used were concerned with *dormant* murine B cell lymphomas (BCL$_1$) [46, 49]. The corresponding non-dimensionalized parameter values used in the numerical simulations of this section are explicitly provided in [37].

The non-dimensionalized model was solved numerically using NAG routine D03PCF, which integrates systems of PDEs via the method of lines and a stiff ODE solver. We are aware of the numerical difficulties that the model poses and special care was taken to specify an appropriate number of grid points used in the numerical scheme.

Figs. 16.3–16.5 show the early evolution of the spatial distributions of TICLs, tumour cells and tumour cell-TICL complexes. More precisely, Fig. 16.4 shows a train of solitary-like waves of tumour cells invading the healthy tissue and eliciting a response by TICLs, as shown in Fig. 16.3. Fig. 16.5 shows the corresponding evolution in time of the spatial distribution of tumour cell-TICL complexes. As can be seen in Figs. 16.6–16.8, for the parameter values chosen, the system exhibits the emergence of a highly dynamic, irregular pattern of cell arrrangement in conjunction with a significant reduction of the tumour bulk as a result of the cytotoxic activity of the TICLs. This behaviour is consistent with several immunomorphological investigations (cf., e.g., [36] and references therein).

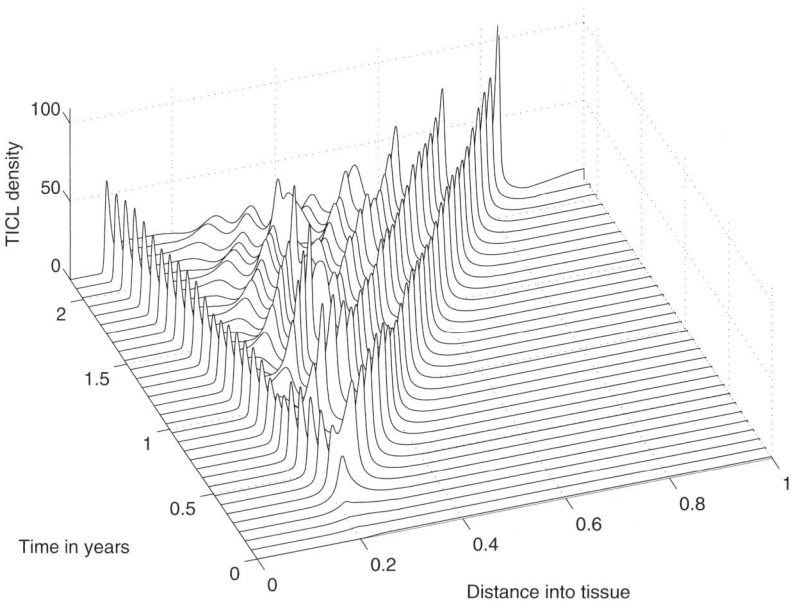

Fig. 16.3. Early dynamics of the spatial distribution of TICL density within the tissue.

In addition to observing the above spatio-temporal distributions of each cell type within the tissue, the temporal dynamics of the overall populations of each cell type (i.e total cell number) was examined. This was achieved by calculating the total number of each cell type within the whole tissue

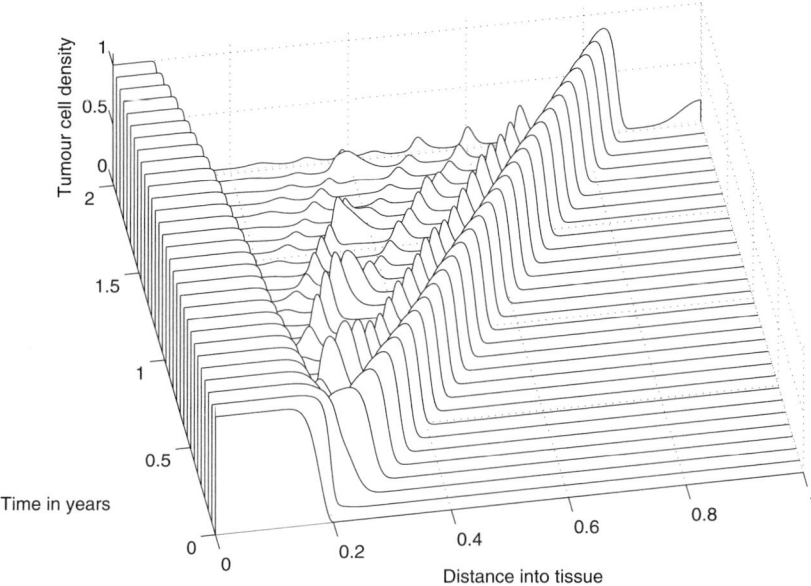

Fig. 16.4. Early dynamics of the spatial distribution of tumour cell density within the tissue.

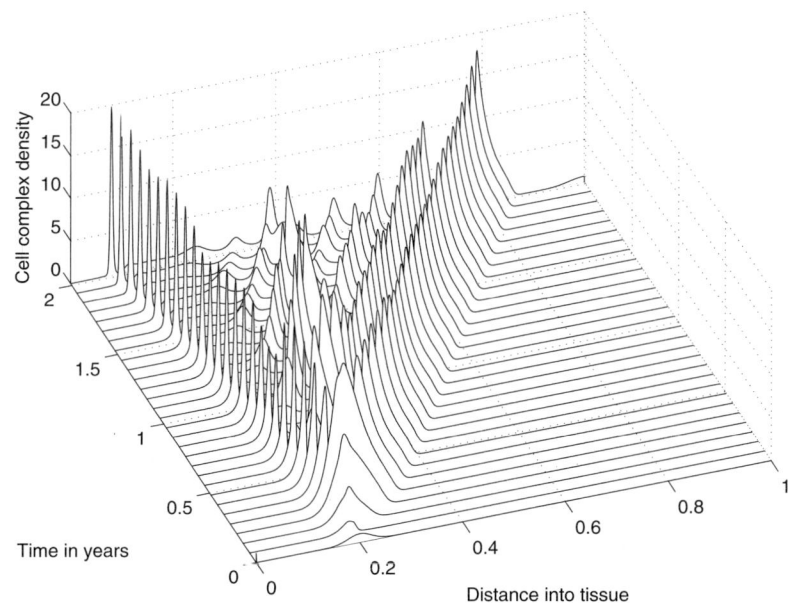

Fig. 16.5. Early dynamics of the spatial distribution of tumour cell-TICL complex density within the tissue.

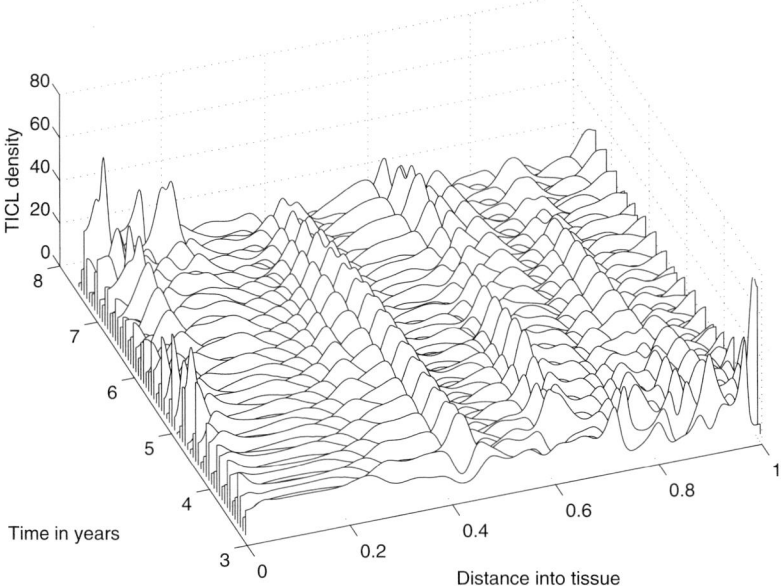

Fig. 16.6. Long-term dynamics of the spatial distribution of TICL density within the tissue.

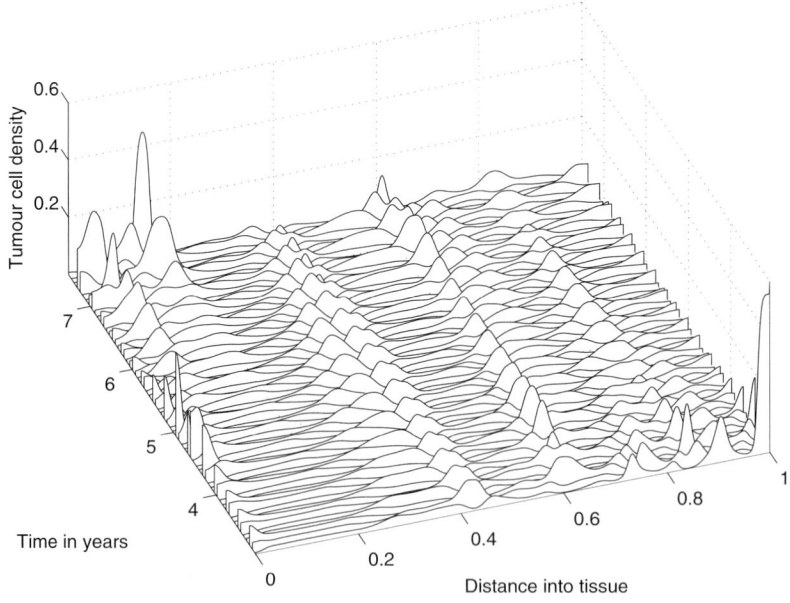

Fig. 16.7. Long-term dynamics of the spatial distribution of tumour cell density within the tissue.

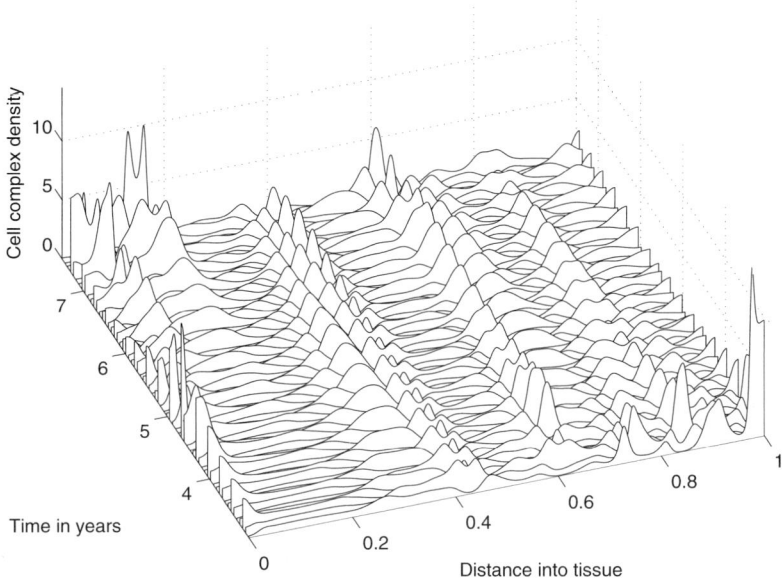

Fig. 16.8. Long-term dynamics of the spatial distribution of tumour cell-TICL complex density within the tissue.

space using numerical quadrature. Fig. 16.9(a) shows the variation in the number of TICLs within the tissue over time (approximately 80 years, an estimated average lifespan). Initially, the total number of TICLs within the tissue increases and then subsequently oscillates around some stationary level (approximately 5.9×10^6 cells). Long-time numerical calculations indicated that this behaviour will persist for all time.

A similar scenario is observed for the tumour cell population. From Fig. 16.9(b), we observe that, initially, the tumour cell population decreases in number before subsequently oscillating around some stationary value (approximately 10^7 cells) for all time. Fig. 16.9(c) gives the corresponding temporal dynamics of the tumour cell-TICL complexes.

The above simulations appear to indicate that eventually the tumour cells develop very small-amplitude oscillations about a "dormant" state, indicating that the TICLs have successfully managed to keep the tumour under control. The numerical simulations demonstrate the existence of cell distributions that are quasi-stationary in time and heterogeneous in space.

Concerning the spatial evolution of cancer dormancy with reference to the aspect of spatial containment, we note that the use of a fixed domain is consistent with various realistic biological settings. BCL_1 lymphomas of the spleen, for instance, are considered to be very good *in vivo* experimental models for investigating the various aspects of tumour development precisely

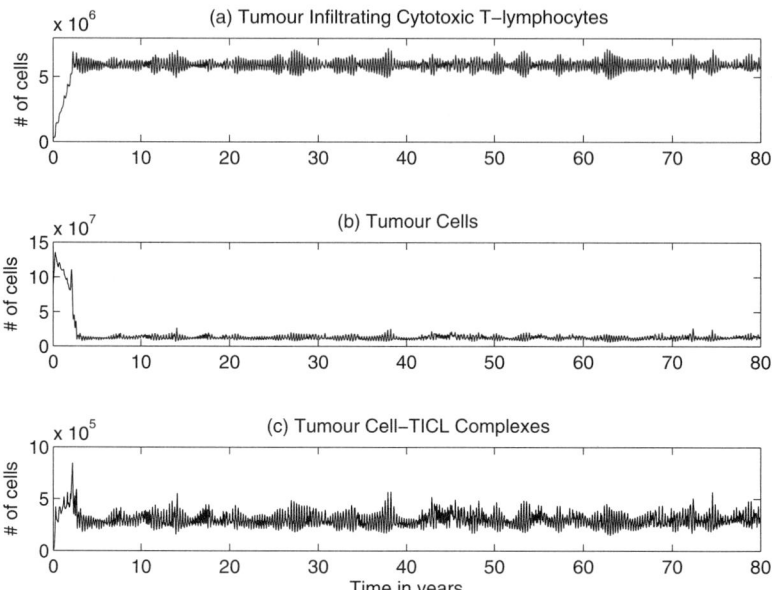

Fig. 16.9. Total number of (a) lymphocytes, (b) tumour cells and (c) tumour cell-TICL complexes within tissue over a period of 80 years.

due to the fact that tumour cells are spatially contained within the lymph tissue of the spleen. Spleens in mice are elongated organs with boundaries defined by very strong basal membranes, which do not permit the tumour cells to escape unless they break these membranes (through well-known invasive processes) and then initiate metastases. However, in our model, we do not consider these cases and this is why we employ a fixed domain and impose zero-flux boundary conditions. Of course, if the domain itself were evolving the tumour cells would not be contained in space, but would rather spread throughout the domain. In the latter case we note that, from a mathematical point of view, it would be trivial to induce some kind of spatial containment of the tumour cells in a subregion of the domain by incorporating some non-autonomous ODE kinetics. However, this is not a realistic approach for the biological settings we consider and our numerical simulations do reflect several temporal as well as spatial aspects of tumour dormancy as they are described in various immunomorphological investigations.

The interesting spatio-temporal dynamics of the system (i.e. the irregular invasive "waves" and the subsequent dynamic patterning) require us to investigate the underlying (spatially homogeneous) kinetics of our system. This is done in the following section.

16.4 Linear Stability Analysis

We consider the following autonomous system of ODEs that describes the underlying spatially homogeneous kinetics of equations (16.9)–(16.12) with $h(x) \equiv 1$:

$$\frac{dE}{dt} = \sigma + \frac{\rho C}{\eta + T} - \sigma E - \mu ET + \epsilon C, \qquad (16.13)$$

$$\frac{dT}{dt} = \beta_1 (1 - \beta_2 T)T - \phi ET + \lambda C, \qquad (16.14)$$

$$\frac{dC}{dt} = \mu ET - \psi C, \qquad (16.15)$$

$$\frac{d\alpha}{dt} = \kappa C - \xi \alpha. \qquad (16.16)$$

We note that since, in the above homogeneous system, the chemokine becomes a "slave variable" we will not consider it in the following analysis and thus we will focus on the three-dimensional dynamical system:

$$\frac{d\mathbf{x}}{dt} = \mathbf{f}(\mathbf{x}), \quad \text{where } \mathbf{x} = \begin{pmatrix} E \\ T \\ C \end{pmatrix} \in \mathbb{R}^3 \qquad (16.17)$$

and

$$\mathbf{f}(\mathbf{x}) = \begin{pmatrix} \sigma + \dfrac{\rho C}{\eta + T} - \sigma E - \mu ET + \varepsilon C \\ \beta_1 (1 - \beta_2 T)T - \phi ET + \lambda C \\ \mu ET - \psi C \end{pmatrix}. \qquad (16.18)$$

Using the parameter values described in the previous chapter, it is straightforward to show that there are four steady states of the system (16.17) given by

$$\mathbf{x}_1 = \begin{pmatrix} 1 \\ 0 \\ 0 \end{pmatrix}, \mathbf{x}_2 \approx \begin{pmatrix} 17.85 \\ 0.02 \\ 0.68 \end{pmatrix}, \mathbf{x}_3 \approx \begin{pmatrix} -0.56 \\ 1.03 \\ -1.2 \end{pmatrix}, \mathbf{x}_4 \approx \begin{pmatrix} -317 \\ 18.4 \\ -12157 \end{pmatrix}.$$

Obviously $\mathbf{x}_3$ and $\mathbf{x}_4$ are biologically unrealistic and so we ignore them for the remainder of this chapter. Now let us define the perturbations

$$\tilde{\mathbf{x}}_i = \mathbf{x} - \mathbf{x}_i, \quad i = 1, 2.$$

By linearizing about each steady state $\mathbf{x}_i$, $i = 1, 2$, we obtain the following linear system for the perturbation $\tilde{\mathbf{x}}_i$:

$$\frac{d\tilde{\mathbf{x}}_i}{dt} = D\mathbf{f}(\mathbf{x}_i)\tilde{\mathbf{x}}_i, \quad i = 1, 2,$$

where, as usual, $D\mathbf{f}(\mathbf{x}_i)$ is the Jacobian matrix of system (16.17) evaluated at the steady state $\mathbf{x}_i$.

It is a straightforward task to show that $D\mathbf{f}(\mathbf{x}_1)$ has three real eigenvalues, two negative and one positive, and thus $\mathbf{x}_1$, which represents the "healthy" steady state, is unstable. Furthermore, $D\mathbf{f}(\mathbf{x}_2)$ has one real eigenvalue that is negative, and two complex (conjugate) eigenvalues with positive real part, and thus $\mathbf{x}_2$, which represents the "tumour dormancy" steady state, is also unstable.

The numerical simulations of the previous chapter indicated that there are non-standard, invasive wave solutions. In order to understand this behaviour we undertook a further numerical investigation looking for some additional structure in the (E, T, C) phase space. The results of numerical computations in this direction are presented in Fig. 16.10(a), where the orbit (trajectory) approaches an isolated closed curve in the phase space, i.e. a limit cycle.

It is well reported in the literature that the spatio-temporal behaviour of reaction-diffusion systems with oscillatory kinetics (i.e. kinetics that exhibit a stable limit cycle) can be quite diverse and complicated. An extensive review of such systems can be found in [13]. In [19] patterns of localized oscillatory regions in reaction-diffusion models for chemical oscillations have been reported. In order for these patterns to appear the kinetics of the PDE systems discussed there must undergo a subcritical Hopf bifurcation and therefore display oscillatory behaviour. We note that we were able to find localized regions of oscillations for a particular choice of initial conditions in our system as well. In [30] the coexistence of a stable stationary solution and a stable limit cycle in a reaction-diffusion model of the Bonhoeffer–van der Pol type has been related to the generation of a self-organized pulse generator and localized oscillatory regions. Also, in [38] the behaviour behind invasive wavefronts in a cubic autocatalysis system has been considered. The model presented there undergoes supercritical Hopf bifurcations and is able to depict a wide range of spatio-temporal behaviours, including, under specific conditions, spatio-temporal chaos. Furthermore, the case of spatio-temporal chaos has been investigated in detail in the framework of predator-prey ecological interactions since there exist experimental/field data which seem to corroborate the presence of chaotic behaviour. In particular, reaction-diffusion systems with oscillatory kinetics have been considered by Sherratt et al. in [44] and [43]. They were able to depict an invasive wave of predators with irregular spatio-temporal oscillations behind the wavefront. In [44], the authors undertook a detailed investigation of that particular behaviour in the framework of simplified reaction-diffusion equations of $\lambda - \omega$ type and were able to relate the appearance of these irregularities with periodic doubling and bifurcations to tori, which are well known routes to chaos. Concerns as to whether this kind of chaotic behaviour is a mathematical artifact rather than a biological reality

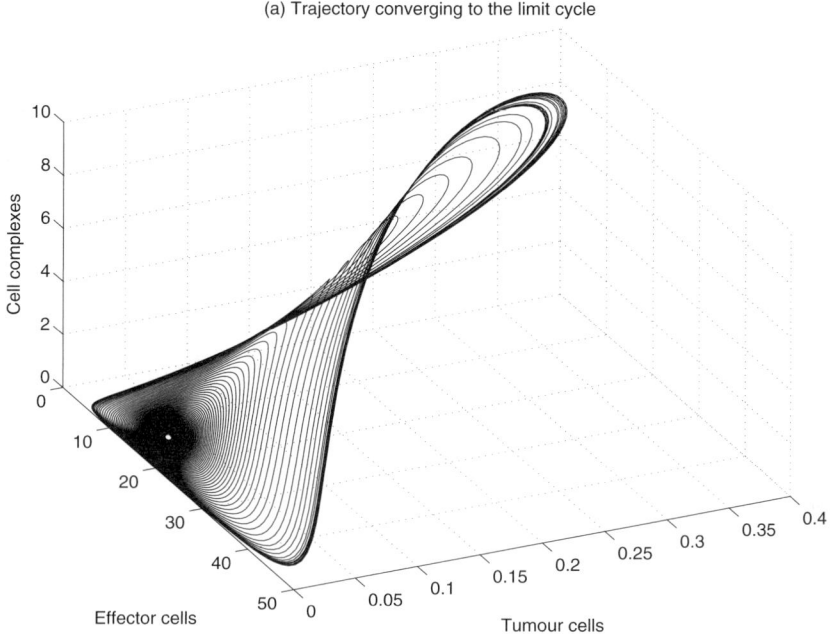

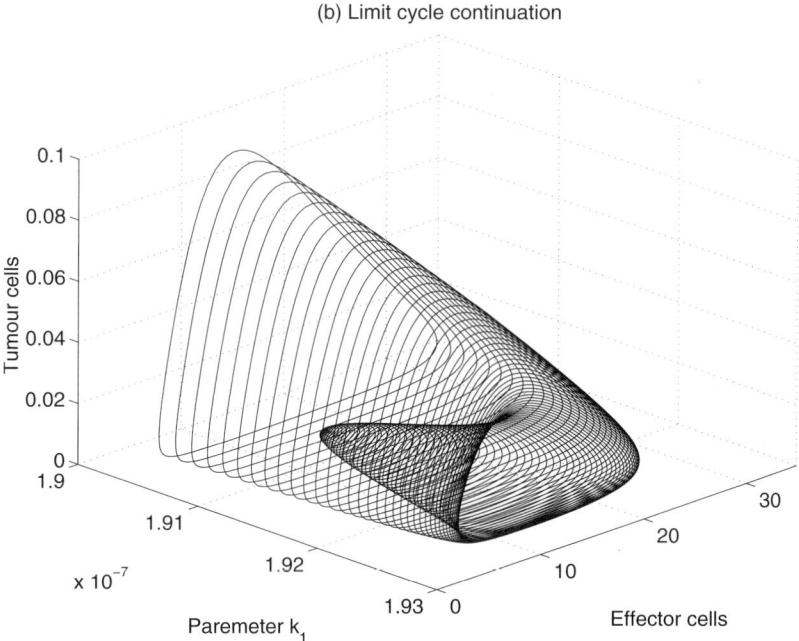

Fig. 16.10. (a) Trajectory of the spatially homogeneous ODE system with initial conditions near the "tumour dormancy" steady state, converging to a limit cycle. (b) Limit-cycle-projection continuation in the coexistence region.

have been raised in [43] where theoretical arguments in favour of the latter were presented.

In the next section we will show that the particular limit cycle appearing in our simulations is a stable one which emerges through a Hopf bifurcation. In addition the heterogeneities appearing in the long-time computations and the non-standard nature of the invading travelling waves will be related to the existence of the limit cycle.

16.5 Bifurcation Analysis

In this section we undertake a numerical bifurcation analysis of system (16.17), that governs the kinetics of our model, first with respect to parameter k_1 and then with respect to parameter p. The bifurcation diagrams presented here have been generated by the numerical continuation package MATCONT [15, 16]. MATCONT provides the implementation of numerical algorithms for tracking Hopf bifurcations and therefore establishing the existence of limit cycles.

In the case of our system MATCONT was able to detect two Hopf bifurcations with respect to parameter k_1; one at $k_1 = 8.421 \times 10^{-8}$ day^{-1}cells^{-1}cm and one at $k_1 = 1.91 \times 10^{-7}$ day^{-1}cells^{-1}cm. The limit cycles that emerge through the first bifurcation, including the one that corresponds to $k_1 = 1.3 \times 10^{-7}$ day^{-1}cells^{-1}cm (the value used for the simulations in Section 16.3), have been characterized by MATCONT as stable. However there is a region around $k_1 = 1.91 \times 10^{-7}$ day^{-1}cells^{-1}cm (the second Hopf bifurcation) where unstable limit cycles coexist with stable ones. Fig. 16.10(b) shows a detailed view of the projections of the limit cycles emerging at the coexistence region to the (E, T) phase plane. The existence of a fold or limit-point cycle (LPC) is evident.

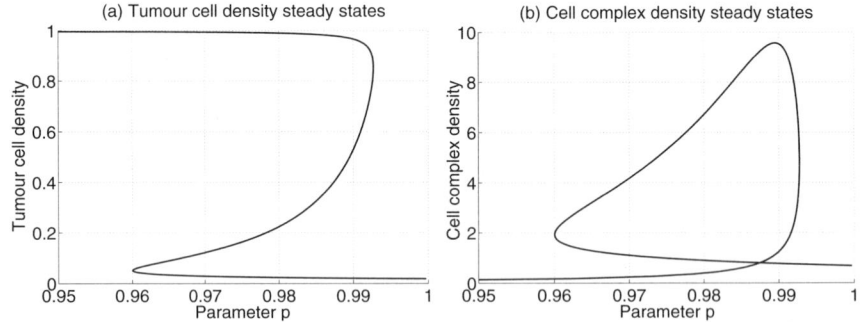

Fig. 16.11. Bifurcation diagrams of (a) tumour cell density T and (b) tumour cell-TICL complex density C versus parameter p.

Next, we consider the bifurcations of the state variables with respect to parameter p. The motivation for the choice of p as a control parameter lies in the heuristic consideration that by reducing the probability of tumour cells being killed by lymphocytes, travelling wave solutions of a more canonical nature should emerge and the special phase space structure related to the existence of the 3D attractor discussed in Section 16.4 should alter.

Figs. 16.11(a) and 16.11(b) show the bifurcation diagrams of the state variables T and C with respect to parameter p. The "healthy" steady state, which does not depend on p, is not included in these diagrams. The appearence of more steady states than the "tumour dormancy" and "healthy" ones for a particular range of p is revealed. The upper part of the bifurcation curve of the tumour cell density T represents the "tumour invasion" steady states, which are stable. By numerically solving the ODE system, we have found that for p less than a critical value (approximately 0.9906) the limit cycle disappears and all the orbits that correspond to non-steady solutions converge to the "tumour invasion" steady state. For p less than 0.96 the "tumour dormancy" steady state disappears. We also carried out simulations of the PDE system (with and without chemotaxis) for values of p less than 0.9906. In this case the solutions concerning E, T and C are of the travelling wave type. Figs. 16.12–16.14 in Section 16.6 depict the evolution of the travelling wave solutions that emerge by setting the parameter p equal to 0.99. According to these numerical observations the existence of the limit cycle in the phase space correlates to the irregular nature of the invasive "wave" of tumour cells. In the next section we focus on the analysis of the travelling wave solutions and their biological implications.

16.6 Travelling Waves: Simulation and Analysis

16.6.1 Simulation of Travelling Wave Solutions

In this section we investigate the travelling wave solutions that arise for a particular range of values of parameter p. For the sake of mathematical simplicity we will not consider the effect of chemotaxis. That is we will investigate the solutions of the system of equations (16.9), (16.11) and (16.12) with $\gamma = 0$. We would like to note here that this is a reasonable simplifying assumption since, according to numerical simulations discussed in [35] (not shown here), the formation and propagation of travelling waves is not affected by the chemotaxis term. Furthermore, we omit the Heaviside function i.e. we set $h(x) \equiv 1$. Specifically then, we will focus on the following non-dimensionalized reaction-diffusion system:

$$\frac{\partial E}{\partial t} = \nabla^2 E + \sigma + \frac{\rho C}{\eta + T} - \sigma E - \mu ET + \varepsilon C, \qquad (16.19)$$

$$\frac{\partial T}{\partial t} = \omega \nabla^2 T + \beta_1 (1 - \beta_2 T)T - \phi ET + \lambda C, \qquad (16.20)$$

$$\frac{\partial C}{\partial t} = \mu ET - \psi C. \qquad (16.21)$$

The dimensional parameter p appearing in the bifurcation analysis of Section 16.5 affects the non-dimensionalized parameters ε and λ and thus the reduction of p leads to different values of ε and λ than the ones used in the tumour-dormancy simulations. In the simulations that follow, parameter p has been set equal to 0.99, whereas in the simulation results depicted in Figs. 16.3–16.8, $p = 0.9997$.

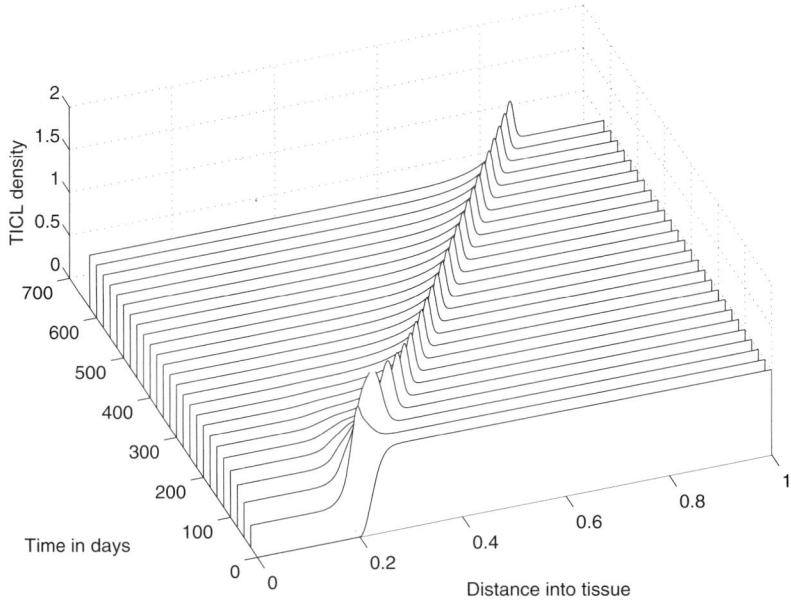

Fig. 16.12. The evolution from the initial conditions of the travelling wave of effector cell density.

The system of equations (16.19), (16.20) and (16.21) has been solved numerically over the interval $[0, 1]$ with zero-flux boundary conditions imposed and the initial conditions given by the non-dimensionalization of equations (16.7). Figs. 16.12, 16.13 and 16.14 show the results of the numerical simulations, which clearly depict the evolution of standard travelling waves from the initial conditions. We note that these travelling waves—and the corresponding travelling waves of the full reaction-diffusion-chemotaxis system—are of

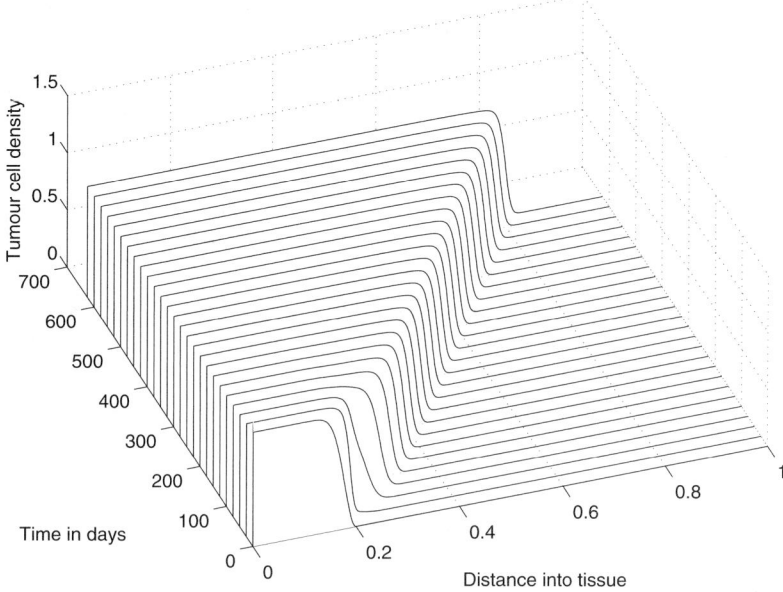

Fig. 16.13. The evolution from the initial conditions of the "invasive" travelling wave of tumour cell density.

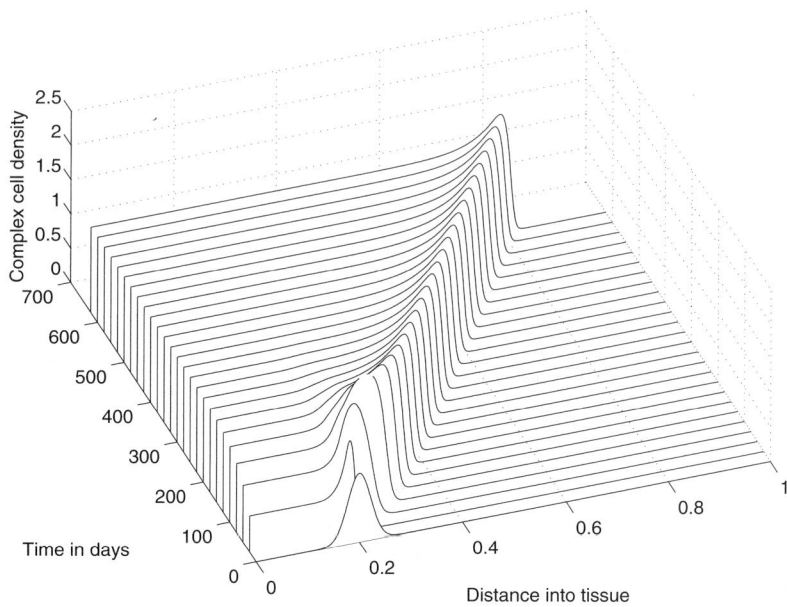

Fig. 16.14. The evolution from the initial conditions of the travelling wave of cell-complex density.

great biological importance because, when they exist, the tumour invades the healthy tissue at its full potential. In the next section we undertake a travelling wave analysis of system (16.19)–(16.21).

16.6.2 Travelling Wave Analysis

The numerical simulations of the previous section indicate that the system of equations (16.19), (16.20) and (16.21) exhibits travelling wave solutions for some choice of parameters. Two of the main approaches for establishing travelling wave solutions for systems of PDEs are (a) the geometric treatment of an appropriate phase space, where one essentially is interested in intersections between unstable and stable manifolds and (b) the Leray–Schauder (degree-theoretic) method, which employs homotopy techniques (see e.g. [9, 50]). From a numerical analysis point of view the former approach is used either in conjuction with a shooting method over a truncated domain or by trying to identify a "trivial" heteroclinic connection for some choice of parameters and then follow its deformation as the parameters are changing using numerical continuation.

In all cases the main purpose is to establish the existence of a travelling wave solution *without* any available information concerning its nature. Our approach, however, is going to be "computer assisted" in the sense that we are going to make use of the information that the numerics of the previous section can provide us.

Since we are interested in waves travelling from the left part of the domain to the right, we specify a travelling coordinate $z = x - ct$, where $c > 0$ and we let

$$\widetilde{E}(z) = E(x,t), \ \widetilde{T}(z) = T(x,t), \ \text{and} \ \widetilde{C}(z) = C(x,t).$$

We note that we assign the same wave velocity c to each variable, as suggested by the numerical simulations. By substituting $\widetilde{E}$, $\widetilde{T}$ and $\widetilde{C}$ into the system of equations (16.19), (16.20) and (16.21) and omitting the tildes for the sake of clarity, we get

$$-c\frac{dE}{dz} = \frac{d^2E}{dz^2} + \sigma + \frac{\rho C}{\eta + T} - \sigma E - \mu ET + \varepsilon C, \qquad (16.22)$$

$$-c\frac{dT}{dz} = \omega\frac{d^2T}{dz^2} + \beta_1(1 - \beta_2 T)T - \phi ET + \lambda C, \qquad (16.23)$$

$$-c\frac{dC}{dz} = \mu ET - \psi C. \qquad (16.24)$$

Our intention is to take advantage of phase-space techniques and thus we formulate the system of equations (16.22), (16.23) and (16.24) as a dynamical system in $\mathbb{R}^5$. In particular, by defining the new variables

$$E_1 = \frac{dE}{dz} \ \text{and} \ T_1 = \frac{dT}{dz},$$

the system of equations (16.22), (16.23) and (16.24) can be formulated as

$$\frac{d\mathbf{x}}{dz} = \mathbf{f}(\mathbf{x}), \quad \text{where} \quad \mathbf{x} = \begin{pmatrix} E_1 \\ E \\ T_1 \\ T \\ C \end{pmatrix} \in \mathbb{R}^5 \qquad (16.25)$$

and

$$\mathbf{f}(\mathbf{x}) = \begin{pmatrix} -cE_1 - \sigma - \dfrac{\rho C}{\eta + T} + \sigma E + \mu ET - \varepsilon C \\ E_1 \\ -\dfrac{c}{\omega}T_1 - \dfrac{\beta_1}{\omega}(1 - \beta_2 T)T + \dfrac{\phi}{\omega}ET - \dfrac{\lambda}{\omega}C \\ T_1 \\ -\dfrac{1}{c}\mu ET + \dfrac{1}{c}\psi C \end{pmatrix}. \qquad (16.26)$$

Since the wave velocity c is unknown, system (16.25) can be regarded as a non-linear eigenvalue problem. Several analytical methods have been developed for estimating c in this framework. However, the numerical solutions of equations (16.19), (16.20) and (16.21) readily yield a value of $c \approx 850$. In the analysis which follows, we therefore use this numerical estimate for c to fix the wave speed at the constant (non-dimensional) value of 850 and hence take c as a fixed parameter.

The steady states of system (16.25) can be found by solving the (non-linear) equation $\mathbf{f}(\mathbf{x}) = \mathbf{0}$. Several numerical optimization methods can be employed for this task. However, for the purposes of the travelling wave analysis, the numerical simulations of the previous section indicate that we should identify a heteroclinic connection between $\mathbf{x}^0$ and $\mathbf{x}^1$, where

$$\mathbf{x}^0 \approx \begin{pmatrix} 0 \\ 0.62 \\ 0 \\ 0.97 \\ 1.24 \end{pmatrix} \quad \text{and} \quad \mathbf{x}^1 = \begin{pmatrix} 0 \\ 1 \\ 0 \\ 0 \\ 0 \end{pmatrix}. \qquad (16.27)$$

One can improve the estimate for $\mathbf{x}^0$ by using the above value as an initial condition in an optimization algorithm. This would also confirm that $\mathbf{x}^0$ is indeed a steady state of system (16.25). The fact that $\mathbf{x}^1$ is also a steady state of (16.25) is trivial.

We are interested in the existence of an orbit $\mathbf{x}_{\mathrm{con}}(z)$ of (16.25) that satisfies

$$\lim_{z \to -\infty} \mathbf{x}_{\mathrm{con}}(z) = \mathbf{x}^0 \quad \text{and} \quad \lim_{z \to \infty} \mathbf{x}_{\mathrm{con}}(z) = \mathbf{x}^1. \qquad (16.28)$$

We consider the linearizations

$$\frac{d\mathbf{x}}{dz} = D\mathbf{f}(\mathbf{x}^0)\mathbf{x} \quad \text{and} \quad \frac{d\mathbf{x}}{dz} = D\mathbf{f}(\mathbf{x}^1)\mathbf{x} \tag{16.29}$$

of the vector field $\mathbf{f}$ at equilibria $\mathbf{x}^0$ and $\mathbf{x}^1$ respectively. It is a straightforward task to determine the spectrum of the Jacobian matrices $D\mathbf{f}(\mathbf{x}^0)$ and $D\mathbf{f}(\mathbf{x}^1)$. Indeed, there are five real eigenvalues of $D\mathbf{f}(\mathbf{x}^0)$, three positive and two negative, with the positive ones implying the existence of a three-dimensional *unstable* manifold $W^u(\mathbf{x}^0)$. Furthermore, there are five real eigenvalues of $D\mathbf{f}(\mathbf{x}^1)$, two positive and three negative, with the negative ones implying the existence of a three-dimensional *stable* manifold $W^s(\mathbf{x}^1)$. We note that

$$\dim(W^u(\mathbf{x}^0)) + \dim(W^s(\mathbf{x}^1)) = \dim \mathbb{R}^5 + 1. \tag{16.30}$$

Equation (16.30) suggests that $W^u(\mathbf{x}^0)$ and $W^s(\mathbf{x}^1)$ probably intersect transversally[1] along a one-dimensional curve in the five-dimensional phase space [5, 24]. If this is the case then this curve would define a (generic) heteroclinic connection.

The values of the parameters of the system under discussion suggest that an approximation of the connecting orbit by perturbing the system of equations (16.22), (16.23) and (16.24) can be feasible. In particular we perturb equations (16.22) and (16.23) by ignoring the effect of the second derivatives on the system (see also [17]). That is we consider the perturbed system

$$-c\frac{dE}{dz} = \sigma + \frac{\rho C}{\eta + T} - \sigma E - \mu ET + \varepsilon C, \tag{16.31}$$

$$-c\frac{dT}{dz} = \beta_1(1 - \beta_2 T)T - \phi ET + \lambda C, \tag{16.32}$$

$$-c\frac{dC}{dz} = \mu ET - \psi C. \tag{16.33}$$

We note here that by ignoring the second derivatives in effect we choose to focus on a *first order* approximation to equations (16.22) and (16.23).

Let $\Pi(\mathbf{x}^0)$ and $\Pi(\mathbf{x}^1)$ be the projections of $\mathbf{x}^0$ and $\mathbf{x}^1$ onto the phase space defined by equations (16.31), (16.32) and (16.33). It is obvious that $\Pi(\mathbf{x}^0)$ and $\Pi(\mathbf{x}^1)$ are steady states of the perturbed system. There is a three-dimensional unstable manifold $W^u(\Pi(\mathbf{x}^0))$ associated with $\Pi(\mathbf{x}^0)$ and a one-dimensional stable manifold $W^s(\Pi(\mathbf{x}^1))$ associated with $\Pi(\mathbf{x}^1)$. We have used XPP (see [18]) to investigate numerically the phase space of the system of equations (16.31), (16.32) and (16.33). XPP provides the implementation of numerical algorithms for tracking one-dimensional invariant manifolds and in the case of $\Pi(\mathbf{x}^1)$ it was able to confirm that $W^s(\Pi(\mathbf{x}^1))$ defines a heteroclinic connection between $\Pi(\mathbf{x}^0)$ and $\Pi(\mathbf{x}^1)$. Figs. 16.15(a) and 16.15(b) show approximations to the connecting orbit defined by $W^s(\Pi(\mathbf{x}^1))$ in the (E, z)- and (T, z)-planes respectively. These compare very well with the results of the spatio-temporal simulations of the full PDE system.

---

[1] See also the discussion on page 120 of [24] concerning what is called the transversality theorem.

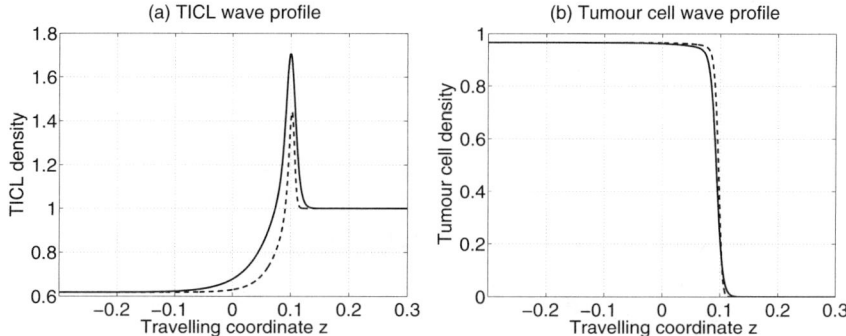

Fig. 16.15. Figures showing the approximation of the connecting orbit (solid line) (a) in the (E, z)-plane and (b) in the (T, z)-plane. The dashed lines correspond to the output of the numerical simulation of the PDE system.

16.7 Finite Element Method Simulations

In this section we undertake an explicit two-dimensional numerical investigation of a restricted version of the model developed in Section 16.2.3. More precisely, the full model is a system of a mixed hyperbolic-parabolic type and as such it poses various difficulties in its numerical approach, especially in a multidimensional framework. Hence, for the sake of computational simplicity, we do not consider the effect of chemotaxis and we omit the Heaviside function in equation (16.9). However, preliminary numerical experimentations with COMSOL Multiphysics[2] on the restricted system over a rectangular two-dimensional domain indicated the necessity for either greatly enhancing the grid or using a stabilizing method, such as streamline diffusion for instance, since several difficulties associated with numerical instabilities emerged. We note here that this was anticipated since the model, even in its restricted form, combines two highly different time scales—the one associated with the slow spatial movement of the cells and the one that underlies the fast reaction kinetics. Nonetheless, the modelling assumptions, and in particular the estimated ranges of values for the random motility coefficients, suggested that we could also modify the system towards a more diffusive setting and thus we have chosen to alter the random motility coefficients in the non-dimensionalized system by multiplying them by a factor of five. Specifically then, in this section, we focus on a modified version of the reaction-diffusion system (16.19)–(16.21), where the Laplacian terms in equations (16.19) and (16.20) have been multiplied by a factor of five.

In what follows, we consider the modified system over the two-dimensional rectangular domain

$$D = [0, 1] \times [0, 1] \subset \mathbb{R}^2,$$

---

[2] See www.comsol.com

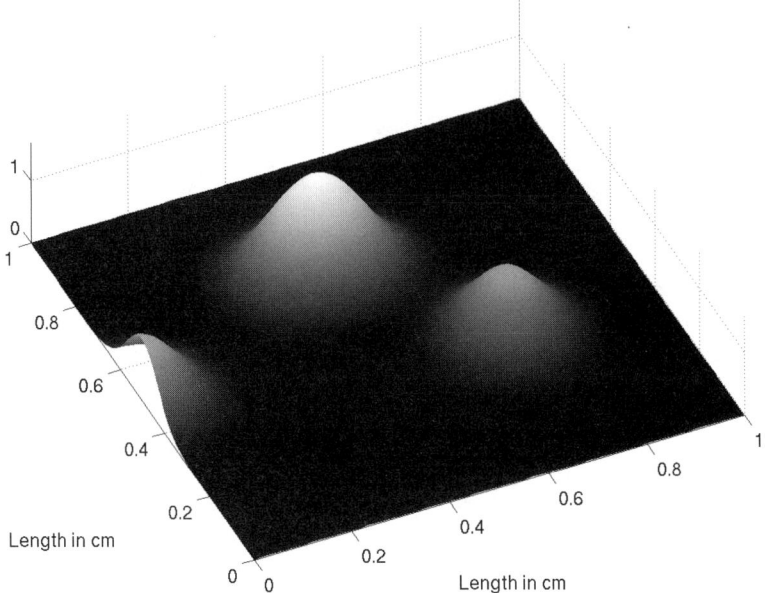

Fig. 16.16. Initial condition for the tumour cell density T.

with zero-flux boundary conditions imposed. Moreover, we assume that initially there are no complexes formed and that there is a homogeneous distribution of effector cells. That is for all $(x, y) \in D$,

$$E(x, y, 0) = 1 \text{ and } C(x, y, 0) = 0.$$

We also assume that three small clumps of tumour cells exist as Fig. 16.16 shows[3].

We have used COMSOL Multiphysics to solve the diffusive version of equations (16.19)–(16.21) with the boundary and initial conditions described. COMSOL provides a number of options to the user concerning the discretization of PDEs and the approximation of solutions. We have specified to the software a finite element space based on triangular linear Lagrange elements. The mesh consisted of $7{,}945$ nodes and $15{,}648$ elements, 240 of which were associated with the boundary of the domain. COMSOL controls the quality of the mesh by assigning to each element a quality measure. More details about the quality of the mesh used in the simulations discussed here can be found in [11].

The above spatial finite element discretization was combined with a finite difference solver in a method-of-lines approach, and the results of the numeri-

---

[3] An explicit algebraic expression for the initial tumour cell distribution can be found in [37].

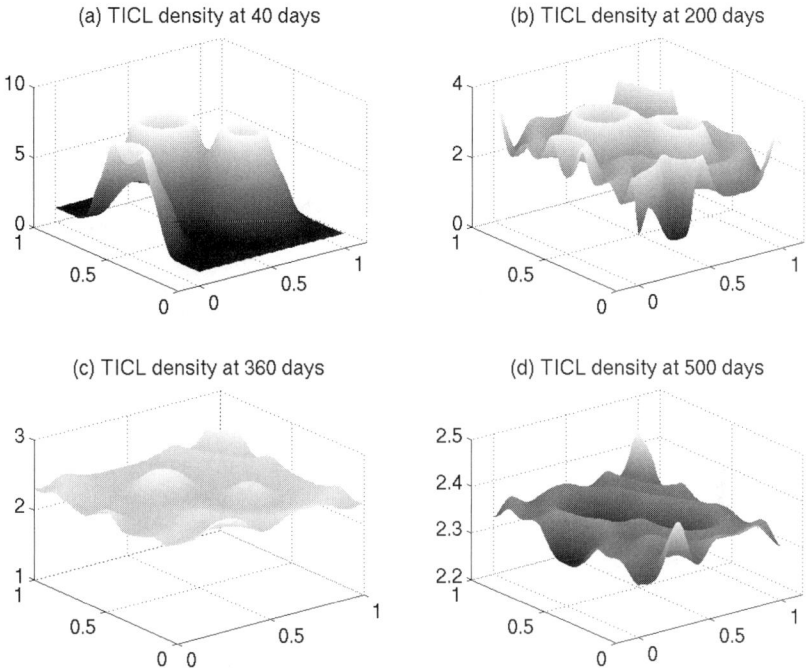

Fig. 16.17. Spatial distribution of TICL density within tissue at times corresponding to 40, 200, 360 and 500 days respectively.

cal computations are shown in Figs. 16.17(a)–(d) and 16.18(a)–(d). In particular, Figs. 16.17(a)–(d) show the evolution of the (non-dimensionalized) spatial distribution of the TICL density within the tissue at times corresponding to 40, 200, 360 and 500 days respectively. The corresponding spatial distribution of tumour cells is shown in Figs. 16.18(a)–(d). Clearly, the simulations depict a reduction of the tumour bulk as a result of the cytotoxic activity of the TICLs, accompanied with the emergence of a highly dynamic, irregular pattern of tumour cell arrangement.

16.8 Discussion and Conclusions

The mathematical analysis and numerical simulations discussed in this chapter were essentially associated with two different models: one was a simplified reaction-diffusion system with no hyperbolic terms and the other was a full reaction-diffusion-chemotaxis system with TICL chemotaxis incorporated. We note here that, for the parameter values employed, the incorporation of chemotaxis does not affect the dynamics qualitatively although, as expected, quantitative differences between the two models do exist. For instance, as the

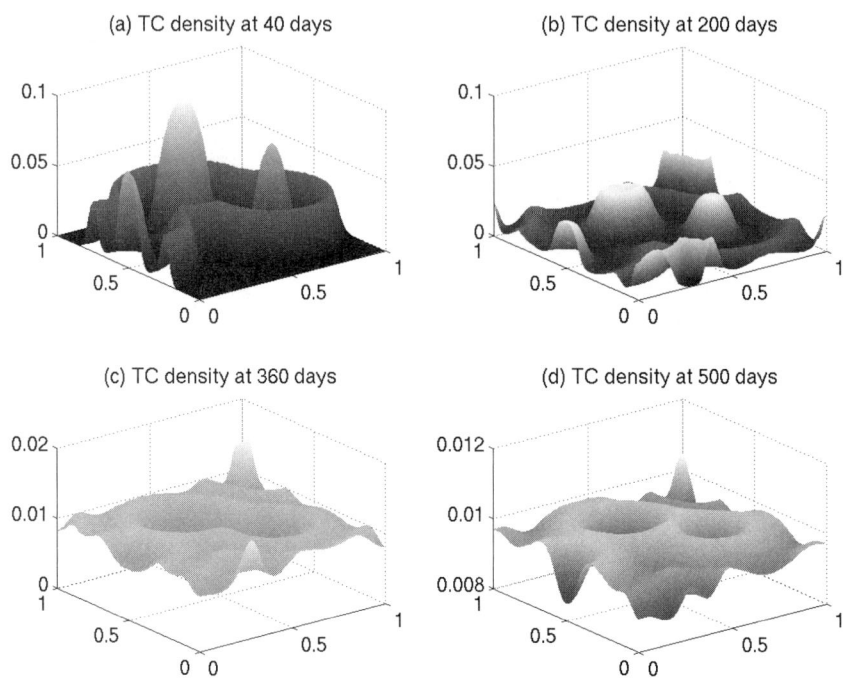

Fig. 16.18. Spatial distribution of tumour cell density within tissue at times corresponding to 40, 200, 360 and 500 days respectively.

numerical simulations discussed in [11, 36] indicate, chemotactic signals from the chemokines localize the TICLs around regions of complex formation. This aggregation phenomenon causes the TICLs to be "slowed down" and unable to fully spread throughout the domain.

The numerical bifurcation analysis of system (16.17) undertaken in this chapter was combined with a systematic investigation of the spatio-temporal dynamics of the PDE model. This study enabled us to correlate numerically the existence of a stable limit cycle in the associated (kinetic) phase space with the irregular spatio-temporal evolution of the "cancer dormancy" solutions for a wide range of parameter values *both* for the reduced reaction-diffusion system *and* for the full reaction-diffusion-chemotaxis model.

Preliminary numerical work, which is not presented in this chapter, has recently shed more light on this issue by indicating that the existence of oscillatory kinetics is a necessary but not a sufficient condition for the development of the irregular spatio-temporal dynamics. More precisely, we have investigated numerically a reduced reaction-diffusion system with zero-flux boundary conditions imposed and two different types of initial conditions: (a) symmetric initial conditions and (b) asymmetric initial conditions, where the asymmetry was defined in terms of the tumour cell distribution. In the first case the system developed *regular* spatio-temporal dynamics and, as a result of the oscillatory kinetics and the presence of symmetry in the initial conditions, the boundaries were oscillating *synchronously*. The highly irregular spatio-temporal dynamics, familiar from Section 16.3, manifested themselves in the simulations associated with the second type of initial conditions. Most interestingly, in this latter case there were indications that the irregular dynamical behaviour was driven by the dynamics of the boundary points, which were oscillating *asynchronously*. These findings seem to indicate that the irregular spatio-temporal dynamics could be driven by a spatial version of coupled asynchronous oscillators, which in turn is a manifestation of the coexistence of the oscillatory kinetics with the presence of asymmetry in the initial conditions. This is to be investigated further.

Finally, we would like to note here that the first order approximation employed in the framework of the travelling wave analysis in this chapter could be further investigated in the context of geometric perturbation theory. More precisely, we believe that Fenichel's invariant manifold theorem [5, 20] has a special role to play here and, as a matter of fact, it seems that one could try to analyze system (16.25) by employing the relevant techniques discussed in [5]. Nonetheless, several problems arise in this direction with perhaps the most prominent of them being the unavailability of simple analytic expressions for the steady states of the system under discussion.

References

1. A. Alsabti. Tumour dormant state. *Tumour Res.*, 13(1):1–13, 1978.
2. D. Ambrosi, N. Bellomo, and L. Preziosi. Modelling tumor progression, heterogeneity, and immune competition. *J. Theor. Medicine*, 4:51–65, 2002.
3. E. de Angelis, M. Delitala, A. Marasco, and A. Romano. Bifurcation analysis for a mean field modelling of tumor and immune system competition. *Math. Comp. Modelling*, 37:1131–1142, 2003.
4. L. Arlotti, A. Gamba, and M. Lachowicz. A kinetic model of tumor/immune system cellular interactions. *J. Theor. Medicine*, 4:39–50, 2002.
5. P.B. Ashwin, M.V. Bartuccelli, T.J. Bridges, and S.A. Gourley. Travelling fronts for the KPP equation with spatio-temporal delay. *Z. Angew. Math. Phys.*, 53:103–122, 2002.
6. N. Bellomo, A. Bellouquid, and E. De Angelis. The modelling of the immune competition by generalized kinetic (Boltzmann) models: review and research perspectives. *Math. Comp. Modelling*, 37:65–86, 2003.
7. N. Bellomo, B. Firmani, and L. Guerri. Bifurcation analysis for a nonlinear system of integro-differential equations modelling tumor-immune cells competition. *Appl. Math. Letters*, 12:39–44, 1999.
8. N. Bellomo and L. Preziosi. Modelling and mathematical problems related to tumor evolution and its interaction with the immune system. *Math. Comp. Modelling*, 32:413–452, 2000.
9. H. Berestycki, B. Larrouturou, and P.L. Lions. Multi-dimensional travelling wave solutions of a flame propagation model. *Arch. Rational Mech. Anal.*, 111:33–49, 1990.

10. N. Breslow, C.W. Chan, G. Dhom, R.A. Drury, L.M. Franks, B. Gellei, Y.S. Lee, S. Lundberg, B. Sparke, N.H. Sternby, and H. Tulinius. Latent carcinoma of prostate at autopsy in seven areas. *Intern. J. Cancer*, 20(5):680–688, 1977.

11. M. Chaplain and A. Matzavinos. Mathematical modelling of spatio-temporal phenomena in tumour immunology. In A. Friedman, editor, *Tutorials in Mathematical Biosciences III: Cell Cycle, Proliferation, and Cancer*, volume 1872 of *Lecture Notes in Mathematics*, pages 131–183. Springer, New York, 2006.

12. P.G. Coulie. Human tumor antigens recognized by T cells: new perspectives for anti-cancer vaccines? *Molecular Medicine Today*, 3:261–268, 1997.

13. M.C. Cross and P.C. Hohenberg. Pattern formation outside equilibrium. *Rev. Mod. Phys.*, 65:851–1112, 1993.

14. R.A. Deweger, B. Wilbrink, R.M.P. Moberts, D. Mans, R. Oskam, and W. den Otten. Immune reactivity in SL2 lymphoma-bearing mice compared with SL2-immunized mice. *Cancer Immun. Immunotherapy*, 24:1191–1192, 1987.

15. A. Dhooge, W. Govaerts, and Yu. A. Kuznetsov. MATCONT: a MATLAB package for numerical bifurcation analysis of ODEs. *ACM Trans. Math. Software*, 29:141–164, 2003.

16. A. Dhooge, W. Govaerts, and Yu. A. Kuznetsov. Numerical continuation of fold bifurcations of limit cycles in MATCONT. In P.M.A. Sloot et al., editors, *Proceedings of the International Conference on Computational Science ICCS 2003, Melbourne, Australia and St Petersburg, Russia, 2-4 June 2003, Part I*, volume 2657 of *Lecture Notes in Computer Science*, pages 701–710. Springer Verlag, Berlin, 2003.

17. S.R. Dunbar. Travelling wave solutions of diffusive Lotka-Volterra equations. *J. Math. Biology*, 17:11–32, 1983.

18. G.B. Ermentrout. *Simulating, Analyzing, and Animating Dynamical Systems: A Guide to XPPAUT for Researchers and Students*, volume 14 of *Software, Environments, and Tools*. SIAM, Philadelphia, 2002.

19. G.B. Ermentrout, X. Chen, and Z. Chen. Transition fronts and localized structures in bistable reaction-diffusion systems. *Physica D*, 108:147–167, 1997.

20. N. Fenichel. Geometric singular perturbation theory for ordinary differential equations. *J. Diff. Eqns.*, 31:53–98, 1979.

21. G. Forni, G. Parmiani, A. Guarini, and R. Foa. Gene transfer in tumour therapy. *Annals Oncol.*, 5:789–794, 1994.

22. U. Foryś. Marchuk's model of immune system dynamics with application to tumour growth. *J. Theor. Medicine*, 4:85–93, 2002.

23. J.A.A. Ghiso. Inhibition of FAK signaling activated by urokinase receptor induces dormancy in human carcinoma cells in vivo. *Oncogene*, 21(16):2513–2524, 2002.

24. J. Guckenheimer and P. Holmes. *Nonlinear Oscillations, Dynamical Systems, and Bifurcations of Vector Fields*, volume 42 of *Applied Mathematical Sciences*. Springer, New York, 1983. Corrected seventh printing, 2002.

25. L. Holmberg and M. Baum. Work on your theories! *Nat. Med.*, 2(8):844–846, 1996.

26. C.G. Ioannides and T.L. Whiteside. T-cell recognition of human tumours–implications for molecular immunotherapy of cancer. *Clin. Immunol. Immunopath.*, 66:91–106, 1993.

27. J. Jaaskelainen, A. Maenpaa, M. Patarroyo, C.G. Gahmberg, K. Somersalo, J. Tarkkanen, M. Kallio, and T. Timonen. Migration of recombinant IL-2-activated T-cells and natural killer cells in the intercellular space of human H-2

glioma spheroids in vitro—a study on adhesion molecules involved. *J. Immunol.*, 149:260–268, 1992.

28. Y. Kawakami, M.I. Nishimura, N.P. Restifo, S.L. Topalian, B.H. O'Neil, J. Shilyansky, J.R. Yannelli, and S.A. Rosenberg. T-cell recognition of human-melanoma antigens. *J. Immunotherapy*, 14:88–93, 1993.

29. C.E. Kelly, R.D. Leek, H.M. Byrne, S.M. Cox, A.L. Harris, and C.E. Lewis. Modelling macrophage infiltration into avascular tumours. *J. Theor. Medicine*, 4:21–38, 2002.

30. R. Kobayashi, T. Ohta, and Y. Hayase. Self-organized pulse generator. *Physica D*, 84:162–170, 1995.

31. V.A. Kuznetsov and G.D. Knott. Modeling tumor regrowth and immunotherapy. *Math. Comp. Modelling*, 33:1275–1287, 2001.

32. V.A. Kuznetsov, I.A. Makalkin, M.A. Taylor, and A.S. Perelson. Nonlinear dynamics of immunogenic tumours: parameter estimation and global bifurcation analysis. *Bull. Math. Biol.*, 56:295–321, 1994.

33. D. Loeffler and S. Ratner. In vivo localization of lymphocytes labeled with low concentrations of HOECHST-33342. *J. Immunol. Meth.*, 119:95–101, 1989.

34. E.M. Lord and G. Burkhardt. Assessment of in situ host immunity to syngeneic tumours utilizing the multicellular spheroid model. *Cell. Immunol.*, 85:340–350, 1984.

35. A. Matzavinos and M.A.J. Chaplain. Travelling-wave analysis of a model of the immune response to cancer. *C.R. Biologies*, 327:995–1008, 2004.

36. A. Matzavinos, M.A.J. Chaplain, and V.A. Kuznetsov. Mathematical modelling of the spatio-temporal response of cytotoxic T-lymphocytes to a solid tumour. *Mathematical Medicine and Biology: A Journal of the IMA*, 21:1–34, 2004.

37. A. Matzavinos-Toumasis. *Mathematical Modelling of the Spatio-temporal Response of Cytotoxic T-lymphocytes to a Solid Tumour*. PhD thesis, University of Dundee, Scotland, 2004.

38. J.H. Merkin and M.A. Sadiq. The propagation of travelling waves in an open cubic autocatalytic chemical system. *IMA J. Appl. Math.*, 57:273–309, 1996.

39. M.R. Owen and J.A. Sherratt. Pattern formation and spatio-temporal irregularity in a model for macrophage-tumour interactions. *J. Theor. Biol.*, 189:63–80, 1997.

40. M.R. Owen and J.A. Sherratt. Modelling the macrophage invasion of tumours: effects on growth and composition. *IMA J. Math. Appl. Med. Biol.*, 15:165–185, 1998.

41. M.R. Owen and J.A. Sherratt. Mathematical modelling of macrophage dynamics in tumours. *Math. Models Meth. Appl. Sci.*, 9:513–539, 1999.

42. V. Schirrmacher. T-cell immunity in the induction and maintenance of a tumour dormant state. *Seminars in Cancer Biology*, 11:285–295, 2001.

43. J.A. Sherratt, B.T. Eagan, and M.A. Lewis. Oscillations and chaos behind predator-prey invasion: mathematical artifact or ecological reality? *Phil. Trans. R. Soc. Lond. B*, 352:21–38, 1997.

44. J.A. Sherratt, M.A. Lewis, and A.C. Fowler. Ecological chaos in the wake of invasion. *Proc. Natl. Acad. Sci. USA*, 92:2524–2528, 1995.

45. J.A. Sherratt, A.J. Perumpanani, and M.R. Owen. Pattern formation in cancer. In M.A.J. Chaplain, G.D. Singh, and J.C. McLachlan, editors, *On Growth and Form: Spatio-temporal Pattern Formation in Biology*. John Wiley & Sons Ltd., Chicester, 1999.

46. H. Siu, E.S. Vitetta, R.D. May, and J.W. Uhr. Tumour dormancy. regression of BCL tumour and induction of a dormant tumour state in mice chimeric at the major histocompatibility complex. *J. Immunol.*, 137:1376–1382, 1986.

47. Z. Szymańska. Analysis of immunotherapy models in the context of cancer dynamics. *Appl. Math. Comp. Sci.*, 13:407–418, 2003.

48. T. Udagawa, A. Fernandez, E.G. Achilles, J. Folkman, and R.J. D'Amato. Persistence of microscopic human cancers in mice: alterations in the angiogenic balance accompanies loss of tumor dormancy. *FASEB J.*, 16(11):1361–1370, 2002.

49. J.W. Uhr and R. Marches. Dormancy in a model of murine B cell lymphoma. *Seminars in Cancer Biology*, 11:277–283, 2001.

50. A.I. Volpert, V.A. Volpert, and V.A. Volpert. *Traveling Wave Solutions of Parabolic Systems*, volume 140 of *Translations of Mathematical Monographs*. American Mathematical Society, Providence, RI, 2000.

51. S.D. Webb, J.A. Sherratt, and R.G. Fish. Cells behaving badly: a theoretical model for the Fas/FasL system in tumour immunology. *Mathematical Biosciences*, 179:113–129, 2002.

52. K.M. Wilson and E.M. Lord. Specific (EMT6) and non-specific (WEHI-164) cytolytic activity by host cells infiltrating tumour spheroids. *Brit. J. Cancer*, 55:141–146, 1987.

53. E. Yefenof. Cancer dormancy: from observation to investigation and onto clinical intervention. *Seminars in Cancer Biology*, 11:269–270, 2001.

Multiscale Modelling of Solid Tumour Growth

Helen M. Byrne,[1] I.M.M. van Leeuwen,[1,2] Markus R. Owen,[1] Tomás Alarcón,[3] and Philip K. Maini[4]

[1] Centre for Mathematical Medicine and Biology, School of Mathematical Sciences, University of Nottingham, Nottingham NG7 2RD, UK
`helen.byrne@nottingham.ac.uk, markus.owen@nottingham.ac.uk`

[2] Department of Surgery and Molecular Oncology, Ninewells Hospital, University of Dundee, Dundee DD1 9SY, Scotland, UK
`ingeborg@maths.dundee.ac.uk`

[3] Department of Mathematics, Imperial College, 180 Queen's Gate, London SW7 2AZ, UK
`a.tomas@imperial.ac.uk`

[4] Centre for Mathematical Biology, Mathematical Institute, University of Oxford, 24-29 St Giles', Oxford OX1 3LB, and Oxford Centre for Integrative Systems Biology, Department of Biochemistry, South Parks Road, Oxford OX1 3QU, UK
`maini@maths.ox.ac.uk`

17.1 Introduction

Biological function arises from complex processes interacting over a large range of spatial and temporal scales. For example, within vascularised tumours, local oxygen levels, determined at the tissue scale by vascular density and blood flow, influence subcellular processes that include progress through the cell cycle and the expression of proteins such as vascular endothelial growth factor (VEGF). Since VEGF is a potent angiogenic factor, its intracellular production, release by the cells and transport through the extracellular space stimulate vascular adaptation at the macroscale. This remodelling, in turn, controls oxygen delivery to the tissue.

Over recent decades, remarkable technological advances within the life sciences have led to the generation of an enormous amount of data relating to phenomena that act at different scales. However, the impressive scientific contributions contained within individual articles are often fragmented and isolated due to the absence of comprehensive conceptual frameworks that allow information to be organised and results integrated. Furthermore, intuitive, verbal reasoning approaches can be inadequate for dealing with such complicated, non-linear dynamical systems. Nor can they keep pace with the vast amount of information being generated. Experience within other areas of science has taught us that quantitative methods are needed to develop com-

N. Bellomo et al. (eds.), *Selected Topics in Cancer Modeling*,
DOI: 10.1007/978-0-8176-4713-1_17, © Springer Science+Business Media, LLC 2008

prehensive theoretical models for interpretation, organisation and integration of these data [GM03].

The challenge for mathematical biology is two-fold: first to develop meaningful mathematical models at each individual scale, then to integrate such models into a computationally tractable multiscale model that allows us to understand how individual processes (for example, binding of a drug to its receptor) at the microscopic level affect the behaviour at the system (macroscopic) level (for example, the effect of a drug on a specific organ).

In addressing this challenge, modelling has two possible roles to play. First, on those rare occasions for which the biological system of interest has been well studied and characterised, it is possible to develop, with a fine degree of accuracy, models capable of replicating the biological observations. Whereas this is of little interest *per se*, exploiting the models to study the effect of different interventions can greatly enhance our understanding of the system's properties and behaviour. Hence, *in silico* techniques provide tools to carry out and iterate experiments that would otherwise be classified as unethical, expensive, time consuming, or simply impossible. Second, most research in biological systems is at a stage where it is impossible to develop accurate, detailed mathematical models. In these cases, modelling also has a vital role to play. Mathematical models essentially translate empirical biological hypotheses into a concrete framework which allows us to compute the outcome of these proposed interactions. By testing against data, this allows hypotheses to be verified or rejected and new hypotheses to be generated. This continual interaction between theoretical and empirical efforts makes it possible to refine the experimental procedure and leads to greater understanding of the complex system. Additionally, it should reduce the need for experimentation.

To exploit the full potential of mathematical modelling in biology, there is an urgent need to develop new theoretical tools for the analysis and synthesis of detailed low-level information into comprehensive, integrative, and quantitative descriptions that span a wide range of spatio-temporal scales. This new research area is viewed as the next "grand challenge" in the life sciences, and is often referred to as the Physiome Project,[5] encompassing the world-wide effort to describe biological function, based on genomic and proteomic mechanisms and their interaction, using qualitative and quantitative mathematical models [Cram04]. The ultimate goal is to transform the wealth of data being generated into a detailed understanding of biological function and, hence, of the complex systems that together form the basis of living organisms.

Within this effort, there is a growing literature devoted to mathematical modelling of different aspects of tumour growth (see, for example, the reviews in [Ad96, AMcE, RCM07]). These models tend to concentrate on processes occurring at one particular scale. Biologists now believe that the complexities of cancer could be explained in terms of a small number of underlying principles, namely, self-sufficiency in growth signals, insensitivity to anti-growth signals,

---

[5] http://www.physiome.org/

evasion of programmed cell death (apoptosis), limitless replication potential, sustained angiogenesis, tissue invasion and metastasis [HW00]. Our long-term goal is to incorporate these features into a multiscale "virtual tumour" model allowing us to organise existing data into an integrative theoretical framework that can clarify the underlying dynamics governing invasive cancers, and lead to the development of therapeutic strategies to combat tumour growth. However, in the shorter term, we can focus on certain aspects of cancer which are already amenable to experimental manipulation with a view to developing clinical strategies to control the disease. Our approach is to develop a multiscale model which can integrate existing models, extending them where appropriate, and be consistently updated by new experimental information. This requires the development of a theoretical framework into which models can be slotted as modules. We anticipate that the resulting model will be similar in scope to the heart models that have been developed by Noble, Hunter and co-workers [Cram04, Nobl06].

By way of illustration we present below three examples of our recent work. In Section 17.2, we present a model for carcinogenesis during the early (avascular) stages of ductal carcinoma *in situ* which focuses on aspects of metabolic changes and somatic evolution. In Section 17.3, we introduce a multiscale model for a vascularised tumour in which the dynamics of the tumour mass are intimately related to those of the blood vessels supplying the tissue with nutrients, and in Section 17.4 we present a model for early colorectal cancer. The common theme underlying these models is the integration of processes occurring on very different spatial and temporal scales. The chapter concludes in Section 17.5 with a summary of our results, a review of related relevant work and a discussion of the challenges that lie ahead for the further development of multiscale models of solid tumour growth in particular and their wider application in biology.

17.2 Metabolic Changes During Carcinogenesis

The pioneering work of Warburg [W30] revealed that tumour cells show an abnormal metabolism, preferentially converting glucose to lactic acid, even in the presence of sufficient oxygen. This is a paradox given that the aerobic glucose metabolic pathway is substantially more energy efficient than anaerobic metabolism, or glycolysis. It also has important clinical implications since a direct correlation between the rate of glucose consumption and tumour aggressiveness has been observed [HSR91]. The reason for this metabolic transition is as yet unclear. It has been proposed that, through factors such as cellular crowding, tumour cells may destroy the native vasculature, the primary mode of oxygen delivery, leading to heterogeneous oxygen perfusion through the tumour tissue. The resulting cyclical periods of hypoxia can initially cause transient adoption of glycolysis. However, the universal adoption of increased glycolysis in human cancer, even under normal conditions, suggests that environmental factors other than hypoxia are involved.

We might expect that the increased acid production associated with the glycolytic phenotype would give rise to a significantly lower intracellular pH. However, magnetic resonance spectroscopy has shown that intracellular tumour pH is higher than that in non-transformed cells [GLB94]. This is due to upregulation of ion transporters which increase the flux of hydrogen ions across the tumour cell membrane into the extracellular space [GRM89]. A combination of this acid transport and the poor tumour vasculature for excess acid removal results in a tumour extracellular pH substantially lower than that of normal tissue. This has led to the acid-mediated tumour invasion hypothesis [GG96].

As the tumour microenvironment becomes more toxic, adaptation becomes essential. Recently a hybrid cellular automaton model has been developed to investigate the cell-microenvironmental interactions that mediate somatic evolution of cancer cells [SGGMG07] during the development of ductal carcinoma *in situ*. We briefly describe the model here, and refer the interested reader to the original paper for full details.

17.2.1 Model Framework

The model builds heavily on work by Gatenby and Gillies [GG04] who hypothesise that evolution of glycolysis is due to environmental constraints imposed by the morphology of the ducts. The blood supply is separated from the interior of the ducts by the basement membrane, so as a pre-malignant lesion grows away from the membrane into the duct it eventually experiences hypoxia. Gatenby and Gillies propose that this leads to an evolutionary sequence consisting of adaptation to hypoxia by upregulation of glycolysis, acidification of the environment (due to anaerobic respiration of glucose) and then cellular adaptation to acid-induced cellular toxicity.

The hybrid cellular automaton model that is used is composed of an $(M \times N)$ array of automaton elements (i, j) with a specific rule set governing their evolution. The distribution of the oxygen, glucose and H^+ fields is also monitored, reaction-diffusion equations being used to characterise their spatio-temporal dynamics. Each automaton element corresponds to a region of size $25\mu m \times 25\mu m$ that is occupied by either a tumour cell or a vacant space. Cells are initially placed as automaton units on the x-axis (the duct membrane). As they divide and undergo genetic alterations, cells move into the duct lumen. Nutrient levels are assumed to be in equilibrium, a reasonable assumption given the time scales associated with cell division, diffusion and their uptake by cells. Cells, in turn, metabolise nutrient into ATP. They are assumed to die if the ATP levels are below a certain threshold; otherwise they divide with a probability that depends on the "excess" amount of ATP. At each division cells can mutate into a different state (*i.e.* hyperplastic, glycolytic, acid-resistant) with a certain probability. During periods of hypoxia, cells revert to anaerobic metabolism, producing lactic acid which is again modelled by a reaction-diffusion equation at equilibrium. This acid can cause cell death, depending on its concentration and the evolutionary state of the cell.

17.2.2 Simulation Results

Results from a typical simulation are presented in Fig. 17.1. The dynamics are, broadly speaking, consistent with those predicted in the verbal model of Gatenby and Gillies [GG04]. First, the hyperplastic cell type predominates, allowing cells to move away from the basement membrane into the duct lumen. Then, as hypoxia becomes important, the glycolytic cell type takes over, creating a highly acidic environment which eventually favours the acid-resistant cell type. However, the model predicts an extra feature, namely the possibility of long-lived transient islands of glycolytic cells surviving in a "sea" of acid-resistant cells. Motivated by this prediction, recent experiments have been carried out which do indeed verify this result [GS07]. The model is currently being extended to include more detailed aspects of the glycolytic pathway, and to investigate how the evolutionary process taking place within the duct may affect the invasiveness of the cell population which eventually breaks through the basement membrane.

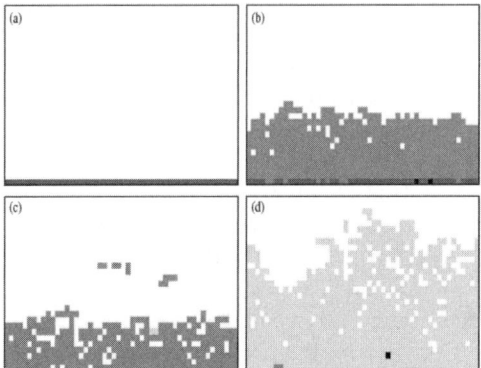

Fig. 17.1. The temporal evolution of a typical cellular automaton at (a) $t = 0$, (b) $t = 100$, (c) $t = 250$ and (d) $t = 300$ generations. Shown are normal epithelial (dark grey), hyperplastic (pink/grey), hyperplastic-glycolytic (green/grey) and hyperplastic-glycolytic-acid resistant (yellow/light grey) cells (colour version online). Cells with other phenotypic patterns are shown as black. Reproduced with permission from [SGGMG07].

17.3 Vascular Tumour Growth

Tumour tissue shares a complex relationship with vasculature. As a growing solid tumour reaches the limits of nutrient diffusion it is believed to secrete tumour angiogenesis factors (TAFs) to promote vascular growth towards and within the tumour. The new vasculature acts as a nutrient supply source and a (toxic) waste product disposal system, and provides access to distant parts of the body via metastatic invasion. At the same time, it allows the host to intensify its immunological response to the tumour cells through, for example, macrophages and neutrophils. As the access to increased nutrient availability allows the tumour to grow, the enhanced pressure of the tumour cells may cause the immature tumour vasculature to collapse [Jain88], creating areas of hypoxia which, in turn, stimulate the cells to secrete TAFs which widen existing blood vessels and create more new vessels. As we illustrate below, an understanding of such complex interactions can be facilitated by formulating, analysing and exploiting multiscale mathematical models.

17.3.1 Model Framework

The modelling framework is outlined in Fig. 17.2 which shows the spatial scales of interest (*e.g.* subcellular, cellular and tissue) and how the processes acting at the different scales interact. As in the model discussed in Section 17.2, nutrients and chemical signals are modelled using reaction-diffusion equations, and cells are modelled as automaton units. While cells can, as in the previous model, be considered as "black boxes" with prescribed parameters, cell properties (*e.g.* proteins associated with the cell cycle) can now be determined by ordinary differential equation (ODE) models operating on the intracellular scale.

The key advances in this model are the consideration of blood flow and vascular adaptation and their coupling to the dynamics of the tumour mass. It is known that normal vasculature is highly dynamic, with vessel radii responding to local mechanical stimuli such as wall shear stress, various biochemical stimuli and longer range stimuli. While this has been studied in great detail in the rat mesentery by Pries, Secomb and co-workers (see, for example, [PSG98]), only recently have similar models been advanced for tumours. In a series of papers, McDougall and co-workers have developed a hybrid model for vascular adaptation, blood flow and angiogenesis in which the tumour is viewed as a fixed source of angiogenic factors that does not grow [MACS02, MAC06]. By adapting an earlier discrete model of angiogenesis due to Anderson and Chaplain [AC98], endothelial cells within a capillary tip are assumed to perform random walks, biased by chemotaxis in response to tumour-derived angiogenic factors and haptotaxis in response to fibronectin gradients generated in the extracellular matrix through which the endothelial cells migrate. McDougall *et al.* used their model to highlight two important phenomena that could be responsible for the failure of blood-borne chemotherapy. First, most

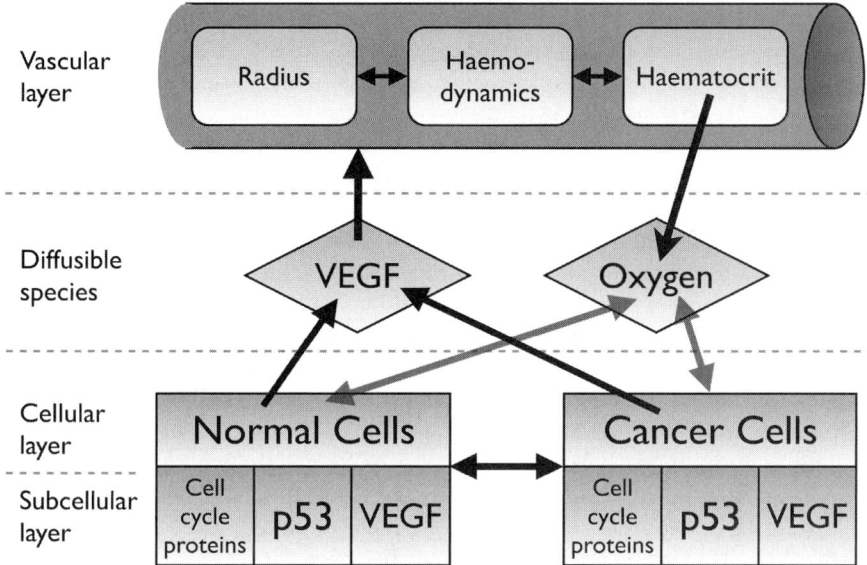

Fig. 17.2. Schematic diagram showing the structure of our multiscale model of vascular tumour growth.

of the drug may be diverted from the tumour by its highly interconnected capillary network. Second, dilution effects as the drug disperses through the vasculature may mean that the concentration reaching the tumour is too low to be effective. Further simulations suggested that increasing the mean radius of capillary vessels and/or decreasing the blood viscosity could substantially increase drug uptake.

In the absence of a detailed flow model for tumour vasculature, we take Pries *et al.*'s model and adapt it to tumours in a reasonable way. The model takes the form

$$R(t + dt) = R(t) + R(t)U(t)\, dt, \tag{17.1}$$

where $R(t)$ is the radius of a blood vessel at time t and dt is the time step. The remodelling function $U(t)$ consists of a number of components, as described above (for details, see [ABM05a, ABM05b, BAOMM]).

For simplicity, we consider a vascular network composed of a regular hexagonal array, with one input and one output, and a pressure drop imposed across it. We use the Poiseuille approximation and Kirchhoff's laws to compute the flow rates through and pressure drops across each vessel. Following [F93], we assume that at branch points the haematocrit, the red blood cells carrying oxygen, splits in proportion to the flow velocities in the daughter vessels. In this way, we can, in a simple first pass, compute the wall shear stresses and metabolic stimuli in each vessel and update their radii using equation (17.1) [ABM05b]. We assume that oxygen (nutrient) diffuses out of the vasculature into the tissue where it is available for metabolism by the normal and cancerous cells that constitute the cellular automata. As in Section 17.2 we use a reaction-diffusion equation to model the distribution of oxygen within the tissue. The cells respond to nutrient levels by dividing, if the concentration is sufficiently high. At lower oxygen concentrations, cancerous cells can survive for a certain period of time by becoming quiescent, but normal cells die. We can phenomenologically take into account the effect of acid production as a by-product of anaerobic metabolism by lowering the threshold of nutrient concentration at which normal cells die if they are surrounded by cancerous cells (an obvious refinement will be to include acid explicitly as a field variable and to model the metabolic biochemistry in more detail [JPCF]).

The basic model can be extended in many ways. For example, we can include, in each cell, equations that caricature the cell cycle [TN01], such detail being important if we wish to consider the effect of cell-cycle-dependent drugs. We can also include the production of VEGF in hypoxic regions and use a reaction-diffusion equation to model its spatio-temporal dynamics. The effect of VEGF on the vasculature can then be included in equation (17.1) where we assume it acts, through the remodelling function $U(t)$, to increase the vessel radius (in effect we are modelling angiogenesis implicitly, an increase in the simulated vessel radius being taken to represent an increase in the number of vessels present in a particular tissue region).

Cell crowding can be included by associating with each element in the automaton a carrying capacity whose value may depend on the number of vessels, tumour cells and normal cells contained within a particular element, to reflect the physical differences between vessels and cells, and the different responses to contact inhibition from normal cells and tumour cells. Cell movement is modelled as a stochastic process, with transition probabilities depending on the space available at neighbouring sites [BAOMM].

17.3.2 Simulation Results

We now summarise some of the key results that we have obtained using our multiscale model of vascular tumour growth.

Haematocrit distribution influences tumour growth

The simulations presented in Fig. 17.3 illustrate the importance of accurately modelling blood flow through the tissue [ABM05a]. In both cases the vascular dynamics are independent of the tumour, but the cellular dynamics are influenced, via oxygen, by behaviour at the macroscale. The upper panels correspond to a case for which the vessels undergo structural adaptation and, hence, the haematocrit and oxygen are distributed non-uniformly across the tissue. The lower panels show how the system evolves when the haematocrit is distributed uniformly throughout the vessels (*i.e.* blood flow is identical in all branches of the vasculature). We see that spatial heterogeneity has a significant effect on the tumour's dynamics and, in this case, actually reduces the tumour burden. We note also that when the oxygen distribution is heterogeneous the tumour develops "finger-like" protrusions similar to those observed in invasive cancers. Here this structure arises because the nutrient distribution is non-uniform.

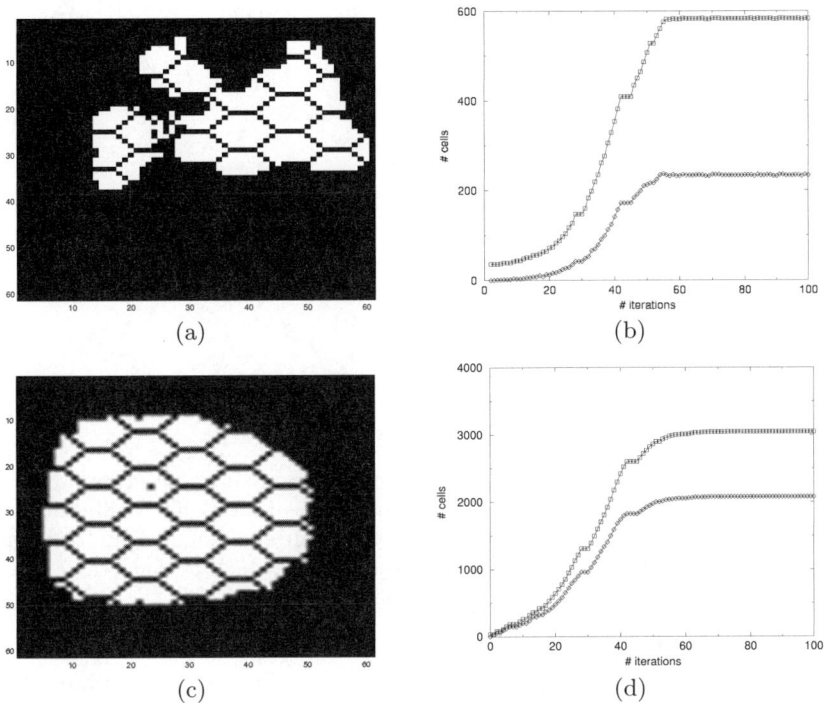

(a)

(b)

(c)

(d)

Fig. 17.3. Series of images showing the spatial distribution of cells for growth in inhomogeneous (panel a), and homogeneous environments (panel c). In panels (a) and (c) cancer cells occupy white spaces and vessels occupy a hexagonal array denoted by black spaces. The other black spaces denote empty spaces. Panels (b) and (d) show the time evolution of the number of (cancer) cells for the heterogeneous and homogeneous cases, respectively: squares denote the total number of cancer cells (proliferating + quiescent); diamonds denote quiescent cells. Reproduced with permission from [ABM03].

VEGF-dependent remodelling may stimulate oscillatory tumour dynamics

The simulation presented in Figs. 17.4 through 17.6 shows how coupling intracellular and macroscale phenomena can influence the dynamics of both the vasculature and the tumour [BAOMM]. In contrast to the results depicted in Fig. 17.3, where vessel adaptation was independent of VEGF, in Figs. 17.4 through 17.6 it is regulated by local VEGF levels. Figs. 17.4 and 17.5 show

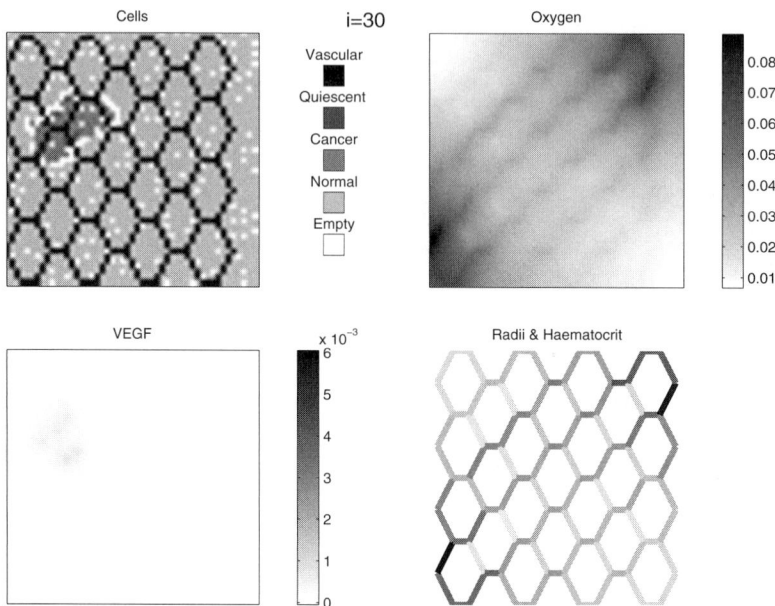

Fig. 17.4. Series of plots showing how a small tumour introduced into a vascular tissue at $t = 0$ has evolved at $t = 30$ (dimensionless time unit). While the oxygen and vessel profiles remain unchanged from their initial configurations, the tumour has increased in size and now contains quiescent cells which produce trace amounts of VEGF. Reproduced with permission from [BAOMM].

how the tumour's spatial composition evolves while Fig. 17.6 summarises its dynamics. Since there is a single inlet (outlet) to the vasculature located in the bottom left (top right) hand corner of the tissue, the incoming blood flow and haematocrit become diluted as they pass through the hexagonal lattice. This creates a heterogeneous oxygen distribution across the domain, with oxygen levels being highest near the inlet and outlet. Over time, the tumour cells proliferate and spread through the tissue towards oxygen-rich regions. As they increase in number, their demand for oxygen outstrips that available from the vasculature, and quiescent regions form. Cells in the quiescent regions produce VEGF which diffuses through the tissue (see Figs. 17.4 and 17.5), stimulating vessel adaptation and biasing blood flow towards low oxygen regions. If the VEGF stimulus is weak then the vasculature does not adapt quickly enough and the quiescent cells die (this is what happens at early times in Fig. 17.6). VEGF levels also decline and blood flow to the remaining tumour cells rises, enabling them to increase in number until the demand for oxygen once again exceeds that being supplied, and so the cycle repeats, with pronounced oscillations in the number of quiescent cells (see Fig. 17.6). In order to highlight the key role played by VEGF in creating these oscillations, also presented in Fig. 17.6 are the results of a simulation which was identical in all respects ex-

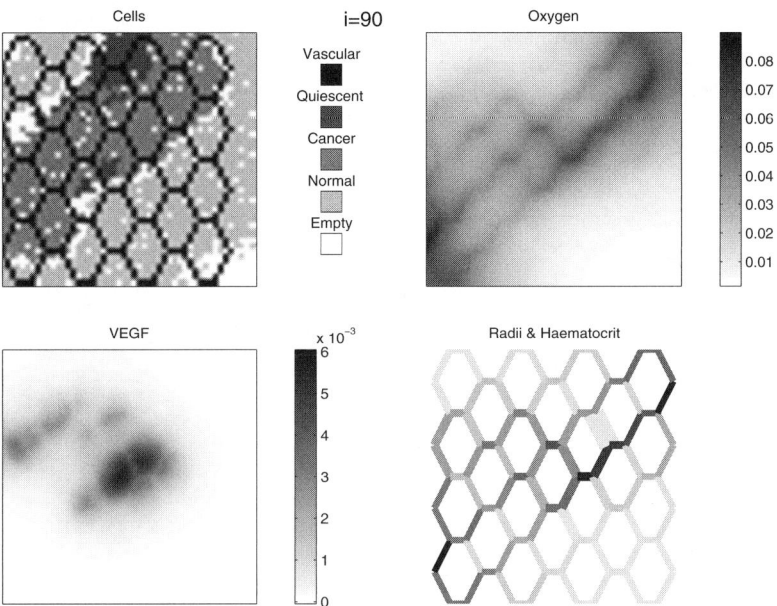

Fig. 17.5. Series of plots showing how the simulation presented in Fig. 17.4 has developed at $t = 90$. The tumour continues to penetrate the tissue region. There are now enough quiescent cells to elicit an angiogenic response. As a result, the vasculature has been remodelled, with blood flow and oxygen supply (haematocrit) being directed primarily towards the tumour mass. Reproduced with permission from [BAOMM].

cept that vascular adaptation was independent of VEGF (as per Fig. 17.3). In both cases, the tumours grow to similar sizes. However, when vascular adaptation is independent of VEGF the evolution is monotonic, the oscillations in the cell populations disappear and the number of quiescent cells is consistently much lower. These results show how coupling between the different spatial scales can effect not only the tumour's growth dynamics but also the proportion of proliferating and quiescent cells that it contains.

Vessel pruning may enhance a tumour's response to radiotherapy

We can use our model to investigate the effects of decreasing the blood vessel number (a primitive way of investigating the effects of anti-angiogenesis treatments). Our results suggest that low levels of vessel pruning may, in certain cases, *enhance* tumour growth by creating a vasculature that allows nutrient to reach tissue more effectively [ABM04b]. It is observed clinically that combination therapy involving anti-angiogenesis treatment and radiotherapy can be more effective than radiotherapy alone and at first glance this seems counter-intuitive. One possible explanation of this observation is provided by

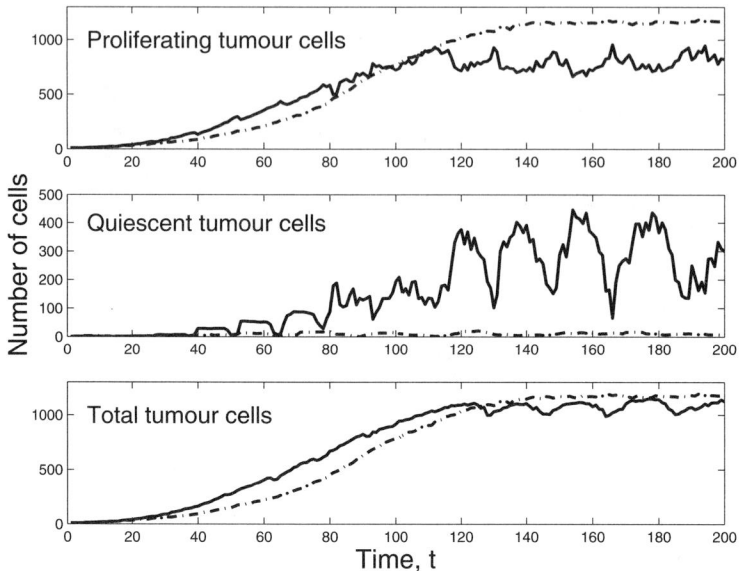

Fig. 17.6. Series of curves showing how, for the simulation in Figs. 17.4 and 17.5, the numbers of proliferating (upper panel), quiescent (middle panel) and total tumour cells (lower panel) change over time. While the number of proliferating cells increases steadily, the number of quiescent cells undergoes oscillations of increasing amplitude until $t \approx 120$. Thereafter, the tumour is sufficiently large that the quiescent cells are never eliminated: quiescent cells that die are replaced by proliferating cells that become quiescent. The dot-dashed lines show the evolution of a tumour which is identical except that its vasculature is not regulated by VEGF. While both tumours reach similar equilibrium sizes, when vascular adaptation is independent of VEGF the oscillations in the cell populations disappear and the number of quiescent cells is much lower. Reproduced with permission from [BAOMM].

the results from our model. An alternative explanation invokes vessel renormalisation [Jain88], and it is now a challenge to the experimental community to devise experiments to distinguish between these possibilities.

Abnormal vascular adaptation alters the tumour's growth dynamics

As mentioned in Section 17.3.1, there is still no good (experimental) model available for vascular adaptation in tumours. It is known, however, that the tumour neovasculature is abnormal in its response mechanisms to signalling cues. Therefore we can use the above model framework to investigate the effects on tumour growth and composition of the failure of different adaptation mechanisms [AOBM06]. This presents the intriguing possibility of being able to determine properties of the vasculature by examination of tumour tissue.

Vessel dematuration reduces the efficacy of chemotherapy

As a further extension of our model, we have incorporated tumour-induced vessel dematuration to assess the effect of vessel structure on the performance of chemotherapeutic agents [RMZAM, AOBM06]. We have found that dematuration can lead to the formation of quiescent regions that are much larger than those observed in simulations with a normal vasculature, thereby hampering the efficacy of cytotoxic drugs designed to target rapidly proliferating (tumour) cells. A further extension has been to include a diffusible anti-VEGFR drug which inhibits the effect of VEGF by competitively binding its receptor [AOBM06]. Our model simulations reproduce two key experimental features: an improved response to cytotoxic drugs following treatment with an anti-VEGFR drug and the emergence of a "window of opportunity," *i.e.* a period of time following treatment with anti-VEGFR during which such improvement is possible. The window opens because the anti-VEGFR drug induces extensive hypoxia within the tumour. This leads to massive VEGF production and a certain amount of cell death caused by oxygen starvation. The surge in VEGF levels stimulates remodelling of the vasculature, bringing oxygen to the hypoxic regions. This effect, coupled with the reduction in oxygen demand caused by cell death there, leads to reoxygenation of the hypoxic regions and a temporary reduction in the size of the quiescent subpopulation. As other regions of the tumour become hypoxic and blood flow undergoes another period of adaptation, the window of opportunity closes.

Explicit incorporation of angiogenesis alters the tumour's growth dynamics

While vessel radii and blood flow within the branches of the vascular network may change over time and, thereby, regulate the supply of nutrients to the tissue, the morphology of the vascular network in the simulations presented above does not change over time. More specifically, the hexagonal symmetry of the network is fixed, angiogenesis is not incorporated explicitly and redundant branches of the network in which blood flow is low do not regress. We have recently modified our model to address these issues [OAMB08], and results from a typical simulation are presented in Fig. 17.7. As the tumour grows and the metabolic demands of the tissue change, VEGF stimulates the ingrowth of new capillary tips towards quiescent regions where VEGF levels are high. Capillary tips that connect successfully to the network alter the morphology of the vasculature and, thereby, alter the pattern of blood flow within, and nutrient supply to, the tissue. As a result of the new connections, the flow through existing vessels may fall and, if low flow (and, hence, low wall shear stress) is maintained for a sufficiently long period, then the vessel is pruned or removed from the system.

For comparison with the basic model, in which angiogenesis is treated implicitly, we present in Fig. 17.8 spatially averaged time-activity curves showing how the coupled dynamics of the tumour and vasculature depend on the way in which vascular adaptation is modelled. The main features to note are the

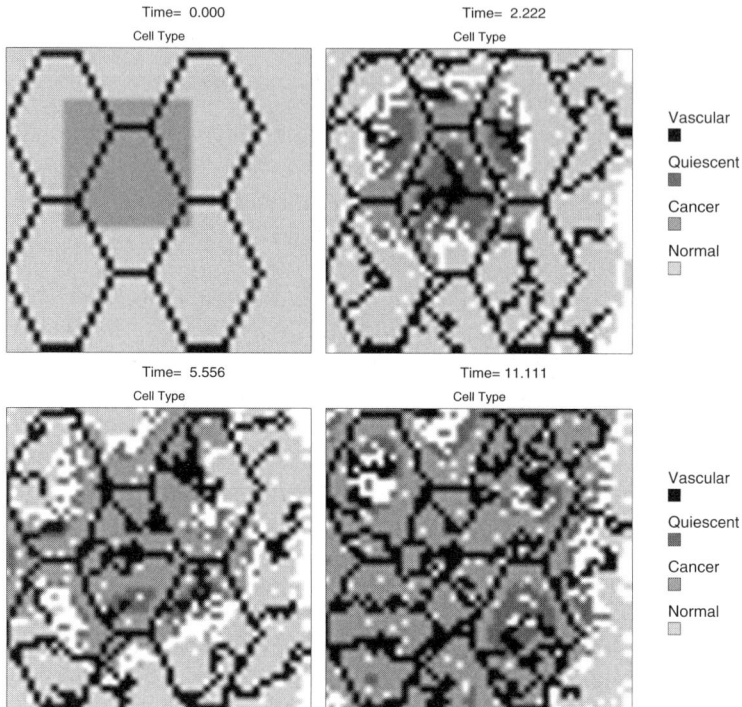

Fig. 17.7. Results from a simulation in which angiogenesis is incorporated explicitly into the vascular remodelling algorithm, thereby allowing the development of arbitrary, asymmetric vascular networks. The plots show the evolution of a small tumour that is embedded, at $t = 0$, into a tissue perfused initially by a hexagonal network of blood vessels. Over time, the structure of the vasculature changes, with existing vessels remodelling and new vessels forming as a result of angiogenesis. The new capillary tips emerge from existing vessels and migrate, via chemotaxis, towards regions of high VEGF concentration. The capillary tips must form connections, and establish a flow, within a fixed period of time; otherwise they regress. The four images show the tissue composition at times $t = 0.00$, $t = 2.22$, $t = 5.55$ and $t = 11.11$.

increase in the number of proliferating tumour cells and the decrease in the number of quiescent tumour cells that occur when angiogenesis is treated explicitly rather than implicitly. These changes are a consequence of the higher spatial resolution that occurs when individual capillary tips are simulated: VEGF produced by quiescent tumour cells will now stimulate the ingrowth of new capillary tips into that region and enable the cells to resume proliferation.

Since our new model distinguishes between blunt-ended capillary tips (in which flow is absent) and vessels which are part of the flow network, it should be possible to generate more detailed predictions concerning the relative efficacy of drugs that target proliferating endothelial cells and those that reduce

blood flow. Additionally, it will be possible to determine whether low levels
of chemotherapy targeted at proliferating tumour cells produce an additional
beneficial effect by destroying angiogenic tumour vessels and, thereby, reducing the supply of nutrients to the tumour mass [Sha06].

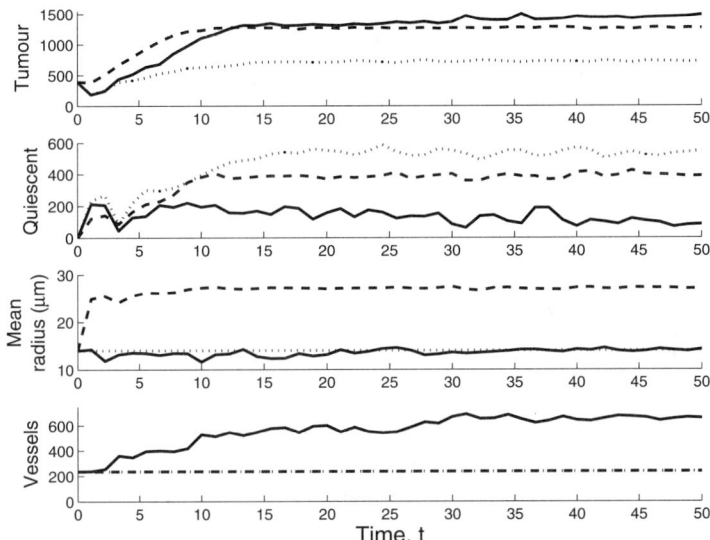

Fig. 17.8. Series of plots showing how the evolution over time of the numbers of
proliferating (upper panel) and quiescent (second panel) tumour cells, mean vessel
radius (third panel) and number of vessels (lowest panel) depends on the mechanisms
that control vascular remodelling. Key: Dotted line, remodelling of the vasculature is
independent of VEGF; Dashed line, VEGF enhances vascular remodelling by stimulating vessel dilation; solid line, VEGF enhances vascular remodelling by stimulating
angiogenesis.

17.4 Colorectal Cancer

Colorectal cancer (CRC) was the second most commonly diagnosed malignancy in Europe in 2006 [Ferl07]; it also ranked second according to cancer
mortality. Most CRCs occur spontaneously, developing from pre-existing, benign polyps (or adenomas), which originate from the epithelial sheet that
lines the luminal surface of the bowel. The intestinal epithelium is characterised by numerous invaginations (Fig. 17.9), or crypts, which drive its rapid
self-renewal. Near the bottom of the crypts, a small number of stem cells proliferate continuously, producing transit cells, which divide several times before
undergoing terminal differentiation. At the same time, cells migrate upwards

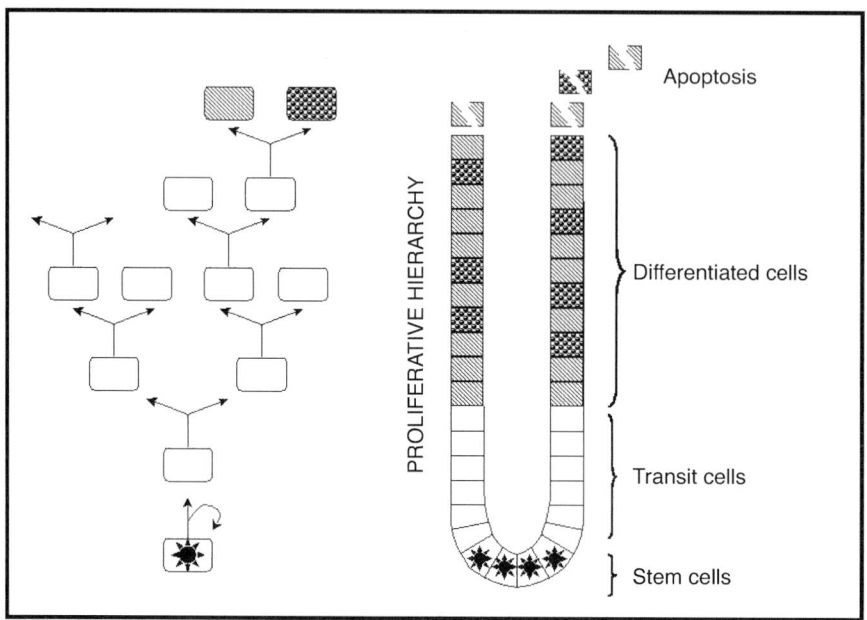

Fig. 17.9. Schematic of the proliferative hierarchy in a normal colonic crypt. Murine crypts contain about 235–250 epithelial cells, which reside on a basement membrane. Proliferating cells (*i.e.* stem and transit cells) occupy the lower third of the crypt. After several divisions, transit cells differentiate into the various cell types that constitute the epithelium (*e.g.* columnar cells and goblet cells).

along the crypt axis and, when they reach the orifice, initiate programmed cell death (apoptosis). Thus a normal crypt can be viewed as a dynamic system in which the processes of cell proliferation, migration, differentiation and death are tightly coordinated by intra-, inter- and extra-cellular cues. Under aberrant conditions genetic and epigenetic alterations cause dysfunctional regulation and loss of homeostasis, eventually leading to the formation of a polyp. Further mutations are required for progression towards a malignant, metastatic carcinoma. Hence, CRC is a multistep, multiscale process in which the progressive accumulation of changes at the molecular level translates into subsequent pathological stages at the macroscale level.

CRC is a natural subject for mathematical investigation because many of the key mutations that arise have been identified and details of their functional effect determined. For example, most CRCs bear inactivating mutations in the *APC* tumour suppressor gene [Ilya05]. This multifunctional protein is a central player in Wingless/Int (Wnt) signalling, a key pathway in the regulation of normal crypt dynamics [Nath04, Sans04]. In the absence of extracellular Wnt, a protein complex that includes Apc marks any free β-catenin molecules for rapid degradation. In contrast, when extracellular Wnt is present, stimulation of specific receptors on the cell's surface inactivates the Apc-complex and β-catenin accumulates. This protein then travels to the nucleus where it induces the expression of a large number of Wnt targets, including genes involved in cell-cycle control, active migration and differentiation. Genetic alterations detected in CRCs generally impede Apc-mediated β-catenin degradation, and, hence, have the same effect as a continuous Wnt signal.

Since CRC has been extensively studied, it is not surprising that a plethora of mathematical models exist that address various aspects of the disease (for a critical review, see [vLBJK06]). For example, as early as 1954, Armitage and Doll [Armi54] developed a stochastic "time to tumour" model, to describe the observed age-dependent CRC incidence. More recently, Komarova and Wang [Koma04] have investigated the likely targets for malignant transformation in the crypt, while d'Onofrio and Tomlinson [dOno07] and Johnston *et al.* [JEBMC] have analysed the cellular changes that can lead to uncontrolled, exponential growth. We introduce here a series of models that simulate different aspects of the normal gut and CRC. Thereafter, we explain how we are adapting, extending and integrating these models to obtain a detailed, mechanistic multiscale model of CRC [vLEIB, Gava05].

17.4.1 Mathematical Modelling

The earliest models of normal crypt dynamics are formulated on simple two-dimensional (2D) grids (the cylindrical crypt is cut open and rolled out to give a surface), with cells assumed to move within predefined rows and columns [Loef86, Paul93]. All cells have the same, constant (rectangular) shape and size, and cell growth is thus ignored. Proliferation and cell-cycle control are modelled by assigning cell-cycle times to daughter cells immediately after division. Cell movement is driven by mitotic pressure: displacements occur naturally when newborn cells are inserted into the grid. Finally, the rules that govern whether a cell differentiates differ for stem and transit cells. After stem cell division, each daughter cell has a certain probability of leaving the stem cell pool and becoming a transit cell. In contrast, transit cells differentiate terminally after a fixed number of divisions. In summary, the 2D grid models can be viewed as basic multiscale models: a 2D tissue is characterised by the behaviour of its cellular constituents, each of which carries its own subcellular cell-cycle time and a record of its differentiation status.

Despite their simplicity, 2D grid models have been successfully used to interpret experimental data concerning cell migration and differentiation in the crypt [Loef86, Paul93]. The main drawback with the 2D approach is that the insertion of newborn cells inevitably shifts a whole column of cells upwards, breaking many cell-cell contacts. This is physically unrealistic as epithelial cells are known to have strong cell-cell connections so that they may form a protective barrier between the body and the contents of the gut. To overcome this deficiency, Meineke *et al.* [Mein01] proposed a 2D lattice-free model in which cell centres are represented as points that can occupy any position on a

2D surface with cylindrical boundary conditions. Polygonal cell shapes, which resemble real epithelial cells, are then determined from the associated Voronoi diagram while cell-cycle control and differentiation are incorporated as in the 2D grid models. Migration and cell-cell adhesion are accounted for by assuming that neighbouring cells are connected by damped springs and balancing the forces due to the spring connections with damping forces associated with cell-substrate binding (see Fig. 17.10). Hence, the position vector x_i for cell i at time $t + \triangle t$ is determined from its position and that of its neighbours at time t as follows:

$$x_i(t + \triangle t) = x_i(t) + \frac{\mu}{\eta} \sum_{\forall j} u_{ij}(t)(d_{ij}(t) - L_{ij}(t))\triangle t, \qquad (17.2)$$

where the summation is over all cells connected to cell i at time t, u_{ij} is a unit vector pointing from cell i to j, L_{ij} is the equilibrium spring length, d_{ij} the distance between i and j, μ the spring constant, and η the damping constant. In contrast to the 2D grid models, cell division now results in local cell rearrangements only.

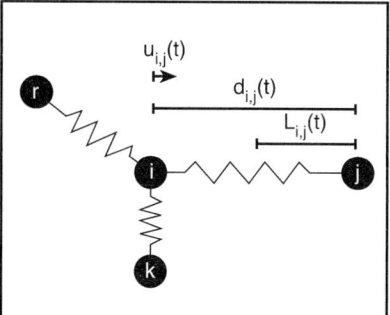 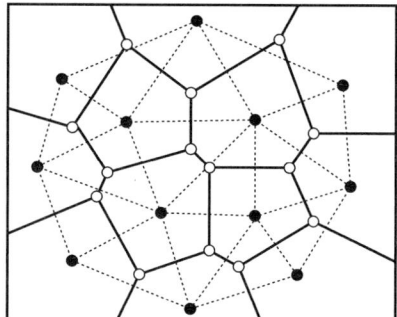

Fig. 17.10. Schematics illustrating the lattice-free approach developed in [Mein01]. (Left) *In silico* cells attached by springs. (Right) *In silico* 2D tissue, showing cell centres (black nodes), vertices (white nodes) and the associated Voronoi tesselation (solid lines). The related Delauney triangulation (dashed lines) is obtained by connecting all neighbouring nodes and defines the network of springs. Reproduced with permission from [vLEIB].

17.4.2 Multiscale Model Assembly

The spatial models described above do not account for subcellular pathways and are, therefore, unable to predict the impact of specific genetic alterations (*e.g.* mutations in the Wnt network) on crypt dynamics. Nor can they be used to explore potential interactions between phenomena occurring at different levels of organisation or to evaluate the impact of cancer drugs on the system. These aims can be achieved by developing a multiscale framework (see Fig. 17.11) that embraces each level of organisation, from molecule to whole organ, in a manner similar to that used to formulate the multiscale model of vascular tumour growth presented in Section 17.3. Building such a framework, and coupling models developed originally to describe phenomena at a single scale, raises many mathematical challenges, four of which we highlight below.

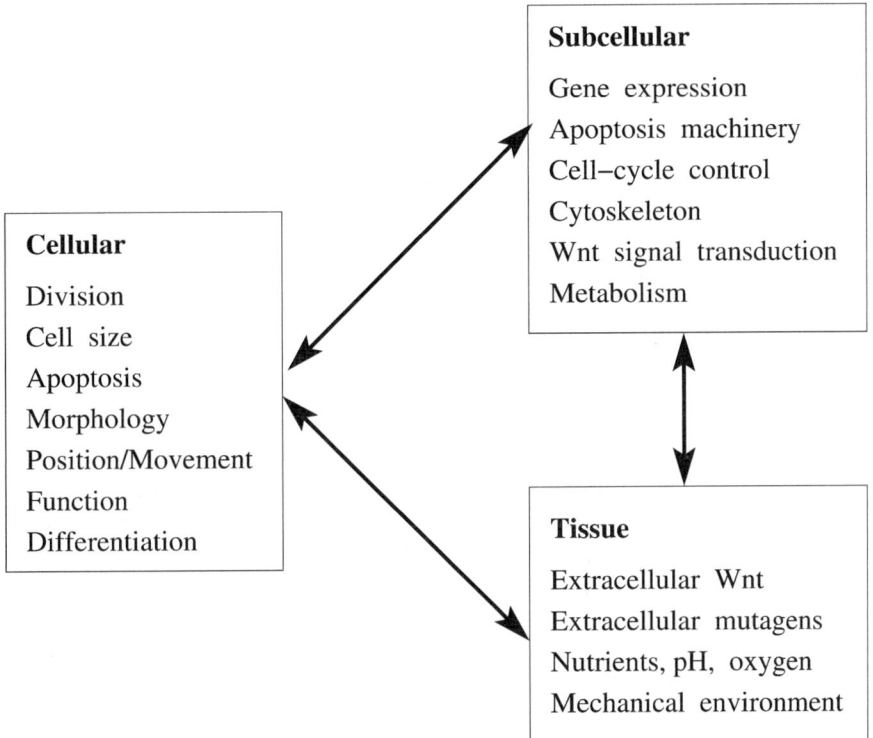

Fig. 17.11. Prototype multiscale model for normal crypt dynamics and CRC. The arrows highlight that the relation between the scales is not simply bottom-up. An extracellular, tissue gradient of Wnt factors, for example, can directly affect subcellular gene expression.

Incorporating extracellular signalling

In the basic model developed in [Mein01] all cellular processes are assumed to be independent of extra- and intra-cellular signals. Experimental evidence suggests, however, that epithelial cells respond to spatial variations in: the composition of the basement membrane; the signals emitted by myofibroblasts; and the level of Wnt factors. By imposing an extracellular Wnt gradient along the vertical crypt axis and using simple models of the (intracellular) Wnt signalling pathway [Lee03, vLBJK07] we are able to predict position-dependent patterns of gene expression. Coupling the Wnt-signalling model with a cell-cycle model (*e.g.* [Swat04, TN01]) provides additional information about how cell-cycle times vary along the crypt axis and how terminally differentiated (*i.e.* non-cycling) cells are generated.

Controlling cell size

In the 2D grid models cell sizes are fixed, whereas in [Mein01] cell size is controlled by the relative spatial position of neighbouring cells. In reality, however, cell size depends on nutrient availability, the cell's metabolic rate, its progress through the cell cycle and contact inhibition. Better control of cell growth and size is thus needed. Cell vertex models, for instance, achieve this goal by associating with the system an energy function which increases as cells deviate from their optimal sizes [Brod04]. Cells are assumed to move in directions that minimise the energy function.

Including cell death

In existing models cell removal occurs only when cells are pushed off the upper edge of the 2D surface. Apoptosis can, however, occur within the crypt at rates which are enhanced by certain experimental manipulations, such as Apc knockout [Sans04] and irradiation [Pott94]. To simulate and explain these results, our model must account for biochemical networks that regulate programmed cell death, biomechanical cell detachment and the resulting changes at the cellular level. At the macroscale, this poses the additional problem of dealing with gaps in the tissue.

Modelling domain growth

In the models described above, the 2D surface remains fixed during the simulation period. Although this may be a good approximation for normal crypts, a more flexible approach is required to describe the changes in crypt size and morphology associated with aberrant crypts and polyp formation. The model of morphogenesis and crypt fission developed in [Dras01] provides one possible resolution to this problem. In [Dras01] Drasdo and Loeffler consider a 1D longitudinal section of a crypt, represent individual cells as deformable circles and assume that migration is driven by cell division. Alternatively, the continuum model of crypt fission developed by Edwards and Chapman [Edwa07] could be adapted to allow for changes in crypt size caused by genetic mutations. In [Edwa07] the epithelial cells are treated as a continuous tissue layer that is attached to a basement membrane by viscoelastic bonds. Model simulations suggest that mutations causing either a net increase in cell proliferation or an increase in the strength of cell bonding can lead to buckling and fission.

17.5 Discussion

We have presented a series of multiscale models of cancer growth, focused on carcinogenesis in early ductal carcinoma *in situ*, vascular tumour growth and colorectal cancer. While we have focused on three particular applications, it is important to note that this is a rapidly growing area of research. For example, Jiang *et al.* [JPCF] have formulated a multicellular model to simulate the growth of multicellular tumour spheroids, using a discrete lattice Monte Carlo model to describe the cellular dynamics and a Boolean network to model the expression of proteins that control the cell cycle. Equally, Patel *et al.* [PGLG] have developed a model for early tumour growth and metabolism that considers the interaction of native tumour vascularity and increased glycolysis. Anderson and colleagues [AWCQ06, GA07] have investigated the effects of heterogeneity in the tissue and nutrient levels on the dynamics of tumour growth and have combined this with mutation and evolution to show mechanisms whereby the classical fingering morphology of a tumour can arise and how the microenvironment can select certain genotypes. Macklin and Lowengrub [ML07] have focused on the biomechanical aspects of a growing tumour mass to predict fingering as a result of microenvironmental factors. Ribba *et al.* [RCS06] have developed a model for colorectal oncogenesis which includes a Boolean description of a genetic model, integrated with a discrete model of the cell cycle and a continuous macroscopic model of tumour growth and invasion. They have used this model to predict the effects of radiotherapy.

While considerable progress has been made in a very short time, many challenges remain ahead. For example, it is impossible (and not desirable) to have a detailed comprehensive model of every process involved in tumour growth. Simplifications need to be made. In modelling a process at one specific spatial scale, we have well-established techniques for determining the errors incurred in making such simplifications. However, when we couple such models into an integrated framework spanning several spatial scales with multiple feedback, as well as feedforward, loops, we have little idea of how errors propagate and grow: to understand this is a huge challenge for the future.

The multiscale approaches outlined in this paper appear to be the natural framework for modelling in this area, but they quickly become computationally infeasible as we try to model a growing tumour consisting of billions of cells. For that we need a continuum approach, but it is not clear how to interface between discrete models (appropriate for small cell numbers) and continuous models, appropriate for large-scale models.

Biological systems are highly robust and therefore we would expect the behaviour of the system to be insensitive to many parameters but crucially dependent on a few select parameters. Therefore, for modelling we may only need crude estimates for most parameters. Model simulations can be performed to identify those parameters to which the system dynamics are most sensitive and thus direct experimental effort to focus on accurate measurements of these parameters. To be successful it is therefore vital that model development be undertaken in close collaboration with experimentalists, and that experimental design and data collection pay attention to the needs of models.

Acknowledgments

PKM was partially supported by a Royal Society-Wolfson Merit Award and NIH grant U56CA113004 from the National Cancer Institute. TA and IMMvL gratefully acknowledge the EPSRC for financial support.

References

[Ad96]   Adam, J.A.: Mathematical models of perivascular spheriod development and catastrophe-theoretic description of rapid metastatic growth/tumor remission, Invasion Metastasis, **16**, 247–267 (1996).

[ABM03]   Alarcón, T., Byrne, H.M., and Maini, P.K.: A cellular automaton model for tumour growth in inhomogeneous environment, J. Theor. Biol., **225**, 257–274 (2003).

[ABM04b]   Alarcón, T., Byrne, H.M., and Maini, P.K.: Towards whole-organ modelling of tumour growth, Prog. Biophys. Mol. Biol., **85**, 451–472 (2004).

[ABM05a]   Alarcón, T., Byrne, H.M., and Maini, P.K.: A multiple scale model for tumour growth, Multiscale Mod. Sim., **3**, 440–475 (2005).

[ABM05b]   Alarcón, T., Byrne, H.M., and Maini, P.K.: A design principle for vascular beds: the effects of complex blood rheology, Microvasc. Res., **69**, 156–172 (2005).

[AOBM06]   Alarcón, T., Owen, M.R., Byrne, H.M., and Maini, P.K.: Multiscale modelling of tumour growth and therapy: the influence of vessel normalisation on chemotherapy, Comp. Math. Methods Med., **7**, 85–119 (2006).

[AC98]   Anderson, A.R.A., and Chaplain, M.A.J.: Continuous and discrete mathematical models of tumour-induced angiogenesis, Bull. Math. Biol., **60**, 857–899 (1998).

[AWCQ06]   Anderson, A.R.A., Weaver, A.M., Cummings, T.M., and Quaranta, V.: Tumor morphology and phenotypic evolution driven by selective pressure from the microenvironment, Cell, **127**, 905–915 (2006).

[AMcE]   Araujo, R.P., and McElwain, D.L.S.: A history of the study of solid tumor growth: the contribution of mathematical modelling, Bull. Math. Biol., **66**, 1039–1091 (2004).

[Armi54]   Armitage, P., and Doll, R.: The age distribution of cancer and a multistage theory of carcinogenesis, Br. J. Cancer, **8**, 1–12 (1954).

[Brod04]   Brodland, G.W.: Computational modeling of cell sorting, tissue engulfment, and related phenomena: a review, Appl. Mech. Rev., **57**, 47–76 (2004).

[BAOMM]   Byrne, H.M., Alarcón, T., Owen, M.R., Murphy, J., and Maini, P.K.: Modelling the response of vascular tumours to chemotherapy: a multiscale approach, Math. Mod. Meth. Appl. Sci., **16**, 1219–1241 Suppl S (2006).

[Cram04]   Crampin, E.J., Halstead, M., Hunter, P., Nielsen, P., Noble, D., Smith, N., and Tawhai, M.: Computational physiology and the Physiome project, Exp. Physiol., **89**, 21–26 (2004).

[Dras01]   Drasdo, D., and Loeffler, M.: Individual-based models to growth and folding in one-layered tissues: intestinal crypts and early development, Nonlinear Analysis, **47**, 245–256 (2001).

[Edwa07]   Edwards, C.M., and Chapman, J.S.: Biomechanical modelling of colorectal crypt budding and fission, Bull. Math. Biol., **69**, 1927–1942, (2007).

[Ferl07]   Ferlay, F., Autier, P., Boniol, M., Heanue, M., Colombet, M., and Boyle, P.: Estimates of the cancer incidence and mortality in Europe in 2006, Ann. Oncol., **18**, 581–592 (2007).

[F93]   Fung, Y.C.: Biomechanics, Springer, New York (1993).

[GG96]   Gatenby, R.A., and Gawlinski, E.T.: A reaction-diffusion model of cancer invasion, Cancer Res., **56**, 5745–5753 (1996).

[GG04]   Gatenby, R.A., and Gillies, R.J.: Why do cancers have high aerobic glycolysis? Nature Rev. Cancer, **4**, 891–899 (2004).

[GM03]   Gatenby, R.A., and Maini, P.K.: Mathematical oncology: cancer summed up, Nature, **421**, 321 (2003).

[GS07]   Gatenby, R.A., Smallbone, K., Maini, P.K., Rose, F., Averill, J., Nagel, R.B., Worrall, L., and Gillies, R.J.: Cellular adaptations to hypoxia and acidosis during somatic evolution of breast cancer, Brit. J. Cancer, **97**, 646–653 (2007).

[Gava05]   Gavaghan, D.J., Simpson, A.C., Lloyd, S., MacRandal, D.F., and Boyd, D.R.: Towards a Grid infrastructure to support integrative approaches to biological research, Philos. Transact. A Math. Phys. Eng. Sci., **363**, 1829–1841 (2005).

[GA07]   Gerlee, P., and Anderson, A.R.A.: An evolutionary hybrid cellular automaton model of solid tumour growth, J. Theor. Biol., **246**, 583–603 (2007).

[GLB94]   Gillies, R.J., Liu, Z., and Bhujwalla, Z.: ^{31}P-MRS measurements of extracellular pH of tumors using 3-aminopropylphosphonate, Am. J. Physiol., **267**, 195–203 (1994).

[GRM89]   Grinstein, S., Rotin, D., and Mason, M.J.: Na^+/H^+ exchange and growth factor-induced cytosolic pH changes: role in cellular proliferation, Biochim. Biophys. Acta, **988**, 73–97 (1989).

[HSR91]   Haberkorn, U., Strauss, L.G., Reisser, C., Hagg, D., Dimitrakopoulu, A., Ziegler, S., Oberdorfe, F., Rudat, V., and van Kaick, G.: Glucose uptake, perfusion, and cell proliferation in head and neck tumours: relation to positron emission tomography and other whole-body applications, Semin. Nuc. Med., **22**, 268–284 (1991).

[HW00]   Hanahan, D., and Weinberg, R.A.: The hallmarks of cancer, Cell, **100**, 57–70 (2000).

[Ilya05]   Ilyas, M.: Wnt signalling and the mechanistic basis of tumour development, J. Pathol., **205**, 130–144 (2005).

[Jain88]   Jain, R.K.: Determinants of tumour blood flow: a review, Cancer Res., **48**, 2641–2658 (1988).

[JPCF]   Jiang, Y., Pjseivac-Grbovic, J., Cantrell, C., and Freyer, J.P.: A multiscale model for avascular tumour growth, Biophys. J., **89**, 3884–3894 (2005).

472   H.M. Byrne et al.

[JEBMC]   Johnston, M.D., Edwards, C.M., Bodmer, W.F., Maini, P.K., and Chapman, S.J.: Mathematical modelling of cell population dynamics in the colonic crypt, Proc. Natl. Acad. Sci., **104**, 4008–4013 (2007).

[Koma04]   Komarova, N.L., and Wang, L.: Initiation of colorectal cancer: where do the two hits hit?, Cell Cycle, **3**, 1558–1565 (2004).

[Lee03]   Lee, E., Salic, A., Kruger, R., Heinrich, R., and Kirschner, M.W.: The roles of APC and Axin derived from experimental and theoretical analysis of the Wnt pathway, PLoS Biol., **1**, E10 (2003).

[vLBJK06]   van Leeuwen, I.M.M., Byrne, H.M., Jensen, O.E., and King, J.R.: Crypt dynamics and colorectal cancer: advances in mathematical modelling, Cell Prolif., **39**, 157–181 (2006).

[vLBJK07]   van Leeuwen, I.M.M., Byrne, H.M., Jensen, O.E., and King, J.R.: Elucidating the interactions between the adhesive and transcriptional functions of beta-catenin in normal and cancerous cells, J. Theor. Biol., **247**, 77–102 (2007).

[vLEIB]   van Leeuwen, I.M.M., Edwards, C.M., Ilyas, M., and Byrne, H.M.: Towards a multiscale model of colorectal cancer, W. J. Gastroenterol., **13**, 1399–1407 (2007).

[Loef86]   Loeffler, M., Stein, R., Wichmann, H.E., Potten, C.S., Kaur, P., and Chwalinski, S.: Intestinal crypt proliferation. I. A comprehensive model of steady-state proliferation in the crypt, Cell Tissue Kinetics, **19**, 627–645 (1986).

[MACS02]   McDougall, S.R., Anderson, A.R.A., Chaplain, M.A.J., and Sherratt, J.A.: Mathematical modelling of flow through vascular networks: implications for tumour-induced angiogenesis and chemotherapy strategies, Bull. Math. Biol., **64**, 673–702 (2002).

[MAC06]   McDougall, S.R., Anderson, A.R.A., and Chaplain, M.A.J.: Mathematical modelling of dynamic adaptive tumour-induced angiogenesis: clinical implications and therapeutic targeting strategies. Bull. Math. Biol., **241**, 564–589 (2006).

[ML07]   Macklin, P., and Lowengrub, J.: Nonlinear simulation of the effect of microenvironment on tumor growth, J. Theor. Biol., **245**, 677–704 (2007).

[Mein01]   Meineke, F.A., Potten, C.S., and Loeffler, M.: Cell migration and organization in the intestinal crypt using a lattice-free model, Cell Prolif., **34**, 253–266 (2001).

[Nath04]   Näthke, I.S.: The adenomatous polyposis coli protein: the Achilles heel of the gut epithelium, Annu. Rev. Dev. Biol., **20**, 337–366 (2004).

[Nobl06]   Noble, D.: Systems biology and the heart, Biosystems, **83**, 75–80 (2005).

[dOno07]   d'Onofrio, A., and Tomlinson, I.P.: A nonlinear mathematical model of cell turnover, differentiation and tumorigenesis in the intestinal crypt, J. Theor. Biol., **244**, 367–374 (2007).

[OAMB08]   Owen, M.R., Alarcón, T., Maini, P.K., and Byrne, H.M.: Angiogenesis and vascular remodelling in normal and cancerous tissues, J. Math. Biol., in press.

[Pan97]   Panetta, J.C.: A mathematical model of breast and ovarian cancer treated with paclitaxel, Math. Biosci., **146**, 89–113 (1997).

[PGLG]   Patel, A.A., Gawlinsky, E.T., Lemieux, S.K., and Gatenby, R.A.: Cellular automaton model of early tumour growth and invasion: the effects of native tissue vascularity and increased anaerobic tumour metabolism, J. Theor. Biol., **213**, 315–331 (2001).

[Paul93]   Paulus, U., Loeffler, M., Zeidler, J., Owen, G., and Potten, C.S.: The differentiation and lineage development of goblet cells in the murine small intestinal crypt: experimental and modelling studies, J. Cell Sci., **106**, 473–484 (1993).

[Pott94]   Potten, C.S., Merritt, A., Hickman, J., Hall, P., and Faranda, A.: Characterization of radiation-induced apoptosis in the small intestine and its biological implications, Int. J. Radiat. Biol., **65**, 71–78 (1994).

[PSG98]   Pries, A.R., Secomb, T.W., and Gaehtgens, P.: Structural adaptation and stability of microvascular networks: theory and simulations, Am. J. Physiol., **275**, H349–H360 (1998).

[RMZAM]   Ribba, B., Marron, K., Agur, Z., Alarcón, T., and Maini, P.K.: A mathematical model of doxorubicin treatment efficacy for non-Hodgkin's lymphoma: investigation of the current protocol through theoretical modelling results, Bull. Math. Biol., **67**, 79–99 (2005).

[RCS06]   Ribba, B., Colin, T., and Schnell, S.: A multiscale mathematical model of cancer and its use in analyzing irradiation therapies, Theor. Biol. Med. Model., **3**, 7 (2006).

[RCM07]   Roose, T., Chapman, S.J., and Maini, P.K.: Mathematical models of avascular tumour growth, SIAM Review, **49**, 179–208 (2007).

[Sans04]   Sansom, O.J., Reed, K.R., Hayes, A.J., Ireland, H., Brinkmann, H., Newton, I.P., Batlle, E., Simon-Assman, P., Clevers, H., Nathke, I.S., Clarke, A.R., and Winton, D.J.: Loss of Apc *in vivo* immediately perturbs Wnt signaling, differentiation, and migration, Genes Dev, **18**, 1385–1390 (2004).

[Sha06]   Shaked, Y., Ciarrocchi, A., Franco, M., Lee, C.R., Man, S., Cheung, A.M., Kicklin, D.J., Chaplin, D., Foster, F.S., Benezra, R., and Kerbel, R.S.: Therapy-induced acute recruitment of circulating endothelial progenitor cells to tumours. Science, **313**, 1785–1787 (2006).

[SGGMG07]   Smallbone, K., Gatenby, R.A., Gillies, R.J., Maini, P.K., and Gavaghan, D.J.: Metabolic changes during carcinogenesis: potential impact on invasiveness. J. Theor. Biol., **244**, 703–713 (2007).

[Swat04]   Swat, M., Kel, A., and Herzel, H.: Bifurcation analysis of the regulatory modules of the mammalian G_1/S transition, Bioinformatics, **20**, 1506–1511 (2004).

[TN01]   Tyson, J.J., and Novak, B.: Regulation of the eukariotic cell-cycle: molecular anatagonism, hysteresis, and irreversible transitions, J. Theor. Biol., **210**, 249–263 (2001).

[W30]   Warburg, O.: The Metabolism of Tumours, Constable Press, London (1930).

Printed in the United States of America